Handbook of
Experimental Pharmacology

Continuation of Handbuch der experimentellen Pharmakologie

Vol. 60

Pyretics and Antipyretics

Contributors

C. G. Van Arman · D. A. J. Armstrong · J. Bligh · B. A. Britt
M. E. Casterlin · K. E. Cooper · B. Cox · M. J. Dascombe
C. A. Dinarello · J. S. Eisenman · G. W. Gander · N. W. Kasting
D. H. Kim · T. F. Lee · A. S. Milton · R. D. Myers · C. Ounsted
R. G. Pertwee · W. W. Reynolds · V. K. Sawhney
J. B. P. Stephenson · M. Székely · Z. Szelényi · J. Szolcsányi
W. L. Veale · S. M. Wolff

Editor

A. S. Milton

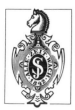

Springer-Verlag Berlin Heidelberg New York 1982

Professor ANTHONY S. MILTON
University of Aberdeen, Marischal College
Department of Pharmacology
Aberdeen AB9 1AS, Scotland, Great Britain

With 82 Figures

ISBN 3-540-11511-0 Springer-Verlag Berlin Heidelberg New York
ISBN 0-387-11511-0 Springer-Verlag New York Heidelberg Berlin

Library of Congress Cataloging in Publication Data. Main entry under title:
Pyretics and antipyretics. (Handbook of experimental pharmacology; v. 60) Includes bibliographies and index.
1. Fever – Chemotherapy. 2. Antipyretics. 3. Pyrogens – Physiological effect. 4. Body temperature – Regulation.
I. Van Arman, C. G. II. Milton A. S. (Anthony Stuart), 1934–. III. Series.
[DNLM: 1. Body temperature regulation – Drug effects. 2. Pyrogens. 3. Fever – Drug therapy. 4. Analgesics,
Anti-inflammatory. W1 HA5IL v. 60/WB 152 P998] QP905.H3 vol. 60 [RB129] 615';.1s 82-5553
ISBN 0-387-11511-0 (U.S.) [616'.04] AACR2

Typesetting, printing, and bookbinding: Brühlsche Universitätsdruckerei, Giessen.
2122/3130-543210

List of Contributors

Dr. C. G. Van Arman, Department of Biological Research, Wyeth Laboratories Inc., P.O. Box 8299, Philadelphia, PA 19101/USA

Dr. D. A. J. Armstrong, Department of Pharmacology, University of Pennsylvania, School of Medicine, Philadelphia, PA 19104/USA

Dr. J. Bligh, Ph.D., D.Sc., Director, Division of Life Sciences and Institute of Arctic Biology, University of Alaska, Fairbanks, AK 99701/USA

Dr. B. A. Britt, M.D., Associate Professor, Departments of Anaesthesia and Pharmacology, University of Toronto, Medical Sciences Building, Toronto, Ontario M5S 1A8, Canada

Dr. M. E. Casterlin, Biothermal Research Institute, Northeast Limnological Laboratory, R. D. 3, Box 10, Wyoming, PA 18644/USA

Dr. K. E. Cooper, Department of Medical Physiology, Faculty of Medicine, The University of Calgary, Calgary, Alberta T2N 1N4, Canada

Dr. B. Cox, D.Sc., Bioscience II Department, ICI Ltd. Pharmaceuticals Division, Alderly Park, Macclesfield, Cheshire SK10 4TG, Great Britain

Dr. M. J. Dascombe, Department of Pharmacology, Materia Medica and Therapeutics, Stopford Building, The Medical School, University of Manchester, Oxford Road, Manchester M13 9PT, Great Britain

Dr. C. A. Dinarello, M.D., Assistant Professor of Medicine and Pediatrics, Division of Experimental Medicine, Tufts University School of Medicine, New England Medical Center, 136 Harrison Avenue, Boston, MA 02111/USA

Dr. J. S. Eisenman, Department of Physiology and Biophysics, Mount Sinai School of Medicine, One Gustave Levy Place, New York, NY 10029/USA

Dr. G. W. Gander, Ph.D., Professor of Pathology, Medical College of Virginia, Virginia Commonwealth University, Box 622, Richmond, VA 23298/USA

Dr. N. W. Kasting, Neuroendocrine Research Lab, 4th Floor Research Building, Massachusetts General Hospital, Boston, MA 02114/USA

Dr. D. H. KIM, Medicinal Chemistry Section, Wyeth Laboratories Inc., P.O. Box 8299, Philadelphia, PA 19101/USA

Dr. T. F. LEE, Department of Pharmacology, Materia Medica and Therapeutics, Stopford Building, The Medical School, Manchester University, Manchester M13 9PT, Great Britain

Professor A. S. MILTON, Department of Pharmacology, Marischal College, University of Aberdeen, Aberdeen AB9 1AS, Scotland, Great Britain

Dr. R. D. MYERS, Professor of Psychiatry and Pharmacology, University of North Carolina, School of Medicine, Chapel Hill, NC 27514/USA

Dr. C. OUNSTED, Consultant Physician, The Park Hospital for Children, Old Road, Headington, Oxford OX3 7LQ, Great Britain

Dr. R. G. PERTWEE, Department of Pharmacology, Marischal College, Aberdeen AB9 1AS, Scotland, Great Britain

Dr. W. W. REYNOLDS, Director, Biothermal Research Institute, Northeast Limnological Laboratory, R. D. 3, Box 10, Wyoming, PA 18644/USA

Miss V. K. SAWHNEY, Department of Pharmacology, University of Aberdeen, Marischal College, Aberdeen AB9 1AS, Scotland, Great Britain

Dr. J. B. P. STEPHENSON, Consultant in Paediatric Neurology, The Royal Hospital for Sick Children, Yorkhill, Glasgow G3 8SJ, Scotland, Great Britain

Dr. M. SZÉKELY, Department of Pathophysiology, University Medical School, Pécs, Szigeti út 12.Pf.99, 7643 Pécs, Hungary

Dr. Z. SZELÉNYI, Department of Pathophysiology, University Medical School, Pécs, Szigeti út 12.Pf.99, 7643 Pécs, Hungary

Dr. J. SZOLCSÁNYI, Department of Pharmacology, University Medical School, Pécs, Szigeti út 12., 7643 Pécs, Hungary

Professor W. L. VEALE, Department of Medical Physiology, Faculty of Medicine, The University of Calgary, 2929 24 Avenue N.W., Calgary Alberta T2N 1N4, Canada

Dr. S. M. WOLFF, M.D., Endicott Professor and Chairman, Department of Medicine, Physician-in-Chief, Tufts University School of Medicine, New England Medical Center Hospital, 171 Harrison Avenue, Boston, MA 02111/USA

To Wilhelm Feldberg

Preface

Fever has always been recognised as the major sign of infectious disease as well as being associated with other illnesses. The suggestion of publishing a volume dedicated exclusively to the subject of fever in the Handbook of Experimental Pharmacology series was one that greatly appealed to me, and I felt very honoured when I was invited to edit it. The first ideas about this volume were conceived in the latter part of 1977 and by the middle of 1978 the first authors had been approached. As is usual with such publications, by the time the first manuscripts were beginning to arrive in the late spring of 1979 there were still a few chapters for which authors had not yet been found. Finally by the end of 1981 the volume was complete. Because of the span of time over which the chapters were written, some refer to more recent work than others; however, I do not feel that this detracts from the overall contribution of all the chapters.

I would like to express my sincere thanks to every one of the authors who have written chapters and thus have made this volume possible. I very much appreciate the help which I have received from the staff of Springer-Verlag, in particular from DORIS WALKER. Last but not least, I wish to thank my secretary Mrs. VALERIE LYON (and her word processor) for not only typing my own chapters but also re-typing chapters from other authors, for keeping a complete tally of the references and for dealing with all the other secretarial work and problems associated with editing this volume.

A. S. MILTON

Contents

CHAPTER 4

Exogenous Pyrogens. C. A. DINARELLO and S. M. WOLFF

CHAPTER 5

Endogenous Pyrogens. G. W. GANDER

CHAPTER 6

Role of Central Neurotransmitters in Fever. B. COX and T. F. LEE

CHAPTER 7

The Role of Ions in Thermoregulation and Fever
R. D. MYERS. With 15 Figures

CHAPTER 8

Electrophysiology of the Anterior Hypothalamus: Thermoregulation and Fever
J. S. EISENMAN. With 5 Figures

CHAPTER 9

Cyclic Nucleotides and Fever. M. J. DASCOMBE. With 6 Figures

CHAPTER 10

Prostaglandins in Fever and the Mode of Action of Antipyretic Drugs
A. S. MILTON. With 8 Figures

CHAPTER 13

Therapeutic Agents Affecting Body Temperature. R. G. PERTWEE

CHAPTER 14

Capsaicin Type Pungent Agents Producing Pyrexia
J. SZOLCSÁNYI. With 4 Figures

CHAPTER 15

The Pathophysiology of Fever in the Neonate
M. SZÉKELY and Z. SZELÉNYI. With 12 Figures

CHAPTER 16

The Treatment of Fever from a Clinical Viewpoint. C. A. DINARELLO

CHAPTER 17

Malignant Hyperthermia: A Review. B. A. BRITT. With 11 Figures

CHAPTER 18

Febrile Convulsions. J. B. P. STEPHENSON and C. OUNSTED. With 1 Figure

CHAPTER 19

The Pyrogenic Responses of Non-mammalian Vertebrates
W. W. REYNOLDS and M. E. CASTERLIN

CHAPTER 20

The Pyrogenic Responses of Invertebrates
M. E. CASTERLIN and W. W. REYNOLDS

CHAPTER 1

Body Heat

A. S. MILTON

If a definition of life were required, it might be most clearly established on that capacity, by which the animal preserves its proper heat under the various degrees of temperature of the medium in which it lives. The most perfect animals possess this power in a superior degree, and to the exercise of their vital functions this is necessary. The inferior animals have it in a lower degree, in a degree however suited to their functions. In vegetables it seems to exist, but in a degree still lower, according to their more limited powers, and humbler destination ···

There is reason to believe, that while the actual temperature of the human body remains unchanged, its health is not permanently interrupted by the variation in the temperature of the medium that surrounds it; but that a few degrees of increase or diminution of the heat of the system, produces disease and death. A knowledge therefore of the laws which regulate the vital heat, seems to be the most important branch of physiology.

JAMES CURRIE, 1808

So wrote James Currie in his book entitled *Medical Reports on the Effects of Water as a Remedy in Fever and Other Diseases*. If ever a justification was needed for research into body temperature regulation and into the mode of action of drugs affecting body temperature then it is contained in those two paragraphs.

Of all the symptoms of disease, fever is the one most easily recognised as being of pathological significance. Why is it that even today body temperature is the first thing that most doctors measure on seeing a sick patient, and temperature is measured daily in every patient in every hospital throughout the land? It is because the course of a disease and the recovery from both disease and surgery can be, in so many cases, most easily monitored by measuring body temperatures.

The symptoms of fever – shivering, cold, and clammy extremities, the burning forehead, profuse sweating and the subjective feeling of heat and cold – have been recorded throughout history. The very words we use stem from the classical languages: fever from the Latin *febris*, and pyrexia and pyretic from the Greek *pyretos*. The folklore of fever is vast, with every culture and civilisation having its own myths and explanations. The most well known of the early explanations come from the works of Empedocles and Hypocrates. Empedocles of Agrigentum in Sicily (504–443 B.C.) proposed the doctrine of the four elements, earth, air, fire, and water, as the "four-fold root of all things." The human body was considered to be composed of these four fundamental elements, with health resulting from a correct balance of all four, and disease an imbalance. Plato and Aristotle introduced the idea of four qualities "dry, cold, hot, and moist," and combined them with the four elements in the following scheme. Cold and dry represented *earth*, hot and moist represented *air*, hot and dry represented *fire*, and cold and moist represented *water*.

Subsequently, Hypocrates (460–370 B.C.) put forward the idea of the four humours, blood, phlegm, yellow bile, and black bile, in which the scheme of the four elements was modified such that cold and dry represented *black bile*, hot and moist, *blood*, hot and dry, *yellow bile*, and cold and moist, *phlegm*. Hypocrates maintained that illness resulted from an overproduction of one of these four humours and that the body destroyed the excess humours, perhaps by increasing the body's heat (i.e. by developing a fever). As Currie says of Hypocrates: "Perceiving the increase of heat to be the most remarkable symptom in fever, he assumed this for the cause and founded his distinctions of fevers, on the different degrees of the intenseness of this heat. He had not an instrument that could measure this exactly, and necessarily trusted to his sensations." Hypocrates obviously believed that fever was necessary for the reduction of disease. Galen (131–201 A.D.), as written in his work *Methodus medendi*, considered that medicines should be classified according to their various humoral contents. Perhaps because of the teachings of Hypocrates and Galen that fever was "beneficial," the use of drugs as antipyretics does not appear in their writings, or indeed the writings of physicians up until the nineteenth century. Any effect on body temperature was purely accidental to their curing of the disease. In the seventeenth century one of the most eminent medical men of his time, Thomas Sydenham (1624–1689), revised the Hypocratic methods of observation and stated "Nature calls in fever as her usual instrument for expelling from the blood any hostile matters that may lurk in it" (LATHAM 1848). Again, quoting from Currie, "It was the postulate of Sydenham that every disease is nothing else but an endeavour of nature to expel morbific matter of one kind or another, by which her healthy operations are impeded." However, in the late nineteenth and in this century physicians have generally regarded fever as being harmful to the body and have made every effort to reduce it. Surprisingly, in spite of these modern views there are those who believe that except in life-threatening situations fever may indeed be beneficial to the organism (see KLUGER 1980).

Modern studies on pyretics and antipyretics and our understanding of fever stem from two important developments. The first was the introduction of the clinical thermometer. The first thermometer is properly attributed to Galileo, who is said to have invented it sometime between the years 1593 and 1597. The first clinical thermometer was described by Sanctorius in 1625, but it was not until the second decade of the eighteenth century that the measuring thermometer was described by Fahrenheit.

The importance of thermometry may be best described in the words of Carl Wunderlich as recorded by Seguin in 1871 (WUNDERLICH and SEGUIN 1871):

Thermometry has truly discovered, according to the vivid expression of Wunderlich, a new world, the one dreamed of by Currie, the law of the action of external upon human temperature. But this therapeutic application of the two relative terms of caloric to the treatment of disease is only the initial impulse of an immense revolution, whose subsequences, hidden to the view of the far-seeing Currie, are hardly traceable in our horizon; I mean, the calorific and frigorific action of all our medicines, vegetables, and their alkaloids, metals, metaloid bodies, and gases. This entirely new field of observation, and of therapeutic action, would vanish like a mirage if thermometry could be suppressed. But, far from this impious impossibility, thermometry will find out even the positivism of empiricism in the law of concordance of the apparently most discording treatments; and will reconcile schools which were divided, only because they did not know that their far diverging means converged to the same action and object – the keeping up of normal temperature, that is to say, life; and the suppressing of the sources of pathological temperatures – that is, death, *in propria persona*.

The second important development was the publication by STONE in 1763 of a paper in the *Philosophical Transactions of the Royal Society of London* on the use of an extract of willow bark in the treatment of fever. This is the first scientific paper to describe the use of an antipyretic drug. However, according to HANZLIK (1927) the use of decoctions of willow bark as a "general febrifuge" goes back to ancient times, and he indicates that this use continued throughout the mediaeval period until the general introduction of salicylates at the end of the nineteenth century. However, according to the teaching of the medical profession based upon the work of Hypocrates and Galen one must assume that somewhere along the line folk medicine and the practice of the medical profession were not as one in the use of drugs to reduce fever. Hanzlik recounts the use of willow bark as a successful substitute for cinchona bark during the Napoleonic Wars (1803–1815) in the treatment of fever. In 1798 LONGMORE wrote a paper on 14 soldiers who were poisoned in Quebec after consuming a "decoction of certain plants" in which he states that an extract of gaultheria (which contains methyl salicylate) "is frequently used by Canadians and is said to be cooling and grateful ptisan in fevers." Until 1874 quinine was the main antipyretic, its use, of course, being primarily in the treatment of malarial fever.

It is interesting to remember that extracts of plants such as willow, which contain substances which we now refer to as salicylates, had been used for centuries in medical treatment, but that no mention of their antipyretic action is recorded until the paper of Stone in 1763. For example, Hypocrates recommended juice of the poplar tree for eye diseases and the leaves of willow trees in childbirth. Celsus, in the first century A.D., used juices of willow trees for removing corns and Discorides recommended their use for earache, skin diseases, and gout. Galen recommended their use for bloody wounds and ulcers. Similarly, one can find mention of many plants containing salicylate in the herbals of the Middle Ages and the Renaissance. Neither Currie nor Wunderlich mention antipyretic drugs in their writings. The former regarded direct cooling of the body as the method of treatment of fever, and Wunderlich was primarily concerned with observations made during various fevers and the progress of the disease.

Just as this chapter began with the words of James Currie, perhaps it is fitting to conclude with the words that he wrote in the Preface to his work and addressed to the Right Honourable Sir Joseph Banks.

About eighteen years ago when I was at Edinburgh I discovered that the accounts given of the temperature of the human body under disease, even by the most approved authors, are, with a few exceptions, founded, not on any exact measurement of heat, but on the sensations of the patient himself, or his attendants.

Impressed with the belief, that till more accurate information should be obtained respecting the acutal temperature in different circumstances of health, and disease, no permanent theory of vital motion could be established, nor any certain progress made in the treatment of those diseases in which the temperature is diminished or increased.

Your faithful and very obedient Servant

Liverpool, 31st October, 1797   JAMES CURRIE

References

Currie J (1808) Medical reports on the effects of water as a remedy in fever and other diseases, 4 th London edn. Philadelphia. Presented for James Humphreys and for Benjamin and Thomas Kite

Hanzlik PJ (1927) Actions and use of salicylates and cinchophen in medicine. In: Medicine monographs, vol 9. Williams and Wilkins, Baltimore

Kluger MJ (1980) Fever. Its biology, evolution, and function. Princeton University Press, Princeton/NJ

Latham RG (1848) The works of Thomas Sydenham, M.D. Printed for the Sydenham Society, vol II, London, p 138

Longmore G (1798) Account of fourteen men of the Royal Artillery at Quebec who were nearly poisoned by drinking a decoction of certain plants. Ann Med Edin 3:364–378

Stone E (1763) An account of the success of the bark of the willow in the cure of agues. Phil Trans 53:195–200

Wunderlich CA,, Seguin E (1871) Medical thermometry and human temperature. William Wood, New York

CHAPTER 2

Fever and Its Role in Disease: Rationale for Antipyretics

N. W. KASTING, W. L. VEALE, and K. E. COOPER

A. Fever

Disease and infection are almost invariably accompanied by the symptom of fever. Indeed, fever may often be the diagnostic sign that such an infection is present and can be used in the diagnosis of specific diseases. In fact, from the detailed descriptions of fevers given by Hippocrates, it is even possible to identify specific ailments (ATKINS and BODEL 1979).

The contention that fever is an important component of disease is attested to by the wide phylogenetic spectrum of vertebrates, and even invertebrates, that are capable of responding to bacterial infection with fever. It was assumed in early times that fever was a disease in itself. Later, as processes of disease began to become understood, it became dogma that fever was beneficial in the body's fight against infection (SYDENHAM 1666, quoted by DE KRUIF and SIMPSON 1940; WELCH 1888), although there was no experimental evidence for or against this assumption.

An evaluation of the role of fever as an integral part of disease necessitates an understanding of the processes involved in the genesis of fever. Furthermore, in an attempt to rationalize the appropriate use of antipyretic drugs, it is essential to attempt to understand the precise role of fever in the disease process.

Fever is a pathological elevation of body temperature caused by any number of agents, called pyrogens. Most naturally occurring fevers result in a moderate increase in body temperature (DUBOIS 1949) which rarely exceeds 3° or 4 °C. The elevation of body temperature in fever is attained by active mechanisms controlled and coordinated by the central nervous system (CNS) and is not due, for instance, to a direct effect of bacteria or their products on heat production or vasoconstriction. Fever may be the result of either an increase in set-point (temperature) around which body temperature is normally regulated (MACPHERSON 1959; COOPER et al. 1964; COOPER 1972; STITT et al. 1974; CABANAC and MASSONNET 1974) or a decrease in thermal sensitivity of central warm-sensitive neurones (MITCHELL et al. 1970; EISENMAN 1974). The elevation in body temperature during fever can be brought about by varying the level of heat production and heat loss, depending on the ambient temperature (PALMES and PARK 1965; ATKINS and BODEL 1972). Fevers produced by a standard dose of bacterial pyrogen (BP) result in a similar increase in body temperature despite wide variations in ambient temperature (GRANT 1949; KERPAL-FRONIUS et al. 1966; COOPER 1972; COOPER and VEALE 1974). That is, fever in the cold may be brought about by intense heat production, whereas in the warm, a simple decrease in heat loss will produce the same degree of fever.

Fever is accompanied by many systemic changes which may be due to the change in body temperature per se or to an event related to fever. These changes include: increases in heart rate (COOPER 1971); increases in renal blood flow (GOLD-RING et al. 1941; CRANSTON et al. 1959; COOPER et al. 1960); increases in hepatic and total splanchnic blood flow (BRADLEY and CONAN 1947); antidiuresis (KRUK and SADOWSKI 1978); effects on cell structure; changes in enzyme levels; modification of the metabolism of carbohydrates, fats, and protein; haemorrhage; increased blood coagulation; changes in gastric secretion and motility; modification of endocrine function (THOMAS 1954; BENNETT and BEESON 1950; BENNETT 1964). To determine the role of fever in disease accurately, it is necessary to take into account these changes that directly or indirectly accompany a fever.

The distinction between fever and hyperthermia is a fundamental one which must be examined (STITT 1979). Fever is an elevated body temperature which is actively produced and actively defended against thermal challenges, hot or cold (MACPHERSON 1959; COOPER et al. 1964). The febrile subject's thermal preferendum is higher than that for the non-febrile subject, indicating the febrile subject feels more comfortable at a higher temperature (CABANAC and MASSONNET 1974). Hyperthermia, such as heat stroke or malignant hyperthermia, is a condition in which heat gain or heat production has exceeded the capacity of the patient to lose heat. The patient has a subjective feeling of being hot but cannot mobilize heat loss mechanisms to a sufficient degree to attain normal body temperature. This distinction is useful, especially when alternative methods to chemically induced antipyresis are used in treatment of fevers. Physical cooling is uncomfortable for the patient who will mobilize heat production and heat conservation effectors to maintain the febrile temperature (STEELE et al. 1970). Antipyretics, however, by virtue of their mode of action, can be thought of as agents which produce a decrease in the setpoint which is elevated during fever; the decrease in body temperature occurs without discomfort or stress.

Pyrogens, the agents responsible for causing a fever, can be divided into two broad classifications; exogenous pyrogens and endogenous pyrogens. Exogenous pyrogens are those substances that are not made by the body and endogenous pyrogens are hormones made by the body. Exogenous pyrogens include Gram-negative and Gram-positive bacteria, viruses, fungi, certain non-microbial antigens, certain steroids, and other pharmacological agents (DINARELLO 1979). Bacterial endotoxin or bacterial pyrogen (BP) is the lipopolysaccharide of the cell wall of Gram-negative bacteria. It is the lipid A moiety that appears to have the pyrogenicity. Endotoxin is the pyrogen used most extensively in experimental studies aimed at determining the mechanisms of the febrile response. This approach only approximates the condition of live, multiplying bacteria but is useful because the febrile responses are repeatable, not lethal, and activated in the same manner as with live bacteria.

These exogenous pyrogens stimulate the cells of the reticulo-endothelial system (RES) to synthesize and release endogenous pyrogen (EP). EP was first demonstrated by BENNETT and BEESON (1953) and has been shown to be a protein with a molecular weight of approximately 15000 daltons (MURPHY et al. 1974; DINARELLO and WOLFF 1977). EP is synthesized de novo (FESSLER et al. 1961; BODEL 1970; NORLUND et al. 1970) or may be changed from an inactive form (HAHN et al. 1970 a, b). It has been shown to be produced in mammals, reptiles, and amphibians (KLUGER 1979). The EP from different species is not identical (DINARELLO et al. 1977) but EP from one species can often produce fevers in another species (DINARELLO et al. 1977; BORSOOK et al. 1978). EP is cleared rapidly from the blood by the kidneys (DINARELLO et al 1978; TOWNSEND and CRANSTON 1979).

EP is produced by blood granulocytes (BEESON 1948), monocytes (BODEL and ATKINS 1967), and eosinophils (MICKENBERG et al. 1972), alveolar macrophages (ATKINS et al. 1967), peritoneal exodate macrophages (HAHN et al. 1967), splenic sinusoidal cells and hepatic Kupffer cells (DINARELLO et al. 1968). The action of EP is not understood fully but it appears to stimulate the neurones in the preoptic area and anterior hypothalamus (PO/AH) which in turn control the events leading to fever. There is no evidence at present, however, that EP actually enters the brain. Therefore, EP may be acting at the level of the vascular endothelium to trigger some intermediary process that in turn stimulates the neurones. EP may, of course, cross into the brain and act directly on the neurones since EP micro-injected onto cells directly stimulates them (SCHOENER and WANG 1975 a).

Several neurotransmitters have been proposed for the pathways regulating fever. There is a large amount of experimental evidence suggesting prostaglandins are an important mediator of fever in the PO/AH; this was first demonstrated by MILTON and WENDLANDT (1970, 1971). This evidence includes:

1) Prostaglandins E_1 or E_2 (PGE_1, PGE_2) had a potent, hyperthermic effect with a short latency when micro-injected directly into the cerebral ventricles or into the tissue of the brain that is sensitive to EP micro-injection in many species (FELDBERG and SAXENA 1971; STITT 1973; LIPTON and FOSSLER 1974; LIPTON et al. 1973; VEALE and WHISHAW 1976).
2) Antipyretic drugs were found to be potent inhibitors of prostaglandin synthesis (VANE 1971; FLOWER and VANE 1972).
3) During fever, PGE levels in the cerebrospinal fluid (CSF) rose and, if the fever was reduced with antipyretic drugs, PGE levels were also reduced (FELDBERG and GUPTA 1973).

There is some evidence against PGE having a role as a mediator in the fever pathway. If the PO/AH was lesioned, PGE no longer caused fever while EP was still capable of inducing a fever (VEALE and COOPER 1975; COOPER et al. 1976). The most convincing evidence is the recent demonstration that a specific PGE antagonist antagonized PGE fevers but arachidonic acid (AA) or EP fevers were unaffected (CRANSTON et al. 1976). This indicates perhaps another AA derivative may be involved or act in conjunction with PGE.

Monoamines may also have a role in CNS connections subserving fever. Micro-injection and depletion studies have yielded conflicting results. Acetylcholine is most certainly involved in the activation of the heat production and heat conservation pathways.

With respect to fever, vasopressin has recently been demonstrated to have a putative role as an endogenous antipyretic in the brain under certain circumstances (KASTING et al. 1979; COOPER et al. 1979).

An anatomical location and a mechanism have been proposed for the set-point around which body temperature is regulated and is elevated during fever. The sodium: calcium ratio in the posterior hypothalamus affects the body temperature around which an animal will regulate its body temperature. An excess of Ca^{+2} caused the animal to regulate at a lower body temperature and an excess of Na^+ caused the animal to regulate at a new higher or "febrile" body temperature (MYERS and VEALE 1970; MYERS and VEALE 1971). The way in which this set-point in the posterior hypothalamus interacts with the pyrogen-sensitive PO/AH and activates the effector pathways is not clear.

The result of the sequence of events described above is the activation of shivering and non-shivering thermogenesis and heat conservation effectors such as vasoconstriction and apnoea, and, consequently, the elevated body temperature called fever. The particular characteristics of the fever are dependent on the particular aetiology of the fever.

B. The Role of Fever in Disease

The question of the use of antipyretics will be discussed in this section. Is fever a beneficial host defence response against infection and does fever render the animal more likely to survive? In theory, it is also possible that fever is beneficial to the infecting micro-organism. In the instance of herpes simplex (fever blisters), this may be true but, except for this example, there is no evidence to support this contention. Fever could also be a neutral side effect of some other process that is of some adaptive value.

The value of fever might be ascertained indirectly by looking at the phylogenetic development of fever. All animals have the ability to thermoregulate behaviourally but ectothermic animals, unlike mammals, lack the physiological effectors for heat production and heat conservation. Thus, behavioural thermoregulation is the principal way in which they regulate their body temperature. This behavioural thermoregulation of ectotherms has been utilized extensively in the study of fever because of the ease with which their body temperature can be experimentally manipulated without stressful intervention, as is the case with mammals. The animals are provided with a thermal gradient which will allow the animal the opportunity to adjust its body temperature by simply moving to a warmer or cooler area of the gradient. The crayfish, an invertebrate, has been shown to respond with a behavioural fever by moving to a warmer ambient temperature when infected with bacteria (CASTERLIN and REYNOLDS 1977a). Fish (REYNOLDS 1977; REYNOLDS et al. 1976), amphibians (CASTERLIN and REYNOLDS 1977b; KLUGER 1977; MYHRE et al. 1977), and reptiles (BERNHEIM and KLUGER 1976a) were capable of responding to live bacteria or BP by behaviourally seeking a warmer ambient temperature and raising their body temperatures to febrile levels. Birds (VAN MIERT and FRENS 1968) and most mammals respond with a fever to live bacteria or BP. The fact that fever has been retained on such a phylogenetically grand scale is tempting evidence for a considerable survival value for the organisms capable of responding to infection with a fever.

Some mammals do not readily get fevers in response to BP or infection and may, in fact, become hypothermic. Rats, mice, and some primates are among those mammals. This unusual circumstance indicates that fever is not absolutely necessary for survival of a species or that intravenously (i.v.) injected BP is not a reliable model for natural infections. If fever has some survival value to the host, then these animals may have developed an alternative mechanisms for dealing effectively with infections.

The question of the beneficial value of fever to an infected animal has been the subject of speculation and investigation for many years. Fevers could be beneficial to an animal in two ways:

1) The high body temperatures of fever could exceed the temperature beyond which the infectious micro-organism could live and thereby directly kill it.

2) Indirectly by affecting one or several biochemical, cellular or humoral components of the body which in turn destroy the micro-organism. This effect could, in turn, involve a change that directly destroyed the micro-organism or a change that depleted an essential substrate for the micro-organism.

The early work which sought to determine the survival value of fever was confused by altering the responses of experimentally infected hyper- or hypothermia. As previously mentioned, these procedures could involve additional stress for the mammals and clearly the response of the animal will involve different mechanisms than those when the animal develops its own fever. It is, therefore, questionable what, if any, meaning such experiments have on the adaptive role of fever in disease. Several of the early studies dealt with the effects of fever on micro-organisms that were directly sensitive to increased temperatures which is a situation now known to represent relatively few infecting micro-organisms.

Thus it is that some micro-organisms may be killed directly by febrile temperatures of the host animal. Indeed, it was known that syphilis and gonorrhea are heat sensitive and are killed directly by increased temperatures. The basis of treatment before the advent of antibiotics consisted of inducing fevers in these patients using artificial fever caused by injections of BP. The high fevers would subsequently arrest the infecting bacteria (CULVER 1917; HENCH 1935; HASLER and SPEKTER 1936). Interestingly enough, these infections seldom produce high fevers (BENNETT and NICASTRI 1960).

Since ectothermic animals can have their body temperatures easily manipulated, they have proven to be an excellent model with which to study survival value of fever. Lizards which are kept at a certain ambient temperature will regulate their body temperature at that level. Lizards were infected with a dose of bacteria which was lethal in 50% of the animals (LD_{50}). Groups of infected lizards were kept at 34° or 36 °C (hypothermic), 38 °C (normothermic), and 40° or 42 °C (febrile). Those lizards allowed to raise their body temperatures above normal or get fevers (40° or 42 °C) had greatly increased survival rates compared with those infected animals with normothermic or hypothermic temperatures (KLUGER et al. 1975). If the infected lizards were allowed to choose the ambient temperature in a thermal gradient, they chose a temperature of about 41 °C that would allow them to raise their body temperatures to febrile levels. The survival rate of these lizards (92%) was much greater than those kept at 38 °C (25%) (BERNHEIM and KLUGER 1976 b).

Similar results were obtained with bacterially infected fish. The survival of infected goldfish is related to their body temperatures. Infected goldfish selected warmer water than normal and consequently their mortality was decreased (COVERT and REYNOLDS 1977).

Fever is clearly beneficial to an infected ectotherm, at least under the conditions studied. The question, then, is how does fever help the host overcome the infecting bacteria? The particular bacteria (*Aeromonas hydrophila*) used in these studies on lizards were found to grow equally well at febrile and normal body temperatures in vitro (GRIEGER and KLUGER 1977). However, if the bacteria were incubated in a low-iron medium, such as occurs in vivo with fevers, then bacterial growth was inhibited at febrile temperatures (41 °C) to a greater extent than at normal temperatures (38 °C). In an attempt to validate these observations, infected lizards were kept at 41 °C (febrile) and given excess iron or saline as control. Mortality was increased in lizards which received the excess iron. Therefore, fever's beneficial effects in the lizard infected with this particular micro-organism result from the integration of fever and low plasma iron. The fever increases the bacteria's need for iron while the serum iron is decreased owing to the bacterial infection (GRIEGER and KLUGER 1978).

Other effects of fever may contribute to its adaptive value as a host defence mechanism. Fever may increase the early response to infection. The same experimental model was used to look at other characteristics of the immunological response (BERNHEIM et al. 1978). Lizards which were allowed to maintain a febrile temperature (41 °C) for 12 h after infection had negative blood cultures compared with positive blood cultures in lizards with body temperatures of 38° or 35 °C. Cultures of other tissues showed febrile lizards contained considerably less live bacteria than afebrile lizards. In vitro experiments indicated no difference in growth rates of bacteria at 35°, 38°, or 41 °C. Histological examination indicated that the injection site for the live bacteria contained considerably more leucocytes in the febrile animals than in afebrile animals despite similar blood counts of white cells in febrile versus afebrile animals. Both in vivo and in vitro tests of granulocyte chemotaxic and phagocytic functions were similar for 41° and 38 °C. Serum antibody levels were similar in febrile and afebrile lizards. The conclusion drawn from this work was that fever enhances the early inflammatory response which causes increased leucocyte emigration to the infected site and containment of the infection.

Thus, it appears that with the lizard and the same pathogenic bacteria, there may be two beneficial effects of fever, and likely more.

The survival or adaptive value of fever in mammals has long been enigmatic (ATKINS and BODEL 1972; BENNETT and NICASTRI 1960; KLASTERSKY and KASS 1970). The clearly beneficial role of fever in other vertebrates suggest it may have a similar, as yet undefined, role in mammals. In an attempt to clarify this issue, rabbits were infected with LD_{50} of a naturally occurring bacterium (*Pasteurella multocida*) and the magnitude of the fever was compared with the mortality. Survival increased as the magnitude of the fever increased up to 2.25 °C. Fevers higher than 2.25 °C were associated with somewhat of a decrease in survival (KLUGER and VAUGHN 1978).

The beneficial integration of reduced plasma iron and fever, as demonstrated in the lizard, was investigated in the rabbit. Plasma iron decreases when the rabbits became infected. In vitro, the bacteria grow less well at febrile temperatures with reduced iron than either normal temperatures with reduced iron or febrile temperatures with high iron (KLUGER and ROTHENBURG 1979). The effects of fever on the early host defence response of mammals has not yet been investigated. The mechanisms by which fever affects other bacteria and infectious agents has not been investigated.

The rat has been used to study the effects of fever on survival. Rats were allowed either to get a normal fever in response to a *Salmonella enteritidis* infection or their preoptic anterior hypothalamic region was cooled while they got the infection. This latter procedure caused that group of rats to maintain a fever of about 1 °C higher than control infected animals. Mortality was considerably greater in the rats with cooled hypothalami and therefore the higher fevers (BANET 1979) This evidence does not allow observations on the survival effect of moderate (normal) fevers in rats but it seems to support the rabbit work which showed a decline in survival with high fevers.

Another model system involved infecting ferrets with influenza viruses and studying the relation between fever and presence of live viruses in their nasal passages. There was a demonstrable negative correlation between fever magnitude and the subsequent presence of live viruses in the nasal passage (TOMS et al. 1977).

Other aspects of the immunological system may be enhanced at febrile temperatures. These include increased breakdown of lysosomal particles thereby releasing hydrolytic enzymes (LWOFF 1969; OVERGAARD 1977), increased interferon production (Ho 1970), increased leucocyte motility (NAHAS et al. 1971; PHELPS and STANISLAW 1969), leucocyte bactericidal activity (SEBAG et al. 1977), and lymphocyte transformation (ROBERTS and STEIGBIGEL 1977; ASHMAN and NAHMIAS 1977).

There is an apparent contradiction to the adaptive theory of fever. There is evidence that fever does not invariably occur in response to BP. Newborn humans may have severe infections without responding with a fever. Of infants infected with SALMONELLA, only 4 out of 26 were febrile (EPSTEIN et al. 1951). Fever occurred in about half of newborn infants with septicaemia and the febrile babies were those at the older end of the age distribution (SMITH et al. 1956). Similarly, infants less than 10 days of age had fewer fevers than infants between 11 and 30 days of age when suffering from urinary tract infections (BERGSTROM et al. 1972). It has also been demonstrated that newborn guinea-pigs (BLATTEIS 1975), rabbits (WATSON and KIM 1963), and sheep (PITTMAN et al. 1973; KASTING et al. 1979) respond with little or no fever to BP under conditions in which the adult animals readily become febrile. This decreased responsiveness has been determined to occur at the level of the CNS since febrile responses to EP were also decreased (BLATTEIS 1977; BLATTEIS and SMITH 1977; KASTING et al. 1979). Thermoregulatory effectors appear to be intact and functional in these animals (BLATTEIS 1975, 1976; ALEXANDER 1975; PITTMAN et al. 1974).

The observation was also made that the female sheep responded to BP with no fever or a fever of lower than normal magnitude for a period of several days before parturition and for several hours afterwards. The fevers were diminished for EP as well, which indicated the effect to be taking place at the level of the CNS, similar to the situation in the newborn lamb (KASTING et al. 1978 a, b).

If fever has a beneficial survival value under normal circumstances of infection, then it is probable that, in the near-term ewe and newborn lamb, fever must have a detrimental effect that is of greater immediate concern than an infection unmodified by fever. If this is the case, then perhaps the ewe and newborn have an alternate mechanism for fighting infection. Conversely, there may be an increased morbidity of near-term ewes and newborn lambs. This has not been investigated to our knowledge.

What the detrimental effect of fever might be in this circumstance is not known. One possibility is that febrile temperatures may adversely affect the maturation of lung surfactant of the foetus in the last few days of intrauterine life. In vitro experiments have demonstrated that lung surfactant was adversely affected by temperatures higher than normal (MEBAN 1978). Higher than normal body temperatures may also increase the consequences of anoxia during parturition.

Whether this afebrile period occurs in human mothers has not been systematically investigated, but anecdotal evidence suggests there may be a similar phenomenon (HIPPOCRATES; KULLANDER, personal communication). Fever and other hyperthermias during certain critical developmental stages of pregnancy have been postulated to cause severe CNS disorders such as microencephaly and spina bifida (SMITH et al. 1978). The teratogenic effects of fever or infection on human foetuses has been disputed, the association between the two variables described as no better than chance (KLEINEBRECHT et al. 1979). This teratogenic effect has been demonstrated experimentally in guinea-pigs (EDWARDS 1967, 1971). Extremely high body temperatures, as occur occasionally during fevers, especially in children can have lethal effects by destroying sensitive tissues, such as occur in the brain. Fever induced by BP in rabbits has been shown to cause disaggregation of polyribosomes in the brain (HEIKKILA and BROWN 1979).

Another problem of significant consequence in children is that of febrile convulsions. Febrile convulsions do not necessarily occur with very high fevers but may be precipitated during any stage of the rise and fall of body temperature during fever (LENNOX-BUCHTHAL 1973). They may, therefore, be caused by some event associated with fever but not caused by absolute temperatures. A child who has had a single febrile convulsion is more likely to have another and is more likely than the non-seizure child to become epileptic (ANNEGERS et al. 1979). Therefore, it is very important to prevent febrile convulsions in children. A detailed review of the literature on febrile convulsions is given in Chap. 7 of this volume.

C. Antipyretic Drugs

BARBOUR (1921) wrote "Substances which reduce the temperature in febrile and similar states but not in normal conditions, unless the dosage be excessive, are termed antipyretics." This description of antipyretics is still an accurate description with regard to what is known of the actions and uses of antipyretics today. Drugs which remove the cause of the infection, such as antibiotics, are not considered antipyretic. Antipyretics can be divided into two major categories, non-steroidal antipyretics and steroidal antipyretics. This chapter will concern itself with the former category, non-steroidal antipyretics. Figure 1 illustrates the chemical structures of some of the important antipyretics employed in the last century.

The earliest antipyretic used was quinine, extracted from Cinchona bark. Quinine has since been found to be effective only against malarial fevers and that effect is principally at the level of the infectious agent, unlike other antipyretics. Short-

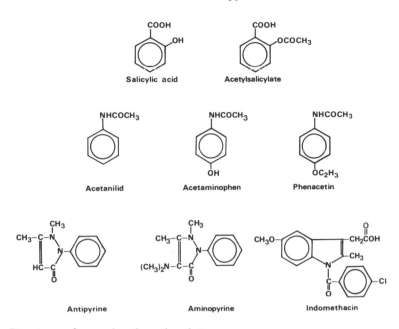

Fig. 1. Structures of several antipyretic substances

ages of Cinchona bark which occurred in England in 1756 prompted the discovery that willow bark extracts had effective antipyretic properties. The isolation of salicin from the willow bark in 1830, and subsequent preparation from salicin of salicylic acid by PIREA in 1838, constituted a major break-through. BUSS first used salicylate clinically in 1875. Acetyl salicylate was first synthesized by VON GER-HARDT in 1853 but was not used clinically until 1899 by DRESSER and WOHLGEMUT.

The p-aminophenol compounds were also discovered quite early. Acetanilid was first prepared in 1886 but was rather toxic. Phenactin and acetophenetidin were also prepared and used as antipyretics. Acetaminophen was prepared and first used in 1893, although it has only recently been reintroduced as a clinical antipyretic. Other antipyretics include pyrazolone derivatives, antipyrine, and aminopyrine, but these compounds have limited used because of toxic side effects. Indomethacin is a potent antipyretic but remains of limited use. Mefanamic acid and other anthranilic acid derivatives have been recently shown to be effective antipyretics (ZIEL and KRUPP 1975).

Recent work has shown evidence for an endogenous antipyretic (KASTING et al. 1978 a, b). Endogenous substances that have been shown to have antipyretic activity include cortisol (CHOWERS et al. 1968), cortisone (ATKINS et al. 1955), and vasopressin (KASTING et al. 1978; COOPER et al. 1979). It is important to realize at which point in the sequence of events between infection and elevation of body temperature that antipyretics act.

1) Antipyretics could interfere with BP–cell interaction and the subsequent synthesis or release of EP.
2) Antipyretics could inactivate EP in the blood.
3) Antipyretics could block EP entry into the brain.

4) Antipyretics could block the action of EP on neurones in the CNS.
5) The antipyretics could effect the thermoregulatory effectors, that is increasing heat loss or decreasing heat production.

Despite the initial report that salicylates decreased EP production (GANDER et al. 1967), most subsequent studies using a variety of antipyretics and cells from different species have shown that antipyretics have no demonstrable effect on BP–cell interaction or EP synthesis and release (LIN and CHAI 1972; VAN MIERT et al. 1971; HOO et al. 1972; CLARK and MOYER 1972). Most in vivo models have also shown little or no effect of antipyretics on circulating EP levels (BENNETT and BEESON 1953; CLARK and CUMBY 1975).

Studies in which antipyretics have been tested indicate that EP is not inactivated nor its potency reduced by incubation with antipyretics (HOO et al. 1972; LIN and CHAI 1972; GRUNDMAN 1969; CLARK and CUMBY 1975).

Initially, it was reported that intracerebroventricular (ICV) salicylate could not antagonize an intravenous EP fever (COOPER et al. 1968). It has subsequently been determined that antipyretics are effective when administered ICV or into the PO/AH and in much smaller quantities than systemic administration (CRANSTON et al. 1971; CRANSTON and RAWLINS 1972; LIN and CHAI 1972; CLARK and ALDERDICE 1972; AVERY and PENN 1974; VAUGHN et al. 1979). In addition, it was shown that acetylsalicylate micro-injected into the PO/AH inhibited the effects of EP micro-injected into the same area (SCHOENER and WANG 1975a). Experiments were performed in which centrally injected EP was antagonized by peripherally administered antipyretics (CRANSTON et al. 1970; LIN and CHAI 1972; CHAI et al. 1971; CLARK and CUMBY 1975). All this evidence makes it unlikely that antipyretics work by preventing the entry of EP into the brain.

Antipyretics, therefore, work in the PO/AH. They could act by antagonizing EP or EP-stimulated events in the PO/AH. The fact that EP and antipyretics act to alter firing patterns of central thermosensitive neurones has been shown repeatedly. Single unit studies demonstrated that IV-injected BP depressed the spontaneous activity and sensitivity of warm-sensitive neurones and increased both spontaneous firing and sensitivity of cold-sensitive neurones (CABANAC et al. 1968; WIT and WANG 1968; EISENMAN 1969). Acetylsalicylate was administered systemically and it reversed the pyrogen-induced changes in neuronal activity but, if no pyrogen was present, these neurones were unaffected by the antipyretic (WIT and WANG 1968). Micro-injected acetylsalicylate antagonized the changes in firing due to micro-injected EP at the same site (SCHOENER and WANG 1975a).

There are several possible ways in which antipyretics could act to antagonize the effects of EP on central neurones. These include:
1) Inhibition of prostaglandin synthesis
2) Antagonism at a specific EP receptor
3) Indirect antagonism of set-point in posterior hypothalamus
4) Indirect antagonism acting through release of an endogenous antipyretic.

There is the possibility that more than one of these mechanisms work in an integrated fashion.

The prostaglandin theory of fever offers a ready explanation for the mechanism of action of antipyretics by virtue of their effects on inhibition of prostaglandins synthesis (VANE 1971). In support of this theory, when antipyretics were administered to reduce fevers, PGE levels decreased in the CSF in parallel. Antipyretic potencies seem to relate well with prostaglandin synthetase inhibition (ZIEL and KRUPP 1975). Of interest is the observation that acetaminophen inhibits only brain synthetase and is antipyretic but not anti-inflammatory.

It is possible that antipyretics compete with EP for a receptor on central neurones. Parallel shifts in a logarithmic dose–response relationship were demonstrated (CLARK and COLDWELL 1972) for salicylate and paracetamol injected ICV on EP fevers. Shifts caused by antipyretics have been demonstrated in other conditions (LIN and CHAI 1972; CLARK and CUMBY 1975). These shifts could be explained by competition for a receptor but other explanations are possible. It was demonstrated that acetylsalicylate could reduce the firing rate of neurones in one side of the hypothalamus that had increased as a result of EP injected on the contralateral side (SCHOENER and WANG 1975 b). Therefore, it seems unlikely that antipyretics work directly by competition for the same receptor as EP.

Antipyretics may function by reducing the set-point as established by $Ca^{2+}:Na^+$ ratio. This would be an indirect effect because of the discrepancies between apparent site of action of antipyretics and the site of the set-point mechanism. It has been shown that efflux of $^{45}Ca^{2+}$ into the third ventricle increased during a fever. During defervescence, increased $^{22}Na^+$ was detected in the ventricle while $^{45}Ca^{2+}$ was retained in the tissue (MYERS 1974).

Evidence has been provided for an endogenous antipyretic in the brain (KASTING et al. 1978 a, b, 1979; COOPER et al. 1979) and the possibility occurs that antipyretics could have their effects directly or indirectly through such a system.

The question of whether antipyretics act by suppressing the effector mechanisms, either in the CNS or the body, has been investigated principally by trying to determine if antipyretics lower body temperatures in normal or cold-exposed animals. The majority of the work investigating this question indicated that cold-exposed animals do not become hypothermic with antipyretics and thus they have no intrinsic activity (CRANSTON et al. 1975; PITTMAN et al. 1976). The rat is an exception to this rule (SATINOFF 1972; FRANCESCONI and MAGER 1975). Therefore, the action of antipyretics does not involve actions on effectors.

It is clear that antipyretics act principally by affecting the activity of hypothalamic neurones disordered by pyrogens. The mechanism of action remains obscure but several theories have been proposed in explanation.

The absorption, metabolism, and toxicity of antipyretic drugs are essential considerations in evaluating possible antipyretic therapy. The antipyretics in most common use clinically are salicylate derivatives, acetaminophen (paracetamol) and, to a lesser extent indomethacin. These substances are administered orally.

Salicylates, after rapid absorption from the stomach and upper intestine, reach a peak plasma level in about two hours. They are distributed throughout body extracellular fluid soon after absorption. Acetylsalicylate is, itself, antipyretic and does not depend on metabolic hydrolysis, although much of it becomes quickly hydrolysed to salicylic acid in the stomach, plasma, liver, and other body sites. Salicylate present in plasma is mostly albumin bound, whereas acetylsalicylate is bound less. Salicylates cross the placenta and they can also penetrate into the brain, reaching tissue concentrations of 3–6 ng/g when plasma concentrations are 20–40 ng/100 ml in the rabbit (GRUNDMAN 1969). Metabolic inactivation is mainly by glycine or glycuronate conjugation in the liver. A small amount is oxidized to a gentisic acid. Most of the salicylate is excreted unaltered in the urine.

Overdose of salicylate may uncouple oxidative phosphorylation and cause severe hyperthermia. Other toxic effects include ringing in the ears, headache and dizziness, and possible skin eruptions. Salicylates have distressing effects on the gastrointestinal tract and may cause vomiting and severe gastric bleeding. Salicylates can cause severe allergic reactions such as asthma or oedema with laryngeal swelling. As well as being antipyretic, salicylate is used extensively as an analgesic and as an anti-inflammatory agent.

Acetaminophen is rapidly absorbed from the intestinal tract, reaching a maximum concentration in the blood in less than an hour. It is bound, to some extent, by plasma proteins. Acetaminophen is conjugated in the liver with glycuronate and excreted in the urine. Phenacetin is metabolized to acetaminophen for its antipyretic effects. Toxic problems include skin eruptions and drug fevers. Kidney and liver damage is a major concern. Phenacetin may have a damaging effect on formed elements in the blood, either by causing haemolytic anaemia, methaemoglobulinaemia or thrombocytopaenia. Acetaminophen is analgesic as well but not anti-inflammatory like the majority of antipyretic drugs.

Indomethacin is rapidly absorbed and reaches a blood maximum after about three hours. Glycuronate-conjugated indomethacin and some unaltered drug are excreted in the urine. There are other minor metabolites. Distressful side effects include gastrointestinal problems, nausea, abdominal pain, and peptic ulceration. Some CNS effects include dizziness, light headedness, confusion, and headache. Circulating blood cell types can be affected. Allergic and hypersensitive reactions are possible side effects. Indomethacin is used for treatment of inflammatory diseases such as arthritis.

Any consideration of antipyretic therapy must take into account the patient's status with respect to the toxic and allergic effects of these drugs.

D. Effects of Antipyresis on Survival

While the effects of fever on survival of lizards were being studied, the effects of antipyresis were examined as well. Antipyresis was accomplished in two ways. The first method was to keep the lizards at their normothermic temperature (38 °C) thus not allowing them the opportunity to raise their body temperatures behaviourally. Alternatively, the lizards were adiministered acetylsalicylate to produce drug-induced antipyresis. In this latter experimental design, the lizards were given the opportunity to move upon a thermal gradient but did not do so (Bernheim and Kluger 1976b). In the case of either form of antipyresis (thermal or chemical), animals infected with bacteria had 75% and 100% mortality respectively, whereas those allowed to get a behavioural fever had a 8% mortality.

In mammals, the evidence for a detrimental effect of antipyresis is not so clear. Rabbits were injected with *Pasteurella multocida* and given a combination of salicylate and acetaminophen intraperitoneally. Antipyretics were ineffective in decreasing the fevers of the rabbits. Depending on the dose of bacteria administered, the antipyretics either decreased the mortality rate or had no effect on mortality rate. This experiment is inconclusive and not easily interpreted because of the lack of effect of antipyretics on fever magnitude (KLUGER and VAUGHN 1978).

Another study has shown much clearer results but, because of the route of administration, the results are not directly analogous to the normal route of antipyretic administration. Salicylate injected directly into the PO/AH of bacterially infected rabbits caused significant antipyresis in the first five hours of the infection. The mortality rate of those rabbits receiving antipyretic therapy was substantially and dramatically greater than control infected rabbits. This effect may have been due to early, rapid growth of bacteria in animals receiving antipyresis (VAUGHN et al. 1980). Thus it may be that fever in the first few hours of infection is critical for survival.

There is no evidence that antipyretics effect survival rate or recovery from infections in humans.

E. Clinical Indications and Contraindications for Antipyretic Therapy

The use of antipyretic drugs in the treatment of febrile diseases involves careful consideration. It must be emphasized that antipyretic therapy does not remove the cause of any fever, it only alleviates some of the symptoms. Previously, indications for antipyretic therapy were not clear. Use of antipyretics can be premised on the simple consideration that antipyretic therapy is called for in circumstances where fevers could have detrimental consequences and antipyretic therapy should not be used in circumstances where antipyretics could be deleterious. The evidence available at present, principally from animal models as described in this chapter, can be used to define guidelines for antipyretic therapy. Especially with modern antibiotic therapy, the adaptive value of fever may be meaningless in most clinically treated infections. However, the evidence does support a beneficial role of fever as a host defence mechanism and, in an uncomplicated infection, antipyretics should not be administered, keeping in mind their potential toxicity and allergic properties. Antipyretics alleviate the malaise and discomfort accompanying fever but, unless these are severe, they should not be considered sufficient cause for the use of antipyretics.

There are, however, several specific circumstances for contraindication of antipyretic therapy. Patients with liver and kidney ailments may be adversely affected by normal therapeutic doses of some antipyretics.

Fevers due to malignancies, unless extremely high, may be beneficial since hyperthermia has been found to be effective in arresting the growth of tumours and hyperthermic treatment is now widely used in conjunction with chemotherapy.

The other circumstance in which fevers should be allowed to occur without antipyretic therapy is when these infections are caused by micro-organisms directly destroyed by high temperatures, such as syphilis and gonococcal infections. However, modern antibiotics usually control these illnesses sufficiently so this circumstance does not often arise.

The administration of antipyretics in conjunction with other drugs should be considered carefully since antipyretics are bound by albumin and other plasma

Table 1. Suggested indications and contraindications for antipyretic therapy

Indications
1. Fevers in patients with cardiovascular limitations
2. Excessively high fevers (e.g. malaria)
3. Fevers in pregnant women 4–6 weeks of gestation owing to possible teratogenic effects of fever, unless contraindicated by possible effects on ductus
4. Fevers in pregnant women near parturition owing to possible effects on foetal lung surfactant or other vital processes – consider effects on ductus
5. Fever in children because they tend to get excessively high fevers and they are also susceptible to febrile convulsions
6. Fevers accompanying schizophrenia

Contraindications
1. Uncomplicated febrile illness in the first day or so
2. Fevers due to malignancies, unless the fever is distressing
3. Fevers due to micro-organisms directly killed by febrile temperatures (e.g. syphilis, gonorrhea) but which are not sensitive to antibiotics
4. Fevers in patients with some kidney or liver ailments
5. Fevers in patients with allergic reactions or toxic side effects from antipyretics
6. Fevers in patients taking other drugs which may interact with antipyretics

proteins and could displace bound drug. Other drug–drug interactions may occur.

There are several circumstances in which antipyretic therapy would be specifically recommended unless any unusual allergic reactions or contraindications previously mentioned co-occur.

Patients in whom increases in cardiac output or heart rate (symptoms that accompany fever) could be dangerous should have fevers controlled with antipyretics. The modifications of renal and hepatic blood flow by endotoxin are not prevented by antipyretics.

Patients in whom fevers tend to reach unusually high levels, such as might occur in malaria, would benefit from antipyretic therapy to prevent direct tissue damage from excessive temperatures.

Pregnant women, particularly at 4–6 weeks of gestation when foetal brain cell proliferation is occurring, should receive antipyretic therapy to prevent any teratogenic rises in body temperature. It should be kept in mind, that antipyretic drugs have been shown to cause ductus arteriosis closure in near-term animals (Coceani et al. 1975) and in premature infants (Heymann and Rudolph 1978) but whether they affect the very early foetus in this respect is not known. Pregnant women in the last few days of gestation should receive antipyretic therapy in the case of fever since there may be reasons to suppress fevers naturally at this time. Fevers may have possible detrimental effects on lung surfactant maturation or exacerbate foetal anoxia. Again, this decision should be weighed against possible detrimental effects of ductus closure as described above.

Young children may get excessively high fevers which could be damaging or lethal and they are also especially susceptible to febrile convulsions which may have serious sequelae. Therefore, antipyretic therapy is called for in treatment of fevers in children, especially those with any personal or family history of febrile convulsions or epilepsy.

It has been reported that fevers are, on numerous occasions, the presenting symptom of schizophrenia and perhaps both may be due to excessive prostaglandin levels in the CNS (FELDBERG 1975). Antipyretic therapy would, therefore, be beneficial in alleviating both conditions.

Fever accompanies such a wide variety of illnesses and disorders that clear-cut guidelines to govern the clinical use of antipyretics are not feasible. However, if the clinician is aware of the basic physiological mechanisms and principles underlying fever and antipyretic therapy, the most intelligent decision can be made.

References

Alexander G (1975) Body temperature control in mammalian young. Br Med Bull 31:62–68

Annegers JF, Hauser WA, Elveback LR, Kurland LT (1979) The risk of epilepsy following febrile convulsions. Neurology (NY) 29:297–303

Ashman RB, Nahmias AJ (1977) Enhancement of human lymphocyte responses to phytomitogens in vitro by incubation at elevated temperatures. Clin Exp Immunol 29:464–467

Atkins E, Bodel P (1972) Fever. N Eng J Med 286:27–34

Atkins E, Bodel P (1979) Clinical fever; its history, manifestations and pathogenesis. Fed Proc 38:57–63

Atkins E, Allison F, Smith MR, Wood WB (1955) Studies on the antipyretic action of cortisone in pyrogen-induced fever. J Exp Med 101:353–366

Atkins E, Bodel P, Francis L (1967) Release of an endogenous pyrogen in vitro from rabbit mononuclear cells. J Exp Med 126:357–386

Avery DD, Penn PE (1974) Blockage of pyrogen induced fever by intrahypothalamic injection of salicylate in the rat. Neuropharmacology 13:1179–1185

Banet M (1979) Fever and survival in the rat. The effect of enhancing fever. Pfluegers Arch 381:35–38

Barbour HG (1921) The heat regulating mechanism of the body. Physiol Rev 1:295–326

Beeson PB (1948) Temperature elevating effect of a substance obtained from polymorphonuclear leukocytes. J Clin Invest 27:525–531

Bennett IL (1964) Introduction: approaches to the mechanisms of endotoxin action. In: Landy M, Brown W (eds) Bacterial endotoxins. Rutgers University Press, New Brunswick, pp xiii–xvi

Bennett IL, Beeson PB (1950) The properties and biological effects of bacterial pyrogens. Medicine (Baltimore) 29:365–400

Bennett IL, Beeson PB (1953) Studies on the pathogenesis of fever II. Characterization of fever-producing substances from polymorphonuclear leukocytes and from the fluid of sterile exudates. J Exp Med 98:493–508

Bennett IL, Nicastri A (1960) Fever as a mechanism of resistance. Bacteriol Rev 24:16–34

Bergstrom T, Larson H, Lincoln K, Winberg J (1972) Studies of urinary tract infections in infancy and childhood. J Pediatr 80:858–866

Bernheim HA, Kluger MJ (1976a) Fever and antipyresis in the lizard Dipsosaurus dorsalis. Am J Physiol 231:298–203

Bernheim HA, Kluger MJ (1976b) Fever: Effects of drug-induced antipyresis on survival. Science 192:237–239

Bernheim HA, Bodel PT, Askenase PW, Atkins E (1978) Effects of fever on host mechanisms after infection in the lizard Dipsosaurus dorsalis. Br J Exp Pathol 59:76–83

Blatteis CM (1975) Postnatal development of pyrogenic sensitivity in guinea pigs. J Appl Physiol 39:251–257

Blatteis CM (1976) Effect of propranolol on endotoxin-induced pyrogenesis in newborn and adult guinea pigs. J Appl Physiol 40:35–39

Blatteis CM (1977) Comparison of endotoxin and leukocytic pyrogen pyrogenicity in newborn guinea pigs. J Appl Physiol 42:355–361

Blatteis CM, Smith KA (1977) Sensitivity of hypothalamic fever mechanisms to locally injected leukocytic pyrogen (LP) in adult and newborn guinea pigs. Physiologist 20:10

Bodel P (1970) Studies on the mechanism of endogenous pyrogen production. I. Investigation of new protein synthesis in stimulated human blood leukoytes. Yale J Biol Med 43:145–163

Bodel P, Atkins E (1967) Release of endogenous pyrogen by human monocytes. N Engl J Med 276:1002–1008

Borsook D, Laburn H, Mitchell D (1978) The febrile responses in rabbits and rats to leukocyte pyrogens of different species. J Physiol (Lond) 279:113–120

Bradley SE, Conan NJ (1947) Estimated hepatic blood flow and bromosulfalen extraction in normal man during pyrogenic reaction. J Clin Invest 26:1175

Cabanac M, Massonnet B (1974) Temperature regulation during fever: change in set-point or change of gain? A tentative answer from a behavioral study in man. J Physiol (Lond) 238:561–568

Cabanac M, Stolwijk JAJ, Hardy JD (1968) Effects of temperature and pyrogens on single unit activity in the rabbit brain stem. J Appl Physiol 24:645–652

Casterlin ME, Reynolds WW (1977a) Behavioral fever in crayfish. Hydrobiologia 56:99–101

Casterlin ME, Reynolds WW (1977b) Behavioral fever in anuran amphibian larvae. Life Sci 20:593–596

Chai LY, Lin MT, Chen NI, Wang SC (1971) The site of action of leukocytic pyrogen and antipyresis of sodium acetyl salicylate in monkeys. Neuropharmacology 10:715–723

Chowers I, Conforti N, Feldman S (1968) Local effects of cortisol in the preoptic area on temperature regulation. Am J Physiol 214:538–542

Clark WG, Alderdice MT (1972) Inhibition of leukocyte pyrogen induced fever by intracerebroventricular administration of salicylate and acetaminophen in the cat. Proc Soc Exp Biol Med 140:399–403

Clark WG, Coldwell BA (1972) Competitive antagonism of leukocyte pyrogen by sodium salicylate and acetaminophen. Proc Soc Exp Biol Med 141:669–672

Clark WG, Cumby HR (1975) The antipyretic effect of indomethacin. J Physiol (Lond) 248:625–638

Clark WG, Moyer SG (1972) The effects of acetaminaphen and sodium salicylate on the release and activity of leucocytic pyrogen in the cat. J Pharmacol Exp Ther 181:183–191

Coceani F, Olley PM, Bodach E (1975) Lamb ductus arteriosus. Effect of prostaglandin synthesis inhibitors on the muscle tone and the response to prostaglandin E_2. Prostaglandins 9:299–308

Cooper KE (1971) Some physiological and clinical aspects of pyrogen. In: Wolstenholme GEW, Birch J (eds) Pyrogens and fever. Churchill Livingstone, Edinburgh London, pp 5–17

Cooper KE (1972) The body temperature set-point during fever. In: Bligh J, Moore RE (eds) Essays on temperature regulation. North Holland, Amsterdam, pp 141–162

Cooper KE, Veale WL (1974) Fever, an abnormal drive to the heat-conserving and producing mechanisms? In: Lederis K, Cooper KE (eds) Recent studies of hypothalamic function. Karger, Basel, pp 391–398

Cooper KE, Cranston WI, Fessler JH (1960) Interactions of a bacterial pyrogen with rabbit leukocytes and plasma. J Physiol (Lond) 154:22–23 P

Cooper KE, Cranston WI, Snell ES (1964) Temperature regulation during fever in man. Clin Sci 27:345–356

Cooper KE, Grundman MJ, Honour AJ (1968) Observations on sodium salicylate as an antipyretic. J Physiol (Lond) 196:56–57

Cooper KE, Veale WL, Pittman QJ (1976) The pathogenesis of fever. In: Brazier MAB, Coceani F (eds) Brain dysfunction in infantile febrile convulsions. Raven, New York, pp 107–115

Cooper KE, Kasting NW, Lederis K, Veale WL (1979) Evidence supporting a role for endogenous vasopressin in natural suppression of fever in the sheep. J Physiol (Lond) 295:33–45

Covert JB, Reynolds WW (1977) Survival value of fever in fish. Nature 267:43–45

Cranston WI, Rawlins MD (1972) Effects of intracerebral microinjections of sodium salicylate on temperature regulation in the rabbit. J Physiol (Lond) 222:257–266

Cranston WI, Vial SV, Wheeler HO (1959) The relationship between pyrogen-induced renal vasodilatation and circulating pyrogenic substances. Clin Sci 18:579–585

Cranston WI, Hellon RF, Luff RH, Rawlins MD, Rosendorff C (1970) Observations on the mechanism of salicylate induced antipyresis. J Physiol (Lond) 210:593–600

Cranston WI, Rawlins MD, Luff RH, Duff GW (1971) Relevance of experimental observations to pyrexia in clinical situation. In: Wolstenholme GEW, Birch J (eds) Pyrogens and fever. Churchill Livingstone, Edinburg London, pp 155–164

Cranston WI, Hollon RF, Mitchell D (1975) Is brain prostaglandin synthesis involved in response to cold. J Physiol (Lond) 249:425–434

Cranston WI, Duff GW, Hellon RF, Mitchell D, Townsend Y (1976) Evidence that brain prostaglandin synthesis is not essential in fever. J Physiol (Lond) 259:239–249

Culver H (1917) The treatment of gonorrheal infections by the intravenous injection of killed gonococci, meningococci and colon bacilli. JAMA 68:362–366

De Kruif P, Simpson WM (1940) Possible significance of the inhibitory effect of fever on anaphylatic phenomena. J Lab Clin Med 26:125–130

Dinarello CA (1979) Production of endogenous pyrogen. Fed Proc 38:52–56

Dinarello CA, Wolff SM (1977) Partial purification of human leukocytic pyrogen. Inflammation 2:179–189

Dinarello CA, Bodel P, Atkins E (1968) The role of the liver in the production of fever and in pyrogenic tolerance. Trans Assoc Am Physicians 81:334–344

Dinarello CA, Renfer L, Wolff SM (1977) The production of antibody against human leukocytic pyrogen. J Clin Invest 60:465–472

Dinarello CA, Weiner P, Wolff SM (1978) Radiolabelling and disposition in rabbits of purified human leukocytic pyrogen. Clin Res 26:522 A

Dubois EF (1949) Why are fever temperatures over 106° F rare? Am J Med Sci 217:361–368

Edwards MJ (1967) Congenital defects in guinea pigs following induced hyperthermia during gestation. Arch Pathol 84:42–48

Edwards MJ (1971) The experimental production of *Arthrogryposis multiplex congenita* in guinea pigs by maternal hypothermia during gestation. J Pathol 104:221–229

Eisenman JS (1969) Pyrogen induced changes in the thermosensitivity of septal and preoptic neurons. Am J Physiol 216:330–334

Eisenman JS (1974) Depression of preoptic thermosensitivity by bacterial pyrogen in rabbits. Am J Physiol 227:1067–1073

Epstein HC, Hochwald A, Ashe R (1951) Salmonella infections of the newborn infant. J Pediatr 38:723–731

Feldberg W (1975) Body temperature and fever: changes in our views during the last decade. Proc R Soc Lond [Biol] 191:199–229

Feldberg W, Gupta KP (1973) Pyrogen fever and prostaglandin activity in cerebrospinal fluid. J Physiol (Lond) 228:41–53

Feldberg W, Saxena PN (1971) Further studies on prostaglandin E_1 fever in cats. J Physiol (Lond) 219:739–745

Fessler JH, Cooper KE, Cranston WI, Vollum RL (1961) Observations on the production of pyrogenic substances by rabbit and human leukocytes. J Exp Med 113:1127–1140

Flower RJ, Vanc JR (1972) Inhibition of prostagladin synthetase in brain explains the antipyretic activity of paracetamol (4-acetamidophenol). Nature 240:410–411

Francesconi RP, Mager M (1975) Salicylate, tryptophan, and tyrosine hypothermia. Am J Physiol 228:1431–1435

Gander GW, Chaffee J, Goodale F (1967) Studies upon the antipyretic action of salicylates. Proc Soc Exp Biol 126:205–209

Goldring H, Chasis H, Ranges HA, Smith HW (1941) Effective renal blood flow in subjects with essential hypertension. J Clin Invest 20:637–653

Grant R (1949) Nature of pyrogen fever: effect of environmental temperature on response to typhoid-paratyphoid vaccine. Am J Physiol 159:511–524

Grieger TA, Kluger MJ (1972) Effects of bacteria and temperature on free serum iron levels in the lizard *Dipsosaurus dorsalis*. Physiologist 20:37

Grieger TA, Kluger MJ (1978) Fever and survival: the role of serum iron. J Physiol (Lond) 279:187–196

Grundman MJ (1969) Studies on the action of antipyretic substances. PhD thesis, Oxford University

Hahn HH, Char DC, Postel WB, Wood WB Jr (1967) Studies on the pathogenesis of fever. XV. The production of endogenous pyrogen by peritoneal macrophages. J Exp Med 126:385–394

Hahn HH, Cheuk SF, Moore DM, Wood WB Jr (1970a) Studies on the pathogenesis of fever. XVII. The cationic control of pyrogen release from exudate granulocytes *in vitro*. J Exp Med 131:165–178

Hahn HH, Cheuk SF, Elfenbein CDS, Wood WB Jr (1970b) Studies on the pathogenesis of fever. XIX. Localization of pyrogen in granulocytes. J Exp Med 131:701–710

Hasler WT, Spekter L (1936) Artificial fever in the treatment of gonorrheal ophthalmia. JAMA 107:102–104

Heikkila JJ, Brown IR (1979) Hyperthermia and disaggregation of brain polysomes induced by bacterial pyrogen. Life Sci 25:347–352

Hench PS (1935) Clinical notes on the results of fever therapy in different diseases. Mayo Clin Proc 10:662–666

Heymann MA, Rudolph AM (1978) Effects of prostaglandins and blockers of prostaglandin synthesis on the ductus arteriosus: animal and human studies. Adv Prostaglandin Thromboxane Res 4:363–372

Hippocrates (1939) The genuine works of Hippocrates, translated by Adams F. Williams and Wilkins, Baltimore, p 114

Ho M (1970) Factors influencing the interferon response. Arch Intern Med 126:135–146

Hoo SL, Lin MT, Wei RD, Chai CV, Wong SC (1972) Effects of sodium acetyl salicylate on the release of pyrogen from leukocytes. Proc Soc Exp Biol 139:1155–1158

Kasting NW, Veale WL, Cooper KE (1978a) Suppression of fever at term of pregnancy. Nature 271:245–246

Kasting NW, Veale WL, Cooper KE (1978b) Evidence for a centrally active endogenous antipyretic near parturition. In: Lederis K, Veale WL (eds) Current studies of hypothalamic function 1978, part II. Metabolism and behavior. Karger, Basel, pp 63–71

Kasting NW, Cooper KE, Veale WL (1979a) Antipyresis following perfusion of brain sites with vasopressin. Experientia 35:208–209

Kasting NW, Veale WL, Cooper KE (1979b) Development of fever in the newborn lamb. Am J Physiol 236:R184–R187

Kerpal-Fronius S, Kiss A, Than G (1966) The effect of pyrogen on body temperature and oxygen consumption in the rat at different environmental temperatures. Acta Physiol Hung 29:267–272

Klastersky J, Kass EH (1970) Is suppression of fever or hypothermia useful in experimental and clinical infectious disease. J Infect Dis 121:81–86

Kleinebrecht J, Michaelis H, Michaelis J, Koller S (1979) Fever in pregnancy and congenital anomalies. Lancet 1:1403

Kluger MJ (1977) Fever in the frog *Hygla cinerea*. Thermobiology 2:79–81

Kluger MJ (1979) Phylogeny of fever. Fed Proc 38:30–34

Kluger MJ, Rothenburg BA (1979) Fever and reduced iron: their interaction as a host defense response to bacterial infection. Science 203:374–376

Kluger MJ, Vaughn LK (1978) Fever and survival in rabbits infected with *Pasteurella multocida*. J Physiol (Lond) 282:243–251

Kluger MJ, Ringler DH, Anver MR (1975) Fever and survival. Science 188:166–168

Kruk B, Sadowski J (1978) Antidiuretic action of intravenous and intracerebral pyrogen in conscious rabbits. J Physiol (Lond) 282:429–435

Lennox-Buchthal MA (1973) Febrile convulsions; a reappraisal. Elsevier, Amsterdam Oxford New York

Lin MT, Chai CV (1972) The antipyretic effect of sodium salicylate on pyrogen induced fever in the rabbit. J Pharmacol Exp Ther 180:603–609

Lipton JM, Fossler DE (1974) Fever produced in the squirrel monkey by intravenous and intracerebral endotoxin. Am J Physiol 226:1022–1027

Lipton JM, Welch JP, Clark WG (1973) Changes in body temperature produced by injecting prostaglandin E_1, EGTA, and bacterial endotoxins into the PO/AH region and the medulla oblongata of the rat. Experientia 29:806–808

Lwoff A (1969) Death and transfiguration of a problem. Bacteriol Rev 33:390–403

MacPherson RK (1959) The effect of fever on temperature regulation in man. Clin Sci 18:281–287

Meban C (1978) Influence of pH and temperature on behavior of surfactant from human neonatal lungs. Biol Neonate 33:106–111

Mickenberg ID, Root RK, Wolff SM (1972) Bactericidal and metabolic properties of human eosinophils. Blood 39:67–80

Milton AS, Wendlandt S (1970) A possible role for prostaglandin E_1 as a modulator for temperature regulation in the central nervous system of the cat. J Physiol (Lond) 207:76–77

Milton AS, Wendlandt S (1971) Effects on body temperature of prostaglandins of the A, E, and F series on injection into the third ventricle of unanesthetized rats and rabbits. J Physiol (Lond) 218:325–336

Mitchell D, Snellen JW, Atkins AR (1970) Thermoregulation during fever: change of set-point or change of gain. Pfluegers Arch Ges Physiol 321:293–302

Murphy PA, Chesney J, Wood WB Jr (1974) Further purification of rabbit leukocyte pyrogen. J Lab Clin Med 83:310–322

Myers RD (1974) Ionic concepts of the set-point for body temperature. In: Lederis K, Cooper KE (eds) Recent studies of hypothalamic function. Karger, Basel, pp 371–390

Myers RD, Veale WL (1970) Body temperature: possible ionic mechanism in the hypothalamus controlling the set point. Science 170:95–97

Myers RD, Veale WL (1971) The role of sodium and calcium ions in the hypothalamus in the control of body temperature of the unanesthetized cat. J Physiol (Lond) 212:411–430

Myhre K, Cabanac M, Myhre G (1977) Fever and behavioral temperature regulation in the frog Ranga esculenta. Acta Physiol Scand 101:219–229

Nahas GG, Tannieres ML, Lennon JF (1971) Direct measurement of leukocyte motility: effects of pH and temperature. Proc Soc Exp Biol Med 138:350–352

Norlund JJ, Root RK, Wolff SM (1970) Studies on the origin of human leukocytic pyrogen. J Exp Med 131:727–743

Overgaard J (1977) Effect of hyperthermia on malignant cells in vivo. Cancer 39:2637–2646

Palmes ED, Park CR (1965) The regulation of body temperature during fever. Arch Environ Health 11:749–759

Phelps P, Stanislaw D (1969) Polymorphonuclear leukocyte mobility in vitro. I. Effect of pH, temperature, ethyl alcohol, and caffeine, using a modified Boyden chamber technique. Arthritis Rheum 12:181–188

Pittman QJ, Cooper KE, Veale WL, Van Petten GR (1973) Fever in newborn lambs. Can J Physiol Pharmacol 51:868–872

Pittman QJ, Cooper KE, Veale WL, Van Petten GR (1974) Observations on the development of the febrile response to pyrogens in sheep. Clin Sci Mol Med 46:591–602

Pittman QJ, Veale WL, Cooper KE (1976) Observations on the effect of salicylate in fever and the regulation of body temperature against the cold. Can J Physiol Pharmacol 54:101–106

Reynolds WW (1977) Fever and antipyresis in the bluegill sunfish, Lepomis macrochinus. Comp Biochem Physiol 57 C:165–167

Reynolds WW, Casterlin ME, Covert JB (1976) Behavioral fever in teleost fishes. Nature 259:41–42

Roberts NJ Jr, Steigbigel RT (1977) Hyperthermia and human leukocyte functions: effects on response of lymphocytes to mitogen and antigen and bactericidal capacity of monocytes and neutrophils. Infect Immun 18:673–679

Satinoff E (1972) Salicylate: action on normal body temperature in rats. Science 176:532–533

Schoener EP, Wang SC (1975 a) Leukocytic pyrogen and sodium acetyl salicylate on hypothalamic neurons in the cat. Am J Physiol 224:185–190

Schoener EP, Wang SC (1975 b) Observations on the central mechanism of acetyl salicylate antipyresis. Life Sci 17:1063–1068

Sebag J, Reed WP, Williams RC Jr (1977) Effect of temperature on bacterial killing by serum and by polymorphonuclear leukocytes. Infect Immun 16:947–954

Smith DW, Clarren SK, Harvey MAS (1978) Hyperthermia as a teratogenic agent. J Pediatr 92:878–883

Smith RT, Platou ES, Good RA (1956) Septicemia of the newborn. Pediatrics 17:549–575

Steele RW, Tanaka PT, Lara RP, Bass JW (1970) Evaluation of sponging and of oral anti-pyretic therapy to reduce fever. J Pediatr 77:824–832

Stitt JT (1973) Prostaglandin E_1 fever induced in rabbits. J Physiol (Lond) 232:163–179

Stitt JT (1979) Fever versus hyperthermia. Fed Proc 38:39–43

Stitt JT, Hardy JD, Stolwijk JAJ (1974) PGE_1 fever: its effect on thermoregulation at different low ambient temperatures. Am J Physiol 227:622–629

Thomas L (1954) The physiological disturbances produced by endotoxins. Ann Rev Physiol 16:467–490

Toms GL, Davies JA, Woodward CG, Sweet C, Smith H (1977) The relation of pyrexia and nasal inflammatory response to virus levels in nasal washings of ferrets infected with influenza viruses of differing virulence. Br J Exp Pathol 58:444–458

Townsend Y, Cranston WI (1979) Sites of clearance of leukocyte pyrogen in the rabbit. Clin Sci 56:265–268

Vane JR (1971) Inhibition of prostaglandin synthesis as a mechanism of action of aspirin-like drugs. Nature 231:232–235

Van Miert AS, Frens J (1968) The reaction of different animal species to bacterial pyrogens. Zentralbl Veterinaermed 15:532–543

Van Miert ASJAM, Van Essen JA, Tromp GA (1971) The antipyretic effect of pyrozalone derivative and salicylates on fever induced with leukocytes or bacterial pyrogen. Arch Int Pharmacodyn Ther 197:288–391

Vaughn LK, Veale WL, Cooper KE (1979) Sensitivity of hypothalamic sites to salicylate and prostaglandin. Can J Physiol Pharmacol 57:118–123

Vaughn LK, Veale WL, Cooper KE (1980) Fever and survival in a mammal: effects of central antipyresis. In: Cox B, Lomax P, Milton AS, Schonbaum E (eds) Thermoregulatory mechanisms and their therapeutic implications. Karger, Basel, pp 115–119

Veale WL, Cooper KE (1975) Comparison of sites of action of prostaglandin and leukocyte pyrogen in brain. In: Lomax P, Schonbaum G, Jacob J (eds) Temperature regulation and drug action. Basel, Karger, pp 218–226

Veale WL, Whishaw LQ (1976) Body temperature responses at different ambient temperatures following injections of prostaglandin E_1 and noradrenaline into the brain. Pharmacol Biochem Behav 4:143–150

Watson DW, Kim YB (1963) Modification of host responses to bacterial endotoxins. I. Specificity of pyrogenic tolerance and the role of hypersensitivity in pyrogenicity, lethality and skin reactivity. J Exp Med 118:425–446

Welch WH (1888) The Cartwright lectures on the general pathology of fever. Med News (Philadelphia) 52:365, 393, 539, 565

Wit A, Wang SC (1968) Temperature-sensitive neurons in preoptic/anterior hypothalamic region: actions of pyrogens and acetyl salicylate. Am J Physiol 215:1160–1169

Ziel R, Krupp P (1975) Effect on prostaglandin synthesis and antiinflammatory drugs. In: Schonbaum E, Lomax P, Jacob J (eds) Temperature regulation and drug action. Karger, Basel, pp 233–241

CHAPTER 3

Thermoregulation: Its Change During Infection with Endotoxin-Producing Micro-organisms

J. BLIGH

A. Introduction

Both historically and practically, fever is associated with pathology, or the abnormal functions of the body, rather than with physiology, or the normal functions of the body. This is because fever does not occur except in association with a pathological condition. Otherwise, the body temperature of humans, and of at least some of the other mammals, remains remarkably constant from birth, or soon after, until death, or shortly before. It may rise above its nychthemeral range of variation during bouts of strenuous exercise, or during exposure of the body to an excessively stressful thermal environment, but a rise in body temperature in any other circumstances is invariably evidence of a pathological condition and is usually evidence of microbial infection.

Whether fever is a *passive* pathological consequence of the infection, or is an *active* component of the physiological defence mechanism by which the body counters such infections, remains unresolved. Some recent evidence supports the view that the elevation of body temperature, alone or in association with other responses, aids the defence against the invasion of micro-organisms.

On the other hand, although the first response of human beings today to a "chill" is to relieve the symptoms with aspirin, or one of the other aspirin-like substances, which has antipyretic as well as anti-inflammatory and mild analgesic properties, there is no evidence that this use of an antipyretic substance adversely affects recovery from an infection.

Perhaps the strongest reason for supposing that fever is a component of the built-in, or acquired, defence mechanisms of the body which is activated only in response to some particular disturbances, is the orderliness of the thermoregulatory changes which occur. Fever is not simply a disruption of the normal processes of homeothermy; it is, as LIEBERMEISTER (1875) implied, and as MACPHERSON (1959) and COOPER et al. (1964) have clearly demonstrated in humans, exactly as if the set-point of normal thermoregulation is temporarily re-set at a higher level (Fig. 1). During the rising phase of the fever the activities of the thermoregulatory effector functions are those consistent with a hypothermic state: heat production is maximized while heat loss is minimized until a steady-state fever is achieved. During the falling phase of fever the activities of the thermoregulatory effector functions are those consistent with a hyperthermic state until the afebrile state of normothermia is restored. During the plateau phase of sustained fever, however, MACPHERSON (1959) found that a febrile human subject, who carried out a patterned series of exercise and rest periods, responded to the heat production of ex-

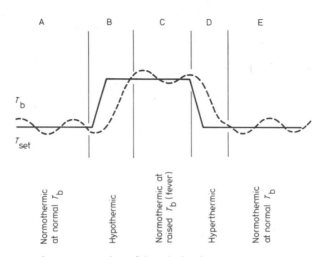

Fig. 1. A diagrammatic representation of the relation between core temperature (T_b) and the set-point temperature (T_{set}). (*A*) before the onset of fever; (*B*) during the rising phase of fever; (*C*) during maintained fever; (*D*) during the subsiding phase; and (*E*) after the return to normal thermoregulation. (From BLIGH 1973)

ercise with essentially the same thermoregulatory changes as those observed in afebrile subjects following the same regime. Thus it was precisely as if the biological thermostat of the febrile man was operating, but at an elevated set-point.

Irrespective of whether fever is a passive consequence or an active response, the basic question to be resolved is: "By what processes does the febrile state result from microbial invasion?" The proposition that fever is part of the capacity of an animal to defend itself against invasion raises a second question: "What role does fever play in the combat between invader and invaded?" Here the emphasis is placed upon the first of these questions, with only a brief consideration of the second.

B. The Elevated Set-Point Concept of Fever

The suggest that in the febrile state the biological thermostat is re-set in an upward direction was made by LIEBERMEISTER (1875) at a time when little if anything was known of pyrogens or of the neurology of homeothermy. That description has now become an orthodoxy, the elaboration of which often involves some fairly definite ideas on how the set-point of body temperature might be achieved by means of endogenous reference-signal generators analogous to or homologous with the processes sometimes used in thermal engineering to establish thermal stability (for example, see MYERS et al. 1976). Precisely what that description of the febrile state really means however, remains uncertain and controversial. Yet despite our persisting ignorance of the nature of the processes involved, both in the creation of a set-point, and in its adjustments, the terms "set-point" and "upward re-setting" are used quite correctly because they describe the *performances* of a system, and imply nothing of the means by which the performances are achieved.

MacPHERSON (1959) amply demonstrated the validity of this description of fever as "an upward re-setting of the thermostat" in humans (see Sect. A) and this was confirmed by COOPER et al. (1964) who noted that when a human is febrile due to illness or the injection of a pyrogen, thermoregulatory responses during the plateau phase of fever are essentially the same as those of an afebrile subject, although during the rising phase of the fever the responses to heat are attenuated.

Neither MacPHERSON (1959) nor COOPER et al. (1964) implied, nor needed to imply, anything about the structures and functions responsible for the existence of the body temperature set-point, or about the perturbations which cause the change in set-point during infection. Their statements were descriptive of *what* happens, not of *how* it happens.

C. The Pyrogens

I. Bacterial Endotoxins

Fever has long been associated with inflammation, and the pyrogenic agent was considered to be a derivative of necrotic cells (WUNDERLICH 1871) which could be those of invading micro-organisms or those from the damaged tissues of the "host." The latter possibility was largely ignored, however after evidence was obtained that micro-organisms can produce and liberate pyrogenic material in vitro (HORT and PENFOLD 1912a, b; SEIBERT 1923, 1925).

The pyrogenic endotoxins of micro-organisms are generally heat-stable lipopolysaccharides, and those produced by Gram-negative bacteria have now been shown to have three distinct molecular regions: a region responsible for their specific immunological properties; a basal polysaccharide core; and a "lipid A" structure which is responsible for the pyrogenic activity (LUDERITZ et al. 1971).

II. Endogenous (Leucocyte) Pyrogens

There was a revival of interest in the possibility of an endogenous pyrogen which may be liberated from damaged cells after it had been demonstrated that fever may accompany non-infectious inflammation. This was confirmed when BEESON (1948) and BENNETT and BEESON (1953a, b) extracted a pyrogenic substance from rabbit polymorph leucocytes, and showed this to be a quite different substance from that obtainable from pyrogenic micro-organisms. SNELL and ATKINS (1967) confirmed that the endogenous pyrogen obtained from leucocytes is distinguishable from bacterial pyrogens by several criteria; it is a heat-labile polypeptide which is not a transformation of a bacterial pyrogen, but is of quite distinct origin (MURPHY 1967a, b).

It was long suspected that the leucocytes were not the sole source of endogenous pyrogen, because fever could still occur in agranulocytic subjects. SNELL and ATKINS (1965) had shown that substances essentially similar to leucocyte pyrogen can be extracted from several other tissues, although in smaller quantities.

Although almost always produced for experimental purposes from polymorphonuclear leucocytes, and therefore frequently referred to as *leucocyte pyrogen*, this *endogenous pyrogen* can also be liberated from monocytes, Kupffer cells, and other fixed cells of the reticular endothelial system (MILTON 1976).

BENNETT and BEESON (1953 b) showed that the endogenous pyrogen (EP) is distinguishable from the bacterial endotoxin (BE) in the time course of the onset of the fever when these substances are injected into a rabbit; while there may be a latency of up to an hour before the onset of fever in response to a BE, the onset of fever after the injection of EP is more prompt.

The obvious working hypothesis derivable from this accumulating evidence was that a BE is not a direct pyrogen, but acts through an influence on some types of reticulo-endothelial cells, causing them first to synthesize and then to release EP into the bloodstream (see ATKINS 1960). From a more recent review of the literature, ATKINS and BODEL (1974) have concluded that the cells capable of producing EP can be caused to do so by either BE, or by some endogenous function of inflammation or tissue damage. The liberated EP is thus considered to be an essential mediator in the genesis of fever (MILTON 1976). This may then pass through the blood-brain barrier and act directly on the central neurones involved in thermoregulation. This sequence of events would explain the correlation between fever and necrosis which may relate to an infectious or a non-infectious condition.

III. The Prostaglandins

Aspirin (acetylsalicylic acid) has long been known to have antipyretic as well as anti-inflammatory and mildly analgesic properties. Salicylic acid is, indeed, the active factor in the extract of the bark of the willow tree (*Salix alba*) which STONE (1763) had found to give relief to malarial fever (ague). Now there is a range of substances which have the same combination of therapeutic properties, indomethacin and acetaminophen, for example. These substances have been shown to have a common biochemical action: the prevention of the formation of prostaglandins from arachidonic acid (VANE 1971). Thus it seemed very likely that the formation of prostaglandins are involved somehow in the processes of pain, inflammation, and fever. The action of aspirin and aspirin-like drugs is said to prevent the action of an enzyme called prostaglandin synthetase, but this is now known to be a misleading description of the enzyme, the action of which is to facilitate the metabolism of arachidonic acid, the products of which includes prostacyclins and thromboxanes as well as prostaglandins. This may be an important distinction since there is evidence that not all the physiological and pathological functions which are altered by aspirin-like drugs are the result of the synthesis of prostaglandins: other products of arachidonic acid breakdown may be involved.

Experiments were soon underway to determine the significance of VANE's discovery of the action of aspirin, in relation to fever. Thus, MILTON and WENDLANDT (1970, 1971 a, b) showed that prostaglandins of the E type caused the same effects as those of a pyrogen when injected into the cerebral ventricles of the cat, rabbit, and rat, and that this effect could be abolished by the aspirin-like drug 4-acetamidophenol (acetaminophen, paracetamol). These essential details have since been thoroughly confirmed and have been found to hold for all placental mammalian species that have been tested. It was then shown that a fever induced in the cat by an intracerebroventricular (i.c.v.) injection of a BE (FELDBERG and GUPTA 1973), and by an i.c.v. injection of physiological saline (DEY et al. 1974), are both accompanied by a rise in the concentration of prostaglandins in the cerebrospinal fluid (CSF). In the latter series of experiments it was shown that the administration of an antipyretic drug (paracetamol or indomethacin) attenuated both the fever response and the PG content of the CSF. Thus the evidence for the view that a prostaglandin E (PGE) is the final causative factor in the genesis of fever was strong: (i) the introduction of PGE into the vicinity of the hypothalamus gives rise to a fever-like hyperthermia, (ii) the fever caused by a pyrogen is attenuated by an aspirin like drug; and (iii) the aspirin-like drug prevents the appearance of PGs in the CSF which normally occurs during pyrogen-induced fever. In the face of this evidence it then seemed that the EP released from leucocytes and other reticulo-endothelial cells is purely intermediary and exerts its effect by activating the metabolism of arachidonic acid.

As will be discussed later, the once near certainty of this interpretation of the evidence has begun to fade. There is now considerable doubt whether prostaglandins are the only pyrogenic products of arachidonic acid metabolism and whether fever is the exclusive consequence of the production of arachidonic acid derivatives. Some evidence indicates that EP, or even a BE, may have a pyrogenic action of its own which is distinguishable from that of arachidonic acid by-products (Fig. 2).

The suspicion that there are at least two terminal activators in a BE-induced fever, stems from the observation that the febrile response is biphasic whereas a prostaglandin-induced fever is monophasic. Furthermore, there is evidence that an aspirin-like antipyretic agent prevents only the first of the two-phase pyrogenic response to a BE.

D. Pyrogen Action

I. Points of Action in the Central Nervous System

Since the physiology of fever must involve some terminal influence on central neurones involved in temperature regulation, a review is now made of the evidence of local and direct effects of bacterial endotoxins, leucocytic pyrogens and PGE on the hypothalmic and related structures in the central nervous system (CNS) known, by ablative and stimulative studies, to be those central structures most intimately involved in thermoregulation.

In the several species of mammals tested, fever occurs when a BE (VILLABLANCA and MYERS 1965; COOPER 1965; MYERS et al. 1971, 1973; LIPTON and FOSSLER 1974), an EP produced from leucocytes (COOPER et al. 1967; JACKSON 1967; REPIN and KRATSKIN 1967; CRANSTON et al. 1970; ROSENDORFF and MOONEY 1971) or PGE (STITT 1973; LIPTON and FOSSLER 1974; CRAWSHAW and STITT 1975; VEALE and COOPER 1975; STITT and HARDY 1975; WILLIAMS et al. 1977) is introduced directly into the preoptic/anterior hypothalamic (PO/AH) part of the brain. The integrity of the PO/AH is necessary for normal processes of thermoregulation, it contains neural structures which are responsive to local temperature changes, and gives rise to appropriate corrective thermoregulatory responses when thermally or electrically stimulated (see BLIGH 1973, for reference to the pertinent literature).

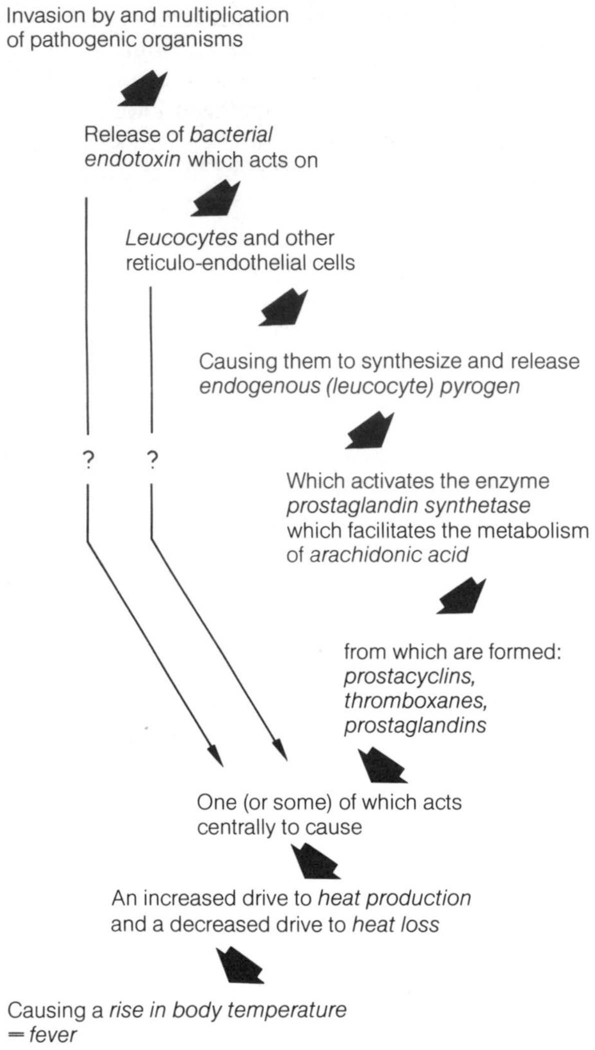

Invasion by and multiplication
of pathogenic organisms

Release of *bacterial
endotoxin* which acts on

Leucocytes and other
reticulo-endothelial cells

?   ?

Causing them to synthesize and release
endogenous (leucocyte) pyrogen

Which activates the enzyme
prostaglandin synthetase
which facilitates the metabolism
of *arachidonic acid*

from which are formed:
*prostacyclins,
thromboxanes,
prostaglandins*

One (or some) of which acts
centrally to cause

An increased drive to *heat production*
and a decreased drive to *heat loss*

Causing a *rise in body temperature*
= *fever*

Fig. 2. A diagrammatic representation of the possible sequence of actions by which an infection can result in fever. The *heavy arrows* indicate the sequence of actions known to occur, but it seems very likely that bacterial endotoxin and/or endogenous (leucocyte) pyrogen has a hyperthermic action which is not dependent on the formation of prostaglandins

In a review of their own evidence, and that of others, Veale and Cooper (1975) noted not only that the PO/AH sites of action of PGE have consistently been found to be the same as those responsive to EP (Feldberg and Milton 1973; Stitt 1973; Veale and Cooper 1974) but also that both these substances cause fever only when they are placed within the PO/AH. Fever has been found to be caused by intracerebral injections of a BE in cats (Villablanca and Myers 1965), and monkeys (Myers et al. 1974); of EP in rabbits (Cooper et al. 1967) and guinea-pigs (Blatteis and Smith 1979), and of PGE in rabbits (Stitt 1973) and monkeys (Simpson et al.

1977) only when injected into the PO/AH region of the brain. The latency of the rise in body temperature in response to such local injections of PGE_1 was found to be less than that to similarly injected EP by STITT and HARDY (1972) and STITT (1973). This distinction has been interpreted as evidence that the action of EP is, in part at least, through the release of PGE_1 in the PO/AH.

Since BE, EP, and PGE will all give rise to fever when introduced directly into the PO/AH region of the brain, it must follow that if a PGE is the sole final causative agent, which acts directly on the PO/AH neurones in a very particular way such as to change the activity of neurones and to raise the set-point, then all stages of the events by which the presence of the BE results in the formation of PGE, can occur locally within this part of the brain. Thus the primary response to BE when injected directly into the PO/AH could be the accumulation of leucocytes or some other mobile reticulo-endothelial cell in the hypothalamic area. Such a response has indeed, been demonstrated by COOPER et al. (1967). This is not to say, of course, that the entire sequence of events normally occurs within the hypothalamus. Since EP can be tranferred from the circulating blood of a febrile animal to an afebrile animal and induce fever in it (ATKINS and WOOD 1955), it might be reasonable to suppose that the production of EP in response to infection is normally a largely extracentral process, the liberated EP passing from the circulating blood into the brain to exert its direct action on specific neurones, or its indirect action by provoking the metabolism of arachidonic acid.

II. Effects on the Electrical Activities of Hypothalamic Neurones

A change in the bioelectrical activity of hypothalamic neurones upon injection of a pyrogen into a rabbit, indicative of a change in central nervous events during fever was reported by KOROLKIEWICZ (1967). Then WIT and WANG (1968 b) recorded a depression of the temperature-related activities of temperature-responsive neurones in the PO/AH of cats in response to changes in local brain temperature after an intravenous (i.v.) injection of a BE. A greater rise in local temperature than normally required to change the firing rate of a temperature-responsive neurone could, however, still elicit an increase in activity, while the intracarotid administration of the antipyretic agent, acetylsalicylate, returned the responsiveness of these PO/AH neurones to their pre-pyrogen level of activity within an hour. EISENMAN (1974) then confirmed the action of a BE on PO/AH neurones in rabbits, by showing that the electrical activities of temperature-responsive neurones were depressed by an i.c.v. injection of BE. Also using rabbits, STITT and HARDY (1975) found that the introduction of PGE_1 directly into the PO/AH also changed the electrical activities of neurones in that part of the brain, and suggested that PGE_1 might modulate the release of a neurotransmitter in the PO/AH.

The majority of thermoresponsive neurones in the PO/AH in cats were found by SCHOENER and WANG (1975) to respond to proximate injections of EP in a manner consistent with the set-point hypothesis: units responding to a rise in local temperature with an increase in firing rate were depressed, while those units responding with a decrease in firing rate were activated by the pyrogenic agent. It was thus concluded that the ultimate action of EP is on PO/AH neurones involved in thermoregulation. In a further study, SCHOENER and WANG (1976) tested the effect of proximate injections of PGE_1 on PO/AH neurones in cats; PGE_1 changed the temperature-related electrical activities of temperature-responsive neurones as if it had caused an upward displacement of the set-point of thermoregulation. JELL and SWEATMAN (1977) have also found that the effect of PGE_1 in cats is specifically on thermoresponsive neurones in the rostral hypothalamus. In the absence of a careful analysis of the time courses of BE, EP, and PGE on PO/AH neurones of one species under standardized experimental conditions, however, the observations provide no clear evidence on whether, in each case, the final effect on the PO/AH neurones is by a common causative agent, and that this is a prostaglandin or some other product of arachidonic acid. The possibility that the EP or, indeed, the BE, have independent effects on PO/AH cells cannot be excluded.

E. Areas of Current Concern and Doubt

At one time the rapidly emerging evidence for a progression from the bacterial invasion to a final action of prostaglandin on preoptic hypothalamic structures in the genesis of fever, was thought to be so strong that a substantial interpretative error seemed exceedingly unlikely. There are, however, three areas of doubt about the validity of this account of the genesis of fever, or at least about whether this is the only sequence of events by which fever can be caused. These areas of doubt are (i) whether the neurones on the PO/AH structures concerned with thermoregulation are the only ones on which pyrogens can act to cause fever; (ii) whether a PGE is the only product, or the principal by-product, of arachidonic acid which is pyrogenic; and (iii) whether the by-products of arachidonic acid are the only substances which can exert a pyrogenic effect.

In addition to these three areas there remain the problems of whether pyrogens have effects other than on thermoregulation and whether fever in of physiological benefit to the host organism.

I. More than One Central Point of Action of Pyrogens?

It is manifestly unsafe to assume that all the disturbances to body temperature occurring during infection derive from the effect (or effects) of pyrogens on hypothalamic structures, since there are several scattered reports of febrile responses to pyrogens after destructive lesions in the PO/AH have disrupted connections between thermosensors and thermoregulatory effectors (RANSON et al. 1939; GUERRA and BARBOUR 1943; LIPTON and TRZCINKA 1976). There is evidence of thermosensitivity in the medulla and spinal cord, and of connections through the CNS at that level between thermosensors and thermoregulatory effectors (see LIPTON 1973; SIMON 1974, for literature). Conceivably, therefore, pyrogens could exert influences on thermoregulation at the levels of these lower thermosensors or sensor–effector connections. This suggestion is, however, unsupported by any direct evidence of fever in response to local injections of pyrogens into these structures. Thus the apparent extrahypothalamic site of action of pyrogens remains unlocated.

Briefly the evidence for suspecting that the PO/AH may not be the sole target of pyrogen action is as follows.

When, in the unanaesthetized goat, the entire preoptic region was destroyed gradually by proton irradiation, there was impairment of the animal's capacity to resist heat and cold, but the animal still responded to a pyrogen with fever (ANDERSSON et al. 1965). It was concluded that another area of the brain, posterior to the hypothalamus could also be concerned in thermoregulation and be acted on by a pyrogen. In the same year, PORTER and KASS (1965) reported that the injection of BE into the posterior hypothalamus of the rat caused fever and that stereotaxic lesions in the posterior hypothalamus rendered the animals more resistant to the lethal effects of an injected BE, while lesions in the anterior hypothalamus increased the sensitivity of the animals to BE. This finding fits the long-standing theory based on the evidence of MEYER (1913), FRAZIER et al. (1936), RANSON and MAGOUN (1939), and CLARK et al. (1939), and still revived from time to time, that the anterior hypothalamus is a site of warm-sensitivity, and that its destruction only inactivates a response to hyperthermia while the posterior hypothalamus is the site of cold-sensitivity and its destruction only inactivates response to hypothermia.

Another indication of a second area of pyrogen activity is that of CABANAC and HARDY (1967) who found that single neuronal units in the thalamus, as well as in the hypothalamus, were temperature responsive, having bell-shaped curves which peaked in either the cold or the warm range. An i.v. injection of BE (typhoid vaccine) was found to cause a decrease in activity in at least some of the thalamic warm units.

After lesions in the preoptic area, VEALE and COOPER (1975) found that rabbits no longer responded to locally (preoptic) applied EP or PGE_1 with a rise in temperature. However, when these two substances were injected into a lateral cerebral ventricle after the lesions had been made in the preoptic area, fever still occurred in response to the EP, but not in response to PGE_1. Intravenous EP also caused fever after the lesions which had stopped the pyrogenic action of centrally administered PGE_1. On the basis of this evidence, VEALE and COOPER (1975) concluded that pyrogen can act at a site other than PO/AH to produce fever, and that this action is independent of the release of PGE_1. That EP can act at more than one site in the brain to cause fever seems very possible, but the reasoning behind the proposition that its action is independent of the release of PGE_1 is less clear: MILTON (1976) has pointed out that VEALE and COOPER did not determine the effect of antipyretic drugs on the fever caused by i.v. or i.c.v. injections of an EP after destruction of the preopticus.

LIPTON and TRZCINKA (1976) have also given evidence that the febrile response to pyrogens in squirrel monkeys persists after destruction of the PO/AH. They conclude that in primates there is either multiple central representation of fever control, or an inherent capacity of central structures to develop sensitivity to pyrogens and to produce coordinated febrile responses. Any secondary centre is unlikely to be in the medulla oblongata since no evidence could be found by LIPTON and TRZCINKA of a response to a pyrogen injected into that area, although LIPTON (1973) had shown the existence of temperature-responsive structures in the medullary region and the possibility that connexions through the CNS from thermosensors to thermoregulatory effectors also exist at this level.

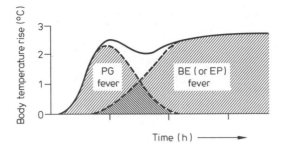

Fig. 3. A diagrammatic representation of the biphasic febrile response to a single intravenous injection of a bacterial endotoxin. Here, the pattern is assumed to be composed of two distinct but overlapping actions, the first of which may depend on the production of endogenous pyrogen (*EP*), and possibly also on the production of prostaglandin (*PG*), and perhaps other metabolites of arachidonic acid, and the second of which may be a direct action of the bacterial endotoxin (*BE*), or through some other transitional process

II. The Biphasic Pattern of Experimentally Induced Fever: Two Causative Factors?

When a fever is induced by a single injection of a BE, there are a first and a second peak in body temperature, divided by a trough (Fig. 3). This has been observed in several species including the rabbit and dog (BENNETT et al. 1957; SZÉKELY 1978 c), the rhesus monkey (MYERS et al. 1973), the guinea-pig (SZÉKELY 1978 b), the goat (FRENS 1974), and the sheep (BLIGH unpublished).

HAAN (1965) attributed the biphasic fever induced in a rabbit by an i.v. injection of a BE to two distinct actions: the first being caused by the BE per se, and the second resulting from the release of an endogenous substance. From evidence then available, it was assumed that the EP, and possibly also the BE, act directly but independently on central nervous structures involved in thermoregulation. From the knowledge that endogenous pyrogen can be derived from the leucocytes from the circulating blood when these are incubated with a BE, it might seem unlikely that the major influence of BE is directly upon CNS structures. However, when BENNETT et al. (1957) introduced a BE into the subarachnoid space, an enormous fever resulted. This was interpreted as evidence that a BE is fully capable of producing fever by a direct action on the CNS. The initial delay in the onset of a BE-induced fever could thus be attributed, in part at least, to the time required for BE, or the lipid A moiety of it, to penetrate the blood-brain barrier.

VEALE et al. (1977) also considered fever to be the result of two mechanisms: the first of which they considered to involve the release of prostaglandin and its action on PO/AH neurones. This component of the fever response to a pyrogen, they suggest, is rapid in its development after an initial latency, and is of relatively short duration. The second phase which develops more gradually but is of greater duration, is supposed by VEALE et al. (1977) to be due to a direct action of EP, at a site other than the PO/AH. FRENS (1974) also concluded that two different processes are involved in the biphasic fever when a BE was injected i.v. into the goat, because with repeated injections of the BE, the second peak rapidly failed to develop, while the initial phase, rapid in its development, and brief in its duration, did not show a pronounced tachyphylaxis.

From a study of the biphasic BE fever in the newborn guinea-pig, SZÉKELY and KOMAROMI (1978) also concluded that the two peaks in the hyperthermia following BE administration are unlikely to be mediated by a single central factor, and postulated a series of two distinct actions in the production of the fever pattern. SZÉKELY (1978a) showed that even a third factor may be involved, since he found the fall in core temperature between the two peaks to be an active phase, dependent upon a central serotonergic function, whereas the two peaks are not so dependent. SZÉKELY (1978b) found that the aspirin-like antipyretic substance indomethacin eliminates the first phase rise in body temperature and the intermediate depression, but does not affect the second peak. From these observations SZÉKELY (1978b) suggests that an arachidonic acid derivative (a prostaglandin and/or a thromboxane) might be responsible for the first-phase rise, but that the second-phase rise in body temperature depends upon the action of another mediator.

In another study, SZÉKELY (1978c) gives evidence of an ontogenetic separation between the development of the mechanism which produces the first phase and the second phase of fever in the rabbit. Whereas in 0- to 3-day-old rabbits an intraperitoneal (i.p.) or i.v. injection of a BE caused only the first peak of the fever response, a 6- to 10-day-old rabbit responded with a biphasic fever.

In an even more recent study HOFFMAN-GOETZ and KLUGER (1979) have found that the first phase, but not the second phase, of a BE-induced fever in the rabbit is attenuated by protein deficiency. Since both normal and protein-deficient rabbits responded to an injected EP with a "first-phase" fever only, HOFFMAN-GOETZ and KLUGER suggest that the probable reason for the interference with fever by protein deficiency is the impairment of the formation of the EP.

Put together, these observations indicate that only the first phase of the two-peak patterned pyrogen-induced hyperthermia is dependent on the production of EP (HOFFMAN-GOETZ and KLUGER 1979) and that it is prevented by pre-treatment with an antipyretic agent which blocks the action of "prostaglandin synthetase" (SZÉKELY 1978b). Thus the first-phase fever appears to be due to a sequence of events involving both EP production and the metabolism of arachidonic acid, while the second-phase fever would seem to involve neither EP nor arachidonic acid metabolism, and could be the result of a direct action of the BE on hypothalamic structures (Fig. 3), as was proposed by HAAN (1965).

This interpretation is apparently compatible with the earlier cited evidence (VEALE and COOPER 1975) of two distinct central nervous sites or structures, a hypothalamic site responsive to both EP and to PGE, and a site responsive to EP but not PGE. Clearly we do not yet know how many central sites responsive to a pyrogen there are nor whether BE, EP, and PGE all have independent pyrogenic effects on the CNS as well as being parts of a chain of events. As is discussed in detail later, whether fever is induced by an i.v. injection of a BE or an i.c.v. injection of PGE_1 the resultant hyperthermia is attributable to the activation of heat production and heat conservation effectors and the inhibition of heat loss effectors. In the sheep the fevers induced by an intravenous injection of an EP and an i.c.v. injection of PGE_1 can both be attenuated by prior i.c.v. injection of atropine, which also blocks the drive from peripheral cold-sensors. This has been interpreted as evidence of a

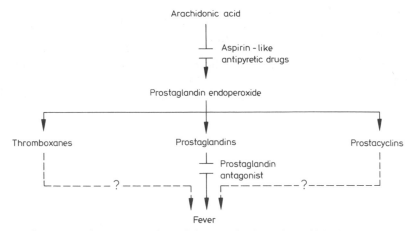

Fig. 4. A diagrammatic representation of the metabolism of arachidonic acid, presumably under the influence of the endogenous (leucocyte) pyrogen, to yield thromboxanes, prostaglandins, and prostacyclins. The prostaglandins of the E series are known to be pyrogenic, but other products of arachidonic acid may also be pyrogenic

common point of action of the two pyrogens. Thus at the moment there is evidence that both EP and PGE_1 act upon the same part of the pathway through the CNS from thermosensors to thermoregulatory effectors. However, any "remnant" fever still caused by EP after i.c.v. atropine, or after arachidonic acid metabolism has been blocked, has not been adequately examined and described.

III. The Pyrogenic Metabolites of Arachidonic Acid

Further doubt as to whether PGE is the terminal, or sole terminal, agent in the genesis of fever arose when CRANSTON et al. (1975) found that although sodium salicylate prevented the increase in PGE concentration in the CSF which had been shown to accompany fever (FELDBERG and GUPTA 1973; FELDBERG et al. 1973), it did not prevent a rise in body temperature. It was then shown that specific prostaglandin antagonists, when injected into the cerebral ventricles, blocked the hyperthermic action of i.c.v.-injected PGE, but did not change the course of a fever induced by i.c.v.-injected EP (CRANSTON et al. 1976) This finding brought into question whether a PGE is, in fact, the sole pyrogenic end-product of arachidonic acid, which metabolizes to produce prostaglandins, thromboxanes, and prostacyclins (Fig. 4) any of which might be pyrogenic and still act after the specific blockage of the pyrogenic action of the prostaglandins. In view of the evidence presented in Sect. E.II this might seem an unnecessary hypothesis, but it was strengthened by the observation of LABURN et al. (1977) that the hyperthermia caused by an i.v. injection of arachidonic acid is unaffected by the presence of prostaglandin antagonists which inhibited fever caused by an i.c.v. injection of PGE.

Stable analogues of prostaglandin endoperoxide were found not to cause a rise in body temperature when injected directly into the PO/AH (HAWKINS and LIPTON 1977), but the possibility remains that naturally occurring products of arachidonic acid other than PGE may be active. CREMADES-CAMPOS and MILTON (1978) have now examined the effects on body temperature of two prostaglandin endoperoxide derivatives, and one of these caused shivering, vasoconstriction of the ears, and a rise in body temperature. Indeed, its effects were essentially the same as those of similarly injected PGE_1 though it was less active. The antipyretic drug, paracetamol, had no effect on an initial hyperthermic response, but suppressed a secondary rise which CREMADES-CAMPOS and MILTON consider to be a more specific effect of the release of endogenous prostaglandin. This comment implies a different interpretation of the biphasic response to a pyrogen from that given by SZÉKELY (1978a), and also indicates that the biphasic response could be the separate effects of two by-products of arachidonic acid. The second prostaglandin endoperoxide derivative tested by CREMADES-CAMPOS and MILTON had the converse effect; it caused panting, peripheral vasodilatation of the ears, and a fall in body temperature. This finding may be of significance in the natural aetiology of fever. Pyrogens have been reported to cause both hyperthermia and hypothermia in rats. This phenomenon has been investigated by SZÉKELY and SZELÉNYI (1977) who have shown that although the hypothermic response to pyrogens is ambient temperature dependent, it is probably an active process. This raises the possibility that not only may there be more than one product of arachidonic acid which acts upon the central processes of thermoregulation, but that different components may act upon it in opposing ways.

SIEGERT et al. (1976) showed that a protein inhibitor, cycloheximide, prevented the febrile response to a BE. Whereas the most obvious reason for this might be a failure to synthesize the polypeptidinous EP, this is unlikely since a rise in the level of PGE in the CSF still occurred, indicative of the stimulated metabolism of arachidonic acid; and because cycloheximide was also found to block the pyrogenic effect of EP. Thus the action of the protein inhibitors would seem to be much nearer to the terminal action, perhaps within the CNS.

CRANSTON et al. (1978) have postulated that if arachidonic acid metabolites other than prostaglandins are involved as mediators of fever, then cycloheximide, which blocks the pyrogenic actions of BE and EP, but which does not block the formation of prostaglandins, should antagonize the hyperthermic response to arachidonic acid. The assumption behind this proposition would seem to be that cycloheximide interferes with a pathway from arachidonic acid to a pyrogenic product other than a prostaglandin. The logic behind this deduction, however, is not made clear. An experiment to test this postulate showed that with rabbits, i.v. cycloheximide attenuated the febrile response to i.v.-injected EP, but failed to interfere with the hyperthermic response to an i.c.v. injection of arachidonic acid. CRANSTON et al. (1978) concluded from this that metabolites of arachidonic acid are unlikely to play any important role in the elevation of body temperature during fever. Their results would seem to indicate, however, only that cycloheximide might act somewhere between the production and liberation of EP and the genesis of the fever, which may or may not involve the metabolism of arachidonic acid. It might, for example, impede the movement of EP across the blood-brain barrier.

The crucial issues at this phase in the study of the processes by which an infection leads to a fever would seem to be whether the antipyretic action of aspirin-like drugs can be attributed to any action other than that of impeding the metabolism of arachidonic acid, and whether the aspirin-like drugs attenuate both components of the biphasic response to a BE. Unequivocal evidence on this issue does not seem to be at hand.

Popular supposition is that the febrile state is the consequence of an additional abnormal influence on the central processes of thermoregulation, rather than the increase in the intensity of some modulatory function that is normally present. Arachidonic acid, the products of which clearly play some role in the genesis of fever, is a natural body constituent. Presumably, it is normally being metabolized at a much slower rate than under febrile conditions since there is now a great deal of evidence of other modulatory functions of the products of arachidonic acid. Thus the question has been asked, whether the products of arachidonic acid metabolism contribute to the normal processes of thermoregulation. An obvious way to seek a reply to this question is to determine whether the blockade of arachidonic acid metabolism with aspirin-like drugs has any influence on thermoregulation in afebrile animals. WOODBURY (1970), SATINOFF (1972), and ROSENDORFF and CRANSTON (1968) have given evidence of a salicylate-induced hypothermia, whereas others have reported no changes in body temperature upon administration of aspirin or aspirin-like drugs.

BECKMAN and ROZKOWSKA-RUTTIMAN (1974) found that in the rat the majority of hypothalamic cells responsive to heat were also affected by salicylate. Whereas this might be interpreted as evidence of some independent pharmacological effect of salicylate, it is also arguable that the products of arachidonic acid serve some physiological function as modulators of the activities of central nervous neurones involved in thermoregulation, and that the action of a pyrogen is to enhance greatly, rather than to instigate, this action.

IV. Are Pyrogens Only Pyrogens?

Many systems of the body are disturbed during infection, or when dead pathogenic organisms or the derived lipopolysaccharide is injected into the body. VAN MIERT (1971), for example, quotes evidence of the inhibition of the reticulo-rumen motility of ruminants, of the release of catecholamines in humans and rabbits, and of hyperglycaemia followed by hypoglycaemia in goats. These are probably only some of the effects of metabolites of the invading organisms which can produce the complex disturbance known as endotoxin shock as well as fever. Thus the preference for the term *bacterial endotoxin* to *bacterial pyrogen* places proper emphasis on the ability of the invading micro-organisms to cause a much more general disturbance to the physiology of the infected subject than just that on thermoregulation.

The purification of the lipopolysaccharide of bacterial origin which gives rise to fever, and the further definition of that part of the lipopolysaccharide molecule which has this property, permits the separation of the effects of this particular endotoxin from other effects of the invading micro-organism. What is not yet clear is how many of them are due to very specific actions on particular cells of the body.

As has been discussed earlier, it now seems fairly well established that while part of the febrile response to a BE may be attributable to an action of the toxin itself on particular cells in the CNS, another part of the response is not due to the direct action of the BE on central neurones concerned in thermoregulation. One primary action of the BE is on leucocytes and possibly other reticulo-endothelial cells, which respond to the presence of the BE with the production and discharge into the blood of a proteinous material. Presumably this can cross the blood-brain barrier and act directly or indirectly on some particular central nervous structure, and that thermoregulation is thereby changed in such a way that the level at which body temperature is regulated is raised. Hence its name: leucocyte pyrogen.

Recent evidence of HOFFMAN-GOETZ and KLUGER (1979) seems to confirm this still rather vague statement about the sequence of events by which the invading micro-organism evokes fever. They have shown that when rabbits are rendered protein deficient, the febrile response to a bacterial infection is much diminished. This, they have attributed to a failure of leucocytes and other reticulo-endothelial cells to produce EP, since the animal will still respond normally to the injection of an EP produced in vitro from the leucocytes of a non-protein-deficient rabbit. HOFFMAN-GOETZ and KLUGER (1979) also observed that not only was there a reduced fever in the protein-deficient rabbits, but also that there was no reduction in plasma iron concentration which accompanies a febrile response to an infection in the ordinary course of events (as discussed in the next paragraph). However, when fever was induced in these animals by the injection of the EP, the plasma iron concentration did fall.

This latter observation fits with other accumulating evidence of effects other than fever of EP, or of other substances produced by the leucocytes at the same time. GARIBALDI (1972) had shown that the EP preparation causes the synthesis of siderophores which have a chelating effect on the iron in extracellular fluids. Hence the explanation for the fall in plasma iron concentration which accompanies fever. Almost at the same time KAMPSCHMIDT et al. (1973) showed that even when partially purified, leucocytic EP retained the ability to exert several effects beside fever: it lowered plasma zinc concentrations as well iron concentrations; it also caused the elevation of particular serum globulins (α_2-acute-phase), and it caused the release of neutrophils from the bone marrow. In further studies MERRIMAN et al. (1977) have found that at every stage in its purification, the pyrogenic material derived from leucocytes had all these other effects. Since the material with all these pyrogenic and other effects migrates as a single factor when subjected to electrophoresis, MERRIMAN et al. (1977) considered it probable that one substance is the common agent.

VAN MIERT and VAN DUIN (1978) have investigated the in vitro antipyretic action of polymyxin B which inactivates a variety of Gram-negative BEs in vitro (COOPERSTOCK 1974), and concluded that it acts primarily by inhibiting EP synthesis and/or its release. Thus it should now be possible to distinguish between the general cellular effects of BE, and those acting specifically through the release of EP, which now clearly needs some functionally less specific name.

Thus it would seem that when we consider fever and its cause or causes, we are looking at only one aspect of a complexity of physiological changes. At least part of the fever response seems to involve the EP-induced metabolism of arachidonic acid, the products of which have many modulatory effects other than that on thermoregulation.

V. Is Fever of Physiological Benefit?

It is now clear that in fever, as in practically all else in the study of the functions of living systems, simplicity can only be discerned in a quite artificial situation, in which the chain of events by which a specific disturbance results in a specific response is considered as if it can operate in isolation from the many other simultaneous and interacting functions involved in the phenomenon of life. Neither the action of a BE, nor that of the so-called EP, or of PGE or of other metabolites of arachidonic acid, are in fact solely associated with the chain of events by which infection results in fever.

Thus it may now be somewhat naive to ask the simple question: "Does the rise in body temperature facilitate the body's defence against infection?" Perhaps the question should be: "Do the many physiological consequences of a BE in the environment of the body's constituent cells, act as a system of defence against infection?" The distinction between these questions can be seen in the different ways in which answers might be sought. To answer the first question one might simply try to prevent the rise in body temperature during the course of an infection, and see if this handicaps the body's defence. To answer the second question one might try to block the specific effects of the BE on the leucocytes and kindred cells, with polymyxin B for example, while leaving the non-specific cellular effects of the BE to run their course. So far, however, only the first of these two questions has been addressed, and as recently as 1978, BERNHEIM et al. concluded that "fever has never been proven beneficial in mammals?" An early suggestion was that the raised body temperature might aid the defence mechanisms through its incremental effect on metabolic processes. The obvious fallacy in this argument was that the elevated temperature would also enhance the growth and multiplication of the invading organisms. Thus, if fever is of survival value there is probably more to the response to BEs than just the induction of hyperthermia.

In mice (CONNOR and KASS 1961), rats (PORTER and KASS 1962), and rabbits (ATWOOD and KASS 1964), the induction of hyperthermia by physical or pharmacological means was found to lower the mortality resulting from administration of a BE. Against this evidence, however, there is now the widespread and apparently harmless use of aspirin-like antipyretic drugs to relieve discomfort during infections. While the principal virtue of these drugs may relate more to their anti-inflammatory and mildly analgesic properties, we may suppose that if the suppression of fever greatly impaired the ability to combat infection, this would soon have been noted clinically and confirmed experimentally. Clearly human beings do no immediate harm to themselves when they swallow even the very considerable quantities of aspirin prescribed in the treatment of rheumatic inflammations, for example. FERREIRA and VANE (1974) thus concluded that whatever the physiological roles of the prostaglandins, these must be modulatory rather than imperative influences on the functions of the body, since the impaired metabolism of arachidonic acid by treatment with aspirin-like drugs is evidently without serious consequences. There must, however, be caution in concluding that the total elimination of the febrile response to infection would be wholly without harmful consequences, since there is no evidence that antipyretic drugs can wholly prevent fever. Evidence discussed earlier now sems to indicate that the pyrogenic by-products of arachidonic acid may be involved only in the first phase of the biphasic febrile response to a single injection of a BE. Thus the second phase of such a fever which does not seem to be mediated by prostaglandins or other products of arachidonic acid metabolism may be unaffected by antipyretic drugs.

Even if this is so, the separation of aspirin-attenuated and non-attenuated components of a fever caused by an infection is difficult because of the continuous liberation of a BE into the circulation. The two or more possible pyrogenic agents may then be acting concurrently rather than phasically as seems to occur after a single injection of a BE. This is evident from a study by CRANSTON et al. (1971) who caused sustained fever in rabbits by means of the continuous infusion of EP after an initial priming injection. The reduction in the induced fever following an i.v. injection of sodium salicylate was greater when given at 4 h into the fever than when given at 3 h, and that at 3 h was greater than at 1 h. If the action of the sodium salicylate is solely on the metabolism of arachidonic acid, then it must be suspected that, contrary to the evidence of the febrile response to single injections of pyrogens, the component of the fever which is attenuated by an antipyretic drug, increases with time when EP is being continuously produced or injected. However, it would seem from the results of CRANSTON et al. (1971) that even the highest doses of sodium salicylate resulted in no more than a 50% attenuation of the fever. Thus, the reduction in the fever resulting from the treatment of the symptoms with aspirin-like drugs, may be insufficient to negate this beneficial effect of the fever completely.

Although the survival value of fever in mammals remains unconfirmed, there is now some evidence that moderate fevers are beneficial to reptiles during bacterial infection (KLUGER et al. 1975; BERNHEIM and KLUGER 1976; COVERT and REYNOLDS 1977; KLUGER and VAUGHN 1978). A mechanism by which this benefit of fever accrues has been proposed: WEINBERG (1974) suggested that the fall in plasma iron concentration which occurs during fever might depress the growth of bacteria. Taking up this suggestion, KLUGER and ROTHENBURG (1978, 1979) and GRIEGER and KLUGER (1978) showed that the growth in vitro of a pathogenic organism is hindered at 41 °C, but not at 38 °C when the iron content of the medium is lowered by means of a chelating agent or by precipitation with magnesium carbonate. Without this reduction in the iron concentration, the growth rate of the bacteria was found to be not very different at the non-febrile (38 °C) and the febrile (41 °C) temperatures. These findings indicate a complex interaction between the chelation of the iron content of the extracellular fluids, and the elevation of both temperatures. Both of these could be consequent upon the production of endogenous pyrogen.

BERNHEIM et al. (1978) have shown by in vivo studies on a lizard, that, when the animal was infected with a micro-organism and then allowed to elevate its body temperature to 41 °C, the blood was virtually sterile after 12 h, whereas the blood from lizards kept at 38 °C ambient temperature, and therefore at a body temperature of 38 °C, for 12 h after infection contained more than a million micro-organisms per ml. BERNHEIM et al. (1978) suggest that the fever enhances some aspect of the early inflammatory response, leading to increased leucocyte immigration at the local site and containment of the infection.

In reptiles the elevation in body temperature in response to a pyrogen results from changes in behavioural thermoregulation, which can be frustrated simply by denying the infected animal the means of selecting an environment which will result in an elevation of body temperature. Since the body temperature of the endothermic mammal cannot be manipulated so easily, and the techniques used to hold down body temperature during infection are somewhat drastic, there is still no clear evidence that these results obtained with reptiles apply also to the mammals. There is, however, at least the indication that if fever is beneficial, the benefit is consequent upon more than one of the actions of EP.

F. Mechanisms of Thermoregulation

I. The Set-Point Machinery: Theory

The statement is frequently made that pyrogens, and the various drugs which cause changes in body temperature, act by inducing changes in the thermoregulatory set-point, but there is remarkably little discussion of what the statement really means. One is left to imagine a little box within the CNS, with a re-set knob which can be turned clockwise or anticlockwise by various chemical substances. We are, of course, dealing with a neuronal complex that somehow relates the input of signals from thermosensors to the output of signals to thermoregulatory effectors, such that whenever body temperature increases or decreases owing to changes in heat production or heat loss, appropriate compensatory adjustments occur in heat production and/or heat loss so as to restore body temperature to a "set" value.

For such a system there must be a sensor, or sensors, of the regulated variable which feeds signals proportional to the regulated variable into the regulator. Both cutaneous and central thermosensors, which presumably are involved in some such function, are known to exist (see BLIGH 1973, for review). There must also be a feedback of the result of the correction–effector activities onto the "regulated variable" sensors; and the circulating blood serves this function. But there must also be the regulator, or the set-point generator. This is assumed to be within the CNS and is, presumably, a function of interacting neurones. There is no firm evidence of how neurones achieve this essential function in a homeostatic system, but some of the theoretical possibilities have been considered by BLIGH (1973, 1978, 1979a).

A popular notion among thermoregulatory physiologists is that for the maintained stability of a quality of quantity, there must be a stable reference-signal generator, the output of which is compared with the signal representative of the regulated variable. It is thus supposed that there are central neurones which perform the role of temperature-insensitive stable reference-signal generators, and that various substances, including the pyrogens, may act upon these reference-signal generator neurones and cause a shift in the signal intensity (that is, in the impulse frequency).

A re-settable reference-signal generator, a sensor of the regulated variable, and a comparator of the two signals giving rise to an "error" or correction–effector activating signal, is a system frequently employed by control-system engineers to achieve a variable "set-point" for a regulating system (Fig. 5a). There is no theoretical difficulty in visualizing how neurons could inter-relate to effect essentially

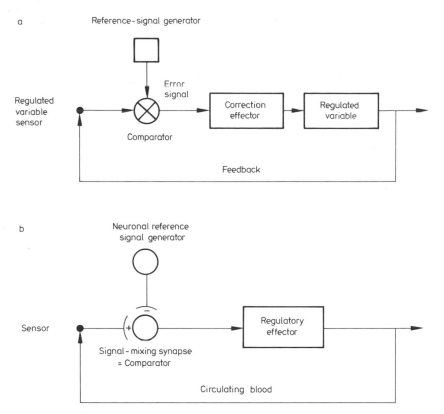

Fig. 5 a, b. A diagrammatic representation of a regulatory system based on the comparison of a signal derived from the sensor of the regulated variable with that derived from a reference-signal generator. The resultant error signal drives the correction effector, the impact of which is fed back onto the sensor of the regulated variable. **a** expressed in terms of control system symbols; **b** expressed in terms of neuronal units and pathways, with the circulating blood functioning as the feedback from correction effector onto sensor

the same regulatory function (Fig. 5 b). Here the synapse functioning as the signal mixer, would be a gate through which signals would pass from sensor to effector only when the excitatory influence exceeded the inhibitory influence of the reference-signal generating neurone.

However, an endogenous reference-signal generator is not an imperative component of homeostatic regulation in an engineered system and therefore does not necessarily exist in analogous biological systems. Differing physical properties of two sensors, or populations of sensors, is an equally common means by which engineers regulate temperature. Indeed, the bimetallic strip, one of the simplest of all thermoregulatory devices, employs this principle. Whether biological homeothermy depends on the opposing influences of two sensor signals, or upon a neuronal reference-signal generator and comparator, the effectors of thermal balance are essentially two opposing and variable corrective functions – those inducing heat production, and those inducing heat loss – each being controlled by efferent neural signals from the CNS.

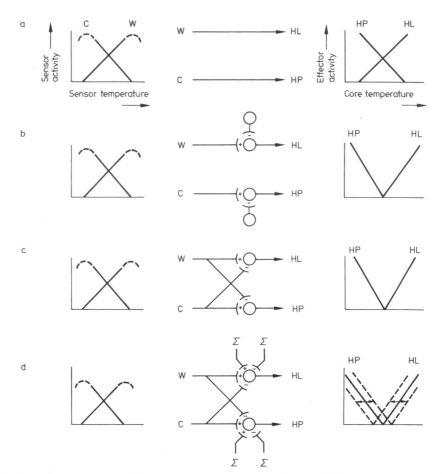

Fig. 6. a If warm-sensors (*W*) link directly to heat loss effectors (*HL*), and cold-sensors (*C*) link directly to heat production effectors (*HP*); and if, over an operational temperature range, the activities of the warm- and cold-sensors are reciprocal, then the balancing activities of the HL and HP effectors could establish thermostability. **b** Stable inhibitory influences (e.g. set-point signal generators) acting on both pathways could create a central null-point between the activities of thermoregulatory heat production and heat loss. **c** Simple crossing inhibition between the two sensor–effector pathways could also create the central null-point. **d** All converging influences from elsewhere in the CNS must be excitatory or inhibitory. Here the many such influences are shown as sums (*Σ*). These influences, by changing the synaptic "gating" on the sensor–effector pathways, will change the core temperature at which heat loss or heat production effectors will be activated

VENDRIK (1959) pointed out that if there are two populations of thermosensors, and if they have converse activity/temperature relations over the operational range of tissue temperatures (see Fig. 6a), then they could function as a set-point generator, and no other special neuronal machinery would be necessary. Others have now also proposed, apparently independently of VENDRIK's thesis, that homeothermy may be based on some such principle (MITCHELL et al. 1970; HOUDAS et al. 1973).

Indeed, as is indicated in Fig. 6a, a functional thermoregulatory system need consist of no more than the opposing signals from warm- and cold-sensors as determinants of the activities of heat loss and heat production effectors respectively, together with the feedback of the thermal consequences of the activities of the heat loss and heat production effectors onto the thermosensors, which the circulating blood inevitably achieves.

Thus, mammalian thermoregulation could be based on a stable reference-signal generator and a comparator; or upon opposing signal changes from two populations of sensors when subjected to temperature changes or, of course, on some as yet totally unrecognized principle. Apart from the evidence of opposing signal changes along the axons of the so-called warm- and cold-thermosensors in response to temperature changes over an operational range, there are many other reasons, some of which have been discussed by BLIGH (1979a, 1980) for suspecting that homeothermy in particular, and perhaps homeostasis generally, may be based on the two-sensor principle of regulation rather than on the endogenous reference-signal generator principle. In the subsequent discussion here, I am assuming that the point (or points) of action of the terminal pyrogenic agent (or agents) is somewhere on the pathways through the CNS from thermosensors to thermoregulatory effectors.

II. The Antiquity of Homeostasis and of Pyrogen Responsiveness

Presumably the central nervous interface between the afferent pathway from a thermosensor and the efferent pathway to a responding thermoregulatory effector, consists of a chain of neurones with intervening synapses at which there are various interactions with other thermally related, and thermally unrelated, activities within the central nervous system, which modulate the relations between the particular sensor and the particular effector. Whether pyrogens act directly or indirectly on the central thermosensor–thermoregulatory effector interface is unknown. Nor is it known whether pyrogens exert their effect (or effects) on primary sensing structures or upon interneurones; nor whether they act upon an entire cell surface or only on a particular structure, such as a specific receptor sites. The overall consequences of pyrogen on thermoregulatory processes, however, are quite specific: there is an increased drive to heat production effectors and/or a decrease in the drive to heat loss effectors, the relative extents of which depend on the prevailing ambient temperature. At high ambient temperature the principal cause of fever is the reduction in heat loss, while at thermoneutral or low ambient temperatures, an increase in heat production may be dominant.

This patterned modulation of the thermoregulatory processes means almost certainly, that pyrogens do not act indiscriminately on nerve cells, but act specifically on particular populations of nerve cells related to thermoregulation so as to effect an orderly change in function. The observed effects of pyrogens on single neurones in the CNS (see Sect. D.II) gives support to this supposition.

Because of these opposing effects of pyrogens on heat loss and heat production effectors (the inhibition of the one, and the excitation of the other), it must follow that if there is only one point of action of a pyrogen on the central nervous interface between thermosensors and thermoregulatory effectors, this must be somewhere before a crossing inhibitory influence between the efferent pathways that control heat loss and heat production effectors, such that the former is attenuated, and the latter is activated by the action of the pyrogen (FRENS 1971). Alternatively, there could be two distinctly different actions of a pyrogen: one to attenuate heat loss effector activities, and the other to activate heat production effector activities.

BLIGH (1979a) has argued that the basic neurology of homeostasis, of which homeothermy is but one component, could be surprisingly simple – at least in its basic principle. The reason for this assertion is that some degree of homeostasis must exist in every multicellular organism that is too large for simple diffusion to and from the external environment to effect the maintenance of the internal environment of the deepest cells of the organism within the limits of variation necessary for their viability. Thus he has supposed that some degree of homeostasis must exist in the larger of the invertebrate marine organisms as a necessary condition for their existence, and that fairly highly developed levels of homeostasis must have existed already at the time of the evolution of the amphibians and the transition of vertebrates from an aqueous to a terrestrial and atmospheric environment. Thermostasis in mammals operates through hypothalamic structures, as do many other of the homeostatic processes, and there is evidence that this is an ancient brain structure that has long been involved in homeostasis. Thus thermostasis could depend on a simple pattern of neuronal activity basic to homeostasis and established long before the evolution of endothermic thermostasis.

Relevant to this argument is the accumulating evidence that pyrogens also cause an elevation in the behaviourally selected (preferred) temperature of reptiles (VAUGHN et al. 1974; REYNOLDS and COVERT 1977), amphibians (KLUGER 1977; MYHRE et al. 1978; REYNOLDS and COVERT 1977), fishes (REYNOLDS et al. 1976; REYNOLDS 1977; REYNOLDS et al. 1978 a, b), and even crustaceans, e.g. the crayfish (CASTERLIN and REYNOLDS 1977a). Thus, however pyrogens act to elevate body temperature, the point of action is manifestly ancient and probably involves relatively simple neurology, since even the preferred temperature of the tadpole is raised in the presence of a pyrogen (CASTERLIN and REYNOLDS 1977b).

III. The Pattern of Neural Connections

In humans at least, and under standardized and steady-state conditions in which non-thermal interferences are minimal, the characteristics of effector functions for thermoregulatory heat production and heat loss, when plotted against core temperature, are near linear (BENZINGER et al. 1963) or linear (CABANAC and MASSONNET 1977) with a central null-point at which both functions are at basal levels (Fig. 7). These relations would seem to imply one of two conditions within the CNS: (i) one in which the linearity of the effector intensity – temperature relation is a consequence of central nervous construction, or (ii) one in which the linearity relates to the pattern of the sensory input, the essential characteristics of which are not lost as the signals pass through the CNS. The first explanation would imply considerable complexity at the central nervous interface, while the second one would imply relative simplicity in the connections between thermosensors and thermoregulatory effectors. I am supposing, as my working hypothesis, that the second condition is the more likely. Indeed, if one accepts that the activity – tem-

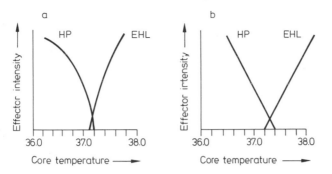

Fig. 7 a, b. The relations between core temperature and the thermoregulatory heat production (*HP*) and evaporative heat loss (*EHL*) activities of humans under stated experimental conditions. **a** the results of BENZINGER et al. (1963); **b** the results of CABANAC and MASSON-NET (1977). The original plots have been re-drawn for easy comparison. The ordinates (*HP* and *EHL*) are not quantitative

perature relations of the warm- and cold-sensors are more-or-less linear over an operational range, and as idealized by VENDRIK (1959), and at least partially supported by electrophysiological studies (NAKAYAMA et al. 1963; HARDY et al. 1964; EISENMAN and JACKSON 1967; EISENMAN 1976), then only quite simple connections between sensors and effectors need exist (Fig. 6). Direct and wholly separate pathways through the CNS from cold-sensors to heat production effectors and from warm-sensors to heat loss effectors could yield relations between thermoregulatory effector activities and core temperature which would be essentially the same as those betwen the activities of the thermosensors and local tissue temperature (Fig. 6a). Such a relation would effect a state of dynamic thermal equilibrium, but uneconomically so, since the thermoregulatory heat loss processes would be continuously acting against the thermoregulatory heat production processes. This, as has been stated above, does not occur, at least in humans (Fig. 7).

The observed pattern of thermoregulatory effector activities with a central null-point could be effected by one of two quite simple neuronal relations. Neurones with continuous temperature-independent activities and exerting an inhibitory influence on the thermosensor–thermoregulatory effector pathways could, as has already been discussed, create synaptic gates which would open at that sensor temperature at which the excitatory activity along the pathways from the sensors just exceeded the inhibitory activity of the temperature-independent neurones (Fig. 6b). Alternatively, simple crossing inhibition between the two thermosensor–thermoregulatory effector pathways would serve equally well to convert the overlap of the cold- and warm-sensor activities, when plotted against temperature, into the non-overlapping curves describing thermoregulatory heat production and heat loss functions in relation to core temperature, with a central null-point (Fig. 6c).

Since the overlapping reciprocal changes in activities of warm- and cold-sensors with changes in body temperature could be the set-point generator, the proposal of reciprocal inhibition of the efferent drives to heat loss and heat production effectors upon each other (Fig. 6c) may seem preferable to the proposal contained in Fig. 6b.

The relations between effector activities and core temperature vary in different physiological and environmental conditions, however, and result in what has been described as upward or downward shifts in the set-point. Whether or not there are spontaneously generated reference signals acting on the thermosensor–thermoregulatory effector pathways, it may be supposed that the variations in thermoregulatory performance in different circumstances are effected largely through converging excitatory and inhibitory influences derived from elsewhere in the CNS and acting on the thermosensor–thermoregulatory effector pathways, and thus moderating thermosensor–thermoregulatory effector relations. There are probably a great number of such influences, but they can be fairly represented by summed excitatory and inhibitory influences acting at an equally representative single synapse on each sensor–effector pathway (Fig. 6 d). This neuronal representation, as has been pointed out by Bligh (1979 a), contains no features that are not recognizable as the bases of organization at the level of the spinal cord.

G. Models for Thermoregulation

I. Point (or Points) of Action of Pyrogens

If Fig. 6 d is a basically real, even though very much simplified, representation of the relations between the input from thermosensors and other neuronal activities on the one hand, and the opposing thermoregulatory effector functions of heat production and heat loss on the other hand, then the possible points of action of pyrogens should be expressible in terms of this representation.

If we suppose that the action of a pyrogen is a single excitatory one, then it must be exerting a direct or indirect excitatory influence somewhere on the pathway from the cold-sensors before the point of origin of the crossing inhibitory influence of heat loss effectors. Such enhancement of the influence of the cold-sensors would cause the synaptic gate on the heat production pathway created by the crossing inhibition to open at a higher than normal body temperature (i.e. at a lower level of true cold-sensor activity), and would also, through the enhancement of the crossing inhibitory influence on the pathway to heat loss effectors, cause the heat loss effectors to be activated at a higher than normal body temperature (i.e. at a higher level of true warm-sensor activity). This point of action, and the theoretical effect of such an action of a pyrogen on the null-point of thermoregulation, is shown in Fig. 8. Obviously this elevated null-point is just another way of expressing an elevation in the set-point of thermoregulation. An *inhibitory* influence of a pyrogen on the pathway from the warm-sensors before the crossing inhibitory influence on heat production effectors might also have the effect of elevating the null-point for thermoregulatory effector functions. Another possibility is that a pyrogen could have two distinct actions and two distinct points of action: an inhibitory one anywhere along the pathway from warm-sensors to heat loss effectors, and an excitatory one anywhere along the pathway from cold-sensors to heat production and conservation effectors.

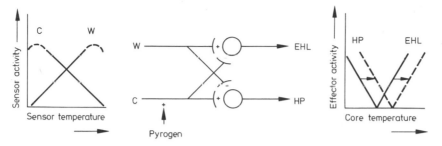

Fig. 8. A theoretical statement of how a pyrogen, by acting on the cold-sensors, or the pathway from them, but before the point of origin of a crossing inhibitory influence on evaporative heat loss, would not only account for the changes in HP and EHL caused by a pyrogen, but would also account for the upward shift in the HP and EHL null-point

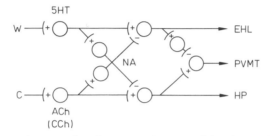

Fig. 9. The diagrammatic expression, in neuronal terms, of the observed thermoregulatory effects of intracerebroventricular injections of 5-hydroxytryptamine (*5-HT*), carbamylcholine (*CCh*) or acetylcholine (*ACh*) and eserine, and noradrenaline (*NA*) in the sheep at high, low, and thermoneutral ambient temperatures. *W*, warm-sensors; *C*, cold-sensors; *EHL*, evaporative heat loss; *PVMT*, peripheral vasomotor tone; *HP*, heat production. (Redrawn from BLIGH et al. 1971)

II. Neuronal Model of Central Thermoregulatory Connections in Sheep

BLIGH et al. (1971) reported that the thermoregulatory effects of 5-hydroxytryptamine (5 HT); acetylcholine (ACh) and eserine, eserine alone or carbamylcholine (CCh); and noradrenaline (NA), when introduced into a lateral cerebral ventricle of the sheep, goat, and rabbit, can be expressed in terms of a simple neuronal model (Fig. 9) which, despite its basic similarity to a model based on the considerations of the central nervous neurology of thermoregulation outlined in Fig. 6c was wholly unrelated to it in conceptual origin. Since then many more studies have been made with the sheep to determine the effects on thermoregulation of other putative transmitter substances, and to attempt to verify or refute the validity of the basic model by means of predictions of the effects of specific synaptic blockades and the comparison of these predictions with the observed effects when such blockades were caused. These studies have been collated and interpreted by BLIGH (1979a), and are summarized in Fig. 10. Some substances have excitatory or inhibitory effects on both heat production and heat loss effectors, while others have opposing actions on the two pathways. Very recent evidence (BLIGH et al. 1979d) indicates the possibility that the crossing inhibitory influence of warm-sensor activity on

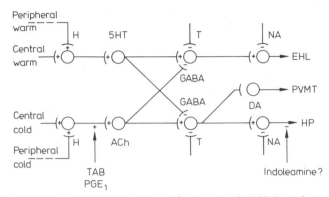

Fig. 10. The extension of the neuronal model of BLIGH et al. (1971) to show the apparent points of action of intracerebroventricular injections into the sheep of histamine (*H*), taurine (*T*), γ-aminobutyric acid (*GABA*), dopamine (*DA*), and prostaglandin E$_1$ (PGE$_1$), as well as of 5-HT, ACh, and NA, and of the intravenous injection of typhoid-paratyphoid A and B vaccine (*TAB*). [Re-drawn from BLIGH (1979b) to show the apparent action of GABA as the tansmitter of crossing inhibition as discussed by BLIGH et al. (1979b)]

heat production and of cold-sensor activity on heat loss may be transmitted through the release of γ-aminobutyric acid (GABA). This finding of a candidate chemical effector of crossing inhibition strengthens the inference of the existence of crossing inhibitory pathways, and allows the possibility that the actions of pyrogenic substances to be expressed in Fig. 10.

III. Point of Action of Bacterial Endotoxin in Sheep

If the final point of action of a BE-induced change in thermoregulation is either on the hypothalamic cold-sensors themselves or on the pathways from the cold-sensors to heat production effectors before the origin of the crossing inhibitory influence on heat loss effectors, many predictions can be made about the effects on a bacterial endotoxin induced fever of the concurrent central (i.c.v.) application of some of the putative transmitter substances (the apparent functions of which are expressed in Fig. 10) or of substances which interfere with the synaptic receptors on which these substances seem to be acting when introduced into the cerebral ventricles.

The first of such predictions to be tested were the interactions of i.v. injections of typhoid–paratyphoid A and B vaccine (TAB-vaccine) and i.c.v. injections of NA and 5HT.

An i.c.v. injection of NA, which has been shown to inhibit both heat production or evaporative heat loss (whichever is being driven at the time) should, if given during the rising phase of fever, inhibit the increased heat production and thus cause a reduction in the rate of rise of body temperature.

An i.c.v. injection of 5HT, which has been shown to activate evaporative heat loss by panting, and inhibit heat production by shivering should, if given during the rising phase of fever, cause the activation of evaporative heat loss by panting, and an attenuation of heat production by shivering. The result of this should be

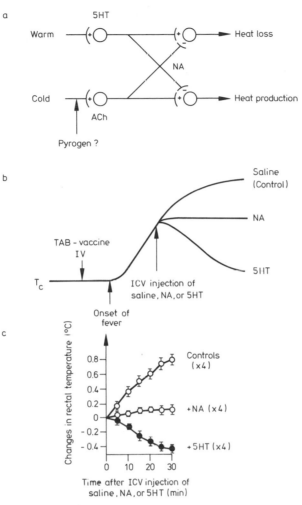

Fig. 11 a–c. A pyrogen-induced fever involves an increase in heat production and a decrease in heat loss, and in terms of the neuronal model of BLIGH et al. (1971) seems to be acting somewhere as indicated in **a**. The predicted effects on the course of an induced fever if 5-HT or NA is injected i.c.v. during the rising phase is shown in **b**. The observed effects of such treatment in sheep during the rising phase of a fever induced by an i.v. injection of TAB vaccine is shown in **c**, where zero time is the point during the rising phase of the fever when NA, 5-HT, or saline (control) was injected i.c.v. (From BLIGH 1975)

not just to attenuate the rise in body temperature, but to cause body temperature to fall.

The predicted effects of NA and 5HT when injected intracerebroventricularly during the rising phase of i.v. TAB-vaccine-induced fever are illustrated in Fig. 11 b. The observed effects on rectal temperature are shown in Fig. 11 c. The accuracy of the prediction is obvious.

An i.c.v. injection or infusion of atropine, which has been shown to attenuate the effects of a peripheral cold stimulus or of an i.c.v. injection of CCh on heat production should, according to Fig. 11 b, also attenuate a BE-induced fever. A prior i.c.v. injection of atropine sulphate did, indeed, greatly reduce the febrile response of the sheep to i.v. TAB-vaccine (BLIGH et al. 1978). The blockade of the serotonergic synapse on the pathways from the warm-sensors with i.c.v. methysergide was found to be without effect on the febrile response to the TAB-vaccine. This accumulating evidence clearly indicates that the action of the pyrogen could, indeed, be on the cold-sensor–heat production and conservation pathway before the cholinergic synapse, before the point of origin of the crossing inhibitory influence on the pathway from warm-sensors to evaporative heat loss effectors, and before the divergence of the pathways to heat production and heat conservation effectors.

When taurine is injected into the cerebral ventricles of the sheep, it exerts an inhibitory influence on heat production, heat conservation, and evaporative heat loss (BLIGH et al. 1979 b). Thus it has an NA-like effect on heat production and evaporative heat loss. However, whereas the effect of i.c.v. injections of NA on heat conservation by peripheral vasomotor constriction is excitatory (TOLLERTON et al. 1978) that of i.c.v. taurine is inhibitory. Thus it was predictable that the effect of i.c.v. taurine on a pyrogen-induced fever would be to attenuate both shivering and peripheral vasoconstriction of the ears, thus reducing the rise, or even reversing the direction of change in rectal temperature. The attenuation of oxygen consumption, and therefore of heat production was, indeed observed when i.v. endotoxin action was compounded with that of i.c.v. taurine, but the anticipated vasodilatation of the ears was not observed. This must be interpreted with caution. At thermoneutrality the tone of the peripheral vasculature of the ears varies spontaneously and quite abruptly between maximum constriction and maximum dilatation. This might indicate that very small changes in the sympathetic drive can cause large changes in the tone of the ear skin blood vessels. If, then, the vasoconstrictive sympathetic drive caused by the action of the pyrogen was not completely blocked by the i.c.v. taurine, a sustained vasoconstriction is readily understandable.

Histamine, when injected i.c.v. into the sheep exerts an excitatory effect on both heat conservation and evaporative heat loss (BLIGH et al. 1980). The direct or indirect influences of histamine on the thermosensor–thermoregulatory effector axes seem to be before the serotonergic synapse on the warm-sensor–evaporative heat loss effector pathway, and before the cholinergic synapse on the cold-sensor–heat production effector pathway, because i.c.v. histamine-induced and ambient-heat-induced panting is attenuated by an i.c.v. injection of the serotonergic receptor blocker, methysergide, while i.c.v. histamine-induced and ambient-cold-induced cutaneous vasoconstriction of the ears is attenuated by an i.c.v. injection of the cholinergic receptor blocker, atropine (BLIGH et al. 1980). Additional evidence in support of this conclusions has come from a further series of experiments in which it has been found that whereas a histamine type I (H_1) receptor blocker, mepyramine, attenuates the effects of ambient heat and cold, and of i.c.v. histamine, on heat production, heat conservation, and evaporative heat loss, it does not interfere with the thermoregulatory effects of i.c.v. injections of 5 HT and CCh (SILVER and BLIGH 1980). Nor, we have found, does pre-treatment with this H_1 receptor blocker attenuate the pyretic response to i.v. TAB-vaccine (BLIGH and SMITH, unpublished).

Because the H_1 receptor blocker attenuates the effects of ambient heat and cold, i.c.v. histamine might be mimicking the role of endogenous histamine as an "on-line" excitatory transmitter on the pathways from both warm- and cold-sensors. In that case, this failure of the H_1 receptor blocker to interfere with the progress of an induced fever might indicate that the action of a pyrogen is not on the cold-sensors, but somewhere on the cold-sensor–heat production pathway efferent to the cold-sensors but afferent to the cholinergic synapse. This interpretation is consistent with the failure of EVANS et al. (1972) to detect any change in the activity–temperature pattern of temperature sensors in the tongue of the rabbit when a bacterial endotoxin was injected i.v. On the other hand, the observed effects of pyrogens on the activity–temperature curves of thermoresponsive neurones in the PO/AH has been interpreted as indicative of an effect of pyrogens on hypothalamic thermosensors in the rabbit (CABANAC and HARDY 1967; EISENMAN 1974) and the cat (WIT and WANG 1968 b).

Our evidence, however, does not justify even a tentative conclusion that the point of action of a pyrogen is on the pathway from cold-sensors and not on the cold-sensors themselves, since the action of i.c.v. and endogenous histamine is not necessarily "on-line" between thermosensors and thermoregulatory effectors and because our experiments only involved changes in ambient temperature but not of hypothalamic temperature. Thus we have no knowledge of whether a histamine receptor blocker would have interfered with an induced drive from hypothalamic thermosensors.

IV. Neuronal Theory of Fever Induction

In the previous section, I have reviewed the studies of the interactions between a fever induced in sheep by an i.v. injection of a BE and specific central nervous synaptic interferences caused by means of i.c.v. injections of putative transmitter substances and other synaptically active substances. All the results are consistent with a point of action of a terminal pyrogen somewhere on the pathway from the cold-sensors efferent to a point of action of i.c.v.-injection histamine; afferent to a point of action of i.c.v.-injected CCh and endogenous ACh, and afferent to the point of origin of a crossing inhibitory influence on heat loss effectors. The predictability of many of the experimental results of these studies, and the virtual absence of effects which are inconsistent with this one point of action are remarkable. However, while the initial observations of the effects on thermoregulation of i.c.v. injections of 5 HT, NA, and CCh, were found by BLIGH et al. (1971) to be essentially the same in sheep, goats, and rabbits, subsequent studies have been confined to one species, the sheep.

One might suppose that in view of the generality of many aspects of mammalian homeothermy, and the febrile response to pyrogens and PGE in the species that have been investigated, there are readily discernible common denominators in mammalian homeothermy and in the genesis of fever. Thus if this neuronal concept is a basically real, although perhaps rudimentary, statement of the processes of thermoregulation and of fever in the sheep, then it should also apply to other species.

The expression of the point of action of a pyrogen in relation to the apparent points of action of particular synaptic functions of putative transmitter substances must face the inevitable objection that the effects of these synaptically active substances, when injected into or near to the PO/AH, vary between species (BLIGH 1963; FELDBERG 1975; HELLON 1975). This might be, and is generally supposed to be, evidence of species differences in the roles of at least some of the putative neurotransmitters in thermoregulation. Even if this is proved to be so, however, it would not, alone, invalidate the basic proposition contained in the neuronal model, since this relates to the neuronal organization at the central interface between the afferent pathways from thermosensors and the efferent pathways to thermoregulatory effectors, and does not relate necessarily to the roles of particular transmitter substances. These, in theory at least, could vary between species without there being any difference in the pattern of the neuronal connections between thermosensors and thermoregulatory effectors. In any case, the essential features of the model have been derived quite independently by others (HAMMEL 1965; WYNDHAM and ATKINS 1968) from the observed relations between thermal disturbances and thermoregulatory responses in man.

There are a number of studies by others of the effects of transmitter-depletor drugs, or of drugs which cause other specific kinds of synaptic interferences, on the course of an induced fever. The majority of these studies has been done on the rabbit which, from the original study of BLIGH et al. (1971) might be expected to be comparable to the sheep, while other studies of this kind have been done on rats which, according to some reports at least, react to intracerebral injections of the monoamines in different ways from sheep and rabbits. The following analysis of these published studies by others has the advantage of countering any bias that inter-specific studies in my own laboratory could entail.

H. Thermoregulatory Agents

I. Central Nervous 5 HT

The earlier studies of the thermoregulatory effects of 5 HT when introduced into the cerebral ventricles of sheep, goats, and rabbits, gave clear evidence of an excitatory influence on the pathway controlling evaporative heat loss, and an inhibitory influence on the pathways controlling heat production and heat conservation. These effects were expressed in the neuronal model of BLIGH et al. (1971) (Fig. 9). From this model one might deduce that the effect on a pyrogen-induced fever of the blockade or inactivation of the serotonergic synapses located on the warm-sensor–evaporative heat loss effectors pathway before a crossing inhibitory influence on the pathways to heat production and conservation, might be to enhance the fever. This is because the pyrogenic action is to cause an increased drive to heat production and an increased inhibition of heat loss with a resultant rise in body temperature which, by increasing the activity of central warm-sensors, would be expected to oppose the influences of the pyrogen. Thus the inactivation of the serotonergic synapse on the pathway from warm-sensors should negate this opposing feedback influence on the progression of the pyrogen-induced hypothermia, which might thus become exaggerated.

Contrary to this expectation, CANAL and ORNESI (1961) observed that pre-treatment of the rabbit with cyproheptadine, which antagonizes the action of 5 HT, interfered with the development of fever induced by a pyrogen. This was interpreted as evidence of a serotonergic mediation of fever. By contrast, however, GIARMAN et al. (1968) and PEINDARIES and JACOB (1971) have reported an increase in a pyrogen-induced fever in the rabbit after pre-treatment with p-chlorophenylalanine (pCPA) to deplete hypothalamic 5 HT. TEDDY (1971) and METCALF and THOMPSON (1975) also noted an increase in the febrile response of the rabbit to intrahypothalamic injection of EP after an earlier intrahypothalamic injection of pCPA. In conflict with these results DES PREZ et al. (1966) found that, whereas depletion of hypothalamic NA of rabbits by means of pre-treatment with α-methyl-p-tyrosine had no effect on the febrile response to a BE, endotoxin, the depletion of both NA and 5 HT by means of reserpine treatment depressed the induced fever. This effect of reserpine was supposed to be the additional effect of 5 HT depletion, but when hypothalamic 5 HT was depleted specifically by means of pCPA there was then no attenuation of the response to the pyrogen (DES PREZ and OATES 1968). Some unidentified third effect of reserpine was therefore suspected. VEALE and COOPER (1974), however, were unable to confirm the depressive effect of pre-treatment of reserpine on induced fevers in rabbits. More recently CARRUBA and BÄCHTOLD (1976) and BORSOOK et al. (1977) both found that in rabbits a reduction in the level of 5 HT in the brain has no appreciable affect the level of the hyperthermia in response to BE or PGE_1. The decrease in a pyrogen-induced fever in the rabbit after i.c.v.-injected 5 HT noted by PEINDARIES and JACOB (1971) is complementary to its effect on endotoxin-induced fever in the sheep (BLIGH 1975). Thus there is quite substantial evidence that in the rabbit, which was found by BLIGH et al. (1971) to respond to i.c.v.-injected 5 HT in the same way as does the sheep, endogenous 5 HT plays no essential role in the induction of fever.

HARVEY and MILTON (1973) found that in cats pre-treatment with pCPA reduced the fever induced by i.c.v.-injected PGE_1. This might indicate a genuine species difference, but this is not the only possible explanation. There is no known reason why there should not be synapses using the same transmitter substance on both of two pathways activating opposing effector processes such as those of heat production and heat loss. It is thus quite possible that with different techniques and different species, a substance potentially able to affect synapses on the pathways to both heat production and heat loss may reach more readily and have a greater effect on the synapse on the one pathway than on the other. It is also possible that a treatment supposed to affect the activity of one particular kind of synapse – say a serotonergic one – also exerts an influence on a synapse at which a related transmitter substance operates – another indoleamine for example. Indeed, some evidence indicates that there could be a serotonergic synapse also on the pathway controlling heat production, as well as on that controlling heat loss, in the sheep: a large i.c.v. dose of norfenfluramine, which causes the release of 5 HT, can cause an increase in heat production at a higher dose level than that which causes an increase in evaporative heat loss (SZÉKELY and BLIGH 1975; SZÉKELY et al. 1976). Further studies (BLIGH et al. 1979 a) now suggest, however, that this observation relates to a tryptaminergic or some other indoleaminergic synapse on the cold-sensor–heat production pathway, since a rise in heat production cannot be induced by large i.c.v. doses of 5 HT.

II. Central Nervous Norepinephrine

COOPER (1965) suggested that the central action of a pyrogen may be the release of NA from nerve terminals in thermoregulatory synapses. Curiously, in the same year, COOPER et al. (1965) found that the depletions of the monoamines (both 5 HT and NA) stored in the hypothalamus of the rabbit by reserpine treatment had no effect on a BE-induced fever, and therefore concluded that the genesis of fever is unrelated to the hypothalamic release of NA, or a failure to release 5 HT.

Later LABURN et al. (1974) and LABURN et al. (1975) again indicated that fever due to the injection of PGE_1 into the anterior hypothalamus of the rabbit is dependent upon an intact noradrenergic system in this region. PRESTON and COOPER (1976) examined this possibility by means of bilateral intrahypothalamic injection of NA into PGE_1-sensitive sites in rabbits and concluded that since the NA did not induce hyperthermia it is unlikely to be a neurotransmitter in the PO/AH mediating either normal or pathological increases in body temperature.

The thermoregulatory effect of interference with a natural role of endogenous NA cannot be predicted from the model of BLIGH et al. (1971), which expressed the view that since i.c.v.-injected NA inhibited either heat production and heat loss (whichever thermoregulatory effector function was active at the time of the injection), and since there was deductive evidence of crossing inhibition, NA could be the terminal inhibitory transmitter of the crossing inhibitory pathways in sheep, goats, and rabbits. There was, however, no direct evidence of this role of NA and the i.c.v.-injected NA could have equally well been mimicking an effect of endogenous NA released from nerve terminals derived from outside the thermosensor–thermoregulatory effector axes. This, indeed, now seems to be the more likely interpretation because: (i) DAHLSTROM and FUXE (1965) could not demonstrate NA-containing cell bodies in the PO/AH area of the brain; (ii) BAUMANN et al. (1977) could detect no loss of crossing inhibition in the presence of α- and β-adrenaline receptor blockers in the sheep; (iii) BLIGH et al. (1977) found no appreciable change in the thermoregulation of sheep after substantial lowering of the NA content of the PO/AH by treatment with i.c.v. injections of 6-hydroxy-dopamine; and (iv) STITT (1976) has provided some functional evidence in support of the proposition that noradrenergic fibres which terminate in the PO/AH may ascend from the reticular-activating system in the rabbit.

If, then, we suppose that endogenous NA exerts an inhibitory influence on the thermoregulatory effector functions arising from elsewhere in the CNS, and that i.c.v.-injected NA mimics these effects, then the removal of this inhibitory influence on the thermensor–thermoregulatory effector axes might increase the thermoregulatory responses to a thermal stimulus. Whether this would actually occur, however, would depend on the extent of the activation of these inhibitory influences under the experimental conditions. It might thus be predicted that the inactivation of a natural noradrenaline-effected inhibitory influence on thermoregulatory effector functions might accentuate a thermal stimulus or the action of a pyrogen, but would not be likely to attenuate the effects of heat or pyrogen.

The substance α-methyl-p-tyrosine can be used to cause the specific depletion of the NA content of central nervous tissues. DES PREZ et al. (1966) used this to lower the NA content of the hypothalamus of the rabbit, and found that this treatment had no effect on the febrile response to BE. Since then METCALF and THOMP-SON (1975) have found that α-methyl-p-tyrosine does cause some reduction in the hyperthermia induced by either BE or EP in the rabbit. The ambient temperatures were 20°–24 °C which is above the thermoneutral temperature of the rabbit. Thus the effect of NA depletion might have been to reduce the inhibitory influence on evaporative heat loss by panting. Without evidence of changes in evaporative heat loss, the significance of this observation by METCALF and THOMPSON (1975) is indeterminate, particularly since it remains unconfirmed.

III. The Central Thermoregulatory Effects of ACh

The effect of i.c.v. injections into sheep and rabbits of eserine alone, eserine plus ACh, or of CCh, was to increase heat production and/or decrease evaporative heat loss. Thus these actions were as if there is a cholinomimetic synapse on the pathway from cold-sensors to heat production effectors before the point of origin of a crossing inhibitory influence on evaporative heat loss (BLIGH et al. 1971 and Fig. 9). In further studies of the sheep alone atropine was found to block the drive of peripheral cold on heat production (MASKREY 1972; BLIGH et al. 1978) and to attenuate the fever induced by an i.v. injection of a bacterial endotoxin.

COOPER and VEALE (1974) have also found that in rabbits the febrile response to EP or PGE is delayed, or reduced by atropine sulphate injected into the cerebral ventricles. The injection of atropine sulphate directly into the PO/AH , however, did not modify the fever caused by an intrahypothalamic injection of PGE_1. Thus the cholinergic synapse which evidently exists on the heat production pathway somewhere efferent to the point of action in the PO/AH of PGE_1, may be outside the PO/AH. Since the revised model of BLIGH et al. (1971) presented here (Fig. 10) is based on i.c.v. injections, it lacks anatomical discrimination, and does not, therefore, in any way run counter to the proposition of COOPER and VEALE (1974).

TANGRI et al. (1975) also reported that with rabbits, the inhibition of acetylcholine synthesis by treatment with hemicholinium blocked BE-induced fever. Pretreatment with blockers of nicotinic receptors (chlorisondamine and +-tubocurarine) reduced the febrile response to the BE, but pre-treatment with atropine did not. This evidence indicates that the cholinergic synapse efferent to the point of action of the pyrogen on the pathway to heat production is nicotinic. COOPER et al. (1976) failed to confirm this finding; the i.c.v. injection of atropine into rabbits was found by them to interfere with the progress of fevers caused by i.v. injections of EP and by i.c.v. and intrahypothalamic injections of PGE_1. The atropine caused the ear skin vessels to dilate, while respiratory frequency increased and shivering ceased; there was, in consequence, an attenuation of the pyrogen-induced rise in body temperature, as well as of the thermoregulatory responses to cold.

Thus there is evidence of a cholinergic synpase between the point of action of EP and of PGE_1 and the thermoregulatory effector pathways by which heat production is augmented, and heat loss minimized in both the sheep and rabbit, but there is conflicting evidence on whether this synapse is muscarinic or nicotinic. Care may be needed however in the designation of central receptors as being of one type or another. A similar lack of clear distinction has been found concerning the classification of histamine receptors involved in thermoregulation in the sheep

(SILVER and BLIGH 1980): an H_1 receptor blocker blocks the effects of i.c.v. histamine and the drives from cold- and warm-sensors, while an H_2 receptor blocker mimics the effects of histamine. We have recently observed that H_1 receptor blocker mempyramine in higher doses, will also simulate the action of histamine.

The only real conflict of evidence of which I am aware, is that of RUDY and VISWANATHAN (1975): intracerebroventricular injections into the rat either of atropine (muscarinic receptor blocker) or mecamyline (nicotinic receptor blocker) were found not to attenuate the hyperthermia induced by PGE_1 when injected into PO/AH. The conclusion was that there is no cholinergic synapse between the point of action of PGE, and the heat production affector pathways in the rat.

J. Other Set-Point Theories

Clearly, from the analysis of studies in other laboratories on other species, mostly with the rabbit, there are areas of uncertainty that have yet to be explored. There is no fundamental conflict of evidence which discounts the hypothesis for the neurological principle of thermoregulation and the action of a pyrogen as expressed in Fig. 10. However, those who try to follow the now confusing literature on the nature of the thermoregulatory set-point and of its change during fever, will be exasperated by yet another concept of the set-point and of its re-setting by a pyrogen. Before concluding this review, I must, therefore, try to establish some kind of bridge between these contending theories, so that students of homeothermy may formulate some judgement on the relative merits of these different concepts, based upon something more substantial than the indoctrinations of one school or another.

I. The Monoamine Balance Set-Point Theory

Prior to the suggestion by FELDBERG and MYERS (1964) that the set-point depends on the relative concentrations or activities of monoamines, thoughts on the nature of the set-point operation were based wholly on engineering concepts, which, while interesting, allowed little opportunity for progress towards understanding the set-point in neuronal terms. Thus the significance of the observation of FELDBERG and MYERS (1964) of the thermoregulatory effects of i.c.v. injections of adrenaline, NA, and 5HT in the cat, and the interpretation placed on those observations cannot be exaggerated: the set-point was thereby brought into the arena of unit neurology. The thesis, however, though magnificent in its simplicity, has not withstood subsequent analysis. If NA and 5HT are endogenous synaptic transmitter substances, presumably they are secondary rather than primary agents, released in response to prior neuronal events. Thus the effects observed by FELDBERG and MYERS in cats in response to i.c.v. or intrahypothalamic injections of monoamines, could relate to "on-line" synaptic activation of thermosensor–thermoregulatory effector pathways *or* to the simulation of converging influences on the thermosensor–thermoregulatory effector pathways from elsewhere in the CNS, and concerned with some modulatory influence upon thermoregulation. As has been pointed out by BLIGH (1979a) in either case the effects on thermoregulation resulting from injections of monoamines into the vicinity of the PO/AH could be very similar. Indeed, in the revised neuronal model of BLIGH (1979a) 5HT is now considered to have an "on-line" role in thermoregulation and NA to have an "off-line" role. Thus the thesis of FELDBERG and MYERS (1964) might now be considered to be a very important stepping stone which has now been left behind as the trail proceeds.

II. The Ionic Balance Set-Point Theory

On the basis of the effects on body temperature of the perfusion of the cerebral ventricules of cats with various physiological salt solutions, FELDBERG et al. (1970) produced a second set-point theory based on the balance of the concentrations of sodium and calcium ions in the anterior hypothalamus. Calcium, they proposed, acts as a "brake" which prevents sodium from exerting its temperature-raising effect. Pyrogen, they supposed, acts by removing the calcium brake. Fever is, therefore, a sodium-induced hyperthermia. It has since been proposed by MYERS and VEALE (1970) that the set-point of body temperature is in the posterior hypothalamus and not in the preoptic/anterior hypothalamic part of the brain, as is often supposed. They proposed further that the basis of the set-point mechanism is the local concentrations of extracellular sodium and calcium ions in the posterior hypothalamus (MYERS and VEALE 1971). Since fever is regarded as a condition in which there is an upward shift in the functional characteristics of the set-point generator, evidence was then sought for the involvement of posterior hypothalamic extracellular ionic shifts in the occurrence of fever. Changes in the flux of injected radio-labelled calcium in the posterior hypothalamus during fever have been demonstrated by MYERS (1971) and MYERS and TYTELL (1972) and interpreted as evidence of a process by which changes in ionic concentrations in the posterior hypothalamus are fundamental to the genesis of fever. The evidence and its interpretation have been discussed in detail by MYERS et al. (1976).

This thesis complies with the fairly orthodox view that the set-point phenomenon results from the operation of a particular and special function not of the thermosensors, but of some component of the neuronal complex lying between the thermosensors and the efferent pathways to the thermoregulatory effectors. Since the balance of sodium and calcium ions influence membrane stability, a non-specific change in synaptic and other neuronal activities when the extracellular ionic concentrations are changed would not be at all surprising. In support of the argument that something more specific is occurring is the specificity of the effects of changes in posterior hypothalamic concentrations of particular ions on body temperature: rise in the extracellular concentration of calcium ions causes a reduction in heat production and a fall in core temperature, while a reduction in the calcium ion concentration, or an increase in the sodium ion concentration, causes an increase in heat production and a rise in body temperature. This would certainly appear to be sound evidence of a specific effect on a particular pathway, but other interpretations of this evidence are possible, and the involvement of the ionic balance in the set-point mechanism as distinct from synaptic gating on the pathway to heat production effectors, is not an inevitable one.

Much earlier evidence of the central neurology of thermoregulation led to the hypothesis that there are two "centres" – one in the anterior hypothalamus concerned in heat loss, and one in the posterior hypothalamus concerned in heat production. That concept is now largely discarded. Currently the evidence indicates that both warm-sensitive and cold-sensitive structures occur specifically in the preopticus/anterior hypothalamus, but the warm-sensitive structures appear to be the more numerous and therefore functionally dominant. The posterior hypothalamus seems to contain a "relay station," which must involve a synapse, on the pathway to heat production effectors. Let us suppose that this is so. If we further suppose that an increase in $[Ca^{2+}]$ in the vicinity of the synapses on that pathway, decreases the efferent activity relative to the afferent activity from cold-sensors by changing the gating properties of the synapse, while a reduction in $[Ca^{2+}]$ or an increase in $[Na^+]$ increases the efferent activity relative to the afferent activity at the synapse on the pathway to heat production effectors, then the one condition would result in a decrease in heat production and a fall in body temperature, while the other condition would result in an increase in heat production and a rise in body temperature.

We can now consider the action of a pyrogen. Whether this acts on cold-sensors in the hypothalamic region, or somewhere on the pathway from the sensors to the heat production effectors, but before the synapse in the posterior hypothalamus, it might be expected that the effect of pyrogen-induced activity in this pathway would increase the frequency of the membrane depolarization at the posterior hypothalamic synapse, and that this change in synaptic activity might influence the flux of calcium ions across the synaptic membranes. Thus the observations of MYERS and his colleagues of increased Ca^{2+} efflux in the posterior hypothalamus in response to PGE, or a pyrogen, could relate to the increased passage of impulses along the cold-sensor–heat production effector pathway through the posterior hypothalamus, while the specific effect of locally injected Ca^{2+} and Na^+ on body temperature could be due the existence of a synapse in the posterior hypothalamic area on the pathway to heat production effectors alone. Clearly I, too, am speculating, but only in order to caution, with CRANSTON (1979), against the assumption that ionic balances *are* the set-point, when they may only be modulators of synaptic events, with pyrogens exerting their influence on body temperature by inducing changes in ionic balances.

K. Concluding Comments

In fever, body temperature is raised by an orderly increase in heat production and decrease in heat loss until it reaches a new elevated level at which it is then regulated very much as it is at its normal level. It is thus precisely "as if" the set-point has been elevated.

If a pyrogen acts at one particular point at the central nervous interface between thermosensors and thermoregulatory effectors, there is some evidence that that point is, in the sheep and rabbit at least, somewhere on the pathway from cold-sensors to heat production and conservation effectors before a cholinergic synapse, and before the point of origin on that pathway, of an inhibitory influence on evaporative heat loss effectors.

BLIGH (1978, 1979a, 1980) has proposed: (i) that the basic neuronal "wiring" through the CNS may consist of two main sensor–effector pathways, one from warm-sensors to heat loss effectors, and the other from cold-sensors to heat pro-duction effectors, with crossing inhibitory influences between them; and (ii) that the set-point may not be the product of the comparison of thermosensor signals with that from a neuronal reference-signal generator, but resides in the different activity temperature characteristics of the warm- and cold-sensors.

The observed effect of pyrogens on the de facto set-point (that is, the level at which body temperature is held stable) is generally consistent with these propo-sitions. An augmentation of the activity in the pathway from cold-sensors, and an inhibition of that from warm-sensors could be expected to raise the body temper-ature at which the rates of heat production and heat loss are equal. Since it is sup-posed that the pathways from sensors to effectors have remained otherwise intact, any further change in body temperature due to a change in heat production or heat loss would be expected to elicit compensatory activity of thermoregulatory effec-tors. In this circumstance body temperature would be defended at an elevated level for so long as the pyrogen was exerting its influence.

There are, however, three aspects of fever for which this model offers no obvi-ous explanation: one is the reported independence of the level of fever from ambi-ent temperature (COOPER and VEALE 1974; VEALE and WHISHAW 1976); another is the upper limit of fever; and the third is that, whether fever is attenuated by a cen-tral cholinergic blockade, by an antipyretic drug which blocks the metabolism of arachidonic acid, or by a condition which prevents the formation of leucocyte pyrogen, the fever is never totally eliminated.

I. The Independence of Fever from the Influence of Ambient Temperature

On this inconsistency, nothing much can be said until more is known of the rela-tions between the thermal information contributed by peripheral and more deeply located thermal sensors. Some evidence, both from synaptic interference studies in my own laboratory (MASKREY and BLIGH 1971; BACON and BLIGH 1976) and from hypothalamic unit activity studies (WIT and WANG 1968a; HELLON 1969, 1970) suggests the convergence of the pathways from peripheral and central thermosen-sors (see BLIGH 1979a). From such an arrangement it would seem that the change in synaptic gating resulting from a change in the activity in the pathways from pe-ripheral temperature sensors should effect the body temperature during fever. However, since quite large changes in ambient temperature do not greatly influence normal thermoregulation either, there is no obvious reason why changes in en-vironmental temperature should greatly effect the level of body temperature during steady-state fever. This relative ineffectiveness of ambient temperature upon either the euthermic or the febrile levels of body temperature may relate to the relative densities of peripheral and deep-body thermosensors.

II. The Upper Limit to the Febrile Response

The apparent upper limit to the re-setting of the physiological "thermostat" during fever featured in the earliest records of temporal patterns of fever during infectious conditions in humans (WUNDERLICH 1871), and was later confirmed by DUBOIS (1949) who asked the highly pertinent question "Why are fevers over 106 °F

(41 °C) rare?" Oddly enough this is not an issue which has attracted much subsequent attention although BLIGH (1966) reviewed the literature and showed that
in addition to the fine control of body temperature, to which the set-point concept
generally relates, there would seem to be a coarse or wide-band control which may
become operational under abnormal circumstances when body temperature rises
well above (41 °C) or falls below (35°–38 °C) the normal range of variation. Some
further evidence for such a phenomenon has been given by LIPTON (1973), who has
also given reasons to suggest that this process may not be dependent on the integrity of the preopticus/anterior hypothalamicus. Earlier studies of KELLER and
McCLASKEY (1964) had also indicated an extrahypothalamic basis for the wide-
band control.

Even if it is proved conclusively that an elevated body temperature is beneficial
in the defence against bacterial invasion, hyperthermia is a potentially dangerous
biological ploy. In the first place, normal body temperature (about 37 °C) is fairly
close to the maximum temperature (about 42 °C) that can be endured for hours
or days without causing permanent injury (see BLIGH 1979 b for discussion). In the
second place, hyperthermia tends to be self-reinforcing because of the van't Hoff/
Arrhenius (or Q_{10}) relation between temperature and metabolic rate. Whatever the
process by which the rise in body temperature during fever is generally limited, it
can be assumed that this process is of great importance to the survival of the individual, and therefore, of a species. This is abundantly evident from the rapidly
fatal consequences of a breakdown of this mechanism when the rise in body temperature is uncontrolled.

The upper limit to fever is conceptually understandable in terms of the gating
functions of synapses between neurones. If a pyrogen acts by adding excitation at
a synapse on the pathways activating heat production and heat conservation, and
adding inhibition at a synapse on the pathways controlling evaporative heat loss,
it may be supposed that the strengths of these additional excitatory and inhibitory
influences are not infinitely large, and that they can be balanced out by countering
synaptic influences. Thus as body temperature rises, the drive from the warm-sensors progressively increases. At some temperature it will exceed the maximum inhibitory influence of a pyrogen on the evaporative heat loss pathway so that sweating occurs and a further rise in core temperature is prevented. Perhaps DuBOIS's
106 °F represents this temperature. What, then, goes wrong in a runaway fever?
There may not be a single cause, but one may be a failure of the secretory processes
of the sweat glands, so that the activating command is ignored.

Viewed in this way, the upper limit of fever could be wholly consistent with the
model presented here, although it must be noted that extrahypothalamic neuronal
functions may be involved.

III. More than One Pathway from Infection to Fever?

After VANE (1971) had shown that aspirin-like antipyretic substances prevent the
formation of prostaglandins from arachidonic acid; MILTON and WENDLANDT
(1970) had shown that the central injection of a prostaglandin E will cause a fever-
like hyperthermia, and FELDBERG et al. (1973) had shown that a pyrogen-induced
hyperthermia is accompanied by a rise in the prostaglandin content of the CSF,

there seemed little doubt that one of the prostaglandins is the terminal activator of fever. The prostaglandin is apparently liberated in response to the presence of leucocyte pyrogen, which in turn is formed and liberated under the influence of endotoxin produced by the invading micro-organism. It has been shown, in the course of this discussion, that many pieces of evidence now indicate that this is considerably less than the whole story. Neither antipyretic medication, nor the blockade of the cholinergic synapse (which, in the sheep at least, seems to be efferent to the point of action of the terminal pyrogen), nor protein deficiency (which seems to impede the formation of leucocyte pyrogen), seems able to prevent a bacterial, or BE-induced fever totally. This could be attributed, in each case, to an incompleteness of the blockade. However, this explanation appears to be unsatisfactory when attention is paid to the temporal pattern of the fever induced by a single application of a BE. In many mammals, the febrile response is usually biphasic. In protein deficiency, there seems to be the preferential loss of the first peak of the biphasic feature, but less impairment or unimpairment of the second phase. If the belief that protein deficiency impedes the production of EP is correct, then it would seem very possible that a BE can cause the second phase of the febrile response by a process other than that of successive formation and liberation of EP and the metabolites of arachidonic acid. This will remain a speculation until careful studies have been made of the whole time course of a fever in response to a single injection of a BE, with the effects of the blockade of EP and synthesis, and of the cholinergic synapse blockage with atropine, superimposed upon the unimpeded response to the BE.

Clearly we do not know which substance or substances do cause fever; there may be more than one terminal action on central neurones, and at more than one location in the CNS. Since we do not know precisely how normal body temperature is regulated by the brain, we cannot yet know how that regulation is changed by pyrogens. However, to my mind the many pieces of information on fever are not as unpatterned and conflicting as might first seem. A pattern can be discerned, although it is somewhat more complex than has been supposed. The pattern which I have discerned here is probably more fantasy than fact, but the virtue of a model may reside not in its proximity to reality but in the way it generates testable hypotheses which lead one away from error and towards a better understanding.

References

Andersson B, Gale CG, Hokfelt B, Larsson BA (1965) Acute and chronic effects of preoptic lesion. Acta Physiol, Scand 65:45 60

Atkins E (1960) Pathogenesis of fever. Physiol Rev 40:580–646

Atkins E, Bodel P (1974) Fever. In: Grant L, McCluskey RT, Zweifach BW (eds) The inflammatory process, vol 3. Academic Press, New York

Atkins E, Wood WB (1955) Studies on the pathogenesis of fever 1. The presence of transferable pyrogen in the blood stream following the injection of typhoid vaccine. J Exp Med 101:519–528

Atwood RP, Kass EH (1964) Relationship of body temperature to the lethal action of bacterial endotoxin. J Clin Invest 43:151–159

Bacon M, Bligh J (1976) Interactions between the effects of spinal heating and cooling and of injections into a lateral cerebral ventricle of noradrenaline, 5-hydroxytryptamine and carbachol on thermoregulation in sheep. J Physiol (Lond) 254:213–227

Baumann IR, Bligh J, Smith CA (1977) Central regulation of temperature in the sheep: the problem of the inhibitory transmitter. In: Cooper KE, Lomax P, Schönbaum E (eds) Drugs, biogenic amines, and body temperature. Karger, Basel, pp 34–36

Beckman AL, Rozkowska-Ruttiman E (1974) Hypothalamic and septal neuronal responses to iontophoretic application of salicylate in rats. Neuropharmacology 13:393–398

Beeson PB (1948) Temperature-elevating effect of a substance obtained from polymorphonuclear leucocytes. J Clin Invest 27:524

Bennett IL, Beeson PB (1953a) Studies on the pathogenesis of fever. I. The effect of injections of extracts and suspensions of uninfected rabbit tissues upon the body temperature of normal rabbits. J Exp Med 98:477–492

Bennett IL, Beeson PB (1953b) Studies on the pathogenesis of fever. II. Characterization of fever-producing substances from polymorphonuclear leukocytes and from the fluid of sterile exudates. J Exp Med 98:493–508

Bennett IL, Petersdorf RG, Keene WR (1957) Pathogenesis of fever: evidence for direct cerebral action of bacterial endotoxins. Trans Assoc Am Physicians 70:64–73

Benzinger TH, Kitzinger C, Pratt AW (1963) The human thermostat. In: Hardy JD (ed) Temperature – its measurement and control in science and industry, vol 3, part 3. Biology and medicine. Reinhold, New York, pp 637–665

Bernheim MA, Kluger MJ (1976) Fever: effect of drug-induced antipyresis on survival. Science 193:237–239

Bernheim MA, Bodel PT, Askenase PW, Atkins E (1978) Effects of fever on host defense mechanisms after infection in the lizard Disposaurus dorsalis. Br J Exp Pathol 59:76–84

Blatteis CM, Smith KA (1979) Hypothalamic sensitivity to leukocytic pyrogen of adult and new-born guinea-pigs. J Physiol (Lond) 296:177–192

Bligh J (1966) The thermosensitivity of the hypothalamus and thermoregulation in mammals. Biol Rev 41:317–367

Bligh J (1973) Temperature regulation in mammals and other vertebrates. Elsevier, North-Holland Amsterdam Oxford New York

Bligh J (1975) Neurotransmitters in temperature regulation. In: Bhatia B, Chhina GS, Singh B (eds) Selected topics in environmental biology. Interprint, New Delhi, pp 3–10

Bligh J (1978) Thermal regulation: what is regulated and how? In: Houdas H, Guieu D (eds) New trends in thermal physiology. Masson, Paris, pp 1–10

Bligh J (1979a) The central neurology of mammalian thermoregulation. Neuroscience 4:1213–1236

Bligh J (1979b) Aspects of thermoregulatory physiology pertinent to hyperthermic treatment of cancer. Cancer Res 39:2307–2312

Bligh J (1980) Have some mammals remained primitive thermoregulators, – or is all thermoregulation based on equally primitive brain functions? In: Schmidt-Nielsen K, Bolis L, Taylor CR (eds) Primitive mammals. Cambridge University Press, Cambridge

Bligh J, Cottle WH, Maskrey MA (1971) Influence of ambient temperature on the thermoregulatory responses to 5-hydroxytryptamine, noradrenaline and acetylcholine injected into the lateral cerebral ventricles of sheep, goats, and rabbits. J Physiol (Lond) 212:377–392

Bligh J, Davis AJ, Sharman DF, Smith CA (1977) Unimpaired thermoregulation in the sheep after depletion of hypothalamic noradrenaline by 6-hydroxydopamine. J Physiol (Lond) 265:51–52P

Bligh J, Silver A, Bacon MJ, Smith CA (1978) The central role of a cholinergic synapse in thermoregulation in the sheep. J Therm Biol 3:147–151

Bligh J, Silver A, Smith CA (1979a) A central serotonergic-like synapse on the pathway to heat production in the sheep. J Therm Biol 4:259–269

Bligh J, Silver A, Smith CA, Bacon MJ (1979b) The effects on thermoregulation in the sheep of intracerebroventricular injections of taurine, glycine, GABA, and muscimol. J Therm Biol 4:9–14

Bligh J, Smith CA, Baumann IR (1979c) Central GABA and thermoregulation in sheep. In: Cox B, Lomax P, Milton AS, Schönbaum E (eds) Thermoregulatory mechanisms and their therapeutic emplications. Karger, Basel, pp 9–11

Bligh J, Silver A, Smith CA (1980) The effects on thermoregulatory mechanisms produced by intracerebroventricular injections of histamine in the sheep. J Therm Biol 4:41–51

Borsook D, Laburn HP, Rosendorff C, Willies GH, Woolf CJ (1977) A dissociation between temperature regulation and fever in the rabbit. J Physiol (Lond) 266:423–433

Cabanac M, Hardy JD (1967) Effect of temperature and pyrogen on unit activity in the rabbit's brain stem. Fed Proc 26:555

Cabanac M, Massonnet B (1977) Thermoregulatory responses as a function of core temperature in humans. J Physiol (Lond) 265:587–596

Canal N, Ornesi A (1961) La serotiniana quale agente ipertermizzante. Atti Accad Med Lomb 16:64–69

Carruba MO, Bächtold HP (1976) Pyrogen fever in rabbits pretreated with p-chlorophenylalanine or 5,6-dihydroxytryptamine. Experientia 32:729–730

Casterlin ME, Reynolds WW (1977a) Behavioral fever in crayfish. Hydrobiologia 56:99–101

Casterlin ME, Reynolds WW (1977b) Behavioral fever in anuran amphibian larvae. Life Sci 20:593–596

Clark G, Magoun HW, Ranson SW (1939) Hypothalamic regulation of body temperature. J Neurophysiol 2:61–80

Connor DG, Kass EH (1961) Effect of artificial fever in increasing susceptibility to bacterial endotoxin. Nature 190:453–454

Cooper KE (1965) The role of the hypothalamus in the genesis of fever. Proc Soc Med 58:740

Cooper KE, Veale WL (1974) Fever, an abnormal drive to the heat conserving and producing mechanisms. In: Lederis K, Cooper KE (eds) Recent studies of hypothalamic function. Karger, Basel, pp 315–322

Cooper KE, Cranston WI, Snell ES (1964) Temperature regulation during fever in man. Clin Sci 27:345–356

Cooper KE, Cranston WI, Honour AJ (1965) Effects of intraventricular and intrahypothalamic injection of noradrenaline and 5-HT on body temperature in conscious rabbits. J Physiol (Lond) 181:852–864

Cooper KE, Cranston WI, Honour AJ (1967) Observations on the site and mode of action of pyrogens in the rabbit brain. J Physiol (Lond) 191:325–337

Cooper KE, Preston E, Veale WL (1976) Effects of atropine, injected into a lateral cerebral ventricle of the rabbit, on fevers due to intravenous leucocyte pyrogen and hypothalamic and intraventricular injections of prostaglandin E_1. J Physiol (Lond) 254:729–741

Cooperstock MS (1974) Inactivation of endotoxin by polymyxin B. Antimicrob Agents Chemother 6:422–425

Covert JB, Reynolds WW (1977) Survival value of fever in fish. Nature 267:43–45

Cranston WI (1979) Central mechanism of fever. Fed Proc 38:49–51

Cranston WI, Hellon RH, Luff RH, Rawlins MD, Rosendorff C (1970) Observations on the mechanism of salicylate-induced antipyresis. J Physiol (Lond) 210:593–600

Cranston WI, Luff RH, Rawlins MD, Wright VΛ (1971) Influence of the duration of experimental fever on salicylate antipyresis in the rabbit. Br J Pharmacol 41:344–351

Cranston WI, Hellon RF, Mitchell D (1975) A dissociation between fever and prostaglandin concentration in cerebrospinal fluid. J Physiol (Lond) 253:583–592

Cranston WI, Duff GW, Hellon RF, Mitchell D, Townsend Y (1976) Evidence that brain prostaglandin synthesis is not essential in fever. J Physiol (Lond) 259:239–249

Cranston WI, Dawson NJ, Hellon RF, Townsend Y (1978) Contrasting actions of cycloheximide on fever caused by arachidonic acid and by pyrogen. J Physiol (Lond) 285:35P

Crawshaw LI, Stitt JT (1975) Behavioural and autonomic induction of prostaglandin E_1 fever in squirrel monkeys. J Physiol (Lond) 244:197–206

Cremades-Campos A, Milton AS (1978) The effect on deep body temperature of the intraventricular injection of two prostaglandin endoperoxide derivatives. J Physiol (Lond) 282:38P

Dahlstrom A, Fuxe K (1965) Evidence for the existence of monoamine containing neurons in the central nervous system. Acta Physiol Scand [Suppl 232] 62:1–55

Des Prez RM, Oates JA (1968) Lack of relationship of febrile response to endotoxin and brain stem 5-hydroxytryptamine. Proc Soc Exp Biol Med 127:793–794

Des Prez R, Helman R, Oates JA (1966) Inhibition of endotoxin fever by reserpine. Proc Soc Exp Biol Med 122:746–749

Dey PK, Feldberg W, Gupta KP, Milton AS, Wendlandt S (1974) Further studies on the role of prostaglandin in fever. J Physiol (Lond) 241:629–646

Dubois EF (1949) Why are fever temperatures over 106 °F rare? Am J Med Sci 217:361–368

Eisenman JS (1974) Depression of preoptic thermosensitivity by bacterial pyrogen in rabbits. Am J Physiol 227:1067–1073

Eisenman JS (1976) Sensory organs and thermogenesis. Isr J Med Sci 12:916–923

Eisenman JS, Jackson DS (1967) Thermal response patterns of septal and preoptic neurons. Exp Neurol 19:33–45

Evans MH, Frens J, Bligh J (1972) Unaltered activity of tongue temperature sensors after administration of pyrogen to rabbit. Eur J Pharmacol 18:333–337

Feldberg W (1975) Body temperature and fever: changes in our views during the last decade. Proc R Soc Lond [Biol] 191:199–229

Feldberg W, Gupta KP (1973) Pyrogen fever and prostaglandin-like activity in cerebrospinal fluid. J Physiol (Lond) 228:41–53

Feldberg W, Milton AS (1973) Prostaglandins in fever. In: Schönbaum E, Lomax P (eds) The pharmacology of temperature regulation. Karger, Basel, pp 302–310

Feldberg W, Myers RD (1964) Effects on temperature of amines injected into the cerebral ventricles. A new concept of temperature regulation. J Physiol (Lond) 173:226–237

Feldberg W, Myers RD, Veale WL (1970) Perfusion from cerebral ventricle to cisterna magna in the unaesthetized cat. Effect of calcium on body temperature. J Physiol (Lond) 207:403–416

Feldberg W, Gupta KP, Milton AS, Wendlandt S (1973) Effect of pyrogen and antipyretics on prostaglandin activity in cisternal c.s.f. of unanaesthetized cats. J Physiol (Lond) 234:279–303

Ferreira SH, Vane JR (1974) Aspirin and prostaglandins. In: Ramwell PW (ed) The prostaglandins, vol 2. Plenum Press, New York, p 38

Frazier CH, Alpers BJ, Lewy EM (1936) The anatomical localization of the hypothalamic centre for the regulation of temperature. Brain 59:122–129

Frens J (1971) Central synaptic interference and experimental fever. Int J Biometeorol 15:313–315

Frens J (1974) Thermoregulation set-point changes during lipopolysaccharide fever. In: Lomax P, Schönbaum E, Jacob J (eds) Temperature regulation and drug action. Karger, Basel, pp 59–64

Garibaldi JA (1972) Influence of temperature on the biosynthesis of iron transport compounds by *Salmonella typhimurium*. J Bacteriol 110:262–265

Giarman NJ, Tanaka C, Mooney J, Atkins E (1968) Serotonin, norepinephrine and fever. Adv Pharmacol Chemother 6 A

Grieger TA, Kluger MJ (1978) Fever and survival: the role of serum iron. J Physiol (Lond) 279:187–196

Guerra (Perez-Carral) F, Barbour HG (1943) The mechanism of aspirin pyresis in monkeys. J Pharmacol Exp Ther 79:55–61

Haan J (1965) Über die zentrale Beeinflußbarkeit des Pyrogen-Fiebers am Kaninchen. Naunyn-Schmiedeberg Arch Exp Pathol Pharmakol 251:138

Hammel HT (1965) Neurones and temperature regulation. In: Yamamoto WS, Brobeck C (eds) Physiological controls and regulations. Saunders, Philadelphia, pp 71–97

Hardy JD, Hellon RF, Sutherland K (1964) Temperature-sensitive neurones in the dog's hypothalamus. J Physiol (Lond) 175:242–253

Harvey CA, Milton AS (1973) The effect of parachlorophenylalanine on the response of the conscious cat to intravenous and intraventricular bacterial pyrogen and to intraventricular prostaglandin E_1. J Physiol (Lond) 234:12–13 P

Hawkins M, Lipton JM (1977) Analogs of endoperoxide precursors of prostaglandins: failure to affect body temperature when injected into primary and secondary central temperature controls. Prostaglandins 13:309–318

Hellon RF (1969) Environmental temperature and firing rate of hypothalamic neurones. Experientia 25:610

Hellon RF (1970) The stimulation of hypothalamic neurones by changes in ambient temperature. Pfluegers Arch 321:56–66

Hellon RF (1975) Monoamines, pyrogens, and cations: their actions of central control of body temperature. Pharmacol Rev 26:289–321

Hoffman-Goetz L, Kluger MJ (1979) Protein deprivation: its effects on fever and plasma iron during bacterial infection in rabbits. J Physiol (Lond) 295:419–430

Hort EC, Penfold WJ (1912a) The relation of salvarsan fever to other forms of injection fever. Proc Soc Med 5:131–139

Hort EC, Penfold WJ (1912b) A critical study of experimental fever. Proc R Soc Lond [Biol] 85:174–186

Houdas Y, Sauvage A, Bonaventure M, Ledru C, Guieu JD (1973) Thermal control in man. Regulation of central temperature or adjustments of heat exchanges by servomechanism. J Dyn Syst Measur Contr G 95:331–335

Jackson DL (1967) A hypothalamic region responsive to localized injection of pyrogens. J Neurophysiol 30:586–602

Jell RM, Sweatman P (1977) Prostaglandin sensitive neurones in cat hypothalamus: relation to thermoregulation and to biogenic amines. Can J Physiol Pharmacol 55:560–567

Kampschmidt RF, Upchurch HF, Eddington CL, Pulliam LA (1973) Multiple biological activities of a partially purified leukocytic endogenous mediator. Am J Physiol 224:530–533

Keller AD, McClaskey EB (1964) Localization, by the brain slicing method, of the level or levels of the cephalic brainstem upon which heat dissipation is dependent. Am J Phys Med 43:181–213

Kluger MJ (1977) Fever in the frog *Hyla cinerea*. J Therm Biol 2:79–81

Kluger MJ, Rothenburg GA (1978) Fever and the reduction in serum iron: An immune response in rabbits infected with *Pasturella multocida*. Physiologist 21:66

Kluger MJ, Rothernburg BA (1979) Fever and reduced iron: their interactions as a host defense response to bacterial infection. Science 203:374–376

Kluger MJ, Vaughn LK (1978) Fever and survival in rabbits infected with *Pasturella multocida*. J Physiol (Lond) 282:243–251

Kluger MJ, Ringler DH, Anver MR (1975) Fever and survival. Science 188:166–168

Korolkiewicz Z (1967) Effect of some pyrogenic substances on bioelectric activity of the rabbit hypothalamus. Acta Physiol Pol 18:783–787

Laburn H, Rosendorff C, Willies G, Woolf C (1974) A role for noradrenaline and cyclic AMP in prostaglandin E_1 fever. J Physiol (Lond) 240:49P–50P

Laburn H, Woolf CJ, Willies GH, Rosendorff C (1975) Pyrogen and prostaglandin fever in the rabbit. II. Effects of noradrenaline depletion and adrenergic receptor blockade. Neuropharmacology 14:405–411

Laburn H, Mitchell D, Rosendorff C (1977) Effects of prostaglandin antagonism on sodium arachidonate fever in rabbits. J Physiol (Lond) 267:559–570

Liebermeister C (1875) Handbuch der Pathologie und Therapie des Fiebers. Vogelwelt, Leipzig

Lipton JM (1973) Thermosensitivity of the medulla oblogata in the control of body temperature. Am J Physiol 224:890–897

Lipton JM, Fossler DE (1974) Fever produced in the squirrel monkey by intravenous and intracerebral endotoxin. Am J Physiol 226:1022–1027

Lipton JM, Trzcinka GP (1976) Persistence of febrile response to pyrogens after PO/AH lesions in squirrel monkeys. Am J Physiol 231:1638–1648

Luderitz O, Westphal O, Staub AM, Nikaido H (1971) Isolation and chemical and immunological characterization of bacterial lipopolysaccharides. In: Weinbaum G, Kadis S, Aji SJ (eds) Bacterial endotoxins, vol 4. Academic Press, New York, pp 145–233

MacPherson RK (1959) The effect of fever on temperature regulation in man. Clin Sci 18:281–287

Maskrey M (1972) Transmitters and modulator substances in the control of body temperature. PhD Thesis, University of Cambridge

Maskrey M, Bligh J (1971) Interactions between the thermoregulatory responses to injection into a lateral cerebral ventricle of the Welsh mountain sheep of putative neurotransmitter substances, and of local changes in anterior hypothalamic temperature. Int J Biometeorol 15, No 2–4:129–133

Merriman C, Pulliam L, Kampschmidt R (1977) Comparison of leukocytic pyrogen and leu-
   kocytic endogenous mediator. Proc Soc Exp Biol Med 156:224–227
Metcalf G, Thompson JW (1975) The effect of various amine-depleting drugs on the fever
   response exhibited by rabbits to bacterial or leucocyte pyrogen. R J Pharmacol 53:21–27
Meyer HH (1913) Theorie des Fiebers und seine Behandlung. Zentralbl Inn Med 6:385–386
Milton AS (1976) Prostaglandins in fever. In: Brasier MAB, Coceani F (eds) Brain dysfunc-
   tion in infantile febrile convulsions. Raven, New York
Milton AS, Wendlandt S (1970) A possible role for prostaglandin E, as a modulator for tem-
   perature regulation in the central nervous system of the cat. J Physiol (Lond) 207:76–
   77 P
Milton AS, Wendlandt S (1971 a) Effects on body temperature of prostaglandins of the A,
   E, and F series on injection into the third ventricle of unanaesthetized cats and rabbits.
   J Physiol (Lond) 218:325–336
Milton AS, Wendlandt S (1971 b) The effects of 4-acetamidophenol (paracatamol) on the
   temperature response of the concious rat to the intracerebral injection of prostagland-
   in E_1, adrenaline and pyrogen. J Physiol (Lond) 217:33–34 P
Mitchell D, Snellen JW, Atkins AR (1970) Thermoregulation during fever: change in set-
   point or change in gain. Pfluegers Arch 321:293–302
Murphy PA (1967 a) Quantitative aspects of the release of leucocyte pyrogens from rabbit
   blood incubated with endotoxin. J Exp Med 126:763–770
Murphy PA (1967 b) The rate of release of leucocyte pyrogen from rabbit blood incubated
   with endotoxin. J Exp Med 126:771–781
Myers RD (1971) Hypothalamic mechanisms of pyrogen action in the cat and monkey. In:
   Wolstenholme GEW, Birch J (eds) Pyrogen and fever. CIBA Foundation Symposium.
   Livingstone, London, pp 131–136
Myers RD, Tytell M (1972) Fever: reciprocal shift in brain sodium to calcium ratio as the
   set point rises. Science 178:765–767
Myers RD, Veale WL (1970) Body temperature: possible ionic mechanism in the hypothal-
   amus controlling the set point. Science 170:95–97
Myers RD, Veale WL (1971) The role of sodium and calcium ions in the hypothalamus in
   the control of body temperature of the unanaesthetized cat. J Physiol (Lond) 212:411–
   430
Myers RD, Rudy TA, Yaksh TL (1971) Fever in the monkey produced by the direct action
   of pyrogen on the hypothalamus. Experientia 27:160–161
Myers RD, Rudy TA, Yaksh TL (1973) Evocation of a biphasic febrile response in the
   rhesus monkey by intracerebral injection of bacterial endotoxins. Neuropharmacol
   12:1195–1198
Myers RD, Rudy TA, Yaksh TL (1974) Fever produced by endotoxin injected into the hypothalamus of the monkey and its antagonism by salicylate. J Physiol (Lond) 243:167–
   193
Myers RD, Simpson CW, Higgins D, Nattermann RA, Rice JC, Redgrave P, Metcalf G
   (1976) Hypothalamic Na^+ and Ca^{++} ions and temperature set-point: new mechanisms
   of action of a central or peripheral thermal challenge and intrahypothalamic 5-HT, NE,
   PGE_1 and pyrogen. Brain Res Bull 1:301–327
Myhre K, Cabanac M, Myhre G (1978) Fever and behavioural temperature regulation in
   the frog Rana esculenta. Acta Physiol Scand 101:219–229
Nakayama T, Hammel HT, Hardy JD, Eisenman JS (1963) Thermal stimulation of electrical activity of single units of preoptic region. Am J Physiol 204:1122–1126
Peindaries R, Jacob J (1971) Interactions between 5-hydroxytryptamine and a purified bacterial pyrogen when injected into the lateral cerebral ventricle of the wake rabbit. Eur
   J Pharmacol 13:347–355
Porter PJ, Kass EH (1962) Mediation by the central nervous system of the lethal action of
   bacterial endotoxin. Clin Res 10:185
Porter PJ, Kass EH (1965) Role of the posterior hypothalamus in mediating the lethal action
   of bacterial endotoxin in the rat. J Immunol 94:641–648
Preston E, Cooper KE (1976) Absence of fever in the rabbit following intrahypothalamic
   injections of noradrenaline into PGE_1-sensitive sites. Neuropharmacology 15:239–244

Ranson SW, Magoun HW (1929) The hypothalamus. Ergeb Physiol Biol Chem Exp Pharmakol 41:56–163

Ranson SW, Clark G, Magoun HW (1939) The effect of hypothalamic lesions on fever induced by intravenous injection of typhoid-paratyphoid vaccine. J Lab Clin Med 25:160–168

Repin IS, Kratskin IL (1967) Analysis of hypothalamic mechanism in the fever reaction. Fiziol Zh SSSR 53:1206–1211

Reynolds WW (1977) Fever and antipyresis in the bluegill sunfish, *Lepomis macrochirus*. Comp Biochem Physiol 57C:165–167

Reynolds WW, Covert JB (1977) Behavioral fever in aquatic endothermic vertebrates. In: Cooper KE, Lomax P, Schönbaum E (eds) Drugs, biogenic amines, and body temperature. Karger, Basel, pp 108–110

Reynolds WW, Casterlin ME, Covert JB (1976) Behavioural fever in telost fishes. Nature 259:41–42

Reynolds WW, Casterlin ME, Covert JB (1978 a) Febrile responses of bluegill *(Lepomis macrochirus)* to bacterial pyrogens. J Therm Biol 3:129–130

Reynolds WW, Covert JB, Casterlin ME (1978 b) Febrile responses of goldfish (*Carassius auratus* L.) to *Aeromonas hydrophila* and to *Escherichia coli* endotoxin. J Fish Dis 1:271–273

Rosendorff C, Cranston WI (1968) Effects of salicylate on human temperature regulation. Clin Sci 35:81–92

Rosendorff C, Mooney JJ (1971) Central nervous system sites of action of a purified leucocyte pyrogen. Am J Physiol 220:597–603

Rudy TA, Viswanathan CT (1975) Effect of central cholinergic blockade on the hyperthermia evoked by prostaglandin E_1 injected in the rostral hypothalamus of the rat. Can J Physiol Pharmacol 53:321–324

Satinoff E (1972) Salicylate action on normal body temperature in rats. Science 176:532–533

Schoener EP, Wang SC (1975) Leukocytic pyrogen and sodium acetylsalicylate on hypothalamic neurons in the cat. Am J Physiol 229:185–190

Schoener EP, Wang SC (1976) Effects of locally administered prostaglandin E_1 on anterior hypothalamic neurons. Brain Res 117:157–162

Seibert FB (1923) Fever-producing substance found in some distilled waters. Am J Physiol 67:90–104

Seibert FB (1925) The cause of many febrile reactions following intravenous injections. Am J Physiol 71:621–651

Siegert R, Philipp-Dormston WK, Radsak K, Menzel H (1976) Mechanism of fever induction in rabbits. Infect Immun 14:1130–1137

Silver A, Bligh J (1980) The use of histamine-receptor blockers in a further investigation of the role of histamine in thermoregulation in the sheep. J Therm Biol 5:131–140

Simon E (1974) Temperature regulation: the spinal cord as a site of extrahypothalamic thermoregulatory functions. Rev Physiol Biochem Pharmacol 71:1–76

Simpson CW, Ruwe WD, Myers RD (1977) Characterization of prostaglandin sensitive sites in the monkey hypothalamus mediating hyperthermia. In: Cooper KE, Lomax P, Schönbaum E (eds) Drugs, biogenic amines, and body temperature. Karger, Basel, pp 142–144

Snell ES, Atkins E (1965) The presence of endogenous pyrogen in normal rabbit tissues. J Exp Med 121:1019–1038

Snell ES, Atkins E (1967) Interactions of gram-negative bacterial endotoxin with rabbit blood in vitro. Am J Physiol 212:1103–1112

Stitt JT (1973) Prostaglandin E_1 fever induced in rabbits. J Physiol (Lond) 232:163–179

Stitt JT (1976) Inhibition of thermoregulatory outflow in conscious rabbits during periods of sustained arousal. J Physiol (Lond) 260:31–32P

Stitt JT, Hardy JD (1972) Evidence that prostaglandin E_1 may be a mediator in pyrogenic fever in rabbits. Biometeorology 5:112

Stitt JT, Hardy JD (1975) Microelectrophoresis of PGE_1 onto single units in the rabbit hypothalamus. Am J Physiol 229:240–245

Stone E (1763) An account of the success of the bark of the willow in the cure of agures. Philos Trans 53:195–200

Székely M (1978a) Endotoxin fever in para-chlorophenylalanine (PCPA) treated newborn guinea pigs and kittens. Life Sci 22:1585–1588

Székely M (1978b) Endotoxin fever in the new-born guinea-pig and the modulating effects of indomethacin and p-chlorophenylalanine. J Physiol (Lond) 281:467–476

Székely M (1978c) Biphasic endotoxin fever in the newborn rabbit. Acta Physiol Acad Sci Hung 51:389–392

Székely M, Bligh J (1975) Effects of intracerebroventricular norfenfluramine on heat production in the sheep. In: Jansky L (ed) Depressed metabolism and cold thermogenesis. Charles University, Prague, pp 188–192

Székely M, Komaromi I (1978) Endotoxin and prostaglandin fever of newborn guinea pigs at different ambient temperatures. Acta Physiol Acad Sci Hung 51:293–298

Székely M, Szelényi Z (1977) The effect of E. coli endotoxin on body temperature in the newborn rabbit, cat, guinea pig, and rat. Acta Physiol Acad Sci Hung 50:293–298

Székely M, Bligh J, Ryan EM, Sümegi I (1976) The ambient temperature dependent effects of norfenfluramine of temperature regulation in the rabbit and sheep. Acta Physiol Acad Sci Hung 48:273

Tangri KK, Bhargava AK, Bhargava KP (1975) Significance of central cholinergic mechanism in pyrexia induced by bacterial pyrogen in rabbits. In: Lomax P, Schönbaum E, Jacob J (eds) Temperature regulation and drug action. Karger, Basel, pp 65–74

Teddy PJ (1971) Discussion contribution. In: Wolstenholme GEW, Birch J (eds) Pyrogens and fever. Churchill, Livingstone Edinburgh London, pp 124–127

Tollerton AJ, Bligh J, Smith CA (1978) Effect of intracerebroventricular injections of noradrenaline on the peripheral vasomotor tone of sheep. J Therm Biol 3:137–142

van Miert ASJPAM (1971) Inhibition of gastric motility by endotoxin (bacterial lipopolysaccharide) in conscious goats and modification of this response by splanchnectomy, adrenalectomy or adrenergic blocking agents. Arch Int Pharmacodyn Ther 193:405–414

van Miert ASJPAM, van Duin CThM (1978) Further studies on the antipyretic action of Polymyxin B in pyrogen-induced fever. Arzneim Forsch/Drug Res 28:2246–2251

Vane JR (1971) Inhibition of prostaglandin synthesis as a mechanism for aspirin-like drugs. Nature New Biol 231:232–235

Vaughn LK, Bernheim HA, Kluger MJ (1974) Fever in the lizard Dipsosaurus dorsalis. Nature Lond 252:473–474

Veale WL, Cooper KE (1974) Evidence for the involvement of prostaglandin in fever. In: Lederis K, Cooper KE (eds) Recent studies of hypothalamic function. Karger, Basel, pp 289–300

Veale WL, Cooper KE (1975) Comparison of sites of action of prostaglandin E and leucocyte pyrogen in brain. In: Lomax P, Schönbaum E, Jacob J (eds) Temperature regulation and drug action. Karger, Basel, pp 218–226

Veale WL, Whishaw IQ (1976) Body temperature responses to different ambient temperatures following injections of prostaglandin E_1 and noradrenaline into the brain. Pharmacol Biochem Behav 4:143–150

Veale WL, Cooper KE, Pittman QJ (1977) The role of prostaglandins in fever and temperature regulation. In: Ramwell P (ed) Prostaglandins, vol 3. Plenum, New York, pp 145–167

Vendrik AJH (1959) The regulation of body temperature in man. Ned Tijdschr Geneesk 103:240–244

Villablanca J, Myers RD (1965) Fever produced by microinjection of typhoid vaccine into hypothalamus of cats. Am J Physiol 208:703–707

Weinberg ED (1974) Iron and susceptibility to infectious disease. Science 184:952–956

Williams JW, Rudy TA, Yaksh TL, Viswanathan CT (1977) An extensive exploration of the rat brain for sites mediating prostaglandin-induced hyperthermia. Brain Res 120:251–262

Wit A, Wang SC (1968a) Temperature-sensitive neurones in preoptic/anterior hypothalamic region: effects of increasing ambient temperature. Am J Physiol 215:1151–1159

Wit A, Wang SC (1968 b) Temperature-sensitve neurons in preoptic/anterior hypothalamic region: actions of pyrogen and acetylsalicylate. Am J Physiol 215:1160–1169
Woodbury DM (1970) Analgesics and antipyretics. In: Goodman LS, Gillman A (eds) The pharmacological basis of therapeutics, 4th edn. Macmillan, New York, pp 314–347
Wunderlich CA (1871) On the temperature in diseases. A manual of medical thermometry. The New Sydenham Society, London
Wyndham CH, Atkins AR (1968) A physiological scheme and mathematical model of temperature regulation in man. Pfluegers Arch 303:14–30

CHAPTER 4

Exogenous Pyrogens*

C. A. DINARELLO and S. M. WOLFF

A. Introduction

The motivation to study the pathogenesis of fever in humans can be traced back to nineteenth century experiments in which human subjects were injected with a variety of materials including milk, bismuth, proteins, sugars, water, saline, and pus. In fact, the term "injection fevers" has been used to characterize these experiments, probably because of the lack of discrimination which scientists exercised by injecting such a multiplicity of agents. Nevertheless, considerable data was generated from these experiments and helped form the basis of our current understanding of the human febrile response. Although the injected substances clearly lacked homogeneity, the response was uniform. Vasoconstriction and chills occurred approximately one to two hours following the injection and most fevers lasted four to five hours. Further interest in this area arose when parenteral fluids were administered for the first time on a large scale and pyrogenic reactions were routinely observed. "Injection fevers" occurred well into the first half of the twentieth century until it was demonstrated that the injected materials were contaminated with Gram-negative bacteria and hence contained bacterial lipopolysaccharide (reviewed in BENNETT and BEESON 1950; ATKINS and BODEL 1974, 1979).

Bacterial lipopolysaccharide (LPS) is a ubiquitous substance. LPS can be found under several conditions because Gram-negative organisms, particularly water-growing *Pseudomonas* spp., are remarkably hardy, can replicate at 4 °C and require few nutrients. For example, certain Gram-negative organisms have been known to contaminate and grow in distilled water at 4 °C. LPS readily leaches off these organisms and is highly soluble in aqueous media. In addition, LPS survives routine autoclaving, organic solvents, acids, ethanol, and sterilizing liquids (ELIN and WOLFF 1973). Since nanogram quantities of bacterial LPS produce fever in humans and rabbits, these substances must be carefully eliminated in research on the pyrogenicity of other agents. Unless the investigator is aware of the potential of LPS to contaminate glassware, water, and laboratory reagents, the pyrogenicity of a particular substance may be due to contaminating bacterial lipopolysaccharide. Although bacterial LPS frequently contaminates materials there are many substances which do not contain this material and yet produce fever in humans and experimental animals. These substances together with LPS are considered exogenous pyrogens.

* This work was supported by funds from the National Institute of Allergy and Infectious Diseases, United States Public Health Service, National Institute of Health

I. General Considerations

The term "exogenous pyrogen" has been used for pyrogenic agents which are derived from outside the host. However, this is somewhat limiting definition, particularly when one takes into consideration the mechanisms which exogenous pyrogens cause fever. It is well established that exogenous pyrogens produce fever by their ability to induce the synthesis and release of endogenous pyrogen (EP) from the host's phagocytic cells (DINARELLO and WOLFF 1978). Furthermore, it is circulating endogenous pyrogen rather than circulating exogenous pyrogen which acts on the thermoregulatory centre to raise the thermostatic setting in the hypothalamus and cause fever. Although there are several reports of exogenous pyrogens producing fever when injected into the cerebral ventricular system or hypothalamic tissue itself, these experiments can hardly be considered physiological or natural. Indeed, investigators have shown that circulating labelled endotoxins do not gain access to the hypothalamus (COOPER and CRANSTON 1963) but rather are rapidly sequestered in the cells of the reticulo-endothelial system (HERION et al. 1964; STARZECKI et al. 1967). Reticulo-endothelial cells have been shown to synthesize and release endogenous pyrogen (DINARELLO et al. 1968; HAESELER et al. 1977) in vitro following the injection of exogenous pyrogens in vivo. With recognition of the essential mediator function of endogenous pyrogen, a more precise definition for "exogenous pyrogen" would be a substance which induces the production of endogenous pyrogen.

For the most part, the majority of exogenous pyrogens are derived from outside the host, but substances of host origin have been demonstrated to cause fever by initiating the production of endogenous pyrogen. Thus, there are endogenous stimulators of endogenous pyrogen. At the present time these include, antigen–antibody complexes, products of lymphocytes (or lymphokines) and androgenic steroid metabolic products.

The ability of any exogenous pyrogen to produce fever lies in the chemicophysical property which enables it to activate a host phagocytic cell. This results in the de-repression of the genome for endogenous pyrogen synthesis which proceeds even after the exogenous stimulus is removed (ROOT et al. 1970; NORDLUND et al. 1970 a; BODEL 1970). Although poorly understood, the action of an exogenous pyrogen on the membrane of phagocytic cells seems to be a critical step in activation and hence, physical modification of exogenous pyrogens which render them non-pyrogenic clearly have altered this interaction. It is the purpose of this chapter to examine the biological and chemical nature of exogenous pyrogens with particular attention to their physical property which enables them to induce EP synthesis.

B. Viruses

Viral infections are unquestionably the most common infectious diseases of humans. Generally speaking, even localized viral infections like the common cold can cause prominent systemic effects such as fever. On the other hand some systemic viral infections produce only fever. Such primary febrile syndromes have been reported, for example, for several of the Coxsackie and ECHO viruses (REED and MCMILLAN 1966; LINNEMANN et al. 1974; ARTENSTEIN et al. 1965). In addition, immunization trials of various viral vaccines have reported fever as a significant side effect of certain vaccine preparations (BUYNAK et al. 1969; YOUNG et al. 1967). Despite the enormous numbers of individuals who experience fever due to viral infections, there are only a few experimental models for viral fevers. Furthermore, the precise physical or biological nature of viruses which allow them to produce fever remains unknown.

I. Experimental Fevers with Viruses

It is clear that influenzal viruses injected intravenously into rabbits cause fever by liberating EP (ATKINS and HUANG 1958 a, b, c). The EP induced by these viral fevers was demonstrated by passive transfer of febrile plasma to normal rabbits. Others have also demonstrated that EP is liberated into the circulation following the injection of materials containing live viruses into rabbits (KING 1964; KANOH et al. 1969; KAWASAKI and KANOH 1974; KANOH and KAWASAKI 1966). Finally, the production of EP was shown in vitro when virus and rabbit blood leucocytes were incubated together (ATKINS et al. 1964; KANOH and KAWASAKI 1966). The mechanism by which viruses bring about the synthesis and release of EP remains unclear. The original experiments on experimental viral fevers in rabbits had shown the requirement for viral particles i.e. soluble substances produced by the virus or viral infected tissue did not cause fever (WAGNER et al. 1949). Further experimentation revealed that temperatures high enough to destroy infectivity without affecting the viral haemagglutinin had no effect on the pyrogenicity. Subsequently, this observation was confirmed when investigators demonstrated that the haemagglutinating property of the virus is necessary to produce fever (KANOH and KAWASAKI 1966). Heating viral suspensions or treatment with ether in order to destroy the haemagglutinative capacity results in loss of pyrogenicity.

Another approach to define the pyrogenic factor of viruses has been neutralization of viral antigens with specific immune sera. In these studies conflicting results have been reported; WAGNER et al. (1949) found that specific antibody would reduce pyrogenicity while KING (1964) reported no effect of specific antibody. In using immune sera to destroy viral antigens, antigen–antibody complexes may be formed which themselves are known to be pyrogenic (ROOT and WOLFF 1968). No studies have been attempted to isolate the haemagglutinating antigen of influenzal viruses and evaluate its ability to induce EP production. There is a single report of a carbohydrate fraction from a parainfluenza virus which activates blood leucocytes to release EP in vitro (ATKINS and BODEL 1974). Although the pyrogenic properties and haemagglutinating capacities of influenza and Newcastle disease viruses are not distinguishable by their thermal sensitivity, ultraviolet irradiation or formaldehyde treatment will completely destroy the pyrogenic activity without impairing the haemagglutinin (SIEGERT and BRAUNE 1964a, b). The treatment of influenzal viral particles with ether results in the separation of G-antigen, haemagglutinin, and lipid substances with a corresponding loss in pyrogenicity. This finding suggests that a spatial relationship of these components is necessary to activate the production of EP since administration of these separated components together in a single injection did not cause fever. However, treating the whole virus with trypsin or pronase has no effect on pyrogenicity (SHU 1974). It can be concluded then that there is an essential lipid and carbohydrate moiety of the haemagglutinin necessary for viral fevers.

II. Interferon

Following the intravenous injection of certain viruses into rabbits, titres of circulating interferon have been noted to coincide with fever. Both EP and interferon appear in the circulation at the same time and reach maximal concentration approximately 4 h following the injection (SIEGERT et al. 1967). Pyrogenic unresponsiveness to a second injection of virus 24 h later also results in failure to increase interferon titres (SIEGERT et al. 1967). Attempts to destroy the pyrogenicity of Newcastle disease virus using heat, lipid solvents, or detergents also eliminated its ability to induce interferon (SHU 1974). Furthermore, both EP and interferon can be induced by the same substances, namely, poly I: poly C (NORDLUND et al. 1970 b) and endotoxin (Ho et al. 1973). Therefore, several investigators have studied the possibility that interferon and EP might be the same molecule. In these experiments, rabbits have been injected with viruses and the febrile serum chromatographed using gel filtration or precipitated with various concentrations of ethanol. Serum interferon and EP commonly co-precipitated and chromatographed together (KOHLHAGE et al. 1968). However, homogeneous preparations of EP and human interferon have been reported and it is clear that these two substances do not share the same physical or chemical characteristics (DINARELLO et al. 1977a, b; STEWART et al. 1977; MOGENSEN and CANTELL 1974). Thus, these two substances are not the same molecule despite the fact that they may be present in the same preparations. On the other hand, these results do suggest that the ability of a virus to induce EP and cause fever may be closely associated with its ability to induce interferon. In the case of non-viral pyrogens which are also interferon inducers, the activation of some unknown cellular process probably leads to the de-repression of the genome for both EP and interferon synthesis. The synthesis and release of both these substances coincide and this accounts for their appearance in the circulation at the same time. However, despite induction, synthesis, and release phenomena, EP and interferon are separate substances for all of the reasons given above.

C. Gram-Positive Organisms

Gram-positive bacterial infections produce some of the most pyrogenic diseases in humans and animals. During the past 20 years, it has become clear that Gram-positive bacteria produce fever by one of three mechanisms: (1) phagocytosis of the intact organisms by leucocytes; (2) production and release of soluble extracellular exotoxins or (3) toxic or host immunological responses to cell wall components. We shall consider each mechanism individually; however, it should be noted that all three may simultaneously be involved in producing fever from Gram-positive bacterial infections as well as in experimentally induced fevers.

I. Intact Organisms

In the most thorough investigation of fever produced from Gram-positive bacterial cells (ATKINS and FREEDMAN 1963), live cells of either *Staphylococcus aureus*, pneumococci, type IV, *S. albus*, *Bacillus subtilis*, or *Listeria monocytogenes* were washed in saline and injected intravenously into rabbits. All bacterial species produced fever after a latent period of approximately 60 min in both normal rabbits as well as rabbits made unresponsive to Gram-negative bacterial lipopolysaccharide. In addition, cell filtrates from *S. albus*, *B. subtilis*, and *L. monocytogenes* did not produce fever, suggesting that the pyrogenic moiety of these bacteria was associated with the bacterial cell itself. Furthermore, the number of bacterial cells necessary to elicit a febrile response was consistently 10^8 organisms or greater with a minimal pyrogenic response observed after the injection of 10^7 organisms. These studies also demonstrated that endogenous pyrogen circulated during these fevers and could be transferred to other rabbits 5 h after the bacteria were injected. Later it was established that rabbits intravenously injected with autoclaved *S. albus* would have fever (ATKINS and FREEDMAN 1963) and that Kupffer cells, splenic or lung macrophages would spontaneously release EP in vitro when removed 1 h following the injection of bacteria (DINARELLO 1969). Thus, it became clear that phagocytosis of Gram-positive bacterial particles was sufficient to initiate EP synthesis, that infection was not necessary and that intravenous injections of Gram-positive bacteria likely represents fever due to particles. Non-microbial particulate substances like colloidal fat, glycogen, gold, silica, and thorium dioxide had previously been shown to produce fever (EISLER et al. 1955; ATKINS and BODEL 1974). Several subsequent studies on the release of EP from phagocytic leucocytes in vitro have confirmed the early in vivo experiments in that a specific ratio of bacterial particles to leucocytes were necessary to initiate EP synthesis (ATKINS et al. 1967; ROOT et al. 1970) and that agents which interfered with the phagocytic ingestion process also prevented EP production (NORDLUND et al. 1970a; BODEL 1970).

II. Extracellular Products

With the exception of group *A* streptococci and some strains of *Staphylococcus aureus* (GIORGIO and 80/81) culture filtrates from Gram-positive bacteria are not pyrogenic. The staphylococcal product which produces fever appears to be protein in nature since it is inactivated by trypsin and precipitates with trichloracetic acid (BODEL and ATKINS 1965). However the pyrogenic staphylococcal product is distinct from the α-, β- or δ-haemolysins as well as leucocidin, hyaluronidase, and coagulase (BODEL and ATKINS 1965). It is possible that this staphylococcal pyrogen is similar to a protein antigen that has been described (VERWEY 1940) and that rabbits having previous infections with pathogenic staphylococci have become sensitized to this antigen (BODEL and ATKINS 1965).

Staphylococci also release a soluble exotoxin called enterotoxin. This enterotoxin has been purified and the biologically active molecule resides in a single polypeptide chain with a molecular weight near 28,000 daltons (SHANTZ et al. 1972). Purified staphylococcal enterotoxin produces fever in normal as well as LPS-unresponsive rabbits (BRUNSON and WATSON 1974) and unlike the protein product described by Bodel and Atkins (1965), the pyrogenicity of the enterotoxin is neutralized by specific antibody. The dose of purified staphylococcal enterotoxin necessary to produce fever in rabbits is 1 μg/kg and hence this material is far less potent than lipopolysaccharides from Gram-negative organisms. Recently, another exotoxin was isolated from *S. aureus*, purified and found to be pyrogenic for mice and rabbits at 1–10 μg/kg (Schlievert et al. 1979). The molecular weight of this material is 12,000 daltons as determined by sodium dodecyl sulphate electrophoresis and had an isoelectric point (pI) of 5.3. In addition, this material was found to be a non-specific mitogen for rabbit and human lymphocytes. It was physically distinct from the staphylococcal enterotoxin. Thus, pathogenic strains of staphylococci produce more than one pyrogenic exotoxin and these exotoxins induce diverse biological effects.

Group *A* streptococci also release several extracellular products which have profound biological and chemical properties. Of these, the scarlet fever toxin (Dick toxin, or erythrogenic toxin) is well known and has been shown to a potent pyrogen. This streptococcal pyrogenic exotoxin (SPE) derived from the classic Dochez NY 5 strain exhibits three antigenically distinct types: type A, an 8,000 dalton glycoprotein with a pI of 4.5; type B, a 22,000 dalton protein with a pI of 8.5, and type C, a 13,000 dalton molecule with a pI of 6.7 (Cunningham et al. 1976; Schlievert et al. 1977; Barsumtan et al. 1978). Each exotoxin type produces fever in rabbits and mice following a latent period of 30 min (Schlievert and Watson 1978). Like the staphylococcal pyrogenic enterotoxin, production of specific antibody to each exotoxin type prevents fever. A fourth erythrogenic toxin, type D, has been described and shown to be pyrogenic for rabbits (Schuh et al. 1970). It was isolated from a mutant strain of streptococci, C 203 U, which produces streptolysin O but not S. Unlike other streptococcal extracellular products, the four pyrogenic erythrogenic toxins are heat resistant (96 °C for 30 min) and withstand change in pH of 1.08 to 11.0. Both the skin activity and pyrogenicity can be neutralized by specific antibody and apparently the antigen–antibody complexes formed when immunized rabbits are challenged in vivo are not sufficient to induce fever themselves.

In addition to producing fever, the streptococcal erythrogenic exotoxin also enhances susceptibility to lethal endotoxin shock, is cytotoxic for splenic macrophages, blocks the clearance of colloidal carbon by the reticulo-endothelial system, and stimulates blast transformation by thymus-dependent lymphocytes (T-lymphocytes) (Watson and Kim 1970; Kanoh and Orgawa 1977; Kanoh and Watson 1977). These data suggest that the varied biological properties of erythrogenic exotoxin may be mediated by another molecule of host origin. The production of EP from leucocytes incubated with the erythrogenic exotoxins suggested that EP mediates the fever produced by these substances (Schuh and Hribalova 1966). In these studies the erythrogenic exotoxin was incubated with polymorphonuclear leucocytes from either normal rabbits or rabbits repeatedly immunized and made unresponsive to the specific streptococcal exotoxin. The leucocytes from immunized rabbits failed to release EP in vitro, suggesting a cytophilic antibody directed against the pyrogenic active site of the exotoxin. Others have failed to demonstrate EP release from rabbit peritoneal leucocytes incubated with the purified exotoxin (Schlievert and Watson 1978). However, in this study the exotoxin was incubated for four hours with the leucocytes and the reported failure might have been due to cell lysis and death during the incubation period. To guard against this, others have exposed the leucocytes to the exotoxin for 30 min, then washed the cells; during subsequent incubation without the toxin, EP was released in vitro (SCHUH and HRIBALOVA 1966).

In a recent study, treatment of rabbits with indomethacin, acetylsalicylate, or cortisone 3 days and 2 h before challenge significantly reduced the febrile response to type C exotoxin (SCHLIEVERT et al. 1978). This suggests that the ability to produce fever is dependent on the cyclo-oxygenase system of prostaglandin synthesis and is consistent with the findings of several other reports on the effects of antipyretics on the febrile responses of essentially all exogenous pyrogens. Despite the fact that these authors have shown that type C streptococcal erythrogenic exotoxin gains access to the cerebrospinal fluid, a very large intravenous dose was used (400 minimal pyrogenic doses) and this finding can hardly be used as evidence that the exotoxin acts directly on the thermoregulatory centre (SCHLIEVERT and WATSON 1978). On the contrary, it seems that the exotoxin, in addition to being pyrogenic and able to elicit other biological changes, also increases the permeability of the blood–brain barrier to itself, bacterial LPS, and whole bacterial organisms like pneumococci and *Haemophilus influenzae*.

III. Cell Wall Components

In addition to the pyrogenicity of the intact Gram-positive bacterial cells and their extracellular products, pyrogenic substances can also be found in disrupted cell wall fragments. This has been shown with staphylococcal as well as streptococcal cell wall homogenates. In general, cell walls are disrupted by sonication and then treated with proteolytic agents like trypsin and pepsin to remove cytoplasmic proteins. Treatment with hot trichloracetic acid (90 °C) removes 95% of the teichoic acid and leaves the peptidoglycan "skeleton" of the cell wall intact. This peptidoglycan fragment represents 75% of the initial cell wall weight (ATKINS and MORSE 1967). Gram-positive as well as Gram-negative bacteria contain the peptidoglycan structure which imparts rigidity to all bacterial cell walls. There are over 70 different types of peptidoglycans, i.e. peptidoglycans with different primary structures found among the Gram-positive bacteria (SCHLEIFER and KANDLER 1972) and within each type there are specific peptide subunits which provide further identity (SCHLEIFER 1975). The basic unit of the peptidoglycan is a repeating sequence of N-acetylglucosamine linked to N-acetylmuramic acid. Attached to the muramic acid is a tetrapeptide composed of alanine, glutamic acid, and lysine in a ratio of 3:1:1 respectively. There is covalent cross-linkage of the tetrapeptides attached to adjacent hexosamine polymers through a L-alanyl-L-alanine bridge and the alanine dipeptide joins the terminal alanine of one peptide to the ε-amino group of the lysine of the adjacent peptide (ROTTA 1974). It should be pointed out that the peptidoglycans of various bacteria have a similar structure, differing mainly in the nature and composition of the interpeptide bridges. Penicillin prevents the formation of the transpeptides between adjacent peptide chains while lysozyme cleaves the repeating polysaccharide units. Lysozmye digestion of *Nocardia* spp. results in a N-acetyloglucosamine-(β-1-4)-N-acetylmuramic acid tetrapeptide monomer (ADAM et al. 1974; ELLOUZ et al. 1974).

The process of sonication, extraction with hot trichloracetic acid and trypsinization results in a peptidoglycan preparation which produces fever indistinguishable from that produced by whole bacterial cell walls or unextracted disrupted cell walls (Atkins and Morse 1967; Rotta 1975; Schleifer 1975). Despite the loss in pyrogenicity, lysozyme treatment of the peptidoglycan has no effect on the adjuvant properties of this substance (Adam et al. 1974). Thus, in these studies the pyrogenic moiety of the peptidoglycan most likely resides in the configuration of either the intact polymer or in the hexosamine–peptide fragment which may be altered by lysozyme degradation (Schleifer 1975). There is a report that a digest of streptococcal cell walls by an enyzme of *Flavobacterium* results in a high molecular weight fraction which retains pyrogenic activity (Hamada 1971) but the chemical nature of this fraction has yet to be determined.

It is unclear whether the biological effects of peptidoglycans are mediated by a toxic or immunological mechanism. Because of the wide variety and similarities of biological effects produced by the peptidoglycans and by bacterial LPS derived from Gram-negative organisms, it has been proposed (Rotta 1975) that these two chemically distinct substances have a similar mechanism of action. Both substances produce fever, elicit the localized Shwartzman reaction, induced non-specific resistance to infection, and produce vascular collapse at high doses (Rotta 1975). Repeated injections of group *A* streptococcal peptidoglycans results in almost complete pyrogenic unresponsiveness, which is similar to that observed with daily injections of bacterial LPS. When rabbits which had been made tolerant to the streptococcal peptidoglycan were challenged with the peptidoglycan from a staphylococcus, they responded with a febrile response comparable to that of normal rabbits (Rotta 1974, 1975). Thus, immunological specificity exists among the different peptidoglycans in producing fever, unlike the pyrogenicity of bacterial LPS which is, in general, non-specific. Moreover, specific antipeptidoglycan serum can neutralize the pyrogenic properties of peptidoglycans in vitro (Rotta 1975; Rotta 1977).

Both the hexosamine polymer and peptide moiety of peptidoglycans are antigenic (Krause 1975) but the biological significance of antibodies to peptidoglycans has yet to be determined. Humans and rabbits have significant quantities of antipeptidoglycan antibodies and in humans the titres are highest in young children and decrease in age (Schachenmayer et al. 1975; Krause 1975). The synthesis of the pentapeptide unit has aided in demonstrating that the C-terminal D-alanyl-D-alanine is the immunodominant determinant of the peptide chain and because of the similarities of the peptidoglycans, cross-reactivity has been shown. In terms of the pyrogenicity of peptidoglycans, these antigenic determinants may be important and play a role in the pathogenesis of febrile diseases like rheumatic fever, although titres to peptidoglycans increase marginally with increasing titres to antistreptolysin O (Schachenmayr et al. 1975).

The varied biological properties of peptidoglycans have led to attempts to unravel the structure–function relationship of these ubiquitous substances. Two areas of research have synthesized the basic subunits of the peptidoglycan: the peptide chains and the hexosamine peptide units. The synthesis of the pentapeptide, L-Ala–γ-D-Glu–L-Lys–D-Ala–D-Ala, represents the immunologically reactive peptide from the group *A*-variant streptococcal peptidoglycan. Intravenous injections of the tetrapeptides, L-alanyl–D-isoglutaminyl–L-lysyl–D-alanine and L-alanyl–D-glutaminyl–L-lysyl–D-alanine, produced fever in rats. Even the dipeptide, L-alanyl–D-isoglutamine produced fever, although the fever from this dipeptide occurred after a prolonged latent period (MASEK et al. 1978). The combination of the hexosamine and dipeptide unit, N-acetylmuramyl–L-alanyl–D-isoglutamine, or muramyl dipeptide (MDP) produce maximal pyrogenic response (KADLECOVA et al. 1977). MDP was also shown to produce fever in rabbits and liberate EP from rabbits and human monocytes in vitro (DINARELLO et al. 1978). There have been no studies on the ability of the synthetic tetrapeptides to induce EP production in vitro. However, studies of these synthetic adjuvants have demonstrated that the pyrogenic moiety of peptidoglycans resides in the small subunits and that the intact polymer produced by sonication may induce fever by a different mechanism, that is, by phagocytosis (ATKINS and MORSE 1967). It is also clear from previous studies that the products of lyzozyme degradation of the peptidoglycan are not pyrogenic, perhaps because the active site is altered in the process.

Teichoic and teichuronic acids are also found in the cell walls of Gram-positive bacteria. These have been shown to produce fever in rabbits but their mechanism of action may be linked to prior antigenic exposure (ATKINS and MORSE 1967). Staphylococcal teichoic acid antibodies have been measured in humans and rise with Gram-positive infections (MARTIN et al. 1979). Other Gram-positive cell wall components are protein and polysaccharide and these substances, unlike the peptidoglycan, may produce fever because they form complexes with specific antibody, which subsequently produce fever (BODEL and ATKINS 1965).

An understandable criticism of the reported work dealing with pyrogenic substances derived from Gram-positive bacteria and synthetic analogues of peptidoglycans is that these preparations may be contaminated with Gram-negative bacteria. Under such circumstances pyrogenicity could be due to the presence of small quantities of LPS. The fact that many of the biological activities of Gram-positive peptidoglycans, exotoxins, and synthesized muramyl peptides are similar to those induced by LPS reinforces this claim. However, the pyrogenic and physical properties of LPS are distinct and separable from substances derived from Gram-positive bacteria. For example, extraction of peptidoglycan with hot (180 °C) formamide for 30 min destroys the pyrogenicity of LPS but has no effect on peptidoglycan activity (ROTTA 1975). Also, rabbits rendered unresponsive to peptidoglycan respond with fever to LPS. Finally, one can neutralize the pyrogenicity of peptidoglycan with specific antiserum. These data support the fact that contaminating LPS is not responsible for the pyrogenicity of peptidoglycan preparations from Gram-positive organisms.

The development of the *Limulus* amoebocyte lysate (LAL) test for the detection of submicrogram quantities of LPS has been a major advance in studies of the possible contamination of exogenous pyrogens by LPS. Depending on preparation and source, the LAL is a highly sensitive in vitro assay for LPS and is generally at least ten times as sensitive as the rabbit pyrogen test (COOPER et al. 1971). However, the LAL may give false positive results; for example, thrombin, poly I: poly C, ribonuclease, and other substances have produced gelation in the LAL which was not due to LPS (ELIN and WOLFF 1973) and others have shown that false negatives can occur; for example, tetracycline, dexamethasone, and $0.34\ M\ Ca^{2+}$

will inhibit the LAL test for LPS (van Noordwijk and de Jong 1977). However, the LAL test remains a highly sensitive method of detecting nanogram quantities of LPS. Products of Gram-positive bacteria have been tested with the LAL and, in general, are a hundred to a thousand times less potent per unit weight than LPS. Peptidoglycan preparations from a variety of Gram-positive bacteria extracted with trichoracetic acid have produced positive LAL at concentrations 10^3–4×10^5 greater than LPS (Wildfeuer et al. 1975). Peptidoglycans obtained by muramidase hydrolysis also caused gelation of the LAL but at a level a hundred times greater than LPS (Kotani et al. 1977). The exotoxins A, B, and C from streptococci produce a positive LAL at concentrations equal to that necessary to produce fever. However, heating the exotoxins to 65 °C for 30 min destroys pyrogenicity and LAL gelation; the pyrogenicity and LAL reactivity for LPS, on the other hand, survive this temperature (Brunson and Watson 1976).

The LAL assay has also been used to test the synthetic adjuvant analogues of the peptidoglycans. The most representative of these synthetic compounds is the muramyl dipeptide, N-acetylmuramyl–L-alanyl–D-isoglutamine (MDP). There is a close correlation between the pyrogenicity and LAL reactivity of MDP and several of its analogues. The concentrations necessary to produce gelation of the LAL are a hundred to a thousand times greater thn that of a reference LPS derived from *Escherichia coli* (Dinarello et al. 1978; Kotani et al. 1977). Moreover, rabbits made unresponsive to LPS will have fever when given MDP (Dinarello et al. 1978). The data suggest that the pyrogenicity of synthetic adjuvants is not due to contamination with LPS.

D. Gram-Negative Bacteria

Like the Gram-positive bacteria, Gram-negative bacteria can produce fever following phagocytosis of intact organisms. However, the LPS which is highly soluble and a very potent pyrogen usually masks the fever produced by phagocytosis of the organisms. For practical purposes, fever produced in Gram-negative infections or from such experimental agents as killed typhoid vaccine or cultures of Gram-negative bacteria represents fever from the LPS of these organisms.

I. Cell Wall Structure

The LPS molecule is an integral part of the cell wall of all Gram-negative bacteria. LPS comprises the outermost layer of the cell wall, being covalently bound to the rigid peptidoglycan which is shared by all bacteria and blue algae. The precise attachment of LPS of the peptidoglycan is unknown but it has been speculated that special lipoprotein molecules are interdispersed between the peptidoglycan and the LPS. For *E. coli* it has been estimated that there are some 250,000 of these lipoprotein units which bind covalently to the hexosamine units of the peptidoglycan. The lipid portion of the lipoprotein units then provides a lipi–lipid interaction for the LPS (Braun 1973). In this manner the orientation of the lipid portion of the LPS molecule is inward and the polysaccharide points outward. This is confirmed by studies which support the fact that the 0-polysaccharide moiety of LPS which provides antigenic specificity occupies the outer surface of the cell wall.

The LPS molecule itself is composed of three-basic subunits; (1) the 0-polysaccharide (or 0-specific chain); (2) the R-core (or core polysaccharide); and (3) the lipid moiety. The polysaccharide portion contains several sugars, mostly hexoses and aminohexoses. The particular sequence and composition of these sugars imparts serospecificity for the Gram-negative bacteria (ELIN and WOLFF 1973). Because of the large numbers and varieties of Gram-negative organisms which colonize the gastrointestinal tract, it is not surprising to detect "natural" antibodies to their 0-polysaccharide antigens. What role these antibodies play in mediating the pyrogenic response to LPS is unclear, but in certain experiments, antibody response to the 0-polysaccharide moiety was shown to mediate the pyrogenic unresponsiveness induced by repeated injections of LPS (WATSON and KIM 1963; GREISMAN et al. 1964). However, other reports using five different serological methods demonstrated that the pyrogenicity of LPS is independent of antibody response (MULHOLLAND et al. 1965). Since recent investigations have focused attention on the importance of the lipid part of the LPS molecule, the role of the 0-polysaccharide and antibody response to these antigens in the production of fever remains unresolved.

The R-core acts as a bridge between the 0-polysaccharide and the lipid. The R-core consists of hexoses, hexosamines, and heptose, the heptoses being cross-linked to adjacent R-core chains by phosphate bonds. The most interesting aspect of the R-core is an eight-carbon ketonic acid, 2-keto-3-deoxyoctonate, or KDO. KDO is unique to LPS and its function in the LPS is unknown. KDO is important because it links the R-core to the glucosamine units of the lipid portion of LPS.

The lipid part of LPS was first isolated by acid hydrolysis (BOIVIN et al. 1933). The term fraction A was given to the lipid soluble moiety and later this was called lipid A. Lipid A is composed of glucosamine units linked covalently to the KDO of the R-core and to each other through phosphate bonds. From each glucosamine unit fatty acids extend in C_{10} to C_{22} units to from the hydrophobic end of the LPS molecule. These fatty acids are palmitic, lauric, myristic, and β-hydroxymyristic acids. The β-hydroxymyristic acid is the major fatty acid and, like KDO, seems to be unique to LPS (RIETSCHEL and LUEDERITZ 1975). The mild acid hydrolysis of LPS cleaves the ketosidic linkage of the KDO to lipid, thus liberating lipid A. The lipid A is insoluble in water and hence biologically inactive. Lipid A can be solubilized by complexing with certain carriers which are water soluble but biologically inert (LUEDERITZ et al. 1973).

II. Pyrogenicity of LPS

LPS has many different biological effects which often reproduce the changes seen in Gram-negative infections. LPS can induce profound changes in the haematological, immune, vascular, and endocrine systems. Of all the biological effects of LPS, the production of fever is perhaps the most commonly observed and studied. Until the development of the AL test for the detection of LPS, fever in rabbits was the most sensitive assay for LPS. Purified LPS in nanogram or smaller quantities elicits fever in rabbits which is dose dependent (WOLFF et al. 1965c). The typical febrile response of rabbits to LPS begins 15–30 min following intravenous injection but this latent period can be shortened if larger doses are given. The fever is usually biphasic, i.e. there are two peak temperature elevations, the first occurring after 90 min and a second, higher peak at 3 h. Decreasing the dose will often result in a monophasic fever.

Humans respond to LPS with a monophasic fever and on a weight basis are more sensitive to the pyrogenic properties of LPS than the rabbit (GREISMAN and HORNICK 1969; WOLFF 1973). In fact, humans seem to be the most sensitive of all animals studied. For example, a purified endotoxin from *Salmonella abortus-equi* (Lipexal) produces a maximal rise in temperature of 2 °C with a dose of 2 ng/kg (WOLFF 1973; DINARELLO and WOLFF 1976). The fever in humans to increasing doses of LPS follows a dose–response relationship. Subsequent to an intravenous injection, there is a latent period of 90–120 min during which time subjects may feel cold. This can be demonstrated by a fall in the peripheral heat flow from the hands and feet (BUSKIRK et al. 1965). With higher doses subjects will experience shaking chills. The decrease in peripheral heat flow represents vasoconstriction and the chills reflect the need to produce more heat or thermogenesis. The peak temperature rise occurs approximately 3–4 h following injection and defervescence is usually noted by 7 h. Human volunteers receiving LPS will have an increase in metabolic rate as reflected by increase in oxygen consumption and it is well recognized that there is a 13% increase in oxygen consumption for every 1 °C rise in human body temperature.

The rhesus monkey, on the other hand, is markedly refractory to the pyrogenicity of LPS and in one study, some monkeys responded with hypothermia while in others 10^3–10^4 more LPS was required to produce fever (SHEAGREN et al. 1967). Monkeys covered with a light blanket, or unrestrained monkeys, responded with fever more regularly. Rhesus monkeys which are trained to sit in a chair will have a monophasic fever following intravenous injection of EP at the same dose per unit weight as the rabbit (PERLOW et al. 1975). Thus, it is unlikely that the hypothalamic response in rhesus monkeys is impaired but rather that experimental and environmental conditions play an important role in the febrile response of rhesus monkeys to LPS. The temperature response of mice and rats to LPS is variable and often hypothermic. This is particularly true of mice, although if mice are warmed to 37 °C 1 h prior to LPS, there is a greater likelihood they will have a febrile response to LPS (BODEL and MILLER 1976).

III. LPS Fever and EP Production

Studies performed some 25 years ago in rabbits established that fever produced by LPS was mediated by a circulating heat-labile substance, endogenous pyrogen (EP) (ATKINS and WOOD 1955a, b; reviewed by ATKINS 1960). Since these experiments, evidence has supported the fact that injection of LPS causes activation of phagocytic leucocytes followed by synthesis and release of EP into the circulation. Following intravenous injection of a moderate pyrogenic dose in rabbits, LPS is rapidly cleared from the circulation. In rabbits and humans, there is an initial leucopenia, mostly a granulocytopenia followed by granulocytosis (WOLFF et al. 1965b; WOLFF 1973) which is due mostly to young granulocytes being released from the marrow (CRADDOCK et al. 1956). Because both LPS and leucocytes disappear from the circulation at approximately the same time, it was postulated that circulating

Table 1. Effect of detoxifications on pyrogenicity of LPS

Treatment	Mechanism	Reduction in pyrogenicity	Reference
Sodium hydroxide	Saponification	10^2–10^6	NETER et al. (1956)
Lithium aluminium hydride	Cleavage of ester bonds	10^3	NOLL and BRAUDE (1961)
Sodium periodate	Oxidation	0	NETER et al. (1956)
Acetic anhydride	Acetylation	10^2	SCHENCK et al. (1969)
Succinic anhydride	Succinylation	10^2–10^3	SCHENCK et al. (1969)
Phthalic anhydride	Alkylation	10^4–10^5	CHEDID et al. (1975) ELIN and WOLFF (personal observation)

leucocytes take up LPS and then leave the vasculature or marginate. Leucocytes have been observed to marginate along the vascular endothelium after LPS, but they do not contain labelled LPS (ROWLEY et al. 1956; HERRING et al. 1963). Moreover, LPS appears to be cleared from the circulation before the leucopenia or significant fever (HERRING et al. 1963). While there is uncertainty about the role of circulating leucocytes in LPS clearance, there is no doubt that the reticulo-endothelial system (RES) contains the highest percentage of LPS following intravenous injection. The rapidity with which LPS leaves the circulation and enters the liver varies from 50% within the first minute to 90% after 5 min (*Rowley* et al. 1956; BRAUDE et al. 1955). Using radio-labelling as well as fluorescein-fixed anti-0 sera, LPS can be seen in the Kupffer cells of the liver. With the report that the Kupffer cells of the liver are potent producers of EP in vitro (DINARELLO et al. 1968), it seems likely that LPS activates these cells to produce EP following intravenous injection.

IV. LPS Structure and Ability to Produce Fever

The mechanism by which LPS activates phagocytic leucocytes to produce EP remains unexplained. During the First International Symposium on Endotoxins held in 1963, discussions centred around the identification of the "toxophore" of LPS which was responsible for the lethal, pyrogenic, vascular, and other properties of the molecule. Early investigation focused on molecular manipulation of LPS by agents which would alter the physical state and configuration of certain groups. This was done in an attempt to "detoxify" LPS. Table 1 lists some of the methods employed and their effects on the pyrogenicity of LPS. Acid hydrolysis results in 10,000–20,000 daltons subcomponents and leads to changes such as random transesterifications in the products of hydrolysis (RIBI et al. 1964; NOWOTNY 1964). Alkaline treatment leads to saponification of the fatty acids esters including O-acyl bonds and represents a major chemical change in the lipid portion of the molecule (NIWA et al. 1969). Alkaline treatment with 0.25 N NaOH at 56 °C for 5 min results in liberation of hydroxymyristic acid without loss of pyrogenicity. Longer treatment (60 min) leads to the loss of all the ester-linked fatty acids and a drastic reduction in pyrogenicity (NETER et al. 1956). Detoxified LPS has also been produced by treatment with $LiAlH_4$ which cleaves ester bonds (NOLL and BRAUDE 1961). It is interesting that treatment with $LiAlH_4$ markedly decreased pyrogenicity for rabbits and lethality for mice while preserving the antigenicity of the preparations. Other experiments have utilized boron trifluoride (BF_3), which causes transesterifications, and potassium methylate (CH_3OK) as a deacylating agent. More recently, detoxified LPS has been produced by acetylation and succinylation using acetic and succinic anhydride (SCHENCK et al. 1969). There is a 1,000-fold decrease in the pyrogenicity of LPS following succinylation while the adjuvanicity of LPS was not affected. The use of phthalic anhydrids as a strong alkylating agent has produced a modification of the LPS so that the ability to induce non-specific resistance to infection is maintained by the detoxified LPS, although a 10^4 reduction in pyrogenicity occurred accompanied by a 10^3 decrease in lethality for mice (CHEDID et al. 1975; ELIN and WOLFF, personal observation). Presumably, alkylation results in a nucleophilic substitution in the glucosamine or ethanolamine residues of the lipid A.

The ability of certain agents to reduce the toxicity and pyrogenicity of LPS while not affecting adjuvanicity suggests there are at least two active sites. Agents which alter the lipid A or its configuration with the R-core result in loss of pyrogenicity. Such results support the contention that the toxic and pyrogenic properties of LPS reside in the lipid A portion. LPS from mutants of *Salmonella minnesota* which do not contain the 0-polysaccharide are pyrogenic and LPS from mutants which lack the heptosephosphate polymer of the R-core are also toxic and pyrogenic (TRIPOLI and NOWOTNY 1966). These studies on mutants confirm the hypothesis that the 0-polysaccharide and R-core are not involved in pyrogenicity. However, the attachment of lipid A to the R-core is important since lipid A is insoluble in water and hence biologically inactive. The genus *Bacteroides* which contributes to the bowel flora of animals and humans produces a LPS with low potency pyrogenicity, toxicity, and gelation in the LAL test (SVEEN et al. 1977). Chemical studies on the LPS extracted from *Bacteroides fragilis* demonstrated that the molecule lacked two essential sugars – KDO and heptose (HOFSTAD and KRISTOFFERSON 1970). Using another strain of *B. fragilis*, this observation has been confirmed (KASPER 1976) and extraction with chloroform–methanol and alcohol indicated that the reduced potency of LPS from *Bacteroides* was due to a loose association between the polysaccharide and lipid moieties.

V. Lipid A and Pyrogenicity

Direct evidence that the pyrogenic property of LPS resides in the lipid A fraction was provided from experiments in which lipid A was complexed to either bovine or human serum albumin. This procedure solubilized the lipid for use in biological fluids while these carrier proteins were shown to be non-pyrogenic and biologically inert. Lipid A, when solubilized with pyridine or triethylamine, produces a typical biphasic fever at 0.2 µg/kg while complexing the same lipid A to proteins produces fever at 2 ng/kg (RIETSCHEL et al. 1973; LUEDERITZ et al. 1973), a concentration similar to that of the parent LPS. Others have reported also that the lipid A fractions contain the pyrogenic moiety (GALANOS et al. 1972). Depending on whether the lipid A is obtained by the original method for hydrolysis using 1 N

HCl (WESTPHAL and LUEDERITZ 1954) or a milder hydrolysis using acetic acid (CHANG and NOWOTNY 1975), recovery of the pyrogenicity in the parent LPS is variable. The original hydrolysis yields a lipid moiety in which only 1% of the activity is recovered. Lipid A complexed to bovine serum albumin (BSA) can also be used to immunize rabbits. After six daily intravenous immunizations, the rabbits had significantly decreased febrile responses when challenged with a hundred times the dose necessary to produce a fever (RIETSCHEL et al. 1973). There was no specificity to the protection afforded to the rabbits using the lipid A–BSA complex since immunized rabbits had similar decreased responses when callenged with the lipid A–BSA obtained from another strain of *Salmonella*. However, transfer of protection to lipid A–BSA could not be accomplished using antiserum (RIETSCHEL and LUEDERITZ 1975). An interesting aspect of this antiserum is that protection could be transfered if the recipient rabbits were given a large dose of lipid A–BSA 24 h before passive transfer of the antiserum. However, these results could also be due to the tolerance induced by a large dose of LPS prior to challenge (SNELL and ATKINS 1967).

More specific identification of the active site for pyrogenicity within the lipid A has been accomplished. These studies have utilized organic solvent partitioning and thin layer and column chromatography in silica gels. Lipid A, which was extracted with 0.5 N sulphuric acid and subjected to organic solvent partitioning chromatography, was separated into three components: neutral, polar I, and polar II lipids. The neutral lipids contained the fatty acids found in lipid A preparations, i.e. lauric, myristic, palmitic, and β-hydroxymyristic acids and these did not produce fever when complexed to BSA. The polar I lipid preparations contained the fatty acids and glucosamine and were a thousand times less pyrogenic than the parent LPS; polar II lipid preparations containing the fatty acids, glucosamine, and phosphorylethanolamine had the highest pyrogenic potency, approximately a hundred times that of the original LPS. These studies confirm the findings reported when the LPS molecule had been detoxified, e.g. the requirement for primary amino groups associated with esterified fatty acids. It is most likely then, that this configuration is critical for activation of phagocytic cells to produce EP.

VI. Pyrogenic Tolerance to LPS

Refractoriness, or tolerance are the terms frequently used to describe a well-known phenomenon of progressive resistance to the biological effects of LPS. This is best demonstrated with daily injections. Although tolerance to the lethal and other toxic manifestations of LPS have been reported (BENNETT and CLUFF 1957), pyrogenic tolerance has been most extensively studied. It is characterized by loss of the second peak of fever in rabbits and a reduction or disappearence of febrile responses in humans (WOOD 1958; ATKINS 1960; ATKINS and SNELL 1965; BEESON 1947 a, b; WOLFF et al. 1965 a, b, c). Pyrogenic tolerance to small doses of a purified LPS did not alter the responses of rabbits to EP (ATKINS and SNELL 1964). In both humans and rabbits receiving continuous infusion of LPS it has been reported that a progressive defervescence takes place after 4 h until body temperature returns to the baseline (GREISMAN and WOODWARD 1965; GREISMAN et al. 1966 b). In this state of tolerance, which persisted for 48 h and could be overcome by a large dose of LPS, the host likewise retained its reactivity to EP.

Both cellular and humoral mechanisms have been proposed to explain tolerance. As mentioned previously, LPS is primarily taken up by the RES, especially the Kupffer cells of the liver; however, in tolerant animals this hepatic uptake is markedly increased (BEESON 1947 b). This is reflected by both a faster rate of clearance from the blood and an absolute increase in the amount of LPS found in the liver (CAREY et al. 1957; SMITH et al. 1957; HERION et al. 1964). Morphological studies in animals treated with LPS have demonstrated hypertrophy and hyperplasia of the RES (BIOZZI et al. 1955; BENACERRAF et al. 1959; AGARWAL and BERRY 1968); furthermore, in such animals, there is also increased clearance of colloidal carbon and trypan blue (FISHER 1967; ARREDONDO and KAMPSCHMIDT 1963; WATNICK and GORDON 1964; AGARWAL and BERRY 1968). However, this hyperphagocytic state the RES also occurs with other agents like glucan, zymosan, thorotrast, BCG, and certain lipids (FISHER 1967; BENACERRAF et al. 1959; LEMPERLE 1966). Since animals given these other agents continue to succumb to the same dose of LPS as do normal controls (LEMPERLE 1966; AGARWAL and BERRY 1968), hypertrophy and hyperplasia of the RES does not, by itself, confer tolerance to LPS. Nevertheless, if RES stimulation is prevented by certain antimitotic drugs (TOBEY et al. 1966), pyrogenic tolerance fails to develop (BERRY and SMYTHE 1965).

It is well established that thorium dioxide (thorotrast) will reverse tolerance ("RES blockade") presumably by preventing the uptake of LPS by the RES (HOWARD et al. 1958; BEESON 1974 b; GARIELI and HOLMGREN 1952). Furthermore, thorotrast reduces the increased uptake of carbon and other colloids often observed in endotoxin tolerance (GREISMAN et al. 1963, 1964). Thorotrast, however, is not the only agent which has this property, for many large molecules which are taken up by the RES produce a comparable affect (FREEDMAN 1960 a, b, c). Although earlier work suggested that thorotrast "reverses" or "abolishes" tolerance (BEESON 1946, 1947 b; BENNETT and CLUFF 1952; ZWEIFACH et al. 1957), it has been shown to produce only partial reversal of tolerance (GREISMAN et al. 1963; WOLFF et al. 1965 c). The explanation for this partial reversal was that the thorotrast resets both the normal and tolerant host's reactivity to LPS (GREISMAN et al. 1964; WOLFF et al. 1965 c). Nevertheless, the hyper-reactivity of the RES in tolerance and the partial reversal of this state by thorotrast, remain the major evidence for the operation of a cellular mechanism in tolerance. There is no evidence that cells other than reticulo-endothelial tissue are changed in the tolerant state. Inflammatory exudate granulocytes from endotoxin-tolerant rabbits release normal amounts of pyrogen when exposed to LPS in vitro (COLLINS and WOOD 1959). This data has been confirmed by others (GREISMAN and HORNICK 1973; DINARELLO 1969). The evidence suggests that the Kupffer cells of tolerant rabbits remove LPS but do not respond by making EP; following RES blockade, LPS is shifted away from the Kupffer cells to the granulocytes where EP is produced.

The other mechanism proposed for tolerance is the development of specific humoral factors evoked by repeated doses of LPS. In his original paper, BEESON was unable to demonstrate transfer of tolerance with serum from rabbits given seven daily injections of typhoid vaccine (BEESON 1947 a). Also, specific anti-O antibodies apparently did not play a role since titres were elevated at a time when tolerance had completely lapsed. Other investigators similarly failed to transfer tolerance passively (CLUFF 1953), and found no correlation between the degree of pyrogenic tolerance and the titre of specific anti-O antibody (RUTENBERG et al. 1965; MORGAN 1948 a, b). Additional arguments against an immune mechanism were the findings that LPS from genus of Enterobacteriaceae would confer tolerance to LPS from immunologically unrelated genera (BEESON 1947 a; MORGAN 1948 a, b) and that tolerance developed readily in patients with agammaglobulinaemia (GOOD 1954; GOOD and VARCO 1955). BOIVIN (BOIVIN and MESROBEANU 1938), the first scientist to extract LPS from Gram-negative bacilli, found immune precipitates were still toxic as did MORGAN (1941), by mixing typhoid vaccine with antiserum in the zone of antibody excess.

However, as these data were being reported, evidence began appearing in favour of a humoral and immune mechanism for tolerance. The first was a well-known finding that after tolerance waned or lapsed, the phenomenon could be rapidly induced with only a few injections. This became known as the "anamnestic" response (NEVA and MORGAN 1950; FARR et al. 1954; WATSON and KIM 1963), although this term was admittedly presumptive. Later, the successful transfer of tolerance with tolerant serum was repeatedly demonstrated (KIM and WATSON 1965 a, b, 1966; GREISMAN et al. 1963; FREEDMAN 1960 a, b, 1959; WOLFF et al. 1964 a, b). Yet there were still experiments in which no correlation was found between the ability of the serum sample to confer tolerance and its anti-O titre (KIM and WATSON 1966; WOLFF et al. 1964 b; MULHOLLAND et al. 1965). But the apparent non-specificity of LPS tolerance was better defined and specific immunological relationships appeared significant in cross-tolerance (WATSON and KIM 1963, 1964).

Results from a small number of experiments support a direct relationship between the anti-O titre and the degree of tolerance. Both early rises in the anti-O antibodies (LANDY et al. 1955) as well as a linear relationship of the anti-O titre to protection against lethality have been demonstrated (LANDY 1953). Also, in a careful study, homologous immune precipitates were non-pyrogenic, ineffective in the Shwartzman reaction, and non-lethal to mice (RADVANY ct al. 1966; NOWOTNY et al. 1965; BERCZI 1967; OGATA and KANAMORI 1978). Furthermore, after absorbing the hyperimmune serum with specific detoxified LPS, there was a moderate return of pyrogenicity (RADVANY et al. 1966). However, these experiments do not rule out the possibility that a serum component which is not anti-O antibody had hence not measured could, nonetheless, be responsible for inactivation of the toxin.

The fraction of tolerant serum which is associated with successful passive transfer against the pyrogenic and lethal properties of LPS has been identified as 19 S or IgM immunoglobulin (KIM and WATSON 1965 a, b). However, this fraction has no detectable anti-O titre and yet transfers 90% of the pyrogenic tolerance. Of the several ways to measure the anti-O antibody in serum, including bactericidal potency, agglutination, passive haemagglutination, and bentonite flocculation, none seems to provide an accurate assay of humoral component which corresponds to the degree of tolerance (MULHOLLAND et al. 1965). In addition, although no specific anti-O antibodies develop in rabbits given immunosuppressive drugs, tolerance develops normally WOLFF et al. 1964 a, b). Also, tolerance can be demonstrated before the titre of anti-O antibody increases (MULHOLLAND et al. 1965; UR-

Table 2. Mechanisms for pyrogenic tolerance to LPS

Cellular	References
Rapid clearance of LPS from blood to RES	Rowley et al. (1956); Howard et al. (1958); Braude et al. (1955); Herring et al. (1963); Herion et al. (1964); Benacerraf and Sebestyen (1957)
Increased uptake and localization of LPS in RES	Smith et al. (1957); Herion et al. (1964); Benacerraf and Sebestyen (1957); Rowley et al. (1956); Braude et al. (1955); Carey et al. (1957)
Hyper-reactivity of RES	Biozzi et al. (1955); Benacerraf et al. (1959)
Hepatosplenomegaly	Agarwal and Berry (1968)
Reversal of tolerance after RES blockade	Beeson (1947b); Garieli and Holmgren (1952); Greisman et al. (1963); Beeson (1946); Wolff et al. (1965c)
Delayed clearance of LPS after RES blockade	Beeson (1947b); Bennett and Cluff (1952); Zweifach et al. (1957)
Less EP produced by Kupffer cells	Dinarello et al. (1969); Greisman and Hornick (1973)

Humoral	References
"Anamnestic" response	Neva and Morgan (1950); Farr et al. (1954); Watson and Kim (1963)
Immune precipitates nonpyrogenic and non-toxic	Radvany et al. (1966); Nowotny et al. (1965); Berczi (1967)
Passive transfer of tolerance with tolerant serum	Greisman et al. (1963); Greisman et al. (1964); Freedman (1959, 1960a, b, c); Wolff et al. (1964a, b, c)
Role of opsonins and natural antibody	Greisman et al. (1963); Rowley (1960)
No transferable factors after splenectomy	Greisman et al. (1966a)
Passive transfer of tolerance with sensitized spleen cells	Young and Greisman (1968)
In vitro neutralization of LPS	Ogata and Kanamori (1978)
Anti-lipid A antibodies	Luederitz et al. (1973)

Baschek and Nowotny 1968). Thus, it is apparent from these data that the factor in tolerant serum which confers tolerance is not anti-O antibody. The concept that the lipid moiety and the polysaccharide O-antigen are separate, first proposed in biochemical investigations of the LPS molecule, could explain the disparity between the antibody titre and the state of tolerance. It has been suggested that the lipid A elicits its own anti-LPS immunoglobulin which has a broad cross-reactivity with LPS of other Gram-negative enteric bacteria (Kim and Watson 1965a, b).

In addition, cellular immunological techniques have been employed to support the immune basis for tolerance. Splenectomy in both humans and rabbits prevented the development of tolerance and plasma from splenectomized rabbits failed to produce a transferable factor (GREISMAN et al. 1966a, b). Also, rapid acquisition of tolerance could be passively transferred with spleen cells from a donor rabbit immunized with LPS (YOUNG and GREISMAN 1968). Yet, thymectomy at birth seemingly does not effect the development of tolerance (CHEDID et al. 1964). Biologically, the responsible factor in tolerant serum has been thought to be an opsonin (GREISMAN et al. 1963; ROWLEY 1960) and IgM, likewise, is associated with the opsonic activity of serum (MICHAEL and ROSEN 1963). However, the opsonic activity in tolerant serum is apparently not reversed by thorotrast since tolerant serum continues to transfer tolerance after such RES blockading agents as thorotrast, trypan blue, or colloidal carbon (FREEDMAN 1960a). Although non-specific opsonic activity for carbon clearance was reported to have been passively transferred with tolerant serum (FREEDMAN 1960c; KAMPSCHMIDT et al. 1965), this observation was not confirmed in later studies and the former results were attributed to possible contamination of the carbon with LPS (GREISMAN et al. 1963; MURRAY 1963).

Natural antibodies to LPS or anti-O antibodies which are present without specific immunization may have a role in tolerance. Thus, the first injection of LPS could induce a secondary rather than a primary immunological response in the host. This would then explain the appearance of tolerance after the first or second injection (CREECH et al. 1949). However, this natural antibody does not seem to mediate LPS's toxicity because colostrum-deprived piglets and mice with no demonstrable IgG or IgM immunoglobins succumb to the lethality of LPS (CHEDID et al. 1964; CREECH et al. 1949; KIM and WATSON 1965a, b). Some investigators maintain that all biological manifestations of toxicity to LPS are secondary to an antibody–antigen interaction, i.e. a hypersensitive host reacting with endotoxin as the antigen (STETSON 1964; KOVATS 1967). Indeed, there has been increasing evidence for the role of "natural" immunization, perhaps from the gastrointestinal tract flora, as a prerequisite for the host's reaction to LPS (SNELL and BRAUDE 1961; SCHAEDLER and DUBOS 1961; BRAUDE and SIEMIENSKI 1961). Re-collection of the preceeding data is often a cumbersome task; Table 2 itemizes the salient arguments for the role of the RES or the immunological mechanism proposed to explain LPS tolerance.

E. Mycobacteria

Tuberculosis is frequently used as a clinical example of an insidious febrile disease. Most individuals with active infections will experience fevers and night sweats before other symptoms are recognized. The source of EP in tuberculosis may come from the interaction between the organism and the phagocytic cell which it parasitizes, the reactive granuloma, or the systemic reaction to products of the mycobacteria. Of these three, the role of soluble products has been the most studied and defined.

I. Febrile Reactions of BCG-Sensitized Animals

Several investigators have infected rabbits and guinea-pigs with BCG (bacillus Cal-
mette-Guérin) and later challenged these animals with intravenous injections of either old tuberculin (OT) or purified protein derivative (PPD) (Hall and Atkins
1959; Allen 1965a, b; Castrova et al. 1966). Following the injection of either OT
or PPD into sensitized animals, EP can be demonstrated in the circulation 3 h after
antigen challenge (Hall and Atkins 1959; Allen 1965a). Some investigators have
found that OT is a better antigen than PPD in inducing fever in animals sensitized
with BCG infections. However, OT, the more complex and heterogeneous of the
two antigenic preparations, is specific and does not produce fever in unsensitized
animals. Skin-test reactivity, which is often correlated with the febrile reaction
(Hall and Atkins 1959), is also more likely to be positive using OT as compared
with PPD. OT is a filtered preparation of autoclaved *Mycobacterium tuberculosis*
and contains cell wall materials, large amounts of polysaccharides and cytoplasmic
proteins; PPD, is a solubilized trichloracetic precipitate of culture supernatants,
may not contain cell wall substances and is mostly protein.

Whatever the physical nature of the exogenous pyrogen in either OT or PPD,
it is clear that its ability to produce fever is related to the state of hypersensitivity
of the host. Daily injections of OT in BCG-sensitized rabbits result in complete
pyrogenic tolerance within five days and can be correlated with disappearance of
the skin test (Hall and Atkins 1959; Moses and Atkins 1961). Rabbits desensitized to OT are not tolerant to viral-induced fevers and respond normally to EP
(Moses and Atkins 1961). Thus, the mechanism in pyrogenic tolerance to OT appears to be related to the ability of this antigen to liberate EP; this is supported by
the fact that tolerance to OT is not reversed by thorotrast (Hall and Atkins 1959)
as is pyrogenic tolerance to LPS.

Sensitivity to OT can be passively transferred to normal rabbits using either
plasma or cells from BCG-infected animals. Between 30 and 60 ml of serum or
plasma was necessary to transfer reactivity and when challenged 2–24 h after the
infusion of plasma from hypersensitive donors, recipient rabbits had small but significant monophasic fevers (Hall et al. 1970). The pyrogenic reactivity in these
normal recipients lasted for 1–3 days. The large quantities of serum used and the
small febrile responses suggest that humoral factors, presumably antibodies, are
not present in high titres or are rapidly excreted. Greater sensitivity to tuberculin
was transferred to normal rabbits with cells from BCG-sensitized donors. Peritoneal mononuclear, spleen, and lymph node cells were able to transfer pyrogenic
reactivity (Hall et al. 1970). Pyrogenic responses to OT were maximal 7–14 days
after transfer and then gradually subsided. These experiments suggest that antibody was being produced during this period and that the decrease in reactivity after
14 days represents either the death of the transferred cells or decreased antibody
production. When granulocytes from sensitized donors were transferred intravenously to normal recipients, responses to OT were maximal after 2 h while granulocytes transferred intraperitoneally were ineffective. From these results, the hypothesis was presented that antibody to tuberculin can passively sensitize the granulocyte which, in turn, releases EP when activated by OT (Atkins and Heijn 1965).

II. Release of EP from Cells Incubated with Tuberculin

Experiments in which phagocytic cells from sensitized or unsensitized donors have been incubated with tuberculin in vitro have confirmed the findings observed in vivo. Cells obtained from sensitized donors included rabbit or guinea-pig circulating blood leucocytes, lung alveolar macrophages, spleen cells, peritoneal granulocytes, and peritoneal macrophages (ATKINS and HEIJN 1965; HALL et al. 1970; ALLEN 1965b; CASTROVA et al. 1966; ATKINS et al. 1967; JOHANOVSKY 1959, 1960; MOORE et al. 1973). When these cells were incubated with either OT or PPD, EP was demonstrated in the culture supernatants 5–20 h later. Like the injection of antigen into sensitized animals, some investigators found OT a more reliable inducer of EP in vitro than PPD. These incubations were carried out in tissue culture buffers and media containing 10%–15% normal rabbit serum or no serum and thus demonstrate the ability of the phagocytic cell to react with tuberculin in the absence of added antibody. However, the role of incubating antibody in mediating the pyrogenic response to OT was supported by results obtained by incubating normal cells with serum from hypersensitive donors. Under these conditions OT was able to stimulate production from normal cells in the presence of hypersensitive, but not normal, rabbit serum (ATKINS and HEIJN 1965). Although the exact interaction of OT with antibody and cells has not been investigated, these experiments indicate that circulatory antibodies to tuberculin are cytophilic and that the antigen (or antigens) induce EP production by stimulating passively sensitized phagocytic leucocytes.

F. Fungi

Disseminated fungal infections are known to cause fever, although some fungal infections producing localized disease are also associated with fever. For example, patients with systemic histoplasmosis or isolated pulmonary infections due to *Coccidioides immitis* experience high fevers. Other fungi, such as cryptococci, ordinarily produce small fevers or no fever at all despite significant infection. The reason for the varied febrile response in fungal infections may be related to the inflammatory response of the host to the fungi. Another explanation for the disparity between the degree of infection and the amount of fever could be related to the degree of host sensitization to fungal products. Studies have suggested that fever to fungal products often requires prior exposure to fungal antigens. Most experiments have focused on the ability of fungal cells themselves or fungal products to produce fever.

I. Pyrogenicity of Fungal Cells

Rabbits have been injected intravenously with a number of live fungal cells; these have included *Candida albicans* (KOBAYASHI and FRIEDMAN 1964; BRAUDE et al. 1960), *Candida tropicals* (SALVIN et al. 1965), *Cryptococcus albidus* (BRIGGS and ATKINS 1966), *Cryptococcus neoformans* (KOBAYASHI and FRIEDMAN 1964), *Blastomyces dermatitidis*, *Histoplasma capsulatum*, and *Sporotrichum schenckii* (BRAUDE et al. 1960). Even the non-pathogenic bread yeast, *Saccharomyces cerevisiae*, has been tested (KOBAYASHI and FRIEDMAN 1964). In all cases fever ensued following the injection of 10^7–10^9 live organisms. In other studies as few as 10^5 cells produced fever. The latent period before onset of fever was usually 60 min or greater, and in most circumstances, the fever was biphasic with the maximal temperature elevation occurring 4–5 h later. In one report, EP was demonstrated to be circulating during the fever (BRAUDE et al. 1960). Autoclaved or formalin-killed yeast cells cells were as pyrogenic as live cells, indicating that fevers occur in the absence of infection and thus is due perhaps to the particulate nature of the cells. There is also a report that spheroblasts obtained by enzymatic degradation of the cell wall of *Candida albicans* are as pyrogenic as untreated cells (KOBAYASHI et al. 1964). The ability of whole yeast cells from several genera to produce fever was not affected by pyrogenic tolerance to LPS (BRIGGS and ATKINS 1966; SALVIN et al. 1965) and supports the contention that yeasts do not synthesize LPS. Furthermore, repeated injections of yeast cells did not result in pyrogenic tolerance but, in some cases, increased febrile responsiveness. This was most often observed in rabbits given live or autoclaved histoplasma or blastomyces organisms in which the fever produced 14 days after the initial injection of yeast cells increased four-fold (BRAUDE et al. 1960). In experiments where live or killed yeast cells are used, the precise mechanisms of their pyrogenicity are difficult to ascertain since there are several fungal antigens associated with the cell walls. Extracting the yeast cells of *Candida* or *Saccharomyces* with ether, phenol, or trichloracetic acid did not reduce their pyrogenicity (KOBAYASHI and FRIEDMAN 1964). Although these data suggest that the fever produced from fungal organisms is due to their particulare nature, the injection of the same number of LPS-free latex particles of similar size as the yeast cells did not produce fever. It is more likely that, even after autoclaving and extraction procedures, antigenic moieties still remain which are necessary for phagocytosis and EP production. Purified cell wall preparations of *C. albicans* devoid of cytoplasmic proteins were as pyrogenic as extracted cell walls (KOBAYASHI and FRIEDMAN 1964).

II. Fever from Fungal Products

Culture broths often contain several fungal products either produced and secreted into the broth or released as yeast cells die. Filtered broths from culture of *Candida* and *Cryptococcus* have been highly pyrogenic in rabbits (BRAUDE et al. 1960; BRIGGS and ATKINS 1966; HALEY et al. 1966). Although rabbits respond to *Candida* soluble products, only rabbits previously exposed to cryptococci had febrile responses to the autologous soluble agent (BRIGGS and ATKINS 1966). Once again, pyrogenic tolerance to LPS had no effect on the response to fungal products. However, despite the finding that daily injections of whole yeast cells do not induce pyrogenic tolerance, repeated injections of soluble extracts result in complete pyrogenic unresponsiveness after three days. These data suggest that pyrogenicity of the soluble agents is related to the state of sensitization of the recipients.

The soluble agent from cryptococci has been fractionated and found to contain two pyrogenic moieties. Using cold ethanol precipitation of the soluble extract, a capsular polysaccharide was isolated and found to be pyrogenic in normal rabbits, i.e. rabbits not previously exposed to cryptococci (HALEY et al. 1966). The mechanism by which this polysaccharide induces fever is unclear and may involve a direct stimulatory effect on the phagocyte membrane in a fashion similar to that of lipid A. Cryptococcal polysaccharide, however, produces fever in LPS-tolerant rabbits. A protein fraction was obtained from ethanol-soluble material and produced fever only in rabbits previously sensitized with soluble products from cryptococci. There was no correlation between fever and skin reactivity to the antigen but with the induction of pyrogenic tolerance, skin-test reactivity similarly waned. Further evidence was presented that the pyrogenicity of the protein fraction from cryptococcal products was mediated by sensitized mononuclear cells and not humoral factors.

G. Non-Microbial Antigens

The study of the pyrogenicity of non-microbial antigens has resulted in a better understanding of certain drug-induced or allergic fevers and has formed the basis for explaining fevers due to immunological diseases. In general, two phenomena have been defined: (1) Antibody-mediated immune fevers where a circulating specific antibody is necessary for the pyrogenicity of the antigen and (2) cell-mediated fevers where sensitized cells are required. Although it has been shown that the pyrogenicity of several microbial antigens is dependent on the state of host sensitization, the use of non-microbial, well-defined specific antigens, free of LPS or other microbial toxins has broadened the concept of immune fevers. Whereas microbial infections induce EP synthesis by several mechanisms, non-microbial antigens seem to cause fever by processes solely related to their antigen structure.

I. Antibody-Mediated Fever

FARR and his colleagues were the first investigators to demonstrate that specific antibody could be passively transferred to normal rabbits and mediate immune fever (GREY et al. 1961). In these studies rabbits which were immunized with BSA and then challenged with specific antigen developed biphasic fevers (FARR 1958, 1959). In other studies, rabbits sensitized to human serum albumin which was free of LPS developed fever when challenged with specific antigen and during the fever, EP was detected in the circulation (ROOT and WOLFF 1968). Not all immunized rabbits developed fever, although circulating antibodies were uniformally present. It appeared that there was a positive correlation between the type of anti-BSA antibody and the febrile response following antigen challenge; rabbits producing non-precipitating antibodies developed fever while those with strong antigen binding capacity had minimal pyrogenic responses (FARR 1959). Others have also made a similar observation using human serum albumin (HSA) in immune fever in rabbits (MOTT and WOLFF 1966). In this latter study 20% of immunized rabbits did not develop fever despite the presence of circulating antibody to the HSA. Thus, it is likely that the type of antibody and its combination with antigen play an important role in mediating these immune fevers. Gel filtration of whole anti-HSA serum demonstrated that the transfer of pyrogenic responses to HSA could be accomplished by fractions containing 7S or IgG antibody (MOTT and WOLFF 1966). Passive transfer of sensitized spleen cells did not impart pyrogenic responsiveness to

BSA and confirms the observation that these fevers are mediated by circulating antibody and not sensitized lymphocytes (GREY et al. 1961). The mechanism by which HSA produces fever in either the actively or passively sensitized host is through the formation of antigen–antibody complexes (ROOT and WOLFF 1968). Five minutes following the intravenous injection of HSA into sensitized rabbits there is a transferable pyrogen in the serum which produces fever in normal rabbits. The fever induced by this pyrogen is similar to that of a sensitized rabbit and most likely represents immune complexes. This was supported by experiments in which soluble immune complexes (HSA–anti-HSA) were made in vitro in ten times antigen excess and, when infused into normal rabbits, produced fevers similar to those exhibited by immunized animals challenged with HSA or normal rabbits receiving the five-minute pyrogen. These soluble complexes were also associated with a decrease in haemolytic complement titres and when total complement was depleted with cobra venom, there was a diminished febrile reaction to the immune complexes (MICKENBERG et al. 1971). From these experiments it is apparent that antibody-mediated immune fever requires the formation of immune complexes associated with the consumption of certain complement components and leads to EP production. Attempts to induce EP synthesis in vitro with normal phygocytic cells and immune complexes have failed (ROOT and WOLFF 1968) but this may be due to cell culture requirements, which are at present unknown.

Tolerance to immune complexes also develops with daily injections and is rapid and often complete. Pyrogenic tolerance to LPS has no effect on immune fever and rabbits made tolerant to immune complexes respond normally to EP or LPS (ROOT and WOLFF 1968; MICKENBERG et al. 1971). Thorotrast blockade of the RES does not reverse pyrogenic tolerance to the antigen in sensitized rabbits, to immune complexes in normal rabbits, or to OT in BCG-infected rabbits and confirms the observations that antibody-mediated immune fever is produced by mechanisms different from that of LPS or other microbial toxins. Complement consumption may play a role in pyrogen tolerance to immune complexes (MICKENBERG et al. 1971). It is possible also that daily injections of antigen induce the formation of special blocking antibodies or antibodies which remove the antigen without inducing EP; however, experiments have failed to transfer pyrogenic immune tolerance with serum from tolerant rabbits (MOTT and WOLFF 1966). There is also the possibility that certain EP-producing cells become "desensitized" to antigens with daily injections and account for pyrogenic tolerance in immune fevers. This has been shown for the streptococcal erythrogenic antigen (SCHUH and HRIBALOVA 1966), LPS (DINARELLO et al. 1968), and OT (DINARELLO 1969) but has not been studied to date with antigens like HSA or BSA.

Other investigators have reported the essential role of antibody in mediating certain immune fevers. Rabbits sensitized to penicillin develop haemagglutinating antibodies to benzylpenicillin and biphasic fevers when challenged with penicillin–protein conjugates (CHUSID and ATKINS 1972). Pyrogenic responsiveness could also be transferred to unsensitized rabbits with serum from immunized rabbits and this antibody-containing serum was also necessary for in vitro EP release by sensitized blood cells incubated with the antigen. In humans, fever developed in subjects who had circulating anti-D-type antibodies when challenged with D-type red blood cells (JANDL and TOMLINSON 1958) and also in patients who had leucoagglutinins when given leucocytes (BRITTINGHAM and CHAPLIN 1957). Thus, from human and animal models there is sufficient evidence that certain immune fevers are mediated by circulating antibodies.

II. Cell-Mediated Immune Fever

Experiments using the antigen OT in BCG-sensitized rabbits had demonstrated that sensitized spleen and lymph node cells could transfer pyrogenic reactions to OT in normal rabbits 7–10 days later (HALL et al. 1970). The interpretation of these experiments suggested that transferred sensitized cells synthesized specific antibody to OT which enabled the unsensitized rabbit to respond to antigenic challenge. More recently, the role of senitized cells in mediating non-microbial immune fever has been studied in rabbits and guinea-pigs. Using the antigens BSA and bovine γ-globulin (BGG) conjugated to dinitrophenol, rabbits responded to antigen challenge with biphasic fevers (ATKINS et al. 1972). When phagocytic blood cells from recently sensitized or unsensitized rabbits were incubated in vitro with antigen, EP was produced only when sensitized draining lymph node cells were present. The requirement for sensitized lymph node cells was also shown using peritoneal macrophages from normal guniea-pigs. These cells produced EP in vitro when incubated with antigen in the presence of sensitized lymph node cells; however, in these studies more EP production occurred during a second harvest of supernatant fluid 42 h after the addition of antigen and indicate a time-dependent mechanism for the interaction of antigen with the sensitized lymphocytes (CHAO et al. 1977). It should be pointed out that lymphocytes, regardless of the species or state of sensitization do not produce EP when stimulated by phagocytic, toxic, or immunological stimuli (ROOT et al. 1970; ATKINS et al. 1972). However, sensitized lymph node cells which are incubated with specific antigen for 18 h do release substances, presumably "lymphokines," into the supernatant and these, in turn, stimulate phagocytic cells to synthesize EP (ATKINS et al. 1972). This pyrogen-inducing lymphokine (PIL) has been demonstrated from rabbit lymph node lymphocytes sensitized to BGG, BSA, and ovalbumin (ATKINS et al. 1972, 1978; ATKINS and FRANCIS 1978) and induces the production of EP from unsensitized mixed blood leucocytes, peritoneal macrophages, monocytes, and Kupffer cells. The peripheral blood neutrophil does not release EP when incubated with either sensitized lymph node cells or PIL (ATKINS et al. 1978). The release of PIL from sensitized lymph node cells incubated with specific antigen correlated with skin-test reactivity of the donor rabbit. In further experiments, no evidence was found that antigen–antibody complexes were responsible for the PIL activity (ATKINS et al. 1978). Since irradiated sensitized lymphocytes and lymph node cells obtained from sensitized rabbits treated with corticosteroids were able to produce PIL, this substance is apparently a product of T-lymphocytes (ATKINS and FRANCIS 1978). It can be concluded from these studies that in some immune fevers, the interaction of antigen with sensitized T-lymphocytes occurs before EP is produced from phagocytic cells, resulting in the release of a pyrogen inducing lymphokine. Why this lymphokine is not produced by peripheral blood lymphocytes from sensitized rabbits and why it does not produce fever when injected into unsensitized animals has not been explained. Nevertheless, it is clear that a model for cell-mediated immune fevers has been developed and can be used to study the production of fever in many immunological diseases.

H. Pyrogenic Steroids

I. Fever in Humans

In 1956, Kappas and co-workers demonstrated that certain steroid metabolites of adrenal and testicular origin produced fever in humans (Kappas et al. 1956). It had been generally assumed that conjugation during their metabolism rendered these substances biologically inactive. Of the several metabolic end-products of steroidal metabolism, etiocholanolone has received the most attention and is considered the prototype of the pyrogenic steroids. Interest in etiocholanolone was heightened in 1958 by reports that plasma levels of unconjugated etiocholanolone increased in certain patients with fever, particularly in patients with "cyclic fevers" (Bondy et al. 1958). Soon thereafter, the syndrome of "etiocholanolone fever" had become synonymous with these and certain other fevers of unknown origin. However, subsequent studies using a double-isotope derivative method demonstrated that levels of etiocholanolone did not correlate with fever and in many patients, etiocholanolone levels fell during fever (George et al. 1969; Wolff et al. 1967).

"Etiocholanolone fever" is no longer recognized as a clinical entity or cause of "periodic fever" but nevertheless, etiocholanolone has been useful as an agent in producing experimental fever and other physiological changes in humans (Wolff et al. 1967). The pyrogenic property of etiocholanolone, like other pyrogenic steroids, is dependent on the steroid configuration of the molecules. For etiocholanolone, the position of the hydrogen on the number 5 carbon atom imparts pyrogenicity to the molecule; the 5-β position corresponds to a pyrogen-active molecule while the 5-α hydrogen molecules produce no fever (Kappas et al. 1960). Etiocholanolone and other pyrogenic steroids produce fever in humans but not in the rabbit; other pyrogenic steroids (including etiocholanolone) have been studied and do not produce fever in the dog, cat, guinea-pig, rat, or mouse (Kappas et al. 1957; Kappas and Ratkovits 1960). This species specificity has not been observed with bacterial lipopolysaccharide. It is interesting that the fever induced by etiocholanolone can only be blocked by the local administration of adrenal corticosteroids at the same site as the etiocholanolone (Wolff et al. 1973). Another interesting property of this pyrogen is the marked differences in febrile responses of the sexes (Kimball et al. 1967). This property may be related to oestrogens and is not seen with endotoxin (Wolff et al. 1973).

After administration of intramuscular etiocholanolone to human subjects, a latent period of 8–12 h ensues and then there is an abrupt increase in temperature, frequently associated with chills, myalgias, headache, and occasional vomiting (Wolff et al. 1967). At this time, pain usually begins at the site of injection. Fever reaches a maximum 12–16 h after the administration of etiocholanolone and then subsides within 24 h.

II. Pyrogenic Steroid-Induced EP

Incubation of etiocholanolone with human peripheral blood leucocytes results in the release of EP (BODEL and DILLARD 1966, 1968; DILLARD and BODEL 1967; WOLFF et al 1967); moreover, human monocytes seem to be the source of EP in these experiments (BODEL and DILLARD 1968). Unlike other activators of EP, 4–8 h exposure of leucocytes to etiocholanolone is required and may reflect the same process observed in human subjects given intramuscular etiocholanolone. Rabbit leucocytes do not synthesize EP when exposed to this steroid and this is consistent with the failure of etiocholanolone to produce fever in rabbits. There was a positive correlation between the ability of pyrogenic C_{19} steroids to produce fever in vivo and cause EP release in vitro (BONDY and BODEL 1971). There was less correlation for the C_{21} steroids, but, in general, the specificity of the chemical configuration required for pyrogenicity was consistent. In addition, a bile acid, lithocholic acid, produced EP in vitro and is reported to cause fever in vivo (BONDY and BODEL 1971).

The release of EP in vitro from leucocytes incubated with etiocholanolone was reduced 50% when the incubation took place in the presence of cortisol (BONDY and BODEL 1971; DILLARD and BODEL 1970). This was not specific for etiocholanolone since a similar reduction in EP production was observed for leucocytes activated by phagocytosis of staphylococci. Oestradiol also produced a significant reduction in EP from these leucocytes but had no effect on etiocholanolone-activated cells (DILLARD and BODEL 1970). Although oestrogens do have anti-inflammatory properties for human leucocytes (BODEL et al. 1972), this is apparently not the mechanism to explain why females exhibit significantly reduced febrile responses to etiocholanolone (KIMBALL et al. 1967).

J. Miscellaneous Exogenous Pyrogens

I. Polynucleotides

Polyinosinic–polycytidylic acid (poly I:C) a synthetic double-stranded RNA, is a well-known stimulator of interferon and in certain animal tumours has been shown to have antitumour activity. Poly I:C is also a potent pyrogen in animals and humans (NORDLUND et al. 1970b; LINDSAY et al. 1969). In rabbits, the intravenous injection of 30–50 µg of poly I:C produces a biphasic fever which has a latent period of one hour and reaches a maximal temperature elevation 4 h later (NORDLUND ct al. 1970b). Other investigators have killed rabbits 1 h after intravenous injection of 0.5 µg/kg poly I:C and found that Kupffer cells of the liver and the splenic cells would spontaneously release EP into the supernatant medium (GANDER and GOODALE 1975). The hepatocytes and circulating blood leucocytes did not release EP under these circumstances.

The pyrogenic properties of poly I:C have also been studied in vitro. Rabbit circulating blood leucocytes (buffy coat cells) will release EP when incubated with 30 µg/ml poly I:C overnight (NORDLUND et al. 1970b; COX and RAFTER 1971), although there is one report in which rabbit leucocytes did not release EP when incubated with concentrations of the polynucleotide as high as 100 µg/ml (FLEETwood et al. 1975). Human peripheral blood leucocytes consistently fail to release EP when stimulated by poly I: C and this has been shown to be due to the presence of double-stranded ribonuclease in human serum (Nordlund et al. 1970 b). Other sera from chickens and foetal calves also contain this ribonuclease and concentrations of human sera as low as 15% completely inactivate the pyrogenicity of the polynucleotide. Evidence was also presented that the pyrogenicity of poly I: C was, in fact, due to the integrity of the long-chain polynucleotides. The inactivation of labelled poly I: C by human serum revealed the generation of single and short oligonucleotides. This inactivation is also associated with the abolition of the capacity of these agents to induce the formation of interferon in both tissue culture and mice (Nordlund et al. 1970 b). Thus, the pyrogenicity and interferon-inducing ability of poly I: C requires the structure of the double-stranded chain.

Recently, poly I: C was shown to produce a positive gelation of the LAL test (Elin and Wolff 1973). When the poly I: C was enzymatically degraded by ribonuclease, it lost its ability to cause the gelation. These studies support other experiments that the pyrogenicity of the polynucleotides is not due to contaminating LPS. Whether the mechanism for poly I: C and LPS to produce the gelation of the LAL and their ability to induce EP synthesis is the same is unknown at this time.

II. Colchicine and Vinblastine

Colchicine and vinblastine are plant alkaloids of known structure which selectively bind to the monomers of microtubular proteins and prevent assembly. Colchicine usually inhibits cells by preventing the formation of microtubules and cell functions like chemotaxis, adhesiveness, degranulation, and phagocytosis are impaired. Although colchicine does not produce fever in rabbits or humans, the drug induces the production of EP from blood phagocytes in vitro (Bodel 1976). Concentrations of 10^{-5} and 10^{-4} M have been shown to induce collagenase and prostaglandin synthesis from human synovial cells in vitro (Harris and Krane 1971; Robinson et al. 1975). Two observations indicate that colchicine is not contaminated with LPS: (a) lumicolchicine, a light-inactivated form, does not induce EP production and (b) colchicine has no effect on rabbit phagocytes. Vinblastine, although not as potent, also caused human cells to release EP. It is not clear whether the ability of these agents to block microtubule formation is related to the induction of EP synthesis. Colchicine in the same concentrations used in the EP studies causes protein synthesis in mouse macrophages (Werb and Gordon 1975).

III. Bleomycin

Bleomycin is an antineoplastic agent isolated from *Streptomyces verticillus* and is highly effective against squamous cell carcinomas and lymphomas (Ichikawa et al. 1969; Rudders 1972). It is thought to exert its antitumour activity by inducing breaks in DNA.

Although bleomycin has no significant bone marrow toxicity, side effects such as acute febrile reactions and hypotension are often reported following intravenous injections (Rudders 1972; Mosher et al. 1972). Although bleomycin is negative in the LAL test, these reactions are similar to those for drugs contaminated with LPS in rabbits (DINARELLO et al. 1973). Even though it is clear that bleomycin is not contaminated with LPS, the drug is pyrogenic in rabbits, producing a prolonged monophasic fever after a latent period of 60 min and lasting 6–12 h which is associated with leucopenia lasting the duration of the fever (DINARELLO et al. 1973). There is no cross-pyrogenic tolerance between the drug and LPS. EP can be produced in vitro when human blood leucocytes are incubated with bleomycin and EP can be transferred in vivo. In rabbits treated with large doses of bleomycin and then challenged 24 h later with LPS, there was no evidence of renal cortical necrosis (generalized Shwartzman reaction). It is not clear whether the antineoplastic function of this drug is responsible for EP induction.

IV. Synthetic Adjuvants

Adjuvants are valuable in the amplification of immune responses. The best-known and certainly most widely used adjuvant in the laboratory is a mixture of non-metabolizable oil and dead mycobacteria (complete Freund's adjuvant). Because of certain toxic side effects of complete adjuvants, attempts have been made to separate the adjuvant responsible moiety of mycobacteria from other cell wall components. This led to the identification of a small water-soluble subunit of the peptidoglycan molecule from *Mycobacterium smegmatis* which enhanced the antibody response to antigens (ADAM et al. 1974). These studies were carried out further and the compound, N-acetylmuramyl–L-alanyl–D-isoglutamine (MDP) was synthesized and found to possess all of the immunogenic properties of the mycobacterial adjuvant (CHEDID et al. 1976). Since MDP effectively increases antibody responses in the absence of oil and also when administered orally, its potential use in human immunization cannot be overstated. However, MDP has been shown to be pyrogenic in rabbits (KOTANI et al. 1976; DINARELLO et al. 1978). MDP is not contaminated with LPS. The synthetic compound produces a positive LAL test in concentrations 10–20 times greater than required to produce fever in rabbits (DINARELLO et al. 1978; KOTANI et al. 1977) and there was no cross-tolerance to the pyrogenicity of LPS (DINARELLO et al. 1978). The fevers produced by MDP and two of its structural analogues, N-acetylmuramyl–L-alanyl–D-glutamic acid (MDPA) or the dimethylester of MDPA, are biphasic with a latent period of 1 h after injection and peak fevers occurring 2–4 h later. The amount of MDP which produced fevers varied from 50 to 200 µg while comparable fevers required 400–1,000 µg of MDPA or its dimethyl ester. Thus, the two structural analogues of MDP were less pyrogenic. The adjuvant properties and potencies of these structural analogues were not diminished from that of parent compound, MDP (AUDIBERT et al. 1976). Thus, the pyrogenic and adjuvant properties of these molecules seem separable.

MDP induces EP synthesis by human and rabbit mononuclear phagocytes (DINARELLO et al. 1978). The concentrations used to induce EP synthesis were 10 µg/ml for rabbit cells while 100–1,000 µg/ml were required to induce human EP. MDPA and dimethyl MDPA were 10–50 times less potent in vitro than MDP. The importance of these studies concerns the precise molecular structure of these synthetic compounds essential for the activation of EP production and the fact that these microbial-derived substances, although synthesized, are able to cause fever and induce EP independent of the presence of specific antibodies or skin-test

Table 3. Exogenous Pyrogens which induce Production of Endogenous Pyrogen

Exogenous pyrogens	Pyrogenic substance	Mechanism of EP-induction
Viruses	Whole virus	Cell infection
	Haemagglutinin	Haemagglutin function?
Gram-positive organisms	Whole organism	Phagocytosis
	Peptidoglycans	Toxicity?
	Teichoic acids	Antigen?, Toxicity?
	Exotoxins	Toxicity
	Enterotoxins	Toxicity
	Proteins	Antigenic
	Erythrogenic toxins	Toxicity
Gram-negative organisms	Whole organism	Phagocytosis
	Peptidoglycans	Toxicity?
	LPS	Toxicity and antigenic
	Lipid A	Toxicity
Mycobacteria	Whole organism	Phagocytosis
	Peptidoglycans	Toxicity?
	Polysaccharides (OT)	Antigenic
	Proteins (OT and PPD)	Antigenic
Fungi	Whole yeast	Phagocytosis
	Capsular polysaccharide	Toxicity
	Proteins	Antigenic
Non-microbial antigens	BSA	Antibody-mediated
	HSA	Antibody-mediated
	BGG	Cell-mediated
	Ovalalbumin	Cell-mediated
	Penicillin	Antibody-mediated
Pyrogenic steroids	Etiocholanolone	?
	5-β-Androstane-3-α-ol-17-one	?
	5-β-pregnane-3-α-ol-20-one	?
	Lithocholic acid	?
Polynucleotides	poly I:C	Double-stranded RNA
Antitumour agents	Bleomycin	DNA breaks ?
Plant alkaloids	Colchicine	Prevention of microtubule formation?
	Vinblastine	Prevention of microtubule formation?
Synthetic adjuvants	MDP	Toxicity?

reactivity. The minimal structure essential for pyrogenicity seems to be the dipeptide, L-alanyl–D-isoglutamine, while the complete molecule containing the muramic acid is a more potent pyrogen (MASEK et al. 1978).

References

Adam A, Ciarbaru R, Ellouz F, Petit JF, Lederer E (1974) Adjuvant activity of monomeric bacterial cell wall peptidoglycans. Biochem Biophys Res Commun 56:561–567

Agarwal MK, Berry LJ (1968) Effect of Actinomycin-D on RES and development of tolerance to endotoxin in mice. RES 5:353–367

Allen IV (1965 a) A study of the liberation of pyrogen by hypersensitive cells in incubation in vitro with specific antigen. J Path Bacterial 90:115–122

Allen IV (1965 b) The pathogenesis of fever in delayed hypersensitivity. Ir J Med Sci 17:207–235

Arredondo MI, Kampschmidt RF (1963) Effect of endotoxins on phagocytic activity of the RES of the rat. Proc Soc Exp Biol Med 112:78–81

Artenstein MS, Cadigan FC Jr, Buescher EL (1965) Clinical and epidemiological features of Coxsackie Group B virus infections. Ann Intern Med 63:597–603

Atkins E (1960) Pathogenesis of fever. Physiol Rev 40:580–605

Atkins E, Bodel P (1974) Fever. In: Zweibach BW, Grant L, McCluskey RT (eds) Academic Press, New York, pp 467–514

Atkins E, Bodel P (1979) Clinical fever: its history, manifestations, and pathogenesis. Fed Proc 38:57–63

Atkins E, Francis L (1978) Pathogenesis of fever in delayed hypersensitivity: factors influencing release of pyrogen-inducing lymphokines. Infect Immun 21:806–812

Atkins E, Freedman LR (1963) Studies in staphylococcal fever. I. Responses to bacterial cells. Yale J Biol Med 35:451–471

Atkins E, Heijn C (1965) Studies on tuberculin fever. III. Mechanism involved in the release of endogenous pyrogen in vitro. J Exp Med 122:207–235

Atkins E, Huang WC (1958 a) Studies on the pathogenesis of fever with influenzal viruses. I. The apperance of an endogenous pyrogen in the blood following intravenous injection of virus. J Exp Med 107:383–435

Atkins E, Huang WC (1958 b) Studies on the pathogenesis of fever with influenzal viruses. II. The effects of endogenous pyrogen in normal and virus-tolerant recipients. J Exp Med 107:403–414

Atkins E, Huang WC (1958) Studies on the pathogenesis of fever with influenzahl viruses. III. The relation of tolerance to the production of endogenous pyrogen. J Exp Med 107:415–453

Atkins E, Morse SI (1967) Studies in staphylococcal fever. VI. Responses induced by cell walls and various fractions of staphylococci and their products. Yale J Biol Med 39:297–311

Atkins E, Snell ES (1964) A comparison of the biological properties of Gram-negative bacterial endotoxin with leukocyte and tissue pyrogens. In: Landy M, Braun W (eds) Bacterial endotoxins. Rutgers University Press, New Brunswick, pp 134–148

Atkins E, Snell ES (1965) Fever. In: Zweibach BW, Grant L, McCluskey RJ (eds) The inflammatory process. Academic Press, New York, pp 495–525

Atkins E, Wood WB Jr (1955 a) Studies on the pathogenesis of fever. I. The presence of transferable pyrogen in the blood stream following the infection of typhoid vaccine. J Exp Med 101:519–528

Atkins E, Wood WB Jr (1955 b) Studies of the pathogenesis of fever. II. Identification of an endogenous pyrogen in the blood stream following the injection of typhoid vaccine. J Exp Med 102:499–516

Atkins E, Cronin M, Isacson P (1964) Endogenous pyrogen release from rabbit blood cells incubated in vitro with parainfluenza virus. Science 146:1469–1470

Atkins E, Bodel P, Francis L (1967) Release of an endogenous pyrogen in vitro from rabbit mononuclear cells. J Exp Med 126:357–386

Atkins E, Feldman JD, Francis L, Hursh E (1972) Studies on the mechanism of fever accompanying delayed hypersensitivity. The role of the sensitized lymphocyte. J Exp Med 135:1113–1132

Atkins E, Francis L, Berheim HA (1978) Pathogenesis of fever in delayed hypersensitivity: role of monocytes. Infect Immun 21:813–820

Audibert F, Chedid L, LeFrancier P, Choay J (1976) Distinctive adjuvanicity of synthetic analogs of myobacterial water – soluble components. Cell Immunol 21:243–249

Barsumian EL, Cunningham CM, Schlievert PM, Watson DW (1978) Heterogeneity of group A streptococcal pyrogenic exotoxin type B. Infect Immun 20:512–518

Beeson PB (1946) Development of tolerance to typhoid bacterial pyrogen and its abolition by reticuloendothelial blockade. Proc Soc Exp Biol Med 61:248–251

Beeson PB (1947a) Tolerance to bacterial pyrogens. I. Factors influencing its development. J Exp Med 86:29–39

Beeson PB (1947b) Tolerance to bacterial pyrogens. II. Role of the reticuloendothelial system. J Exp Med 86:39–48

Benacerraf B, Sebestyen MM (1957) The effect of bacterial endotoxins on the reticuloendothelial system. Fed Proc 16:860–867

Benacerraf B, Thorbecke GJ, Jacoby D (1959) Effect of zymosan on endotoxin toxicity in mice. Proc Soc Exp Biol Med 100:796–799

Bennett IL Jr, Beeson PB (1950) The properties of biologic effects of bacterial pyrogens. Medicine 29:365–400

Bennett IL Jr, Cluff LE (1952) Influence of nitrogen mustard upon reactions to bacterial endotoxin. Shwartzman phenomenon and fever. Proc Soc Exp Biol Med 81:304–308

Bennett IL Jr, Cluff LE (1957) Bacterial pyrogens. Pharmacol Rev 9:427–458

Berczi I (1967) Endotoxin neutralizing effect of antisera to E. coli endotoxins. Immun Forsch 132:303–318

Berry LJ, Smythe DS (1965) Some metabolic aspects of tolerance to bacterial endotoxin. J Bacteriol 90:970–977

Biozzi G, Benacerraf B, Halpern BN (1955) The effect of Salmonella typhi and its endotoxin on the phagocytic activity of the reticulo-endothelial system in mice. Br J Exp Pathol 36:226–239

Bodel P (1970) Studies on the mechanism of endogenous pyrogen production. I. Investigation of new protein synthesis by stimulated human blood leukocytes. Yale J Biol Med 43:145–163

Bodel P (1974) Studies on the mechanism of endogenous pyrogen production. II. Role of cell products in the regulation of pyrogen release from blood leukocytes. Infect Immun 10:451–457

Bodel P (1976) Colchicine stimulation of pyrogen production by human blood monocytes. J Exp Med 143:1015–1056

Bodel P, Atkins E (1965) Studies in staphylococcal fever. V. Staphylococcal filtrate pyrogen. Yale J Biol Med 38:282–298

Bodel P, Dillard M (1966) Studies on the mechanisms of steroid fever. Excerpta Med Int Congr Ser 137:132–141

Bodel P, Dillard M (1968) Studies on steroid fever. I. Production of leukocyte pyrogen in vitro by etiocholanolone. J Clin Invest 48:107–117

Bodel P, Miller H (1976) Pyrogen from mouse macrophages causes fever in mice. Proc Soc Exp Biol Med 151:93–96

Bodel P, Dillard M, Kaplan SS, Malawista SE (1972) Anti-inflammatory effects of estradiol on human blood. J Lab Clin Med 80:373–384

Boivin A, Mesrobeanu L (1938) Recherches sur les antigénes somatiques et sur les endoxines des bacteries. IV. Sur l'action anti-endotoxique de l'anticorps. Rev Immunol 4:40–56

Boivin A, Mesrobeanu I, Mesrobeanu L (1933) Technique pour la préparation des polysaccharides microbians spécifiques. C R Soc Biol (Paris) 113:490–492

Bondy PK, Bodel P (1971) Mechanism of action of pyrogenic and antipyrogenic steroids in vitro. In: Wolstenholme GE, Birch J (eds) Pyrogens and fever. Churchill Livingstone, Edinburgh, pp 101–113

Bondy PK, Cohn GL, Herrmann W (1958) The possible relationship of etiocholanolone to periodic fever. Yale J Biol Med 30:495–501

Braude AI, Siemienski J (1961) The influence of endotoxin on resistance to infection. Bull NY Acad Med 37:448–462

Braude AI, Carey FJ, Salesky M (1955) Studies with radioactive endotoxin. J Clin Invest 43:858–865

Braude AI, McConnell J, Douglas H (1960) Fever from pathogenic fungi. J Clin Invest 39:1266–1276

Braun V (1973) Molecular organization of the rigid layer and the cell wall of Escherichia coli. J Infect Dis [Suppl] 128:1–8

Briggs RS, Atkins E (1966) Studies in cryptococcal fever. I. Responses to a soluble agent derived from cryptococci. Yale J Biol Med 38:431–448

Brittingham TE, Chaplin H Jr (1957) Febrile transfusion reactions caused by sensitivity of donor leukocytes and platelets. JAMA 165:819–823

Brunson KW, Watson DW (1974) Pyrogenic specificity of staphylococcal exotoxins, staphylococcal enterotoxin and Gram-negative endotoxin. Infect Immun 10:347–351

Brunson KW, Watson DW (1976) Limulus amebocyte lysate reaction with streptococcal pyrogenic exotoxin. Infect Immun 14:1256–1258

Buskirk ER, Thompson RH, Rubenstein M, Wolff SM (1965) Heat exchange in men and women following intravenous injection of endotoxin. J Appl Physiol 19:907–913

Buynak EB, Weibel RE, Whitman JE, Stokes J, Hilleman MR (1969) Combined live measles, mumps, and rubella virus vaccines. JAMA 207:2259–2262

Carey FJ, Braude AI, Zalesky M (1957) Studies with radioactive endotoxin. III. The effect of tolerance on the distribution of radioactivity after intravenous injection of *Escherichia coli* endotoxin labeled with Cr^{51}. J Clin Invest 37:441–445

Castrova A, Pekarek J, Johanovsky J, Svejcan B (1966) Study on systemic reaction of delayed hypersensitivity. Folia Microbiol (Praha) 11:123–133

Chang CM, Nowotny A (1975) Relation of structure to function in bacterial O-antigens. Endotoxicity of Lipid A. Immunochemistry 12:19–20

Chao P, Francis L, Atkins E (1977) The release of an endogenous pyrogen from guinea pig leukocytes in vitro. J Exp Med 145:1288–1298

Chedid L, Parant M, Boyer F, Skarnes RC (1964) Nonspecific host responses in tolerance to the lethal effect of endotoxins. In: Landy M, Braun W (eds) Bacterial endotoxins. Rutgers University Press, New Brunswick, pp 500–516

Chedid L, Audibert F, Bona C, Damais C, Parant F, Parant M (1975) Biological activities of endotoxins detoxified by alkylation. Infect Immun 12:714–721

Chedid L, Audibert F, Le Francier P, Choay J, Lederer E (1976) Modification of the immune response by a synthetic adjuvant and analogs. Proc Natl Acad Sci USA 73:2472–2475

Chusid MJ, Atkins E (1972) Studies in the mechanisms of penicillin-induced fever. J Exp Med 136:227–240

Cluff LE (1953) Studies on the effect of bacterial endotoxins on rabbit leucocytes. II. Development of acquired resistance. J Exp Med 98:349–358

Collins RD, Wood WB Jr (1959) Studies on the pathogenesis of fever. VI. The interaction of leukocytes and endotoxin in vitro. J Exp Med 110:1005–1016

Cooper KE, Cranston WI (1963) Clearance of radioactive bacterial pyrogen from the circulation. J Physiol (Lond) 166:41–42P

Cooper JF, Levin J, Wagner HN Jr (1971) Quantitative comparison of in vitro and in vivo methods for the detection of endotoxin. J Exp Med 78:138–148

Cox CG, Rafter GW (1971) Pyrogen and enzyme release from rabbit blood leukocytes promoted by endotoxin and polyinosinic polycytidylic acid. Biochem Med 5:2227–2236

Craddock CG Jr, Perry S, Lawrence JS (1956) The dynamics of leukocytosis, as studied by leukopheresis and isotopic techniques. J Clin Invest 35:285–294

Creech HJ, Hankwitz RF Jr, Wharton DRA (1949) Further studies of the immunological properties of polysaccharides from *Serratia marcescens*. I. The effects of passive and active immunization on the lethal activity of the polysaccharides. Cancer Res 9:150–159

Cunningham CM, Barsumian EL, Watson DW (1976) Further purification of group streptococcal pyrogenic exotoxin and characterization of purified toxin. Infect Immun 14:767–775

Dillard M, Bodel P (1967) Release of leukocyte pyrogen by etiocholanolone. J Clin Invest 46:1050

Dillard GM, Bodel P (1970) Studies on steroid fever. II. Pyrogenic and anti-pyrogenic activity in vitro of some endogenous steroids of man. J Clin Invest 49:2418–2426

Dinarello CA (1969) PhD thesis. Yale University, New Haven, pp 30–41

Dinarello CA, Wolff SM (1976) Exogenous and endogenous pyrogens. In: Brazier MAB, Coceani F (eds) Brain dysfunction in infantile febrile convulstions. Raven, New York, pp 117–128

Dinarello CA, Wolff SM (1978) Pathogenesis of fever in man. N Engl J Med 298:607–612

Dinarello CA, Bodel P, Atkins E (1968) The role of the liver in the production of fever and in pyrogenic tolerance. Trans Assoc Am Physicians 81:334–344

Dinarello CA, Ward SB, Wolff SM (1973) Pyrogenic properties of bleomycin. Cancer Chemother Rep 57:393–398

Dinarello CA, Renfer L, Wolff SM (1977a) The production of antibody against human leukocytic pyrogen. J Clin Invest 60:465–472

Dinarello CA, Renfer L, Wolff SM (1977) Human leukocytic pyrogen: purification and development of a radioimmunoassay. Proc Natl Acad Sci USA 74:4624–4627

Dinarello CA, Elin RJ, Chedid L, Wolff SM (1978) The pyrogenicity of synthetic adjuvants. J Infect Dis 138:760–767

Eisler R, Moeller HC, Grossman MI (1955) Febrile responses of rabbits to intravenous injection of colloidal substances. US Army Medical Nutritional Laboratory Report Denver, Colorado 9937 TU, No 167

Elin RJ, Wolff SM (1973a) Nonspecificity of the Limulus amebocyte lysate test: positive reactions with polynucleotides and proteins. J Infect Dis 128:349–352

Elin R, Wolff SM (1973b) Bacterial endotoxins. In: Laskin AI, Lechevalier HA (eds) CRC handbook on microbiology. CRC Press, Cleveland, pp 215–239

Ellouz F, Adams A, Cirobaru R, Lederer E (1974) Minimal structural requirements for adjuvant activity of bacterial peptidoglycan derivatives. Biochem Biophys Res Commun 59:1317–1325

Farr RS (1958) The febrile response upon injection of bovine alumin into previously sensitized rabbits. J Clin Invest 37:894–899

Farr RS (1959) Fever as a manifestation of an experimental allergy. J Allergy 30:268–269

Farr RS, Clark SJ Jr, Proffitt JE, Campbell DH (1954) Some humoral aspects of the development of tolerance to bacterial pyrogens in rabbits. Am J Physiol 177:269–275

Fisher S (1967) Localization of radioiodinated endotoxin in organs of mice and rabbits: Effect of thorotrast, trypan blue, endotoxin, and carbon administered intravenously. Nature 213:511–512

Fleetwood MK, Gander GW, Goodale F (1975) Effect of metabolic inhibitors on pyrogen production by rabbit leukocytes. Proc Soc Exp Biol Med 149:336–339

Freedman HH (1959) Passive transfer of protection against lethality of homologous and heterologous endotoxins. Proc Soc Exp Biol Med 102:504–506

Freedman HH (1960a) Passive transfer of tolerance to the pyrogenicity of bacterial endotoxin. J Exp Med 111:453–464

Freedman HH (1960b) Further studies on the passive transfer of tolerance to pyrogenicity of bacterial endotoxin. The febrile and leukopenic responses. J Exp Med 112:619

Freedman HH (1960c) Reticuloendothelial system and passive transfer of endotoxin tolerance. Ann NY Acad Sci 88:99–115

Galanos C, Rietschel FT, Luederitz O, Westphal O, Kim YB, Watson DW (1972) Biological activities of Lipid A complexed with bovine-serum albumin. Eur J Biochem 31:230–239

Gander GW, Goodale F (1975) The role of granulocytes and mononuclear leukocytes in fever. In: Temperature regulation and drug action. Karger, Basel, pp 51–58

Garieli ER, Holmgren H (1952) Studies in the blockade of the reticuloendothelial system. Acta Pathol Microbiol Scand 31:205–215

George JM, Wolf SM, Diller E, Bartter FC (1969) Recurrent fever of unknown etiology: failure to demonstrate association between fever and plasma unconjugated etiocholanolone. J Clin Invest 48:558–563

Good RA (1954) Clinical investigations on patient with agammaglobulinemia. J Lab Clin Med 44:803–807

Good RA, Varco RL (1955) A clinical and experimental study of agammaglobulinemia. Lancet 75:245–246

Greisman SE, Hornick RB (1969) Comparative pyrogenic reactivity of rabbit and man to bacterial endotoxin. Proc Soc Exp Biol Med 131:1154–1158

Greisman SE, Hornick RB (1973) Mechanisms of endotoxin tolerance with special reference to man. J Infect Dis 128:257–268

Greisman SE, Woodward WE (1965) Mechanisms of endotoxin tolerance. III. The refractory state during continuous intravenous infusions of endotoxin. J Exp Med 121:911–933

Greisman SE, Carozza FA, Dixon Hills H Jr (1963) Mechanisms of endotoxin tolerance. Relationship between tolerance and reticuloendothelial system phagocytic activity in the rabbit. J Exp Med 117:663 674

Greisman SE, Wagner HN, Iio M, Hornick RB, Carozza FA, Woodward WE (1964) Mechanisms of endotoxin tolerance in man. In: Landy M, Braun W (eds) Bacterial endotoxins. Rutgers University Press, New Brunswick, pp 537–545

Greisman SE, Young EJ, Carozza FA Jr (1966a) Immunosuppression and endotoxin tolerance. Clin Res 14:332

Greisman SE, Young EJ, Woodward WE (1966b) Mechanisms of tolerance. IV. Specificity of the pyrogenic refractory state during continuous intravenous infusions of endoxotin. J Exp Med 124:983–1000

Grey HM, Briggs W, Farr RS (1961) The passive transfer of sensitivity to antigen induced fever. J Clin Invest 40:703–706

Haeseler F, Bodel P, Atkins E (1977) Characteristics of pyrogen by isolated rabbit Kupffer cells in vitro. RES 22:569–581

Haley LD, Meyer R, Atkins E (1966) Studies in cryptococcal fever. II. Responses of sensitized and unsensitized rabbits to various substances derived from cryptococcal cells. Yale J Biol Med 39:165–185

Hall CH Jr, Atkins E (1959) Studies on tuberculin fever. I. The mechanism of fever in tuberculin hypersensitivity. J Exp Med 109:339–359

Hall WJ, Francis L, Atkins E (1970) Studies on tuberculin fever. IV. The passive transfer of reactivity with various tissues of sensitized donor rabbits. J Exp Med 131:483–498

Hamada S (1971) Studies on cell walls of group A Streptococcus pyogens, type 12. Biken J 14:214–220

Harris ED Jr, Krane SM (1971) The effect of colchicine on collagenase production in cultures of rheumatoid synovium. Arthrititis Rheum 14:669–673

Herion JC, Walker RI, Palmer JG (1960) Relation of leukocyte and fever responses to bacterial endotoxin. Am J Physiol 199:809–815

Herion JC, Herring WB, Palmer JG, Walker RI (1964) Cr^{51}-labeled endotoxin distribution in granulocytopenic animals. Am J Physiol 206:947–950

Herring WB, Herion JC, Walker RT, Palmer JG (1963) Distribution and clearance of circulating endotoxin. J Clin Invest 42:79–87

Ho M, KE YH, Armstrong JA (1973) Mechanism of interferon induction by endotoxin. J Infect Dis 128:212–219

Hofstad R, Kristoffersen J (1970) Chemical characteristics of endotoxin from Bacteroides fragilis. J Gen Microbiol 61:15–19

Howard JG, Rowley D, Wardlaw AC (1958) Investigations on the mechanism of stimulation of non-specific immunity by bacterial lipopolysaccharides. Immunology 1:181–203

Ichikawa T, Nakano I, Hirokawa I (1969) Bleomycin treatment of the tumors of penis and scrotum. J Urol 102:699–707

Jandl JH, Tomlinson AS (1958) The destruction of red cells by antibodies in man. II. Pyrogenic, leukocytic, and dermal responses to immune hemolysis. J Clin Invest 37:1202–1228

Johanovsky J (1959) The mechanism of the delayed type of hypersensitivity. IV. The formation of pyrogenic substances during incubation of cells of hypersensitive rabbits with tuberculin in vitro. Folia Microbiol (Praha) 4:286–291

Johanovsky J (1960) Production of pyrogenic substances in the reaction of cells of hypersensitive guinea pigs with antigen in vitro. Immunology 3:179–184

Kadlecova O, Masek K, Petrovick YP (1977) A possible site of action of bacterial peptidoglycan in the CNS. Neuropharmacology 16:699–702

Kampschmidt RF, Upchurch HF, Park A (1965) Further studies on carbon clearance after endotoxin in the rat. RES 2:256–262

Kanoh S, Kawasaki H (1966) Studies on myxovirus pyrogen. I. Interaction of myxovirus and rabbit polymorphonuclear leukocytes. Biken J 9:177–184

Kanoh S, Ogawa Y (1977) Studies on the interaction between proteolipid and bacterial pyrogen. Jpn J Med Sci Biol 30:67–70

Kanoh S, Watson DW (1977) Pyrogenic specificity of endotoxin and exotoxin A. Jpn J Med Sci Biol 30:64–67

Kanoh S, Kawasaki H, Nishio A (1969) Studies on myxovirus pyrogen. II. Some factors affecting fever tolerance in rabbits. Biken J 12:169–180

Kappas A, Ratkovits B (1960) Species specificity of steroid-induced fever. J Clin Endocrinol 20:898–900

Kappas A, Hellman L, Fukushima DK, Gallagher TE (1956) The pyrogenic effect of etiocholanolone. J Clin Endocrinol 16:948–952

Kappas A, Hellman L, Fukushima DN, Gallagher TF (1957) The pyrogenic effect of etiocholanolone. J Clin Endocrinol Metab 17:451–457

Kappas A, Soybel W, Glickman P, Fukushima DK (1960) Fever-producing steroids of endogenous origin in man. AMA Arch Intern Med 105:701–708

Kasper DL (1976) Chemical and biological characterization of the lipopolysaccharide of *Bacteroides fragilis* subspecies *fragilis*. J Infect Dis 134:59–66

Kawasaki H, Kanoh S (1974) Studies on the myxovirus pyrogen. III. Comparative studies on the leucocytic pyrogens induced by influenza virus and bacterial pyrogen in vitro (author's translation). Virus (Tokyo) 24:51–56

Kim YB, Watson DW (1965a) Role of antibody in reactions to gram-negative bacterial endotoxin. Fed Proc 24:457

Kim YB, Watson DW (1965b) Modification of host response to bacterial endotoxins. II. Passive transfer of immunity to bacterial endotoxins with fractions containing 19 S antibodies. J Exp Med 121:751–759

Kim YB, Watson DW (1966) Role of antibodies in reactions to gram-negative bacterial endotoxin. Ann NY Acad Sci 133:727–745

Kimball HR, Vogel JM, Perry S, Wolff SM (1967) Quantitative aspects of pyrogenic and hematologic responses to etiocholanolone in man. J Lab Clin Med 69:415–427

King MK (1964) Pathogenesis of fever in rabbits following intravenous injection of Coxsackie virus. J Lab Clin Med 63:23–29

Kobayashi GS, Friedman L (1964) Characterization of the pyrogenicity of *Candida albicans*, *Saccharomyces cerevisiae*, and *Cryptococcus neoformans*. J Bacteriol 88:660–666

Kobayashi GS, Friedman L, Kofroth JF (1964) Some cytological and pathogenic properties of pheroplasts of *Candida albicans*. J Bacteriol 88:795–801

Kohlhage H, Pollmann W Siegert R (1968) Studies on the differentiation of myxoviruses induced interferon and endogenous pyrogen from rabbits. Life Sci 7:627–633

Kotani S, Watanabe Y, Shimono T et al. (1976) Correlation between the immunoadjuvant activities and pyrogenicities of synthetic N-acetylmurmamyl peptides or amino acids. Biken J 19:9–13

Kotani S, Watanbe Y, Kinoshita F et al. (1977) Gelation of the amoebocyte lysate of *Tachypleus tridentatus* by cell wall digest of several Gram-positive bacteria and synthetic peptidoglycan subunits of natural and unnatural configurations. Biken J 20:5–10

Kovats TG, (1967) Endotoxin susceptibility and hypersensitivity. Medical University Szeged, Szeged

Krause RM (1975) Immunological activity of the peptidoglycan. Z Immunitaetsforsch Immunbiol 149:136–150

Landy M (1953) Enhancement of the immunogenicity of typhoid vaccine by retention of the V. antigen. Am J Hyg 58:148–159

Landy M, Johnson AG, Webster ME, Sagin JF (1955) Studies on the O antigen of *Salmonella typhosa*. II. Immunological properties of the purified antigen. J Immunol 74:466–473

Lemperle G (1966) Effect of RES stimulation on endotoxin shock in mice. Proc Soc Exp Biol Med 122:1012–1015

Lindsay HL, Trown PW, Brandt J, Forbes M (1969) Pyrogenicity of Poly 1. Poly C in rabbits. Nature 223:717–718

Linnemann CC, Steichen J, Sherman WG, Schiff GM (1974) Febrile illness in early infancy associated with ECHO virus infection. Pediatrics 84:49–54

Luederitz O, Galanos C, Lehmann V et al. (1973) Lipid A: chemical structure and biological activity. J Infect Dis 128:9–21

Martin RR, Greenberg SB, Wallace RJ (1979) Staphylococcal teichoic acid antibodies. Lancet 1:731

Masek K, Kadlecova O, Petrovicky P (1978) Pharmacological activity of bacterial peptidoglycan: the effect on temperature and sleep in the rat. Toxicon [Suppl] 1:991–1003

Michael JG, Rosen FS (1963) Association of "natural" antibodies to gram-negative bacteria with the gamma-macroglobulins. J Exp Med 118:619–628

Mickenberg ID, Snyderman R, Root RK, Mergenhagen SE, Wolff SM (1971) The relationship of complement consumption to immune fever. J Immunol 107:1466–1476

Mogensen KE, Cantell K (1974) Human leukocyte interferon: a role for disulphide bonds. J Gen Virol 22:95–103

Moore DM, Murphy PA, Chesney JP, Wood WB Jr (1973) Synthesis of endogenous pyrogen by rabbit leukocytes. J Exp Med 137:1263–1274

Morgan HR (1941) Immunologic properties of an antigenic material isolated from E. typhosa. J Immunol 41:161–175

Morgan HR (1948a) Resistance to the action of the endotoxins of enteric bacilli in man. J Clin Invest 27:706–712

Morgan HR (1948b) Tolerance to the toxic action of somatic antigens of enteric bacteria. J Immunol 59:129–134

Moses JM, Atkins E (1961) Studies on tuberculin fever. II. Observations on the role of endogenous pyrogen in tolerance. J Exp Med 114:939–959

Mosher MB, De Conti RC, Bertino JR (1972) Bleomycin therapy in advanced Hodgkin's disease and epidermoid cancer. Cancer 30:56–60

Mott PD, Wolff SM (1966) The association of fever and antibody response in rabbits immunized with human serum albumin. J Clin Invest 45:372–379

Mulholland JH, Wolff SM, Jackson A, Landy M (1965) Quantitative studies of febrile tolerance and levels of specific antibody evoked by bacterial endotoxin. J Clin Invest 44:920–926

Murray IM (1963) The mechanism of blockade of the reticuloendothelial system. J Exp Med 117:139–152

Neter E, Westphal O, Luederitz O, Gorzynski SA, Eichenberger E (1956) Studies of enterbacterial lipopolysaccharides. Effects of heat and chemicals on erythrocyte modifying, antigenic, toxic, and pyrogenic properties. J Immunol 76:377–385

Neva FA, Morgan HR (1950) Tolerance to the actions of endotoxins of enteric bacilli in patients convalescent from typhoid and paratyphoid fevers. J Lab Clin Med 35:911–919

Niwa M, Milner KC, Ribi E, Rudbach JA (1969) Alteration of physical, chemical, and biological properties of endotoxin by treatment with mild alkali. J Bacteriol 97:1069–1077

Noll H, Braude AI (1961) Preparation and biological properties of a chemically modified E. coli endotoxin of high immunogenic potency and/or toxicity. J Clin Invest 40:1935–1951

Nordlund JJ, Root RK, Wolff SM (1970a) Studies on the origin of human leukocytic pyrogen. J Exp Med 131:727–743

Nordlund JJ, Wolff SM, Levy HB (1970b) Inhibition of biologic activity of Poly I: Poly C by human plasma. Proc Soc Exp Biol Med 133:439–444

Nowotny A (1964) Chemical detoxification of bacterial endotoxin. In: Landy M, Braun W (eds) Bacterial endotoxins. Rutgers University Press, New Brunswick, pp 29–37

Nowotny A, Radvany R, Neale N (1965) Neutralization of toxic bacterial O-antigens with O-antibodies while maintaining their stimulus on non-specific resistance. Life Sci 4:1107–1110

Ogata S, Kanamori M (1978) Effects of homologous O-antibody on host responses to lipopolysaccharide from Yersinia enterocolitica: neutralization of its pyrogenicity. Microbiol Immunol 22:485–494

Perlow M, Dinarello CA, Wolff SM (1975) A primate model for the study of human fever. J Infect Dis 132:157–164

Radvany R, Neale NL, Nowotny A (1966) Relation of structure to function in bacterial O-antigens. VI. Neutralization of endotoxic O-antigens by homologous O-antibody. Ann NY Acad Sci 133:763–786

Reed RW, McMillan GC (1966) Coxsackie and echo viruses. Am J Med Sci 251:141–155

Ribi E, Anacker RL, Kukushi K, Haskin WT, Landy M, Mulner KC (1964) Relationship of chemical composition to biological activity. In: Landy M, Braun W (eds) Bacterial endotoxins. Rutgers University Press, New Brunswick, pp 16–28

Rietschel ET, Luederitz O (1975) Chemical structure of lypopolysaccharides and endotoxin immunity. Z Immunitaetsforsch Immunbiol 149:201–213

Rietschel ET, Kim YB, Watson DW, Galanos C, Luederitz O, Westphal O (1973) Pyrogenicity and immunogenicity of lipid A complexed with bovine serum albumin or human serum albumin. Infect Immun 8:173–177

Robinson DR, Smith H, McGuire MB, Levine L (1975) Prostaglandin synthesis by rheumatoid synovium and its stimulation by colchicine. Prostaglandins 10:67–85

Root RK, Wolff SM (1968) Pathogenetic mechanisms in experimental immune fever. J Exp Med 128:309–323

Root RK, Nordlund JJ, Wolff SM (1970) Factors affecting the quantitative production and assay of human leukocytic pyrogen. J Lab Clin Med 75:679–693

Rotta J (1974) Biologically active components of the cells of Gram-positive bacteria. J Hyg Epidemiol Microbiol Immunol (Praha) 18:353–358

Rotta J (1975) Endotoxin-like properties of the peptidoglycan. Z Immunitaetsforsch Immunbiol 149:230–244

Rotta A (1977) Biological characteristics of peptidoglycans of Group A Streptococcus and some other bacterial species. I. Tolerance and effect of antibody in fever response, and heart damaging effect in rabbits. J Hyg Epidemiol Microbiol Immunol (Praha) 21:433–440

Rowley D (1960) The role of opsonins in non-specific immunity. J Exp Med 111:137–149

Rowley D, Howard JG, Jenkins CR (1956) The fate of ^{32}P-labeled bacterial lipopolysaccharide in laboratory animals. Lancet 270:366–368

Rudders RA (1972) Treatment of advanced malignant lymphomas with bleomycin. Blood 40:317–332

Rutenberg SH, Rutenberg AM, Smith EE, Fine J (1965) On the nature of tolerance to endotoxin. Proc Soc Exp Biol Med 118:620–623

Salvin SB, Peterson RDA, Good RA (1965) The role of the thymus in resistance to infection and endotoxin toxicity. J Lab Clin Med 65:1004–1022

Schachenmayr W, Heymar B, Haferkamp O (1975) Antibodies to peptidoglycan in sera from population studies. Z Immunitaetsforsch Immunbiol 149:179–186

Schaedler RW, Dubos RJ (1961) The susceptibility of mice to bacterial endotoxins. J Exp Med 113:559–565

Schenck JR, Hargie MP, Brown MS, Evert DS, Yoo AL, McIntire FC (1969) The enhancement of antibody formation by E. coli lipopolysaccharide and detoxified derivative. J Immunol 102:1411–1422

Schleifer KH (1975) Chemical structure of the peptidoglycan, its modifiability and relation to biological activity. Z Immunitätsforsch Immunbiol 149:104–117

Schleifer KH, Kandler O (1972) Peptidoglycan types of bacterial cell walls and their toxonomic implications. Bacteriol Rev 36:407–426

Schlievert PM, Watson DW (1978) Group A streptococcal pyrogenic exotoxin: pyrogenicity, alteration of blood-brain barrier and separation of sites for pyrogenicity and enhancement of lethal endotoxin shock. Infect Immun 21:753–763

Schlievert PM, Bettin KM, Watson DW (1977) Purification and characterization of group A streptococcal pyrogenic exotoxin type C. Infect Immun 16:673–679

Schlievert PM, Bettin KM, Watson DW (1978) Effect of antipyretics on group A streptococcal pyrogenic exotoxin fever production and ability to enhance lethal endotoxin shock. Proc Soc Exp Biol Med 157:472–475

Schlievert PM, Schoettle DJ, Watson DW (1979) Purification and physiochemical and biological characterization of a staphylococcal pyrogenic exotoxin. Infect Immun 23:609–617

Schuh V, Hribalova V (1966) The pyrogenic effect of scarlet fever toxin. II. Leukocytic pyrogen formation induced by scarlet fever toxin or Salmonella paratyphi B endotoxin. Folia Microbiol (Praha) 11:112–122

Schuh V, Hribalova V, Atkins E (1970) The pyrogenic effect of scarlet fever toxin. IV. Pyrogenicity of strain C 203 U filtrates: comparison with some basic characteristics of the known types of scarlet fever toxin. Yale Y Biol Med 43:31–42

Snell S, Braude AI (1961) Intradermal reactions in man to autologous erythrocytes sensitized with tuberculin or endotoxin. J Immunol 87:119–124

Snell ES, Atkins E (1967) Interactions of Gram-negative bacterial endotoxin with rabbit blood in vitro. Am J Physiol 212:1103–1112

Shantz ES, Roessler WG, Woodburn MJ et al. (1972) Purification and some chemical and physical properties of staphylococcal enterotoxin A. Biochemistry 11:360–366

Sheagren JN, Wolff SM, Shulman NR (1967) Febrile and hematologic responses of rhesus monkeys to bacterial endotoxin. Am J Physiol 212:884–890

Shu HL (1979) Interfering and interferon-inducing capacity of NDV. II. Relationship between pyrogenic, interfering, and interferon-inducing activities. Arch Gesamte Virusforsch 46:191–197

Siegert R, Braune P (1964a) The pyrogens of myxoviruses. I. Induction of hyperthermia and its tolerance. Virology 24:209–217

Siegert R, Braune P (1964b) The pyrogens of myxoviruses. II. Resistance of influenza A pyrogen to heat, ultraviolet, and chemical treatment. Virology 24:218–224

Siegert R, Shu HL, Kohlhage H (1967) Correlation between fever and interferon titer in rabbits after induction with myxoviruses. Life Sci 6:615–620

Smith RT, Braude AI, Carey FJ (1957) The distribution of Cr^{51}-labeled *E. coli* endotoxin in the generalized Shwartzman reaction. J Clin Invest 36:695–699

Starzecki B, Reddin JL, Gran A, Spink WW (1967) Distribution of endotoxin Cr^{51} in normal and endotoxin resistant dogs. Am J Physiol 213:1065–1071

Stetson CA (1964) Role of hypersensitivity in reactions to endotoxin. In: Land M, Braun W (eds) Bacterial endotoxins. Rutgers University Press, New Brunswick, pp 658–664

Stewart WE, Lin LS, Wiranswska-Stewart M, Cantell K (1977) Elimination of size and change heterogeneities of human leukocyte interferons by chemical cleavage. Proc Natl Acad Sci USA 74:4200–4204

Sveen K, Hofstad T, Milner KC (1977) Lethality for mice and chick embryos, pyrogenicity in rabbits and ability to gelate lysate from amoebocytes of *Limulus polyphemus* by lipopolysaccharides from *Bacteroides*, *Fusobacterium*, and *Veillonella*. Acta Pathol Microbiol Scand 85:388–396

Tobey RA, Peterson DF, Anderson EC, Puck TT (1966) Life cycle analysis of mammalian cells. II. The inhibition of division in Chinese hamster cells by puromycin and actinomycin. Biophys J 6:567–581

Tripoli D, Nowotny A (1966) Relation of structure to function in bacterial O-antigens. Ann NY Acad Sci 133:604–619

Urbaschek B, Nowotny A (1968) Endotoxin tolerance induced by detoxified endotoxin. Proc Soc Exp Biol Med 127:650–654

Van Noordwijk J, De Jong Y (1977) Comparison of the Limulus amebocyte lysate (LAL) test with the rabbit test: false positives and false negatives. Dev Biol Stand 34:39–43

Verwey WF (1940) A type-specific antigenic protein derived from the Staphylococcus. J Exp Med 71:635–644

Wagner RR, Bennett IL, Le Quire VS (1949) The production of fever by influenzal viruses. I. Factors influencing the febrile response to single injections of virus. J Exp Med 90:321–333

Watnick AS, Gordon AS (1964) Endotoxin influences on carbon clearance and resistance to bacterial infection. RES 1:170–184

Watson DW, Kim YB (1963) Modification of host responses to bacterial endotoxins. J Exp Med 118:425–432

Watson DW, Kim YB (1964) Immunological aspects of pyrogenic tolerance. In: Landy M, Braun W (eds) Bacterial endotoxins. Rutgers University Press, New Brunswick, pp 522–536

Watson DW, Kim YB (1970) Erythrogenic toxins. In: Montie TC, Kadis S, Ajl SJ (eds) Microbial toxins. Academic Press, New York, pp 173–187

Werb Z, Gordon S (1975) Secretion of a specific collagenase by stimulated macrophages. J Exp Med 142:346–354

Westphal O, Luederitz O (1954) Chemische Erforschung von Lipopolysacchariden gramnegativen Bakterien. Angew Chemie 66:407–417

Wildfeuer A, Heymer B, Spiler D, Scheifer KH, Vaneh E, Haferkamp O (1975) Use of Limulus assay to compare the biological activity of peptidoglycan and endotoxin. Z Immunitätsforsch Immunbiol 149:258–264

Wolff SM (1973) Biological effects of bacterial endotoxins in man. J Infect Dis 128:251–256

Wolff SM, Mulholland JH, Rubenstein M (1964a) Suppression of the immune response to bacterial endotoxins. In: Landy M, Braun W (eds) Bacterial Endotoxins. Rutgers University Press, New Brunswick, pp 319–325

Wolff SM, Mulholland JH, Rubenstein M (1964b) Effect of 6-mercaptopurine on endotoxin tolerance. Clin Res 12:455

Wolff SM, Adler RC, Buskirk ER, Thompson RH (1964c) A syndrome of periodic hypothalamic discharge. Am J Med 36:956–967

Wolff SM, Mulholland JH, Ward SB, Rubenstein M, Mott PD (1965a) Effect of 6-mercaptopurine on endotoxin tolerance. J Clin Invest 44:1402–1409

Wolff SM, Rubenstein M, Mulholland JH, Alling DW (1965b) Comparison of hematologic and febrile response to endotoxin in man. Blood 26:190–201

Wolff SM, Mulholland JH, Ward SB (1965c) Quantitative aspects of the pyrogenic responses to rabbits to endotoxin. J Clin Med 65:268–276

Wolff SM, Kimball HR, Perry S, Root R, Kappas A (1967) The biological properties of etiocholanolone. Ann Intern Med 67:1268–1295

Wolff SM, Kimball HR, Marshall JR (1973) The effects of hydrocortisone and estrogen on experimental fever induced by etiocholanolone. J Infect Dis 128:243–247

Wood WB Jr (1958) Studies on the cause of fever. N Engl J Med 258:1023–1027

Young EJ, Greisman SE (1968) Transfer of "anamnestic" tolerant responses to endotoxin with spleen cells. Clin Res 16:337

Young ML, Dickstein B, Weibel RE, Stokes JH, Buynak EB, Hilleman MR (1967) Experiences with Heryl Lynn strain live attentuated mumps virus vaccine in a pediatric outpatient clinic. Pediatrics 40:798–803

Zweifach B, Benacerraf B, Thomas L (1957) The relationship between the vascular manifestations of shock produced by endotoxin, trauma, and hemorrhage. II. The possible role of the reticulo-endothelial system in resistance to each type of shock. J Exp Med 106:403–420

CHAPTER 5

Endogenous Pyrogens

G. W. GANDER

A. Introduction

In the last few years there has been increasing interest in the polymorphonuclear leucocyte (PMN), primarily because immunologists have found that PMNs play an important role in immune reactions. Consequently, many of the functions of PMNs are being viewed from a new perspective. These new perspectives almost always lead to new insights in understanding. The role of endogenous pyrogen (EP) in the pathogenesis of fever is no exception.

The purpose of this chapter is to briefly describe the nature of EP, discuss factors affecting release and finally describe some recent findings which, if corroborated, will facilitate immensely the study of EP.

This review is intended to provide a modern perspective on the nature of EP. This perspective obviously will reflect certain of the author's biases. For further information on endogenous pyrogen, a number of good reviews are available: HAHN (1974), CRANSTON (1976), DINARELLO and WOLFF (1978), DINARELLO (1980), BEISEL (1980), and LIPTON (1980).

B. Nomenclature

In the past years, there has been considerable controversy over nomenclature. However, at present, two terms are used to refer to the endogenous proteins produced by leucocytes; either leucocytic pyrogen (LP), or endogenous pyrogen (EP). The use of both of these terms will permit access to most of the recent world literature when using the various literature retrieval techniques. As this review will show, these terms are being used collectively for the multiple endogenous peptides of the reticuloendothelial system (RES) cell origin that participate in the development of fever.

C. Assay of Endogenous Pyrogen

Progress in understanding the role of EP in fever development has been slow principally because of the difficulty in assaying EP in a quantitative fashion. Not only was EP relatively recently discovered but its distinction from endotoxins or lipopolysaccharide (LPS) has continued to be a major source of confusion. Even investigators experienced in distinguishing between LPS and EP can sometimes be misled.

The first methods for measuring EP (KAISER and WOOD 1962) were derived from the well-established methods for measuring exogenous pyrogens (endotoxin) in drugs and parenteral fluids (U. S. PHARMACOPEIA 1970). It was shown that the febrile response to endotoxin exhibits proportionality between the amount of pyrogen and the magnitude of the fever. Consequently, measuring the area under the fever curve became the accepted procedure for measuring pyrogens. A dose response relationship was established between EP injected and both the areas under the fever curve and the maximum temperature rise (BORNSTEIN et al. 1963). However, the narrow dose range over which the response remains linear was often overlooked. Since that time, more and more investigators have begun to measure the maximum temperature elevation during the febrile episode following intravenous injection of EP. It is much easier to recognize when too large a dose of pyrogen has been given and thus exceeds the linear range. Rabbits will not respond to EP with more than about 1.5 °C temperature rise no matter how much pyrogen has been given.

This bioassay for EP, although reliable and specific, is subject to many pitfalls and is a rather difficult and demanding procedure. One must use so-called trained rabbits, i.e. rabbits that have experienced being held for 3–4 h per day in a restrained box with a rectal probe inserted 3–4 cm into the rectum. After 3 or 4 days these animals are considered trained. BORNSTEIN et al. (1963) found that among trained rabbits, a certain number gave variable responses to a constant dose of EP given on consecutive days. Therefore, those rabbits giving unacceptable responses need to be removed from the group of rabbits used for EP assays.

It is difficult to do comparative studies because the mean response to a given dose of EP will vary among groups of trained recipients. Therefore, it is difficult to compare different preparations of EP during purification or to compare results from different laboratories.

A final and perhaps the most serious problem concerns endotoxin contamination of EP samples. Stringent precautions against LPS contamination must be taken because LPS will also induce fevers in rabbits at doses as low as 5 ng. The problem is particularly insidious because endotoxin in the presence of serum becomes heat labile and takes on many of the properties of EP (ATKINS et al. 1974). Unfortunately, many of the reagents used for tissue culture, although sterile, may contain traces of LPS.

Biological assays, although perhaps very sensitive, may not be very accurate, and multiple determinations of a single sample are necessary to obtain meaningful data.

Although EP from one species is active in other species, usually higher doses are needed when crossing species in order to obtain a response (ALLISON et al. 1973; BODEL and ATKINS 1966). In spite of these problems, human LP is routinely assayed in rabbits in many laboratories.

In order to circumvent the problem of using so much human LP in the rabbit assay, BODEL and MILLER (1978) used the mouse for bioassay of human LP. They claim an increase of 100-fold in sensitivity over the rabbit assay, with pyrogen released from 100,000 granulocytes being sufficient to obtain a positive response.

This method is not without deficiencies. The mice are held at 35 °C ambient temperature and their rectal temperatures must be taken manually every 10 min for

30 min. Six to eight animals are used for each sample, presumably because of variability of response. A dose response curve is not included in this paper either.

DINARELLO et al. (1977 a, b) have attempted to eliminate most of the problems with bioassay of LP by developing a radioimmunoassay. The radioimmunoassay is dependent on the availability of purified antiserum. DINARELLO has made the assumption that all antigens in his LP preparation contain free amino groups which will react with the Bolton-Hunter reagent, thus giving rise to radioactive antigens (BOLTON and HUNTER 1973). During purification, radioactivity associated with pyrogenic activity indicated LP while radioactivity not associated with pyrogenicity was taken to be contaminating protein. Although this assumption would not rule out contaminating endotoxin, other data such as elution volume of the pyrogenic fraction makes this possibility unlikely. However, HATTINGH et al. (1979) reported recently that most preparations of serum albumin were pyrogenic after a number of stages of purification; unfortunately, he did not test his preparations for LPS using the Limulus assay. One can conclude as he did either that albumin is a pyrogen or, alternatively and I believe more likely; that endotoxin or perhaps lipid A is binding to the albumin molecule, rendering it pyrogenic. If it can be shown that lipid A alone will bind to hydrophobic regions of protein molecules, the problem of pyrogen assay becomes even more problematic. I know of no experiments which provide any direct evidence either for or against this hypothesis. These problems need to be considered when developing an assay for LP, even for a radioimmunoassay. If the antibody preparation contains antibody to lipid A then radioimmunoassay will not necessarily distinguish between LP, LPS, and lipid A bound to protein. Since endotoxin can be assumed to be present unless extreme precautions have been taken to remove it, it is essential to demonstrate that there is no competition between LP and either LPS or lipid A bound to protein in any assay including radioimmunoassay. Now that it has been demonstrated that radioimmunoassay of LP is feasible, great strides should be made rapidly in understanding the mechanism of fever production.

D. Sources of LP

I. Cells Capable of Pyrogen Release

The PMN leucocyte was implicated early in the study of endogenous pyrogen. Much emphasis was placed on the important role of the PMN in clinical fevers; however, fevers which commonly occur in neutropaenic or agranulocytic patients or in patients with granulomatous diseases were not easily explained.

At the same time ATKINS et al. (1967) and HAHN et al. (1967) reported that peritoneal exudate, lymph node, and lung macrophages can produce an endogenous pyrogen. Since that time Kupffer cells have also been shown to release EP (DINARELLO et al. 1968; HAESELER et al. 1977). However, hepatocytes were unable to release EP. Later the inability of hepatocytes to release EP was confirmed in another laboratory (GANDER and GOODALE 1975).

The lymphocyte does not appear able to elaborate EP (ATKINS et al. 1972), although it has been shown that lymphocytes in response to antigen release a "lymphokine" or activator which induces macrophages to produce EP (ATKINS and

BODEL 1974; ATKINS and FRANCIS 1977; ATKINS and FRANCIS 1973; ATKINS and FRANCIS 1978; ATKINS et al. 1978).

It has been observed that only so-called professional phagocytes, i.e. phagocytes that have receptors for immunoglobulins and complement, are capable of releasing EP (ATKINS and BODEL 1974). BODEL and MILLER (1977) tested this hypothesis by comparing EP production in mouse macrophages with that of "non-professional" phagocytes. Human fibroblasts, He-La cells and mouse L cells did not release any detectable EP after phagocytosing considerable numbers of either erythrocytes or latex particles. Mouse peritoneal macrophages on the other hand released significant quantities of EP on similar treatment. No EP was released when 3×10^7 He-La or fibroblast cells were permitted to phagocytose either erythrocytes or latex particles. More than a 100-fold more He-La than macrophage cells are required to give detectable EP. Since phagocytosed bacteria such as the *Staphylococci* induce greater release of EP than do latex particles in macrophages, it would be of interest to use this system to study release of EP from non-professional phagocytes. The presence of IgG and complement receptors on these cells suggests that these receptors may play some role in the activation process.

Although it has been suggested that some tumour cells may produce EP, no proof has been forthcoming (CRANSTON et al. 1972, 1973; BODEL 1974 b, c). CRANSTON et al. (1973) found that slices of renal carcinoma tissue removed from febrile patients released EP-like material when incubated in vitro. They were, quite properly, careful to point out that EP is released from the tumour and could originate from either the tumour cells or from inflammatory cells present within the tumour. However, tumour slices from non-febrile patients did not release EP on incubation in vitro. EP release from active tumour slices was inhibited by cycloheximide. The release of EP from macrophages is also inhibited by cycloheximide; however, in PMN's only the activation step is inhibited by cycloheximide. These observations suggest that macrophages present within the tumour are probably the source of the EP. However, it is not clear why tumours from afebrile patients do not release EP in vitro. If macrophages are responsible, then presumably they have not been activated in the afebrile patients. Alternately the tumour cells conceivably could be producing EP as BODEL and WENC (1978) suggest, since it is not uncommon for tumour cells to release hormones and other inappropriate endogenous proteins.

II. Animal Species Releasing EP

Almost all warm-blooded animals will, under certain circumstances, develop fever sometime during the course of an infectious disease. One would speculate that an endogenous pyrogen must therefore appear in the animal's circulation. Leucocytic pyrogen has been prepared from the blood of man (CRANSTON et al. 1956), rat, pig, ox, baboon (BORSOOK et al. 1978), dog (PETERSDORF and BENNETT 1957), guineapig (CHAO et al. 1977; BLATTEIS 1977), mouse (BODEL and MILLER 1976), goat (VANMIERT and ATMAKUSUMA 1970), and the monkey (CHAI et al. 1971; PERLOW et al. 1975). An EP-like substances has also been prepared from the blood of the lizard (*Dipsosaurus dorsalis*). This substance when reinjected into the lizard induces a behavioral fever (BERNHEIM and KLUGER 1977). These authors have concluded that because lizards produce an endogenous pyrogen-like substance and respond to rabbit EP, reptilian, avian and mammalian fevers may have had a common phylogeny. It is clear now that EP from different species is similar, i.e. there is cross reaction between many species, but EP probably is not identical among all species because the dosage varies greatly between species (BORSOOK et al. 1978).

It appears likely that birds also possess a similar mechanism for fevers, i.e. formation of EP by leucocytes in response to exogenous pyrogens, since it has been shown that pigeons become febrile when given heat-killed gram negative bacteria. Their fevers, like mammals and reptiles, defervesce in response to salicylate (D'ALECY and KLUGER 1975). PITTMAN et al. (1975) have shown that chickens become febrile when given bacterial products derived from many enteric bacteria.

The lack of absolute species specificity is not very surprising in the light of experiments reported by KLUGER and his associates which suggest that reptiles have a similar mechanism for pyrogen production. BERNHEIM and KLUGER (1977) have shown that lizards *Dipsosaurus dorsalis* develop a behavioural fever when given lizard endogenous pyrogen. Furthermore, lizards also developed behavioural fever in response to rabbit EP. D'ALECY and KLUGER (1975) have also shown that pigeons become febrile when given gram-negative heat-killed bacteria and that this fever defervesces in response to salicylate. REYNOLDS et al. (1976) have shown that blue gills (*Lepomis macrochirus*), small-mouth bass (*Micropterus salmoides*), and goldfish (*Carassius auratus*) (REYNOLDS et al. 1977) develop behavioural fevers in response to heat killed gram-negative bacteria. These authors also showed that acetaminophen induced antipyresis in febrile fishes. The similarity in response of fishes, reptiles, birds, and mammals suggests that mechanisms for fever production evolved early in the development of vertebrates.

E. Cellular Events

The so-called activation process in granulocytes for EP production has been partially elucidated through the work of many investigators but most notably by WOOD and co-workers and more recently by ATKINS, BODEL, and MURPHY (KAISER and WOOD 1962; BODEL 1970; HAHN et al. 1970a; ATKINS and BODEL 1974; MURPHY et al. 1974). As a result of these and other studies it is now generally agreed that in granulocytes production of pyrogen is a two-step process. The first step, activation by agents such as endotoxin, bacteria or even phagocytosis of inert particles, is presumed to be induced when these agents interact with the cell membrane. At this time protein synthesis appears to be a requirement for subsequent pyrogen release, since several investigators have shown that either cycloheximide, puromycin or actinomycin D when added with the activator blocks subsequent release of EP (NORDLUND et al. 1970; BODEL 1970; HAHN et al. 1970; TABORSKY 1972; MOORE et al. 1973; SIERGERT et al. 1975, 1976). However, if these inhibitors are added after 1–2 h of activation there is no effect on subsequent production and release of EP (HAHN et al. 1970; NORDLUND et al. 1970). Therefore, the production of EP has been divided into several stages: first, activation occurs by interaction of the activating agent with the cell; secondly, early production begins with the cell synthesizing RNA in preparation for new protein synthesis and perhaps an EP precursor is being converted to active EP. The final phase begins about 2 h after activation, when EP is continuously produced for 8–12 h and production is insensitive to in-hibitors of either protein or RNA synthesis.

Recent studies have helped to resolve some of these apparently contradictory steps. It appears that much confusion existed because of the assumption that granulocytes were responsible for EP production. This is a reasonable assumption since EP is produced in abundance from rabbit peritoneal exudate cells. These cells usually are more than 95% granulocytes. However, it is not too unusual for mac-rophages to make up as much as 30% of the total cell population GANDER (unpub-lished). At any rate, very recently HANSON et al. (1980) have reported that rabbit neutrophils do not secrete EP when stimulated with *Staphylococcus epidermidis*. They suggest that macrophages may be the only source of EP. However, they admit that other known stimuli of EP release must be tested with pure preparations of PMN before we can conclude that EP is derived solely from macrophages. How-ever, further evidence is produced by the observation made by MURPHY et al. (1980) that lymphocyte activating factor (LAF) produced by alveolar macrophages appears to be identical to EP prepared from peritoneal exudate cells. Both preparations showed the same microheterogeneity.

Because of this discovery, attempts to better understand the cellular events in EP production should be forthcoming, since macrophages are relatively easy to harvest and to maintain in culture. One should keep in mind that there are many clear differences reported for release of EP between exudate cells and mononuclear leucocytes. For example, the release phase is said to last about 12–14 h for PMN's (MURPHY 1967) and lasts about 36 h in blood monocytes (DINARELLO 1968; BODEL 1974 a; SOROKIN 1980).

The results obtained using inhibitors of both RNA and protein synthesis have lead to the concept that the activation phase consists of a period of RNA synthesis followed by protein synthesis. The idea of a pro-pyrogen has been repeatedly pro-posed because of the apparent lack of effect of protein inhibitors during the release phase (BODEL 1974 a; DINARELLO 1980). It is now recognized that many if not most secreted proteins undergo post-translational modification (STEINER et al. 1980). It has been proposed that the multiple forms of EP now known to exist are formed by post-translational changes. Alternatively, many have said that the different forms represent the products from different kinds of cells. For example, at one time it appeared that the 38,000-dalton EP was produced by macrophages and the smaller 15,000-dalton molecule was synthesized by granulocytes. This hypothesis has not held up; however, if monocytic cells are the only cells capable of EP pro-duction, then another explanation seems more likely. DINARELLO (1980) has pro-posed that the 38,000-dalton EP is an aggregate of the 15,000-dalton monomer. It appears to the author that the EP molecule may become active during its transport across the cell membrane as occurs with other proteins such as procollagen and blood-clotting factors (STEINER 1980). This idea is especially compelling because it has been observed by many investigators that little pyrogen is present within the cell at the time when active release is occurring (HAHN et al. 1970; BODEL 1970). The observation that interference with membrane ion flux by treatment of cells with ouabain (HAHN et al. 1970) is further suggestive evidence that the cell mem-brane plays an active role in the release process.

It is repeatedly stated that most substances which activate leucocytes for pyrogen production also induce lysosomal enzyme release and induce "the respiratory burst." KLEMPNER et al. (1978) have shown that human blood neutrophils are stimulated to release superoxide and undergo a "respiratory burst in response to small amounts (as little as 1 or 2 rabbit pyrogenic doses) of human EP." No attempt was made in these studies to determine whether there was additional EP produced by these cells. However, other investigators have been unable to demonstrate either activation or inhibition of leucocytes by EP present in the incubation medium (BODEL 1974a).

BODEL (1976) reported a small but persistent enhancement of pyrogen release by cytocholasen B and colchicine. MITCHELL et al. (1975) also observed a similar modest stimulation in pyrogen release from leucocytes phagocytosing E. coli. All of these observations suggest that the leucocyte membrane is the appropriate site for studying the details of pyrogen release.

The early phases of the process, although not clearly understood, appear to involve the now well-understood process of gene derepression, RNA synthesis and finally new protein synthesis (DINARELLO 1980).

The details of the very early process, i.e. activation, and the late process, i.e. secretion, are largely unknown at this time. If the recent observation that only mononuclear leucocytes synthesize EP is correct then progress on understanding the cellular events of EP formation should come more easily.

F. Isolation and Characterization of EP

Endogenous pyrogen, like many biologically active substances, has eluded detailed characterization since its first discovery in 1948 by Beeson. Because of its hormone-like activity it has been exceedingly difficult to obtain any chemically significant quantity for characterization. Furthermore, because the only method available for following activity during purification has been the bioassay in rabbits, most of the material purified has been used during the purification for assay purposes. In spite of these major problems considerable progress has been made since the first attempts around 1960 by several laboratories (RAFTER et al. 1960; GANDER and GOODALE 1965).

In those early studies EP was thought to be a single molecular species, to be heat labile and perhaps to contain a lipid moiety. Through the work of a number of investigators, especially Atkins and Bodel, Wood and Murphy and Dinarello, the biochemical nature of EP is much more clearly defined today.

I. Methods for Purification

The methods used for purification have followed, in general, the advances in methodology for purification of proteins. With the advent of gel filtration it was soon found that EP consisted of more than one molecular component (BODEL et al. 1968; MURPHY et al. 1974; DINARELLO et al. 1974).

The observation that loses in activity during purification (presumably because of oxidation occurring under alkaline conditions) could be regenerated by treat-

ment with mercaptoethanol suggested the presence of free sulfhydryl groups necessary for activity (BODEL et al. 1969; MURPHY et al. 1974). However, only the
15,000-dalton species from rabbits appears to exhibit these properties. Isoelectric
focussing of EP partially purified by gel filtration and affinity chromatography has
provided the most pure preparations (DINARELLO 1980).

II. Heterogeneity of EP

Endogenous pyrogen from either rabbits or man contains at least two pyrogenic
molecular species. One of these is a 15,000-dalton protein and the other, a 45,000-
dalton protein. In some preparations, notably those from rabbit peritoneal exudate
cells, the 15,000-dalton form predominates. In contrast, pyrogen isolated from human monocytes consists predominately of the 45,000-dalton form (BODEL 1970;
DINARELLO 1974). Consequently, it is usually claimed that neutrophils release the
15,000-dalton species and monocytes release 45,000-dalton species. However, if in
fact neutrophils do not release any pyrogens as Murphy claims, then the monocytes
may be responsible for all of the molecular species produced. DINARELLO (1980)
has proposed that the 45,000-dalton molecule is an aggregate of the 15,000-dalton
molecule. RIECK and KOHLHAGE (1970) and SIEGERT et al. (1966) have shown that
viruses induce release of the 45,000-dalton EP, and several investigators have
shown that circulating EP in febrile rabbits consists primarily of the 45,000-dalton
pyrogen (RIECK and KOHLHAGE 1970).

It seems obvious that within the next few years the role of EP in host defence
processes will become more clearly understood. If this peptide does in fact have
multiple biological activities, i.e. as lymphocyte activator, acute phase reactant
stimulator (leucocyte endogenous mediator) and pyrogen, then EP can take its
rightful place as one of many products of acute inflammation.

References

Allison ES, Cranston WI, Duff GW, Luff RH, Rawlins MD (1973) The bioassay of human
    endogenous pyrogen. Clin Sci Mol Med 45:449–458
Anonymous (1970) United States Pharmacopia, U.S. Government Printing Office,
    Washington, D.C.
Atkins E, Bodel P (1974) Fever. In: Zweifach, Grant, McClusky (eds) The inflammatory
    process. Acad Press, New York
Atkins E, Francis L (1973) Role of lymphocytes in the pyrogenic response comparison of
    endotoxin with specific antigen and the nonspecific mitogen concanavalin A. J Infect
    Dis [Suppl] 128:S 277–S 283
Atkins E, Francis L (1977) Additional studies on the role of a lymphokine in the genesis
    of antigen induced fever in delayed hypersensitivity. In: Cooper KE, Lomax P, Schoen-
    baum E (eds) Drugs, biogenic amines, and body temperature. Proceedings of the Third
    Symposium on the Pharmacology of Thermoregulation. Banff, Alberta, Canada (1976).
    S. Karger, Basel, Switzerland; New York, N.Y. USA, pp 118–121
Atkins E, Francis L (1978) Pathogenesis of fever in delayed hypersensitivity: factors in-
    fluencing release of pyrogen inducing lymphokines. Infect Immun 21:806–812
Atkins E, Bodel P, Francis L (1967) Release of an endogenous pyrogen in vitro from rabbit
    mononuclear cells. J Exp Med 126:357–384
Atkins E, Feldman JD, Francis L, Hursh E (1972) Studies on the mechanism of fever ac-
    companying delayed hypersensitivity. The role of the sensitized lymphocyte. J Exp Med
    135:1113–1132

Atkins E, Francis L, Bernheim HA (1978) Pathogenesis of fever in delayed hypersensitivity: role of monocytes. Infect Immun 21:813–820

Beisel WR (1980) Endogenous pyrogen physiology. Physiol 23:38–42

Bernheim HA, Kluger MJ (1977) Endogenous pyrogen-like substance produced by reptiles. J Physiol (Lond) 267:659–666

Blatteis CM (1977) Comparison of endotoxin and leukocytic pyrogen pyrogenicity in new-born Guinea pigs. J Appl Physiol 42:355–361

Bodel P (1970) Studies on the mechanism of endogenous pyrogen production. I. Investigation of new protein synthesis in stimulated human blood leukocytes. Yale J Biol Med 43:145–163

Bodel P (1974a) Studies on the mechanism of endogenous pyrogen production. Part 2. Role of cell products in the regulation of pyrogen release from blood leukocytes. Infect Immun 10:451–457

Bodel P (1974b) Pyrogen release in-vitro by lymphoid tissues from patients with Hodkins disease. Yale J Biol Med 47:101–112

Bodel P (1974c) Part I. Generalized perturbations in host physiology caused by localized tumors and fever. Ann NY Acad Sci 230:6–13

Bodel P (1976) Colchicine stimulation of pyrogen production by human blood leukocytes. J Exp Med 143:1015–1026

Bodel P, Atkins E (1966) Human leukocyte pyrogen producing fever in rabbits. Proc Soc Exp Biol Med 121:943–946

Bodel P, Miller H (1976) Pyrogen from mouse macrophages causes fever in mice. Proc Soc Exp Biol Med 151:93–96

Bodel P, Miller H (1977) Differences in pyrogen production by mononuclear phagocytes and by fibroblasts or HeLa cells. J Exp Med 145:607–617

Bodel P, Miller II (1978) A new sensitive method for detecting human endogenous (leukocyte) pyrogen. Inflammation 3:103–110

Bodel P, Wenc K (1978) Spontaneous pyrogen production by mouse histiocytic and myelomonocytic tumor cell lines in-vitro. J Exp Med 147:1503–1516

Bodel PT, Wechsler A, Atkins EA (1969) Comparison of endogenous pyrogens from human rabbit leukocytes utilizing Sephadex filtration. Yale J Biol Med 41:376–387

Bolton AE, Hunter WM (1973) The labelling of proteins to high specific radioactivities by conjugation to a ^{125}I-containing acylating agent. Biochem J 133:529–539

Bornstein DL, Bredenberg C, Wood WB Jr (1963) Studies on the pathogenesis of fever – XI quantitative features of the febrile response to leucocytic pyrogen. J Exp Med 117:349–364

Borsook D, Laburn H, Mitchell D (1978) The febrile responses in rabbits and rats to leucocyte pyrogens of different species. J Physiol (Lond) 279:113–120

Chai CY, Lin MT, Chen HI, Wang SC (1971) The site of action of leukocytic pyrogen and antipyresis of sodium acetylsalicylate in monkeys. Neuropharmacology 10:715–723

Chao P, Francis L, Atkins E (1977) The release of an endogenous pyrogen from guinea pig leukocytes in vitro: A new model for investigating the role of lymphocytes in fevers induced by antigen in hosts with delayed hypersensitivity. J Exp Med 145:1288–1298

Cranston WI (1976) Fever and leukocyte pyrogen. Isr J Med Sci 12:951–954

Cranston WI, Goodale F, Snell ES, Wendt F (1956) The role of leukocytes in the initial action of bacterial pyrogens in man. Clin Sci 15:219–226

Cranston WI, Luff RH, Rawlins MD (1972) The pathogenesis of fever in renal carcinoma. Clin Sci 42:18–19

Cranston WI, Luff RH, Owen D, Rawlins MD (1973) Studies on the pathogenesis of fever in renal carcinoma. Clin Sci Mol Med 45:459–467

D'Alecy L, Kluger M (1975) Avian febrile response. J Physiol London 253:223–232

Dinarello CA (1980) Endogenous pyrogens in fever. In: Lipton JM (ed). Raven Press, New York

Dinarello CA, Wolff SM (1978) Pathogenesis of fever in man. N Engl J Med 298:607–612

Dinarello CA, Bodel PT, Atkins E (1968) The role of the liver in the production of fever and in pyrogenic tolerance. Trans Assoc Am Phys 81:334–344

Dinarello CA, Goldin NP, Wolff SM (1974) Demonstration and characterization of 2 distinct human leukocytic pyrogens. J Exp Med 139:1369–1381

Dinarello CA, Renfer L, Wolff SM (1977 a) The production of antibody against human leukocytic pyrogen. J Clin Invest 60:465–472

Dinarello CA, Renfer L, Wolff SM (1977 b) Human leukocytic pyrogen: purification and development of a radioimmunoassay. Proc Natl Acad Sci USA 74:4624–4627

Gander GW, Goodale F (1965) Chemical properties of leucocytic pyrogen I. Partial purification of rabbit leucocytic pyrogen. Exp Mol Path 1:417–426

Gander GW, Goodale F (1975) The role of granulocytes and mononuclear leukocytes in fever. In: Lomax P, Schoenbaum E, Jacob J (eds). Temperature regulation and drug action. Proceedings of a Symposium. Paris, France (1974); S. Karger, Basel, Switzerland; New York, NY USA, pp 51–58

Haeseler F, Bodel P, Atkins E (1977) Characteristics of pyrogen production by isolated rabbit kupffer cells in vitro. J Reticuloendothel Soc 22:569–581

Hahn H (1974) Fieber. Immun Infekt 2:69–72

Hahn HH, Chas DC, Pastel WB, Wood WB Jr (1967) Studies on the pathogenesis of fever XV. The production of endogenous pyrogen by peritoneal macrophages. J Exp Med 126:385–394

Hahn HH, Cheuk SF, Elfenbein CD, Wood WB (1970) Studies on the pathogenesis of fever XIX. Localization of pyrogen in granulocytes. J Exp Med 131:701–709

Hahn HH, Cheuk SF, Moore DM, Wood WB Jr (1970) Studies on the pathogenesis of fever. XVII. The cationic control of pyrogen release from exudate granulocytes in vitro. J Exp Med 131:165–178

Hanson DF, Murphy PA, Windle BE (1980) Failure of rabbit neutrophils to secrete endogenous pyrogen when stimulated with staphylococci. J Exp Med 151:1360–1370

Hattingh J, Laburn H, Mitchell D (1979) Fever induced in rabbits by intravenous injection of bovine serum albumin. J Physiol (Lond) 290:69–77

Kaiser HK, Wood WB (1962) Studies on the pathogenesis of fever X. The effect of certain enzyme inhibitors on the production and activity of leukocytic pyrogen. J Exp Med 115:37–47

Klempner MS, Dinarello CA, Gallin JI (1978) Human leukocytic pyrogen induces release of specific granule contents from human neutrophils. J Clin Invest 61:1330–1336

Lipton JM (1980) Fever. Raven Press, New York

Mitchell RH, Gander GW, Goodale F (1975) Relationship between phagocytosis and the production of leukocytic pyrogen. Adv Exp Biol Med 73 A:257–266

Moore DM, Cheuck SF, Morton JD, Berlin RD, Wood WB Jr (1970) Studies on the pathogenesis of fever XVIII. Activation of leukocytes for pyrogen production. J Exp Med 131:179–188

Moore DM, Murphy PA, Chesney PJ, Wood WB Jr (1973) Synthesis of endogenous pyrogen by rabbit leukocytes. J Exp Med 137:1263–1274

Murphy PA (1967) The rate of release of leukocyte pyrogen from rabbit blood incubated with endotoxin. J Exp Med 126:771–781

Murphy PA, Chesney PJ, Wood WB Jr (1974) Further purification of rabbit leukocyte pyrogen. J Lab Clin Med 83:310–322

Murphy PA, Simon PL, Willoughby WF (1980) Endogenous pyrogens made by rabbit peritoneal exudate cells are identical with lymphocyte-activating factors by rabbit alveolar macrophages. J Immunol 124:2498–2501

Nordlund JJ, Root RK, Wolf SM (1970) Studies on the origin of human leukocytic pyrogen. J Exp Med 131:727–743

Petersdorf RG, Bennett IL Jr (1957) Studies on the pathogenesis of fever VII. Comparative observations on the production of fever by inflammatory exudates in rabbits and dogs. Bull Johns Hopkins Hosp 100:277–286

Perlow M, Dinarello CA, Wolf SM (1975) A primate model for the study of human fever. The J Inf Dis 132:157–164

Pittman QJ, Veale WL, Cooper KE (1975) Effect of prostaglandin E, and bacterial pyrogen on body temperature in the chicken. Proc Can Physiol Soc 6:45

Rafter WS, Collins RD, Wood WB Jr (1960) Studies in the pathogenesis of fever VII. Preliminary chemical characterization of leucocytic pyrogen. J Exp Med 111:831–840

Reynolds WM, Covert JB (1977) Behavioral fever in aquatic ectothermic vertebrates. In: Cooper KE, Lomax P, Schoenbaum E (eds) Drugs, biogenic amines, and body temperature. Karger, Basel

Reynolds WM, Casterlin MC, Covert JB (1976) Behavioral fever in teleost fishes. Nature, London 259:41–42

Rieck T, Kohlhage H (1970) Behavior of different endogenous pyrogens in a biogel column. Life Sci 9:985–989

Siegert R, Pollmann W, Shu HL (1967) Zur chemischen Natur des Endogenen durch Myxoviren induzierten Pyrogens. Z Naturforsch 22 B:320–323

Siegert R, Philipp-Dormstom WK, Radsak K, Menzel H (1975) Inhibition of Newcastle disease virus induced fever in rabbits by cycloheximide. Arch Virol 48:367–373

Siegert R, Philipp-Dormston WK, Radsak K, Menzel H (1976) Mechanism of fever induction in rabbits. Infect Immun 14:1130–1137

Sorokin AV, Agasarov LG, Efremov OM (1980) Conditions favoring production and mechanism of action of macrophage pyrogen. Biull Eksp Biol Med 89:278–281

Steiner DF, Quinn PS, Chan SJ, Marsh J, Tager H (1980) Processing mechanisms in the biosynthesis of proteins. Ann NY Acad Sci 343:1–16

Taborsky I (1972) Effect of cycloheximide on in vitro formation of rabbit granulocyte pyrogen induced with influenza A/PR 8 virus or endotoxin. Acta Virol 16:376–381

Van Miert ASJPAM, Atmakusuma A (1970) Comparative observations on the production of fever by bacterial pyrogens and leucocytic pyrogens in goats and rabbits. Zentbl Vet Med 17:174–178

CHAPTER 6

Role of Central Neurotransmitters in Fever

B. Cox and T. F. Lee

A. Introduction

The aim of this chapter is to review the published evidence which suggests that central neurotransmitters play a role in fever. As such it relies heavily on two basic assumptions. Firstly that thermoregulation involves central neurotransmitter pathways and secondly that fever is a disturbance of thermoregulation. The second assumption will be discussed in full in other chapters of this book; the first has been the subject of a number of recent reviews and symposia (Cox and Lomax 1977; Milton 1978; Lomax and Schönbaum 1979; Cox et al. 1980).

Much of the work on central transmitters and fever stems from the publication in 1963 of the "new concept of temperature regulation" based on a balance between noradrenaline and 5-hydroxytryptamine in the hypothalamus (Feldberg and Myers 1963) and it is no coincidence therefore that these two amines have received the greatest attention. However, these have not been the only two neurotransmitters studied as this chapter will show. Indeed some of the work predates that of Feldberg and Myers when apparently the tacit assumption was made that neurotransmitters played some role in the mediation of the febrile response (Göing 1959; Kroneberg and Kerbjuweit 1959; Canal and Ornesi 1961).

Thus accepting that central neurotransmitters play an important role in thermoregulation, we shall attempt to evaluate critically the evidence for and against the involvement of any particular neurotransmitter in the febrile response. Our task is not aided by the fact that there appears to be both species and even strain differences in the response of animals to centrally applied neurotransmitters and also that any one neurotransmitter may exist at more than one point in the central thermoregulatory pathways. In an ideal world those investigating the role of neurotransmitters in fever would have taken this into account and considered species, strain, site of effect and specificity of the drugs or agents used. As the reader will know the world is far from ideal.

In the following sections we will deal with the three neurotransmitters which have been investigated in most detail. These are noradrenaline, 5-hydroxytryptamine, and acetylcholine and we shall consider how the evidence for their possible role in fever has been collected from experiments involving depleting agents, antagonists, and agonists and also biochemical studies. The evidence for a role of other neurotransmitters, as yet poorly investigated, will also be presented in so far as any evidence is available.

B. Noradrenaline

I. Depleting Agents

Most of the work investigating the possible involvement of brain amines in the febrile response has been carried out in the rabbit. The first suggestion that noradrenaline acted as a mediator was based on experiments with reserpine (Göing 1959; Kroneberg and Kerbjuweit 1959) when the febrile response to bacterial pyrogen was shown to be absent after intravenous reserpine pretreatment (Table 1). Further, the effect of reserpine could be prevented by the monoamine oxidase inhibitor iproniazid provided it was given before and not after the reserpine (Göing 1959; Kroneberg and Kerbjuweit 1959). This suggested that intact endogenous amine stores were important for the production of a febrile response. This effect of reserpine was subsequently confirmed by a number of workers (see Table 1), who used a variety of pyrogenic agents. The important site for the reserpine-induced depletion is not clear since an intracerebroventricular injection of reserpine has been found to be ineffective against pyrogen-induced fever (Cooper et al. 1967; Veale and Cooper 1975). Thus it would appear that there is either a peripheral component in reserpine's action or that some central extrahypothalamic area is involved which reserpine cannot reach after intracerebroventricular injection (Veale and Cooper 1975), since intracerebroventricular reserpine would be expected to reach the hypothalamus. There have been some reports indicating the ineffectiveness of reserpine pretreatment. Yasuda (1962) showed that although reserpine could prevent the febrile response to *E. coli* endotoxin it was ineffective against both typhoid vaccine and *P. fluorescens* pyrogen. The reason for this discrepancy is unclear. Another negative result was obtained by Tangri et al. (1975). However, these workers used a different route and pretreatment time for reserpine, an intramuscular injection 72 h before pyrogen challenge compared with either intravenous or intraperitoneal pretreatment for between 17 and 24 h as used by most other workers in the field.

The experiments with reserpine must of course be interpreted with caution since it is a nonspecific depleting agent, and 5-hydroxytryptamine as well as the catecholamines are known to be depleted following reserpine injection (Des Prez et al. 1966; Mašek et al. 1968, 1972; Metcalf and Thompson 1975). More direct evidence for noradrenaline as a mediator of the febrile response comes from experiments with α-methyl-p-tyrosine, which depletes catecholamines but not 5-hydroxytryptamine (Moore and Dominic 1971). As with reserpine, febrile responses to various pyrogens have been shown to be attenuated by pretreatment with α-methyl-p-tyrosine (Table 2). Some workers have, however, been unable to confirm these observations. Tangri et al. (1975) used an intracerebroventricular route of injection and the lack of an effect of α-methyl-p-tyrosine may be explained in an analogous manner to that used for reserpine. The failure of α-methyl-p-tyrosine to work in the experiments of Des Prez et al. (1966) is more difficult to explain. They showed that guanethidine (10 mg/kg i.p.) and α-methyl-p-tyrosine, both of which markedly depleted brainstem and hypothalamic noradrenaline without an effect on 5-hydroxytryptamine, were unable to modify the febrile response to pyrogen. However, since these authors also showed that p-chlorophenylalanine failed to pre-

Table 1. Effect of reserpine on pyrogen fever in rabbits

Dose (route)	Time schedule	Pyrogen (dose, route)	Effect on response to pyrogen	References
1 mg/kg (i.v.)	Daily for 3 days	S. abortus equi lipopolysaccharide (0.001–100 µg/kg, i.v.)	Attenuation	GÖING (1959)
1 mg/kg (i.v.)	21 h	E. coli lipopolysaccharide (1 µg/kg, i.v.)	Attenuation	KRONEBERG and KURBJUWEIT (1959)
1 mg/kg (i.v.)	21 h	E. coli lipopolysaccharide (1.5 µg/kg, i.v.)	Attenuation	YASUDA (1962)
1–1.5 mg/kg	24 h	E. coli endotoxin (25 µg/kg)	Attenuation	DES PREZ et al. (1966)
1 mg/kg (i.p.)	21 h	Streptococcal mucopeptide (25–50 µg, i.c.v.)	Attenuation	MAŠEK et al. (1968, 1972)
1 mg/kg (i.p.)	17 h	TAB vaccine (0.1 ml/kg i.v.)	Attenuation	METCALF and THOMPSON (1975)
1 mg/kg (i.p.)	17 h	Leucocyte pyrogen: (10 ml i.v. followed by a continuous i.v. infusion at 0.08 ml min^{-1})	Attenuation	METCALF and THOMPSON (1975)
1 mg/kg (i.v.)	21 h	Typhoid vaccine (0.05 mg/kg, i.v.)	Potentiation	YASUDA (1962)
1 mg/kg (i.v.)	21 h	P. fluorescens pyrogen (10 µg/kg, i.v.)	No effect	YASUDA (1962)
1.5 mg/kg (i.m.)	72 h	S. typhi "0" cell (10^5 organisms, i.c.v.)	No effect	TANGRI et al. (1975)
0.35–0.75 mg (i.c.v.)	12 h	S. abortus equi lipopolysaccharide (0.25–0.9 µg, i.v.)	No effect	COOPER et al. (1969)
0.5 mg (i.c.v.)	24 h	Leucocyte pyrogen (unspecified dose i.v.)	No effect	VEALE and COOPER (1975)

Table 2. Effect of α-methyl-p-tyrosine on pyrogen fever in rabbits

Dose (route)	Time schedule	Pyrogen (dose, route)	Effect on response to pyrogen	References
100 mg/kg (i.p.)	8 h	Leucocyte pyrogen (2 × 10^8 organisms, i.v.)	Attenuation	GIARMAN et al. (1968)
200 mg/kg (i.p.)	21 h	Streptococcal mucopeptide (25–50 µg i.c.v.)	Attenuation	MAŠEK et al. (1968, 1972)
?	?	Leucocyte pyrogen (?)	Attenuation	TEDDY (1969)[a]
200 mg/kg (i.p.)	17 h	TAB vaccine (0.1 ml/kg, i.v.)	Attenuation	METCALF and THOMPSON (1975)
200 mg/kg (i.p.)	17 h	Leucocyte pyrogen (10 ml i.v. followed by a continuous i.v. infusion at 0.08 ml min^{-1})	Attenuation	METCALF and THOMPSON (1975)
100 mg/kg (i.p.)	12 h	Streptococcal exotoxin (20 mg/kg, i.v.)	Attenuation	SCHLIEVERT and WATSON (1979)
200 mg/kg (i.p.)	8 h	E. coli endotoxin (25 µg, i.v.)	No effect	DES PREZ et al. (1966)
10 mg (i.c.v.)	24 h	S. typhi "0" cell (10^5 organisms, i.c.v.)	Attenuation	TANGRI et al. (1975)

[a] Unspecified dose and time schedule

vent the febrile response (see 5-hydroxytryptamine section), their work is at odds with most others in this field.

A role for noradrenaline in the febrile response in rabbits receives further support from studies with the more specific catecholamine-depleting agent, 6-hydroxydopamine (Kostrzewa and Jacobowitz 1974). The febrile responses to either "E" pyrogen from *P. vulgaris* (0.02 µg, i.v.) or prostaglandin E_1 (PGE_1) (500 ng, i.h.) were attenuated by both intracerebroventricular (600 µg, 5–7 days before pyrogen injection) and intrahypothalamic (150 µg, 3–5 days before pyrogen injection) pretreatment with 6-hydroxydopamine (Laburn et al. 1974, 1975) and similar results have been obtained by other workers. Thus Kandasamy (1977) showed that intracerebroventricular pretreatment with 6-hydroxydopamine (three doses of 500 µg/kg given 1,4 and 7 days before arachidonic acid injection) prevented the febrile response to arachidonic acid (100 µg/kg, i.v.) and Lin (1980) also demonstrated that PGE_1-induced fever could be attenuated by 15–40 days intracerebroventricular pretreatment with 6-hydroxydopamine (750 µg). However, in other species, 6-hydroxydopamine has been reported to produce opposite effects. Thus the febrile response to O-somatic antigen (2 µg/kg, i.v.) in cats was potentiated after intracerebroventricular 6-hydroxydopamine pretreatment when it was given as three doses of 500 µg, 1, 4, and 7 days before antigen injection (Harvey and Milton 1974 b; Milton and Harvey 1975). In rats, a similar potentiation was observed in the febrile response to *E. coli* pyrogen, prostaglandin (E_2 and $F_{2\alpha}$) or arachidonic acid after intrahypothalamic pretreatment with 6-hydroxdopamine (two doses of 100 µg with a 2-day interval) (Splawinski et al. 1976). More recently, Ford and Klugman (1980) also found that the febrile response to *S. typhosa* endotoxin (20 mg/kg, i.p.) or bovine leucocyte pyrogen (2 ml, i.p.) was enhanced after pretreatment with 6-hydroxydopamine (200 µg, i.c.v.). These contrasting results with 6-hydroxydopamine may be best explained by a species difference. Thus in rabbits, intracerebral injection of noradrenaline usually causes hyperthermia whereas hypothermia has been reported in rats and cats after central noradrenaline injection (for review see Bruinvels 1979). Thus it is possible that central noradrenaline plays different roles in the febrile response dependent on species. It may actually be a mediator in the rabbit, but in the rat and cat central noradrenaline may function to reduce the severity of the febrile response.

II. Sympathomimetic Agents and Monoamine Oxidase Inhibitors

Another approach in the attempt to examine the role of noradrenaline in fever has been to increase central sympathetic activity. In rabbits, intracerebral injection of noradrenaline enhanced the fever induced by streptococcal exotoxin (Schlievert and Watson 1979) (Table 3). In addition these workers also showed that the febrile response was not affected by isoprenaline. These findings were in agreement with the results from antagonist studies (see adrenoceptor antagonists section) suggesting that α- but not β-adrenoceptors may be involved in the febrile response. However, some work has thrown doubt on the involvement of noradrenaline in the febrile response in the rabbit (Preston and Cooper 1976). These workers could find no effect of noradrenaline when it was injected into a PGE-sensitive site within the rabbit hypothalamus. However, their studies only rule out an interaction at one

particular site. The possibility still remains that noradrenaline is involved in the febrile response but not at the point where the prostaglandins are acting. In other
species, pyrogen or PGE-induced fever was attenuated by central noradrenaline injection (Table 3), which is consistent with the observations made with 6-hydroxy-
dopamine above. Unfortunately in most of the studies referred to in Table 3 the
effect of noradrenaline on its own was not mentioned and synergism between two
hyperthermic effects remains a possibility.

Another way to increase central sympathetic activity is to prevent noradrenaline metabolism by inhibition of monoamine oxidase enzymes. Results obtained by
studying the effects of monoamine oxidase inhibitors on the fever induced by different pyrogens seem less consistent than other studies (Table 3). Both potentiation
(GÖING 1959; YASUDA 1962) and a lack of effect (KRONEBERG and KERBJUWEIT
1959; GARDEY-LEVASSORT et al. 1970a; CRANSTON and LUFF 1972) have been reported. COOPER and CRANSTON (1966) found that pargyline only slightly prolonged
the duration of the febrile response. However, this study was complicated by the
finding that two out of nine rabbits died of hyperpyrexia after pargyline, whereas
none of the animals died after the pyrogen treatment on its own. The lack of specificity of the monoamine oxidase inhibitors and their differing effects on the sub-
types of monoamine oxidase enzyme means that a much more careful analysis of
the effects of a variety of inhibitors is required.

III. Adrenoceptor Antagonists

The role of various neurotransmitters in normal thermoregulation has been frequently investigated by the use of specific receptor antagonists. Similar methods
have been used in the study of pyrogen- or PGE-induced fever. Most workers have
found that the febrile response is less after blockade of α-adrenoceptors (Table 4).
In contrast, β-adrenoceptor antagonists appear to be ineffective against the febrile
response (Table 4). However, it is difficult to draw a firm conclusion on the involvement of α-adrenoceptors in the febrile response since some workers have
failed to confirm an effect of α-adrenoceptor antagonists (BURKS and VAN INWE-
GEN 1975; TANGRI et al. 1975; SZEKELY 1979a, b). The most striking result was obtained by KANDASAMY et al. (1975), who reported that pyrogen- or PGE-induced
fever was only antagonized by phenoxybenzamine, but not by phentolamine. Indeed in most cases, where a positive result was obtained the result came from studies with phenoxybenzamine, a drug which is also known to have anticholinergic,
antihistamine, and antiserotonergic (anti-5-HT) properties (NICKERSON and COL-
LIER 1975). Thus the possibility of the involvement of α-adrenoceptors in febrile responses still requires further investigation, particularly in the use of selective α-ad-
renoceptor antagonists.

IV. Brain Catecholamine Levels

Another approach is to measure the content of amines in the brain before and during fever. The results obtained from this approach have lacked any apparent pattern and made the situation less clear. The apparent inconsistencies may due to a
number of factors. In most studies, the amine levels were only measured at the peak

Table 3. Effects of sympathomimetics and MAOI on fever

Species	Drug (dose, route, time schedule)	Fever induced by (dose, route)	Effect on febrile response	References
Sympathomimetics				
Rabbits	NA (50 μg, i.c.)	Streptococcal exotoxin (20 mg/kg, i.v.)	Potentiation	SCHLIEVERT and WATSON (1979)
	Isoproterenol (50 μg, i.c.)	Streptococcal exotoxin (20 mg/kg, i.v.)	No effect	SCHLIEVERT and WATSON (1979)
Sheep	NA (200–300 μg, i.c.v.)	TAB vaccine (?)	Attenuation	BLIGH and MASKREY (1971)
Rats	NA (4 μg, i.c.v., 10 min after)	PGE_2 (2 μg, i.c.v.)	Attenuation	GURIN et al. (1979)
Fowl	NA (1 μmol, i.c.v., 0.2 μmol, i.h.)	PGE_1 or PGE_2 (140 nmol, i.c.v., 56 nmol i.h.)	Attenuation	NISTICO and MARMO (1979)
	α-methyl-NA (0.5 μmol, i.c.v., 0.1 μmol i.h.)	PGE_1 or PGE_2 (140 nmol, i.c.v., 56 nmol i.h.)	Attenuation	NISTICO and MARMO (1979)
Chicks	NA (0.05 μmol, i.h.)	"0"-somatic antigen of S. dysenteriae (1 μg, i.h.)	Attenuation	ARTUNKAL et al. (1977)[a]
Monoamine oxidase inhibitors				
Rabbits	Iproniazid (100 μg/kg, i.v., 24 h before)	S. abortus equi lipopolysaccharide (0.001 ~ 100 μg/kg, i.v.)	Potentiation	GÖING (1959)
	Iproniazid (100 mg/kg, s.c., 26 h before)	E. coli lipopolysaccharide (1 μg/kg, i.v.)	No effect	KRONEBERG and KURBJUWEIT (1959)
	Iproniazid (100 mg/kg, i.v., 24 h before)	E. coli lipopolysaccharide (0.25 or 0.5 μg/kg, i.v.)	No effect	GARDEY-LEVASSORT et al. (1970a)
	Iproniazid (100 mg/kg, i.v., 24 h before)	Gonococcus vaccine (10^8 organisms/kg, i.v.)	No effect	GARDEY-LEVASSORT et al. (1970a)
	β-phenylisopropylhydrazine (3 mg/kg, i.v., 26 h before)	E. coli lipopolysaccharide (1.5 mg/kg, i.v.)	Potentiation	YASUDA (1962)
	β-phenylisopropylhydrazine (3 mg/kg, i.v., 26 h before)	P. fluorescens pyrogens (10 μg/kg, i.v.)	Potentiation	YASUDA (1962)
	Pargyline (25 mg/kg, i.v., 90 min before)	Leucocyte pyrogen (0.25 ~ 0.5 ml, i.v.)	No effect	COOPER and CRANSTON (1966b)
	Pargyline (25 mg/kg, i.v., 24 h before)	E. coli lipopolysaccharide (0.25 or 0.5 μg/kg, i.v.)	No effect	GARDEY-LEVASSORT et al. (1970a)

Pargyline (25 mg/kg, i.v., 24 h before)	Gonococcus vaccine (10^8 organisms/kg, i.v.)	No effect	GARDEY-LEVASSORT et al. (1970a)
Desimipramine (625 μg, i.c.v., 4 h after)	Leucocyte pyrogen (?)	No effect	CRANSTON and LUFF (1972)

[a] Drug produced hypothermia on its own
[b] See text

Table 4. Effect of adrenoceptor antagonists on fever

Species	Drug (dose, route, time schedule)	Fever induced by (dose, route)	Effect on febrile response	References
α-Adrenoceptor antagonists				
Rabbits	Phenoxybenzamine (50 μg, i.h.)	PGE_1 (500 ng, i.h.)	Attenuation	LABURN et al. (1974, 1975)
	Phenoxybenzamine (25 μg + 15 μg 15 min after pyrogen, i.h., bilaterally)	P. vulgaris "E" pyrogen (0.02 μg, i.v.)	Attenuation	LABURN et al. (1975)
	Phenoxybenzamine (1 mg/kg, i.v., 30 min before)	S. typhi lipopolysaccharide (100 pg, i.c.v.) and PGE_1 (1 μg, i.c.v.)	Attenuation	KANDASAMY et al. (1975)
	Phenoxybenzamine (1 mg/kg, i.v., 30 min before)	Arachnoid acid (100 μg/kg, i.v.)	Attenuation	KANDASAMY (1977)
	Phenoxybenzamine (1 mg/kg, i.v., 1 h before)	Streptococcal exotoxin (20 mg/kg, i.v.)	Attenuation	SCHLIEVERT and WATSON (1979)
	Phenoxybenzamine (50 μg, i.c.v., before)	S. typhi "0" (10^5 organism, i.c.v.)	No effect	TANGRI et al. (1975)
	Phentolamine (10 mg/kg, i.v., 30 min before)	S. typhi lipopolysaccharide (100 pg, i.c.v.) and PGE_1 (1 μg, i.c.v.)	No effect	KANDASAMY et al. (1975)
Monkeys	Phentolamine (1.5–3.6 μg, i.h., 20 min before)	PGE_1 (100 ng, i.h.)	Attenuation	SIMPSON et al. (1977)
Guinea pigs (newborn)	Phentolamine (30 μg, i.c.v., 30 min before)	E. coli lipopolysaccharide (0.2 or 0.002 μg, i.c.v.)	No effect	SZEKELY (1979a)
Cats	Phentolamine (100 μg, i.v., 5 min before)	PGE_1 (100 μg, i.v.)	No effect	BURKS and VAN INWEGEN (1975)

B. Cox and T. F. Lee

Table 4. (continued)

Species	Drug (dose, route, time schedule)	Fever induced by (dose, route)	Effect on febrile response	References
Kittens	Phentolamine (30 µg, i.c.v., 30 min before)	E. coli lipopolysaccharide (0.2 or 0.002 µg, i.c.v.)	No effect	Szekely (1979 b)
β-Adrenoceptor antagonists				
Rabbits	Propranolol (50 µg, i.h.)	PGE$_1$ (500 ng, i.h.)	No effect	Laburn et al. (1974, 1975)
	Propranolol (25 µg + 15 µg 15 min after pyrogen, i.h., bilaterally)	P. vulgaris "E" pyrogen (0.02 µg, i.v.)	No effect	Laburn et al. (1975)
Monkeys	Propranolol (7 µg, i.h., 20 min before)	PGE$_1$ (100 ng, i.h.)	No effect	Simpson et al. (1977)
	Practolol (7 µg, i.h., 20 min before)	PGE$_1$ (100 ng, i.h.)	No effect	Simpson et al. (1977)
	Sotalol (1.6~7 µg, i.h., 20 min before)	PGE$_1$ (100 ng, i.h.)	No effect	Simpson et al. (1977)
Guinea pigs	Propranolol (6 mg/kg, i.p., 2 min before)	S. enteritidis endotoxin (2 µg/kg, i.v.)	No effect	Blatteis (1976)
Guinea pigs (newborn)	Propranolol (6 mg/kg, i.p., 2 min before)	S. enteritidis endotoxin (2 µg/kg, i.v.)	Attenuation	Blatteis (1976)[a]
Kittens	Propranolol (30 µg, i.c.v., 30 min before)	E. coli lipopolysaccharide (0.2 or 0.002 µg, i.c.v.)	No effect	Szekely (1979 a)
Kittens	Propranolol (30 µg, i.c.v., 30 min before)	E. coli lipopolysaccharide (0.2 or 0.002 µg, i.c.v.)	No effect	Szekely (1979 b)

[a] The dose of propranolol produced a significant fall in core temperature on its own

time of the fever. Thus it was not possible to determine whether the changes were causative or consequent on the fever. Further, different workers used different brain regions when determining the change in amines, making comparisons difficult. In rabbits no change in brainstem noradrenaline levels was observed either at the peak time after *E. coli* lipopolysaccharide injection (TAKAGI and KURUMA 1966) or during the fever induced by pyrexial (KURUMA et al. 1964). In contrast, a decrease in noradrenaline was found in the midbrain and pons when measured at the peak of the fever induced by pyrogen injection (METCALF and THOMPSON 1975). A similar decrease was shown to occur in the hypothalamus after *E. coli* endotoxin (5 µg/kg, i.v.) or leucocyte pyrogen (2×10^8 organisms, i.v.) (GIARMAN et al. 1964). There have also been reports of a decrease in noradrenaline levels accompanied by an increase in noradrenaline metabolites in the hypothalamus and brainstem at the second peak and during defervescence after *E. coli* lipopolysaccharide (1.5 µg/kg, i.v.) or gonococcus vaccine injections (10^8 organisms/kg, i.v.) (GARDEY-LEVASSORT 1977; GARDEY-LEVASSORT et al. 1977).

Measurement of amine levels within the brain are not sufficient to indicate the activity of the amine system during fever, and turnover studies are of more value. Therefore several experiments have been carried out to measure the turnover of noradrenaline during fever. No change in noradrenaline turnover rate was observed in either the brainstem or the hypothalamus of rats at the time of peak fever after streptococcal mucopeptide injections (2 mg/kg i.v., MAŠEK et al. 1973; 500 µg/kg i.v., MAŠEK et al. 1980). Similar results were obtained when studying the hypothalamus of kittens and newborn guinea pigs during fever induced by *E. coli* endotoxin (0.2 µg/kg, i.c.v.) (HAHN and SZEKELY 1979). MYERS and WALLER (1976) also investigated the activity of adrenergic systems during fever by using a push-pull cannula technique and could find no consistent release of [^{3}H]-noradrenaline in the hypothalamus of the monkey during PGE-induced fever. Thus except on a few occasions in the rabbit, the results obtained from the measurement of either amine levels or amine turnover do not support the hypothesis of the involvement of noradrenaline in the febrile responses.

V. Conclusion

Consideration of the above results suggests that central adrenergic systems are possibly involved in fever. However, noradrenaline may play a different role in different species. In rabbits, it seems to act as a mediator of the febrile response; since (1) the fever can be attenuated by selective noradrenaline depletion or blockade of central adrenergic transmission; (2) the fever can be potentiated by increasing central adrenergic activity either by monoamine oxidase inhibition or by direct injection of noradrenaline. In other species, noradrenaline may act to reduce the febrile response rather than as a mediator. However, in all species, noradrenaline seems to produce its effects via α-adrenoceptors and even though there is some controversy, at least no evidence has been presented which suggests the involvement of β-adrenoceptors. This may not be surprising as it has also been demonstrated that it is the α-adrenoceptor which is important in normal thermoregulation (for review see BRUINVELS 1979). Unfortunately most of the biochemical data do not support the pharmacology in the suggestion of a possible involvement of noradrenaline in the febrile response. The differences may, however, be due to the methods employed, more studies involving turnover and more detailed time course studies are required before firm conclusions can be made. It is obvious therefore that there is a need for further work in this area.

C. 5-Hydroxytryptamine

I. Depleting Agents

As with noradrenaline, attempts have been made to examine the possibility of the involvement of 5-hydroxytryptamine (5-HT) in the febrile response by the use of depleting agents. The work with reserpine has been discussed in full in the previous section and limitations due to its lack of specificity noted. However, the discovery of a selective 5-HT depleting agent, p-chlorophenylalanine (PCPA) (KOE and WEISSMAN 1966), opened up new possibilities. As a result of this discovery, numerous experiments have been carried out to attempt to determine the role of 5-HT in fever and these are summarised in Table 5. In rats and cats, pretreatment with PCPA resulted in attenuation of the fever induced by either pyrogen or PGE injection. In contrast, in guinea pigs, pyrogen-induced fever was unaffected by PCPA pretreatment. As might be anticipated from the result with 6-OHDA and noradrenaline, PCPA produced different effects in the rabbit. Thus, in this species, pyrogen-induced fever was potentiated after PCPA pretreatment, which suggests that 5-HT acts to reduce the febrile response rather than promote it. However, there is not total agreement on the role of 5-HT since other workers have reported that PCPA has no effect on either pyrogen- or PGE-induced fever in rabbits (Table 5). This discrepancy may due to variation in the dose and pretreatment time. In general PCPA has been reported to be active when a dose higher than 300 mg/kg i.p. is used with a pretreatment time of less than 48 h. If these conditions are not met then the 5-HT stores, even though low, may be sufficient to maintain an adequate physiological function.

Involvement of 5-HT in the febrile response has also been indicated in experiments where the relatively selective 5-HT depleting agents 5,6- or 5,7-dihydroxytryptamine (DHT) have been used (BJÖRKLUND et al. 1974). The fever induced by intracerebroventricular injection of either PGF_2 (1–10 µg) or PGE_2 (10 µg) was reduced after intracerebroventricular pretreatment with 5,6-DHT (75 µg, 10 days before PGE injection) in rats (BRUS et al. 1979). A similar attenuation of PGE_1-induced fever (500 ng, i.c.v.) in rabbits has also been reported after 5,7-DHT pretreatment (300 µg, i.c.v., 2–15 days before PGE injection) (LIN 1980). However, in this case the effect may be due to a nonspecific effect of 5,7-DHT, since under the conditions of the experiment it could also cause depletion of central noradrenaline stores (BJÖRKLUND et al. 1975; LORDEN et al. 1979). LIN (1978) also found that the fever induced by the same amount of PGE_1 was not affected by PCPA pretreatment (Table 5) arguing against 5-HT involvement. The work of CARRUBA and BÄCHTOLD (1976) also argues against 5-HT involvement in the febrile response. They showed that the fever induced by Pyrifer VII (0.5 µl/kg, i.v.) was not affected by a 72-h pretreatment with 5,6-DHT (50 µg, i.c.v.). However, before ruling out a role for 5-HT from these studies, the following possibilities must

Table 5. Effect of PCPA on pyrogen- or PGE-induced fever

Species	Dose of PCPA (route, time schedule)	Fever induced by (dose, route)	Effects on febrile response	References
Rabbits	300 mg/kg (i.p., 48 h)	Leucocyte pyrogen (2 × 10^8 organisms, i.v.)	Potentiation	GIARMAN et al. (1968)
	?	Leucocyte pyrogen (?)	Potentiation	TEDDY (1969)[a]
	300 mg/kg (i.p., 21 h)	Streptococcal mucopeptide (25 µg, i.c.v.)	Potentiation	MAŠEK et al. (1972)
	300 mg/kg (i.p., 12 h)	Streptococcal pyrogen exotoxin (20 mg/kg, i.v.)	Potentiation	SCHLIEVERT and WATSON (1979)
	250 mg/kg (i.p., 72 h)	E. coli endotoxin (25 µg, i.v.)	No effect	DES PREZ and OATES (1968)
	125 mg/kg × 3 (i.p.; 18, 42, 66 h)	PGE$_1$ (5 µg, i.c.v.)	No effect	SINCLAIR and CHAPLIN (1974)
	300 mg/kg (i.p., 72 h)	TAB vaccine (0.1 ml/kg, i.v.)	No effect	METCALF and THOMPSON (1975)
	300 mg/kg (i.p., 72 h)	Leucocyte pyrogen (10 ml i.v. followed by a continuous i.v. infusion at 0.08 ml/min)	No effect	METCALF and THOMPSON (1975)
	100 mg/kg × 4 (i.p., 1, 2, 3, 4 days)	Pyrifer VII (0.5 µl/kg, i.v.)	No effect	CARRUBA and BÄCHTOLD (1976)
	75 nmol/kg × 3 (i.p., 7, 8, 9 days)	P. vulgaris "E" pyrogen (0.02 µg, i.v.)	No effect	BORSOOK et al. (1977)
	300 mg/kg × 2 (p.o., 24, 48 h)	Arachnoid acid (100 µg/kg, i.c.v.)	No effect	KANDASAMY (1977)
	300 mg/kg (i.p., 72 h)	PGE (500 ng, i.c.v.)	No effect	LIN (1978)
Cats	300 mg/kg × 2 (p.o., 24, 48 h)	0-somatin antigen (2–4 µg/kg, i.v. 75 ng, i.c.v.)	Attenuation	HARVEY and MILTON (1974a), MILTON and HARVEY (1975)
	300 mg/kg × 2 (p.o., 24, 48 h)	PGE$_1$ (50~500 mg, i.c.v.)	Attenuation[b]	HARVEY and MILTON (1974a), MILTON and HARVEY (1975)
	?	PGE$_1$ (100 ng, i.h. bilaterally) or pyrogen (?, i.v.)	No effect	VEALE and COOPER (1975)
Kittens	300 mg/kg × 2 (i.p., 24, 48 h)	E. coli endotoxin (0.2 µg, i.c.v.)	Attenuation[c]	SZEKELY (1978a, 1979b)
Rats	316 mg/kg (i.p., 72 h)	S. typhosa endotoxin (20 µg/kg, i.p.)	Attenuation	FORD and KLUGMAN (1980)
	316 mg/kg (i.p., 72 h)	Bovine leucocyte pyrogen (2 ml, i.p.)	Attenuation	FORD and KLUGMAN (1980)
Guinea pigs	300 mg/kg × 2 (i.p., 24, 48 h)	E. coli endotoxin (0.2 µg, i.c.v.)	No effect	SZEKELY (1978b)
Guinea pigs (newborn)	300 mg/kg × 2 (i.p., 24, 48 h)	E. coli endotoxin (0.2 µg, i.c.v.)	No effect[d]	SZEKELY (1978a, b)

[a] Unspecified doses

[b] Attenuated low doses (50~150 ng) only

[c] Attenuated the early phase only

[d] The transient fall in core temperature between two peaks was attenuated

be taken into consideration: (1) different mechanisms may be involved in PGE-and Pyrifer VII-induced fever; (2) residual 5-HT stores may be adequate and allow the febrile response to occur. This second possibility seems reasonable since there was only 30%–40% depletion of 5-HT in the hypothalamus and brainstem after administration of this dose of 5,6-DHT.

An entirely different approach, which lends support to the concept of a role of 5-HT in the febrile response in the rat, has been used by other workers (KADLECOVÁ et al. 1977; MAŠEK et al. 1980). This group found that the fever induced by the peptidoglycan of *A. streptococcus* (2 mg/kg i.v. or 500 µg/kg i.v.) could be abolished by electrical lesions of the raphé nuclei. It is not possible to totally exclude the involvement of other neurotransmitters from these experiments since non-5-HT neurones have also been shown to be present within the raphé nuclei regions and these workers also showed that the fever could be abolished by producing a lesion in other brain regions. However, since in the raphé nuclei there are a large number of 5-HT containing cell bodies then 5-HT must be considered as a prime candidate.

II. 5-Hydroxytryptamine Agonists and Uptake Inhibitors

The confusion that exists when the studies with depleting agents are considered is not helped when one considers studies in which agonists are used. In all cases central injections of 5-HT have been reported to attenuate the febrile response due to either pyrogen or PGE injection (Table 6). However, these experiments are very difficult to interpret since 5-HT on its own usually caused a significant change in core temperature. In rabbits, two groups have reported potentiation of the febrile response after systemic injection with the 5-HT precursor, 5-hydroxytryptophan (5-HTP) (Table 6). In contrast, LIN et al. (1979) reported that 5-HTP produced an attenuation of the febrile response in rabbits pretreated with the peripheral decarboxylase inhibitor, Ro 4-4602. The major problem in interpreting this data is that the 5-HTP may be exerting peripheral as well as central effects. At least in the experiments of LIN et al. a peripheral decarboxylase inhibitor was used and in their study the results agreed with those where 5-HT was injected centrally.

Another way to enhance central 5-HT availability is to prevent its inactivation by uptake into nerve terminals. LIN et al. (1979) reported that the PGE_1-induced fever could be attenuated by either systemic or central pretreatment with 5-HT uptake inhibitors (Table 6). This result may once again suggest that 5-HT acts to reduce fever in rabbits. However, some controversy remains since others have found uptake inhibitors to be ineffective (Table 6). In one case a short pretreatment time of 15 min was used (SINCLAIR and CHAPLIN 1974) and in the other there was a species difference (SIMPSON et al. 1977).

III. Indoleamine Antagonists

The first suggestion that 5-HT was involved in the febrile response came as early as 1961 when CANAL and ORNESI found that typhoid vaccine-induced fever was attenuated by cyproheptadine (Table 7). These workers also showed that the febrile response could be potentiated by the monoamine oxidase inhibitor phenyl-isopyl-hydrazine (5 mg/kg, i.v., 12 h before vaccine injection). Attenuation of fever by cy-

Table 6. Effect of serotonergic agonists and uptake inhibitors on pyrogen- or PGE-induced fever

Species	Drug (Dose, route, time schedule)	Fever induced by (dose, route)	Effect on febrile response	References
Serotonergic agonists				
Rabbits	5HT (0.1 mg/kg, i.c.v.)	S. typhi "T$_2$" lipopolysaccharide (1 pg–1 µg/kg i.c.v.)	Attenuation	PEIDARIES and JACOB (1971)[a]
	5HT (50 µg, i.c.)	Streptococcal exotoxin (20 mg/kg, i.c.v.)	Attenuation	SCHLIEVERT and WATSON (1979)
	5HTP (20 mg/kg, i.p.)	Leucocyte pyrogen (2 × 10^8 organisms, i.v.)	Prolonged fever	GAIRMAN et al. (1968)[a]
	5HTP (25 mg/kg, i.v., 2 h)	Streptococcal mucopeptide (25~50 µg, i.v.)	Potentiation	MAŠEK et al. (1968)
	5HTP (5–20 mg/kg, i.p.)[b]	PGE$_1$ (500 ng, i.c.v.)	Attenuation	LIN et al. (1979)
Sheep	5HT (200 µg, i.c.v.)	TAB vaccine (0.7–1 ml, i.v.)	Attenuation	BLIGH and MASKREY (1971)
Goats	5HT (800 µg, i.c.v.)	E. coli lipopolysaccharide (0.1 µg/kg, i.v.)	Attenuation	FRENS (1975)[a]
Rats	5HT (25 µg, i.c.v., 10 min after PGE$_2$)	PGE$_2$ (2 µg, i.c.v.)	Attenuation	GURIN et al. (1979)
Chicks	5HT (0.05 µmol, i.h.)	"O"-somatic antigen of S. dysenteriae (1 µg, i.h.)	Attenuation	ARTUNKAL et al. (1977)[a]
Uptake inhibitors				
Rabbits	Chlorimipramine (5 mg/kg, i.v., 15 min)	PGE$_1$ (5 µg, i.c.v.)	No effect	SINCLAIR and CHAPLIN (1974)
	Chlorimipramine (1–20 mg/kg, i.p. or 0.15–0.5 mg, i.c.v., 120–150 min)	PGE$_1$ (500 ng, i.c.v.)	Attenuation	LIN et al. (1979)
	Fluoxetine (1.2–10 mg/kg, i.p. or 0.16–0.4 mg, i.c.v., 60–120 min)	PGE$_1$ (500 ng, i.c.v.)	Attenuation	LIN et al. (1979)
Monkeys	Fluoxetine (5 µg, i.h., 20 min)	PGE$_1$ (100 ng, i.h.)	No effect	SIMPSON et al. (1977)

[a] Drug by itself caused significant temperature changes
[b] With R04–4602 pretreatment (15–30 mg/kg, 30 min)

proheptadine has subsequently been confirmed by others (KANDASAMY et al. 1975; KANDASAMY 1977) (Table 5). However, it may be necessary to take into consideration that this effect may be due to some property of cyproheptadine other than 5-HT antagonism since other classical 5-HT antagonists have been reported to be ineffective against pyrogen-induced fever in the rabbit (Table 7). KANDASAMY (1977) has suggested that cyproheptadine may act as a prostaglandin synthetase inhibitor rather than as a 5-HT antagonist and that this property explains its ability to inhibit the febrile response. However, this suggestion does not explain some results obtained in other species in which methysergide has been shown to be effective against either pyrogen- or PGE-induced fever (Table 7). The discrepancy may of course be due to species differences, but at present studies with 5-HT antagonists have been equivocal and have not allowed any firm conclusions to be drawn.

IV. Brain 5-Hydroxytryptamine Levels and Turnover

Since the first reports by CANAL and ORNESI (1961) that a decline in whole brain 5-HT level occurred during typhoid vaccine-induced fever, there have been numerous experiments to determine the levels of 5-HT or its metabolite, 5-hydroxyindoleacetic acid (5-HIAA), during the febrile response. In general when the rabbit was the experimental animal, a decrease in 5-HT levels in either the hypothalamus or the brainstem has been observed at the peak of fever and this was accompanied by an increase in 5-HIAA levels both during the fever and during defervescence (Table 8). On the other hand, either no change in 5-HT level in various brain regions during fever (GARDEY-LEVASSORT et al. 1977) or only slight fall in 5-HT levels in the hypothalamus during defervescence (GIARMAN et al. 1968) has been reported by others (Table 8). The reasons for these discrepancies are unclear. HAHN and SZEKELY (1979) found an increase in 5-HIAA levels in the hypothalamus of kittens and newborn guinea pigs. The inconsistent results obtained in these biochemical studies may due to the fact that the amine levels were usually only determined at the peak time of the fever. Further it is possible that different mechanisms may be involved in the fever induced by different pyrogens (i.e. TAB vaccine compared with pyrogen leucocyte, METCALF and THOMPSON 1975; E. coli lipopolysaccharide compared with antigonococcus vaccine, GARDEY-LEVASSORT et al. 1977) (Table 8).

In order to obtain more information on the role of 5-HT, turnover rate rather than absolute level has been studied. This was usually done by measuring the accumulation of 5-HT after pargyline pretreatment. In rabbits, OLIVE et al. (1971) observed no change in 5-HT turnover during antigonococcus vaccine-induced fever. However, MAŠEK et al. (1973, 1980) reported an increase in 5-HT turnover in the rat hypothalamus and brainstem at the peak time of the fever induced by streptococcal mucopeptide (2 mg/kg, i.v., 1973; 500 µg/kg i.v., 1980). These workers also found that the increase in 5-HT turnover could be reduced by salicylate (120 mg/kg, i.p.) pretreatment (MAŠEK et al. 1973). Thus once again there appears to be a species difference in the response to pyrogen.

This species difference in the febrile response was also noted by MYERS. He found an increase in $[^3H]$-5-HT release from the cat hypothalamus during S. typhosa perfusion (10^7 organisms/ml at the rate of 50 µl/min) (MYERS 1977), whereas

Table 7. Effect of indoleamine antagonists on pyrogen- or PGE-induced fever

Species	Drug (dose, route, time schedule)	Fever induced by (dose, route)	Effect on febrile response	References
Rabbits	Cyproheptadine (1 μg/kg, i.v., 15 min)	Typhoid vaccine (0.1–1 ml/kg, i.v.)	Attenuation	CANAL and ORNESI (1961)
	Cyproheptadine (3 mg/kg, i.v., 30 min)	S. typhi lipopolysaccharide (100 pg, i.c.v.)	Attenuation	KANDASAMY et al. (1975)
	Cyproheptadine (3 mg/kg, i.v., 30 min)	PGE₁ (1 μg, i.c.v.)	Attenuation	KANDASAMY et al. (1975)
	Cyproheptadine (3 mg/kg, i.v., 30 min)	Arachnoid acid (100 μg/kg, i.c.v.)	Attenuation	KANDASAMY (1977)
	Methysergide (1 mg/kg, i.v., 15 min)	PGE₁ (5 μg, i.c.v.)	No effect	SINCLAIR and CHAPLIN (1974)
	Cinanserin (3 mg/kg, i.v., 30 min)	PGE₁ (1 μg, i.c.v.)	No effect	KANDASAMY et al. (1975)
	Cinanserin (3 mg/kg, i.v., 30 min)	S. typhi lipopolysaccharide (100 pg, i.c.v.)	No effect	KANDASAMY et al. (1975)
	UML-491 (1 mg, i.c.v., 1 h)	S. typhi "0" cells (10⁵ organisms, i.v.)	No effect	TANGRI et al. (1975)
Cats	Methysergide (300–500 μg, i.c.v.)	TAB vaccine (0.1 ml, i.c.v.)	Attenuation	MILTON and HARVEY (1975)
	Methysergide (300–500 μg, i.c.v.)	"0" somatic antigen (0.1 μg, i.v.)	Attenuation	MILTON and HARVEY (1975)
Monkeys	Methysergide (1.5–5 μg, i.h., 20 min)	PGE₁ (100 ng, i.h.)	Attenuation	SIMPSON et al. (1977)

Table 8. Effects of pyrogen on brain 5 HT and 5 HIAA levels in rabbits

Fever induced by	Site of study	Change in amine level	References
Change in 5 HT level			
Typhoid vaccine (0.1–1 ml/kg, i.v.)	Whole brain	Decrease[a]	CANAL and ORNESI (1961)
Typhoid vaccine (0.05 mg/kg, i.v.)	Brainstem	Decrease[a]	KURUMA et al. (1964)
Pyrexal (1 μg/kg, i.v.)	Brainstem	Decrease[a]	KURUMA et al. (1964)
E. coli lipopolysaccharide (0.2–0.5 μg/kg, i.v.)	Brainstem	Decrease[a]	TAKAGI and KURUMA (1966)
E. coli lipopolysaccharide (5 μg/kg, i.v.)	Hypothalamus	Slight decrease[b]	GIARMAN et al. (1968)
Leucocyte pyrogen (2×10^8 organisms, i.v.)	Hypothalamus	Slight increase[c]	GIARMAN et al. (1968)
E. coli lipopolysaccharide (1.5 μg/kg, i.v.)	Hypothalamus	No change[a]	OLIVE et al. (1969)
Antigonococcus vaccine (10^8 organisms/kg, i.v.)	Hypothalamus	No change[a]	OLIVE et al. (1969)
Antigonococcus vaccine (10^8 organisms/kg, i.v.)	Hypothalamus	No change	GARDEY-LEVASSORT et al. (1970b)
	Brainstem	Decrease[b]	GARDEY-LEVASSORT et al. (1970b)
Leucocyte pyrogen (10 ml i.v. followed by a continuous i.v. infusion at 0.08 ml/min)	Midbrain and pons/medulla hypothalamus	Decrease No change[a]	METCALF and THOMPSON (1975)
E. coli lipopolysaccharide (1.5 μg/kg, i.v.)	Hypothalamus, brainstem, CSF	No change	GARDEY-LEVASSORT et al. (1977)
TAB vaccine (0.1 mg/kg, i.v.)	Hypothalamus	Decrease	METCALF and THOMPSON (1975)
Change in 5 HIAA level			
Antigonococcus vaccine (10^8 organisms/kg, i.v.)	Hypothalamus, brainstem	Increase[b,c]	GARDEY-LEVASSORT et al. (1970b)
	CSF	Increase[c]	
E. coli lipopolysaccharide (1.5 μg/kg, i.v.)	CSF	Increase[c]	GARDEY-LEVASSORT et al. (1977)
	Hypothalamus, brainstem	No change	

[a] Amine levels only measured at peak time of fever
[b] During fever
[c] During defervescence

no consistent release of $[^3H]$-5-HT was observed from monkey hypothalamus after PGE perfusion.

V. Conclusion

The results obtained from investigations into the possible involvement of 5-HT in febrile responses have been far more controversial than those for noradrenaline. In general, 5-HT seems most likely to be a mediator of the febrile response in rats and cats. Thus the fever induced by either PGE or pyrogens in these species can be reduced by either 5-HT antagonists or by reducing central 5-HT transmission with specific depleting agents or electrolytic lesions of 5-HT neurones. Also a significant increase in 5-HT turnover or release has been reported during fever in these species. On the other hand, in rabbits, 5-HT may play a modulatory role in febrile responses, since, firstly, only potentiation of febrile responses has been reported after PCPA treatment never inhibition, even though some studies have claimed that PCPA has no effect on febrile response, these negative findings may be due to insufficient reduction of 5-HT stores. Secondly, fever has been shown to be reduced after facilitation of 5-HT transmission by specific 5-HT uptake blockade. In addition, studies of 5-HT levels in rabbits have noted a significant decrease in 5-HT during peak fever and an increase in 5-HIAA during defervescence. This would be consistent with an increased activity in 5-HT neurones in an attempt to reduce the fever. If it is accepted that 5-HT acts as a mediator of the fever in cats and rats and as a modulator in the rabbit, then this would be consistent with the amine hypothesis of thermoregulation proposed by FELDBERG and MYERS (1963). These workers proposed opposite roles for 5-HT and noradrenaline in thermoregulation, a situation that also appears to apply in fever. However, it must be accepted that there remains a good deal of controversy, which can only be resolved by further careful experimentation.

D. Acetylcholine

I. Cholinergic Antagonists

Although there have been some reports that acetylcholine (ACh) has a role in the control of body temperature (CRAWSHAW 1979), there have been suprisingly few attempts to determine if it has any significance in the febrile response. TANGRI et al. (1975) reported that the fever induced by S. typhi "0" cells in rabbits could be reduced by pretreatment with nicotinic antagonists but not by pretreatment with muscarinic antagonists (Table 9). The inability of muscarinic antagonists to affect the febrile response was apparently confirmed by the observation that benztropine had no effect on PGE$_1$-induced fever in rabbits (SINCLAIR and CHAPLAIN 1974). Since benztropine also has antihistaminic properties then this finding would also argue against a role for histamine in this response. There is not total agreement that muscarinic antagonists are ineffective against fever in the rabbit since COOPER et al. (1976) showed that atropine almost completely abolished the febrile response when it was induced by either leucocyte pyrogen or PGE$_1$. This latter group suggested that the discrepancy between their observations and those of TANGRI et al.

Table 9. Effects of cholinergic antagonists on pyrogen- or PGE-induced fever

Species	Drug (dose, route, time schedule)	Fever induced by (dose, route)	Effect on febrile response	References
Muscarinic antagonists				
Rabbits	Atropine (500 μg, i.c.v., 1 h before)	S. typhi "0" cells (10^5 organisms, i.v.)	No effect	TANGRI et al. (1975)
	Atropine (200 μg, i.c.v., 15 min before and after pyrogen injection)	PGE_1 (100 ng, i.h. bilaterally) or leucocyte pyrogen	Attenuation	COOPER et al. (1976)
	Benztropine (0.2 mg/kg, i.v., 15 min before)	PGE_1 (5 μg, i.c.v.)	No effect	SINCLAIR and CHAPLIN (1974)
Rats	Atropine (40 μg, i.h. or 80 mg/kg, i.p.)	PGE_1 (50–100 ng, i.h.)	No effect	VISHWANATHAN and RUDY (1974)
	Atropine (34 μg, i.h., 1 h before)	PGE_1 (100 ng, i.h.)	No effect	RUDY and VISHWANATHAN (1975)
Sheep	Atropine (200 nmol/kg, i.c.v., 30 min before)	PGE_1 (70 nmol, i.c.v.) or TAB vaccine (1 ml, i.v.)	Attenuation	BLIGH et al. (1978)
Monkeys	Atropine (5–10 μg, i.h., 20 min before)	PGE_1 (100 ng, i.h.)	Attenuation	SIMPSON et al., (1977)
Nicotinic antagonists				
Rabbits	Chlorisondamine (100 μg, i.c.v., 1 h before)	S. typhi "0" cells (10^5 organisms, i.v.)	Attenuation	TANGRI et al. (1975)
Rats	Tubocurarine (25 μg, i.c.v., 1 h before)	S. typhi "0" cells (10^5 organisms, i.v.)	Attenuation	TANGRI et al. (1975)
	Mecamylamine (18 μg, i.h., 1 h before)	PGE_1 (100 ng, i.h.)	No effect	RUDY and VISHWANATHAN (1975)

(1975) could be explained in differences in pretreatment times. TANGRI et al. used a 1-h pretreatment whereas COOPER et al. used only 15 min. Unfortunately there were no controls that would allow determination of duration of antagonistic effect in these experiments.

There have been other reports that atropine can attenuate the febrile response in other species including sheep and monkey (Table 9) but these await confirmation. In the rat, atropine has been reported to be ineffective against PGE_1-induced fever (RUDY and VISHWANATHAN 1975), which argued against a possible role of ACh in fever in this species. Since these workers also reported that mecamylamine was ineffective then neither muscarinic nor nicotinic receptors appear to be involved.

II. Cholinomimetics and Anticholinesterases

Experiments using anticholinesterase drugs provide evidence that ACh is involved in mediation of the febrile response in rabbits, since TANGRI et al. (1975) have shown that physostigmine (50 µg, i.c.v.) potentiates the fever induced by *S. typhi* "0" cells. However, in rats physostigmine (0.3 mg/kg, i.p.) has been reported to reduce the febrile response to either PGE_1 (0.5 µg, i.c.v.) or dihomo-γ-linolenic acid (2.5 µg, i.c.v.) (BODZENTA and WISNIEWSKI 1977). This could argue in favour of a role for ACh in the rat in contrast to the findings with antagonists. However, the findings with anticholinesterases need to be interpreted with caution since these drugs on their own can lower core temperature. A similar criticism can be levelled against the use of muscarinic agonists, where arecoline (10 µg, i.c.v.) has been reported to attenuate PGE_2-induced fever in the rat (GURIN et al. 1979).

III. Conclusion

The results obtained from the above experiments suggest that ACh is unlikely to be involved in the febrile response in rats. In contrast, it does appear that ACh may play an important role in the febrile response in rabbits, since the PGE- or pyrogen-induced fever can be attenuated by cholinergic antagonists and potentiated by anticholinesterases.

E. Other Amines

I. Dopamine

In comparison with what is known about the involvement of 5-HT and noradrenaline in the febrile response, there is very little known about the role of dopamine. PELA et al. (1977) showed that the magnitude of febrile response to *E. coli* lipopolysaccharide (1.5 ng, i.c.v.) in rabbits could be attenuated by pretreatment with the dopamine antagonist pimozide (1–4 µg, i.c.v.). However, KANDASAMY (1977) reported that pimozide (1 mg/kg, i.v.) injected 30 min before pyrogen challenge had no effect on the fever induced by arachidonic acid (100 µg/kg, i.v.) in the same species. Since different pyrogenic agents were used in these two studies, then no firm conclusions can be drawn at present. GARDEY-LEVASSORT et al. (1977) investigated the changes in dopamine and its metabolites in different brain tissues of rabbits during fever induced by either *E. coli* lipopolysaccharide (1.5 µg/kg, i.v.) or antigonococcal vaccine (10^8 organisms/kg, i.v.). In *E. coli*-induced fever, 3,4-dihydroxyphenylacetic acid (DOPAC) and homovanillic acid (HVA) levels were low in the hypothalamus, brainstem and caudate nucleus before the first peak of fever and were high in the hypothalamus, brainstem and cerebrospinal fluid during the second peak of fever and during defervescence. In contrast only slight changes in HVA and DOPAC levels were observed in antigonococcal-induced fever. In neither case was there any change in dopamine levels. Thus there is some evidence to suggest that central dopaminergic systems may be involved in certain febrile responses. The best evidence comes from studies involving *E. coli*-induced fever in rabbits, where both the antagonist and the biochemical data are consistent. However, it is not possible as yet to suggest any general role for dopamine. More experiments using different pyrogens and species other than the rabbit are required.

II. γ-Aminobutyric Acid

Recently γ-aminobutyric acid (GABA) has been shown to be a neurotransmitter within the central nervous system and has been reported to cause hyperthermia in some species (CLARK 1979). In the anaesthetised dog, the hyperthermic response to intracerebroventricular injection of GABA (0.3 mg) could be attenuated by sodium salicylate perfusion (250 µg/µl) (DHUMAL et al. 1974), indicating the possible involvement of prostaglandins. These authors also reported attenuation of GABA (20 µg, i.c.v.)-induced hyperthermia by sodium salicylate (150 mg/kg, i.p., 1 h before) in the rat (DHUMAL et al. 1976), thus confirming, it seems, a prostaglandin involvement in GABA-induced hyperthermia. However, these results do not imply that GABA mediates a general febrile response. One possible interpretation is that pyrogen could activate prostaglandin release via a central GABA-ergic system. However, this postulate requires a greater depth of investigation and it is more likely that the GABA effect is simply pharmacological.

III. Histamine and Taurine

Of the other putative amine neurotransmitters, only histamine and taurine have been studied for their possible involvement in the febrile response. However, histamine seems unlikely to be involved in the fever, since neither histamine H_1 nor histamine H_2 antagonists (mepyramine, metiamide, diphenhydramine) have been reported to change the febrile response induced by either pyrogen or PGE (BURKS 1976; OKEN and LOCH 1979; BLIGH 1980). In addition, central injections of histamine cause hypothermia rather than hyperthermia in most species (CLARK and CLARK 1980).

In rabbits, taurine, infused intracerebroventricularly after intravenous injection of either leucocyte pyrogen or *S. typhosa* endotoxin, firstly inhibited the initial rise in body temperature and then prolonged the fever when the infusion was stopped (HARRIS and LIPTON 1977; LIPTON and TICKNOR 1979). However, modification of the febrile response by taurine seems likely to be nonspecific since the apparent inhibition of the pyrogen-induced rise in body temperature could be due to the hypothermic effect of taurine (HARRIS and LIPTON 1977). In addition, the prolongation of fever by taurine may be nonspecific due to interference with active transport processes that terminate the effects of pyrogen. It has been previously reported that intracerebroventricular injection of probenecid, a drug which blocks transport of organic acids (SPECTOR and LORENZO 1974), also produced a similar effect on pyrogen-induced fever (CRAWFORD et al. 1979). Thus taurine would not appear to be specifically involved in febrile response.

F. Peptides

I. Kinins

An involvement of kinins in the febrile response was first suggested by PELA et al. (1975), who found that the levels of kinin-like substances in the rabbit hypothalamus decreased after *E. coli* lipopolysaccharide (1.5 µg/kg, i.v.) injection. Later, ALMEIDA E SILVA and PELA (1978) demonstrated a dose-related hyperthermia by bradykinin and its analogues after i.c.v. injection. The hyperthermia induced by bradykinin (5 µg, i.c.v.) was attenuated by a 30-min pretreatment with either indomethacin (2 mg/kg, i.v.) or paracetamol (30 mg/kg, i.v.). These results could argue for the participation of kinins in the febrile response. However, no firm conclusion can be drawn until many more detailed experiments have been performed.

II. Thyroid-Releasing Hormone

Thyroid-releasing hormone (TRH) is a tripeptide that causes hyperthermia in most species (CLARK 1979). In rats, the hyperthermia induced by central injections of TRH has been reported to be attenuated by prostaglandin synthetase inhibitors (COHN et al. 1980), suggesting an involvement of prostaglandins. However, as with GABA, this does not necessarily imply that TRH is involved in general febrile responses. Experiments by MYERS et al. (1977) do not support a role for TRH in fever since no temperature changes were observed when TRH was injected into the thermosensitive regions of cat brain (both preoptic and posterior hypothalamus). More recently, BOSCHI and RIPS (1981) reported that a hyperthermia occurred after TRH was injected into the nucleus accumbens, a structure which is usually regarded as not being involved in thermoregulation. In addition to the change in body temperature, stereotyped behaviour and "wet-body" shakes were also observed. Thus the hyperthermia could be secondary to the behavioural effects. In contrast, sedation is usually observed after PGE or pyrogen injection. Thus the role, if any, of TRH in the febrile response remains obscure.

III. Opioids

Even though it is known the injection of morphine or the enkephalins can cause hyperthermia in most species (CLARK 1979; CLARK and CLARK 1980), it seems unlikely that endogenous opioids are involved in the febrile response. In cats, injection of morphine or enkephalin into the PGE_1-sensitive site has been shown to induce a rise in body temperature. However, this hyperthermia differed from the PGE_1-induced hyperthermia in two ways. Firstly PGE_1 caused an immediate rise in body temperature after injection, whereas the peak effect with opiates occurred at least 1 h after injection (MILTON 1975; MYERS and RUWE 1980). Secondly an increase in motor activity was observed after morphine injection, whereas sedation occurred after PGE injection (MILTON 1975). In addition, the hyperthermia induced by opiates was not blocked by prostaglandin synthetase inhibitors suggesting that prostaglandins were not involved (MILTON 1975; CLARK and CUMBY 1978).

G. Conclusion

Only two of the known neurotransmitters (noradrenaline and 5-HT) have been extensively investigated for a possible role in the febrile response and even though there is good evidence that these two are involved, their exact role is poorly understood.

Attempts to determine a specific role have been hampered by the wide species and strain differences, which has meant that few, if any, generalisations can be made. Further it is by no means certain that all pyrogenic agents act through a common neurotransmitter pathway even when a single strain of animal is used.

Thus a large number of carefully controlled experiments are required to provide further information. Studies with specific neurotransmitter agonists and antagonists would be helpful in this respect as would investigations comparing the time course of the febrile with the time course of changes in neurotransmitter turnover in specific brain regions. Until such work is carried out our knowledge of the role of central neurotransmitters in fever must remain at a very superficial level.

References

Almeida e Silva TC, Pela IR (1978) Changes in rectal temperature of the rabbit by intracerebroventricular injection of bradykinin and related kinins. Agents Actions 8:102–107

Artunkal AA, Marley E, Stephenson JD (1977) Some effects of prostaglandin E_1 and E_2 and of endotoxin injected into the hypothalamus of young chicks: Dissociation between endotoxin fever and the effects of prostaglandins. Br J Pharmac 61:39–46

Björklund A, Baumgarten H-G, Nobin A (1974) Chemical lesioning of central monoamine axons by means of 5,6-dihydroxytryptamine and 5,7-dihydroxytryptamine. Adv Biochem Psychopharmac 10:13–33

Björklund A, Baumgarten H-G, Rensch A (1975) 5,7-dihydroxytryptamine: improvement of its selectivity for serotonin neurons in the CNS by pretreatment with desipramine. J Neurochem 24:833–835

Blatteis CM (1976) Effect of propranolol on endotoxin-induced pyrogenesis in newborn and adult guinea pigs. J Appl Physiol 40:35–39

Bligh J (1980) Central neurology of homeothermy and fever. In: Lipton JM (ed) Fever. Raven Press, New York, pp 81–89

Bligh J, Maskrey M (1971) The interaction between the effects on thermoregulation of TAB vaccine injected intravenously and monoamines injected into a lateral cerebral ventricle of the Welsh mountain sheep. J Physiol (Lond) 213:60–62p

Bligh J, Silver A, Bacon MJ, Smith CA (1978) The central role of a cholinergic synapse in thermoregulation in the sheep. J Thermal Biol 3:147–151

Bodzenta A, Wisniewski K (1977) The effect of prostaglandin E_1 on central cholinergic mechanisms. Pharmacol 15:143–151

Borsook D, Laburn HP, Rosendorff C, Willies GH, Woolf CJ (1977) A dissociation between temperature regulation and fever in the rabbit. J Physiol (Lond) 266:423–433

Boschi G, Rips R (1981) Effects of thyrotropin releasing hormone injections into different areas of rat brain on core temperature. Neurosci Lett 23:93 98

Bruinvels J (1979) Norepinephrine. In: Lomax P, Schönbaum E (eds) Body temperature regulation, drug effects, and therapeutic implications. Marcel Dekker, New York, pp 257–288

Brus R, Herman ZS, Szkilnik R, Zabawska J (1979) Mediation of central prostaglandin effect by serotoninergic neurons. Psychopharmacol 64:113–120

Burks TF (1976) Antiadrenergic actions of metiamide in cat thermoregulatory mechanisms. Proc West Pharmacol Soc 19:75–78

Burks TF, van Inwegen RG (1975) Phentolamine inhibition of morphine induced hyperthermia in cats. Proc West Pharmacol Soc 18:199–203

Canal N, Ornesi A (1961) Serotonina encefalica e ipertermia da vaccino. Atti Accad Med Lomb 16:69–73

Carruba MO, Bachtold HP (1976) Pyrogen fever in rabbits pretreated with p-chlorophenylalanine or 5,6-dihydroxytryptamine. Experientia 32:729–730

Clark WG (1979) Changes in body temperature after administration of amino acids, peptides, dopamine, neuroleptics, and related agents. Neurosci Biobehav Rev 3:179–231

Clark WG, Clark YL (1980) Changes in body temperature after administration of acetylcholine, histamine, morphine, prostaglandins, and related agents. Neurosci Biobehav Rev 4:175–240

Clark WG, Cumby HR (1978) Hyperthermia responses to central and peripheral injections of morphine sulphate in the cat. Br J Pharmac 63:65–71

Cohn ML, Cohn M, Taube D (1980) Thyrotropin releasing hormone induced hyperthermia in the rat inhibited by lysine acetyl-salicylate and indomethacin. In: Cox B, Lomax P, Milton AS, Schönbaum E (eds) Thermoregulatory mechanisms and their therapeutic implications. Karger, Basel, pp 198–201

Cooper KE, Cranston WI (1966) Pyrogens and monoamine oxidase inhibitors. Nature 210:203–204

Cooper KE, Cranston WI, Honour AJ (1967) Observations on the site and mode of action of pyrogens in the rabbit brain. J Physiol (Lond) 191:325–337

Cooper KE, Preston E, Veale WL (1976) Effects of atropine, injected into a lateral cerebral ventricle of the rabbit, on fever due to intravenous leucocyte pyrogen and hypothalamic and intraventricular injections of prostaglandin E_1. J Physiol (Lond) 254:729–741

Cox B, Lomax P (1977) Pharmacologic control of temperature regulation. Ann Rev Pharmacol Toxicol 17:341–353

Cox B, Lomax P, Milton AS, Schönbaum E (1980) Thermoregulatory mechanisms and their therapeutic implications. Karger, Basel

Cranston WI, Luff RH (1972) The role of noradrenaline in the rabbit brain during pyrogen-induced fever. J Physiol (Lond) 225:66–67p

Crawshaw LI (1979) Acetylcholine. In: Lomax P, Schönbaum E (eds) Body temperature regulation, drug effects, and therapeutic implications. Marcel Dekker, New York, pp 305–335

Crawford IL, Kennedy JI, Lipton JM, Ojeda SR (1979) Effects of central administration of probenecid on fever produced by leukocytic pyrogen and PGE_2 in the rabbit. J Physiol (Lond) 287:519–533

Des Prez RM, Helman R, Oates JA (1966) Inhibition of endotoxin fever by reserpine. Proc Soc Exp Biol Med 122:746–749

Dhumal VR, Gulati OD, Raghunath PR, Sivaramakrishna N (1974) Analysis of the effects on body temperature of intracerebroventricular injection in anaesthetized dogs of gamma-aminobutyric acid. Br J Pharmac 50:513–524

Dhumal VR, Gulati OD, Shan NS (1976) Effects on rectal temperature in rats of γ-aminobutyric acid; possible mediation through putative transmitters. Eur J Pharmac 35:341–347

Feldberg W, Myers RD (1963) A new concept of temperature regulation by amines in the hypothalamus. Nature 200:1325

Ford DM, Klugman KP (1980) Constrasting roles of 5-hydroxytryptamine and noradrenaline in fever in rats. J Physiol (Lond) 304:51–57

Frens J (1975) Thermoregulation set-point changes during lipopolysaccharide fever. In: Lomax P, Schönbaum E (eds) Temperature regulation and drug action. Karger, Basel, pp 59–64

Gardey-Levassort C (1977) Brain amine metabolism during pyrogen fever: the role of stress. In: Cooper KE, Lomax P, Schönbaum E (eds) Drugs, biogenic amines and body temperature. Karger, Basel, pp 153–159

Gardey-Levassort C, Olive G, Fontagne J, Szafranowa H, Lechat P (1970a) Réponse fébrile du Lapin aux pyrogènes bactériens et teneur de l'hypothalamus en sérotonine et noradrénaline après un pré-treatment aux I.M.A.O. J Pharmac (Paris) 1:57–64

Gardey-Levassort C, Olive G, Szafranowa H, Sadeghi D, Lechat P (1970b) Détermination simultaneé des taux de 5-hydroxytryptamine et d'acide 5-hydroxyindolacétique dans le liquide céphalorachidien, l'hypothalamus et la tronc cérébral du Lapin au cours de la fièvre induite par un pyrogène bacterien. CR Soc Biol (Paris) 164:1946–1951

Gardey-Levassort C, Tanguy O, Lechat P (1977) Brain concentrations of biogenic amines and their metabolites in two types of pyrogen-induced fever in rabbits. J Neurochem 28:177–182

Giarman NJ, Tanaka C, Mooney J, Atkins E (1964) Serotonin, norepinephrine, and fever. Adv Pharmacol 6A:307–317

Göing H (1959) Beeinflussung der Fieber-erzeugenden Wirkung bakterieller Pyrogene durch Iproniacid, Reserpine, und Dibenamin. Arzneim Forsch 9:793–794

Gurin VN, Tsaryuk VV, Tret'yakovich AG (1979) Weakening of the hyperthermic effect of prostaglandin E_2 by cholinomimetics, monoamines, and calcium ions. Bull Exp Biol Med 87:151–154

Hahn Z, Szekely M (1979) Hypothalamic monoamine contents in endotoxin fever of newborn guinea pigs and kittens. Neurosci Lett 11:279–282

Harris WS, Lipton JM (1977) Intracerebroventricular taurine in rabbits: Effects on normal body temperature, endotoxin fever, and hyperthermia produced by PGE_1 and amphetamine. J Physiol (Lond) 266:397–410

Harvey CA, Milton AS (1974a) The effect of parachlorophenylalanine on the response of the conscious cat to intravenous and intraventricular bacterial pyrogen and to intraventricular prostaglandin E_1. J Physiol (Lond) 236:14–15p

Harvey CA, Milton AS (1974b) The effect of intraventricular 6-hydroxydopamine on the response of the conscious cat to pyrogen. Br J Pharmac 52:134–135p

Kadlecová O, Mǎsek K, Petrovický P (1977) A possible site of action of bacterial peptidoglycan in the CNS. Neuropharmacol 16:699–702

Kandasamy SB (1977) Central effect of 5,8,11,14-eicosatetraenoic acid (arachidonic acid) on the temperature in the conscious rabbits. Experientia 33:1626–1627

Kandasamy B, Girault J-M, Jacob J (1975) Central effects of a purified bacterial pyrogen, prostaglandin E_1 and biogenic amines on the temperature in the awake rabbit. In: Lomax P, Schönbaum E (eds) Temperature regulation and drug action. Karger, Basel, pp 124–132

Koe BK, Weissman A (1966) p-Chlorophenylalanine: a specific depletor of brain serotonin. J Pharmac exp Ther 154:499–516

Kostrzewa RN, Jacobowitz DM (1974) Pharmacological action of 6-hydroxydopamine. Pharmac Rev 26:199–288

Kroneberg G, Kurbjuweit HG (1959) Die Beeinflussung von experimentellem Fieber durch Reserpin und Sympathicolytica am Kaninchen. Arzneim Forsch 9:556–558

Kuruma D, Takagi H, Yamada H (1964) Changes in serotonin and catecholamine contents in the brains of febrile rabbits I. The fever induced by pyrexal and changes in serotonin and catecholamine contents in the brain stem (in Japanese). Folia Pharmacol 60:563–568

Laburn HP, Rosendorff C, Willies G, Woolf C (1974) A role for noradrenaline and cyclic AMP in prostaglandin E_1 fever. J Physiol (Lond) 240:49–50p

Laburn H, Woolf CJ, Willies GH, Rosendorff C (1975) Pyrogen and prostaglandin fever in the rabbit-II: Effects of noradrenaline depletion and adrenergic receptor blockade. Neuropharmacol 14:405–411

Lin MT (1978) Prostaglandin E_1-induced fever in rabbits pretreated with p-chlorophenylalanine. Experientia 34:59–60

Lin MT (1980) Effects of brain monoamine depletions on thermoregulation in rabbits. Am J Physiol 238:R364–371

Lin MT, Pang IH, Chern SI, Chern YF (1979) Effects of increasing serotonergic receptor activity in brain on prostaglandin E_1-induced fever in rabbits. Pharmacol 18:188–194

Lipton JM, Ticknor CB (1979) Central effect of taurine and its analogues on fever caused by intravenous leukocytic pyrogen in rabbits. J Physiol (Lond) 287:535–543

Lomax P, Schönbaum E (1979) Body temperature regulation, drug effects, and therapeutic implications. Marcel Dekker, New York

Lorden JF, Ottmas GA, Dawson R Jr, Callaham H (1979) Evaluation of the non-specific effects of catecholamine and serotonin neurotoxins by injection into the median forebrain bundle of the rat. Pharmac Biochem Behav 10:79–86

Mašek K, Kadlecová O, Petrovický P (1980) A possible site of action and mechanism involved in peptidoglycan fever in rats. In: Lipton JM (ed) Fever. Raven Press, New York, pp 123–130

Mašek K, Kadlecová O, Rašková H (1973) Brain amines in fever and sleep cycle changes caused by streptococcal mucopeptide. Neuropharmacol 12:1039–1047

Mašek K, Rašková H, Rotta J (1968) The mechanism of the pyrogenic effect of streptococcus cell wall mucopeptide. J Physiol (Lond) 198:345–353

Mašek K, Rašková H, Rotta J (1972) On the mechanism of fever caused by the mucopeptide of group A streptococcus. Naunyn-Schmiedeberg's Arch Pharmac 274:138–145

Metcalf G, Thompson JW (1975) The effect of various aminedepleting drugs on the fever response exhibited by rabbits to bacterial or leucocyte pyrogen. Br J Pharmac 53:21–27

Milton AS (1975) Morphine hyperthermia, prostaglandin synthetase inhibitors and naloxone. J Physiol (Lond) 251:27–28p

Milton AS (1978) The hypothalamus and the pharmacology of thermoregulation. In: Cox B, Morris ID, Weston AH (eds) Pharmacology of the hypothalamus. Macmillan, London, pp 105–134

Milton AS, Harvey CA (1975) Prostaglandins and monoamines in fever. In: Lomax P, Schönbaum E (eds) Temperature regulation and drug action. Karger, Basel, pp 133–142

Moore KE, Dominic JA (1971) Tyrosine hydroxylase inhibitors. Fed Proc Fed Am Soc Exp Biol 30:859–870

Myers RD (1977) New aspects of the role of hypothalamic calcium ions, 5-HT and PGE during normal thermoregulation and pyrogen fever. In: Cooper KE, Lomax P, Schönbaum E (eds) Drugs, biogenic amines, and body temperature. Karger, Basel, pp 51–53

Myers RD, Ruwe WD (1980) Fever: Intermediary neurohumoral factors serving the hypothalamic mechanism underlying hyperthermia. In: Lipton JM (ed) Fever. Raven Press, New York, pp 99–110

Myers RD, Waller MB (1976) Is prostaglandin fever mediated by the presynaptic release of hypothalamic 5-HT or norepinephrine? Brain Res Bull 1:47–56

Myers RD, Metcalf G, Rice JC (1977) Identification by microinjection of TRH-sensitive sites in the cat's brainstem that mediate respiratory, temperature, and other autonomic changes. Brain Res 126:105–115

Nickerson M, Collier C (1975) Drugs inhibiting adrenergic nerves and structures innervated by them. In: Goodman LS, Gilman A (eds) The pharmacological basis of therapeutics, 5th edn. Macmillan, New York, p 536

Nistico G, Marmo E (1979) Antagonism of prostaglandin E_1 and E_2 fever by catecholamines. Res Comm Chem Pathol Pharmacol 23:89–95

Oken MM, Loch J (1979) Corticosteroid and antihistamine modification of bleomycin-induced fever. Proc Soc Exp Biol Med 161:594–596

Olive G, Gardey-Levassort C, Lechat P (1971) Détermination du turnover de la sérotonin dans l'hypothalamus et le tronc cérébral du Lapin à l'acmé de la fièvre provoquée par un pyrogène bactérien. J Pharmacol (Paris) 2:61–70

Olive G, Gardey-Levassort C, Szafranowa H, Lechat P (1969) Teneur de l'hypothalamus en sérotonin et noradrénaline à l'acme de la fièvre provoquée chez le Lapin par des pyrogènes bacteriens. CR Soc Biol (Paris) 163:1062–1065

Pela IR, Gardey-Levassort C, Lechat P (1977) Pimozide and pyrogen induced fever in rabbits. Experientia 33:63–64

Pela IR, Gardey-Levassort C, Lechat P, Rocha e Silva M (1975) Brain kinins and fever induced by bacterial pyrogens in rabbits. J Pharm Pharmac 27:793–794

Peindaries R, Jacob J (1971) Interactions between 5-hydroxytryptamine and a purified bacterial pyrogen when injected into the lateral cerebral ventricle of the wake rabbit. Eur J Pharmacol 13:347–355

Preston E, Cooper KE (1976) Absence of fever in the rabbit following intrahypothalamic injections of noradrenaline into PGE_1-sensitive sites. Neuropharmacol 15:239–244

Rudy TA, Viswanathan CT (1975) Effect of central cholinergic blockade on the hyperthermia evoked by prostaglandin E_1 into the rostral hypothalamus of the rat. Can J Physiol Pharmacol 53:321–324

Schlievert PM, Watson DW (1979) Biogenic amine involvement in pyrogenicity and enhancement of lethal endotoxin shock by group A streptococcal pyrogenic exotoxin. Proc Soc Exp Biol Med 162:269–274

Simpson CW, Ruwe WD, Myers RD (1977) Characterization of prostaglandin sensitive sites in the monkey hypothalamus mediating hyperthermia. In: Cooper KE, Lomax P, Schönbaum E (eds) Drugs, biogenic amines, and body temperature. Karger, Basel, pp 142–144

Sinclair JG, Chaplin MF (1974) Effects of p-chlorophenylalanine, α-methyl-p-tyrosine, morphine, and chlorpromazine on prostaglandin E_1 hyperthermia in the rabbit. Prostaglandins 8:117–124

Spector R, Lorenzo AV (1974) The effects of salicylate and probenecid on the cerebrospinal fluid transport of penicillin, aminosalicylic acid, and iodide. J Pharmac exp Ther 188:55–65

Splawinski JA, Gorka Z, Suder E, Kaluza J (1976) The effect of 6-hydroxydopamine on pyrogen, prostaglandins (E_2 and $F_{2\alpha}$) and arachidonic acid fever in rats. In: Samuelsson B, Paoletti R (eds) Advances in prostaglandin and thromboxane research, Vol 2. Raven Press, New York, pp 834–835

Szekely M (1978 a) Endotoxin fever in parachlorophenylalanine (PCPA) treated newborn guinea pigs and kittens. Life Sci 22:1585–1588

Szekely M (1978 b) Endotoxin fever in the new-born guinea-pig and the modulating effects of indomethacin and p-chlorophenylalanine. J Physiol (Lond) 281:467–476

Szekely M (1979 a) Central and peripheral adrenergic mechanisms in endotoxin fever of newborn guinea pigs. Acta Physiol Acad Sci Hung 54:257–263

Szekely M (1979 b) Endotoxin fever in the newborn kitten. The role of prostaglandins and monoamines. Acta Physiol Acad Sci Hung 54:265–276

Takagi H, Kuruma I (1966) Effect of bacterial lipopolysaccharide on the content of serotonin and norepinephrine in rabbit brain. Jap J Pharmacol 16:478–479

Tangri KK, Bhargava AK, Bhargava KP (1975) Significance of central cholinergic mechanism in pyrexia induced by bacterial pyrogen in rabbits. In: Lomax P, Schönbaum E (eds) Temperature regulation and drug action. Karger, Basel, pp 65–74

Teddy PJ (1969) The effects of alternations in hypothalamic monoamines content on fever in the rabbit. J Physiol (Lond) 204:140–141 p

Veale WL, Cooper KE (1975) Comparison of sites of action of prostaglandin E and leucocytic pyrogen in brain. In: Lomax P, Schönbaum E (eds) Temperature regulation and drug action. Karger, Basel, pp 218–226

Yasuda M (1962) Effect of reserpine on febrile responses induced by pyrogenic substances. Jap J Pharmacol 11:114–125

CHAPTER 7

The Role of Ions in Thermoregulation and Fever*

R. D. MYERS

A. Introduction

The enormous significance of cation involvement in all of the vital functions of the body has become increasingly recognized in the last decade. The dynamic characteristics of the transmembrane exchange, metabolism, and other biological activity of essential cations are now clearly established experimentally. Of particular note is the fact that in the central nervous system (CNS), as in other organs, certain cations do much more physiologically than simply provide a balanced, osmotic fluid milieu for the tissue within which cells live and prosper.

At the structural level, Ca^{2+} ions play a fundamental role in the excitation and contraction of both cardiac and striated muscles (ANDERSON et al. 1978). The activity of this cation in the brain is thought now to be involved in the intricate processes of the cerebral cortex (e.g. ADEY 1971), and is believed also to influence differential states of sleep selectively (e.g. TÓSZEGHI et al. 1978; BORBÉLY and TOBLER 1979), the emotional stability of the animal (VEALE and MYERS 1971), the feeding behaviour of the normally satiated animal (GISOLFI et al. 1977), as well as blood pressure regulation and even hypertension (BLAUSTEIN 1977).

At the cellular level, certain dynamic characteristics of cation exchange have been identified; for example, when stimulated electrically, autonomic ganglion cells actively take up Ca^{2+} ions (BLAUSTEIN 1971). What is equally fascinating is the functional interaction of cations as illustrated by an interdependence of Na^+ and Ca^{2+} ions in the release of both transmitter substance in muscle (COLOMO and RAHAMIMOFF 1968) and neurosecretory hormones (DREIFUSS et al. 1971). That certain cations are also highly labile is well known. In brain tissue, Ca^{2+} is readily accumulated in mitochondria (COOK and ROBINSON (1971) and bound to perikarya and synaptosomes (LAZAREWICZ et al. 1974). The transmembrane flux of Ca^{2+} ions is likewise remarkable (JUNDT et al. 1975) in that the cation passes easily through the ependymal lining from the brain to cerebrospinal fluid (CSF) (GRAZIANI et al. 1967). Calcium is also unbound and released from cells in the cerebral cortex by electrical current or by other modes of stimulation, including drugs and other chemical substances (STAHL and SWANSON 1971; KACZMAREK and ADEY 1973; BAWIN et al. 1978).

* The author is grateful for the research support of the National Science Foundation, U.S. Office of Naval Research, National Institutes of Health and of the U.N.C. Center for Alcohol Studies, J.A. Ewing, Director. A very special indebtedness is also acknowledged to Professors W. Feldberg, W.L. Veale, and C.V. Gisolfi, with whom many of the ideas contained herein were germinated and enjoyably shared

In this chapter, the physiological role of the essential cations in fever and in the regulation of an animal's normal body temperature will be considered. Although potassium, calcium, and other species of ion have been studied in relation to peripheral thermal receptors (e.g. SHEA et al. 1969; HENSEL and SCHÄFER 1974), this review will be devoted principally to those actions of the cations on thermoregulatory and temperature "set-point" mechanisms thought to be mediated by cellular processes located anatomically within the diencephalon (MYERS 1978).

B. Systemic Effects of Altered Ion Levels

Although *Kochsalzfieber* (common salt fever) had been recognized in pediatric practice as a clinical problem as early as 1907, a young clinic assistant in Heidelberg was the first to explore the problem in an animal. Injecting solutions into the ear vein of the rabbit, FREUND (1911) found that normal saline (0.85%) induced an intense rise in the body temperature. Interestingly, when adrenaline was added to the sodium chloride solution infused intravenously, the sodium fever was enhanced, suggesting calorigenic synergism of the amine with the monovalent cation (FREUND 1911). Later SCHÜTZ (1916) described a set of narcosis-like symptoms observed after an injection of a high dose of magnesium in the rabbit. These responses were accompanied by a hypothermia, an effect which was reported also by SCHÜTZ when a calcium chloride solution was administered to the animal.

As reviewed lucidly by GREENLEAF (1979), many early workers in Europe and North America believed that sodium and other fevers were due to imbalances in fluid-electrolyte levels in the body. A sharp change in osmotic pressure, even when caused by an excess in plasma sugar concentration or a large negative water balance, induced an increase in temperature of up to 6 °C. When water was administered therapeutically to offset the fluid deficit, the hyperpyrexic response of the human subject or animal usually abated (GREENLEAF 1979).

In more recent years, it has been demonstrated in several ways that plasma osmolarity can influence body temperature. In the human subject, a decline in temperature is caused by the ingestion of water, whereas an increase in osmolarity following NaCl ingestion raises core temperature (NIELSEN et al. 1971; SNELLEN et al. 1972). The early work of FREUND and SCHÜTZ was confirmed with exactitude by NIELSEN (1974a) who also found that a cold environment enhances a Ca^{2+}-induced hypothermia in the rabbit with a peripheral vasomotor response accounting for the temperature change. When the rat is fed a diet deficient in calcium, the body temperature as well as blood pressure tend to increase (ITOKAWA et al. 1974); conversely, a prolonged dietary deficiency in magnesium leads to a concurrent decline in both temperature and blood pressure. Since the changes are less significant when the rat's diet is deficient in both cations, any drastic alteration in the systemic concentration of a single ion could influence the core temperature of an animal over the long term. In the chicken kept at 24 °C, Ca^{2+} ions infused intravenously cause a significant reduction in cloacal temperature. This does not occur if the bird is heated in a chamber maintained at 45 °C (EDENS 1976). Na^+ is without effect at the 24 °C ambient temperature. When a 4- to 8-week-old chick is exposed to 5 °C, either Na^+ or K^+ given intramuscularly suppresses the cold-induced hypothermia;

on the other hand, Ca^{2+} enhances the fall in temperature (DENBOW and EDENS 1978, 1980). In humans at rest, the oral ingestion of a hypertonic solution of either Na^+ or Ca^{2+} ions has very little if any effect on body temperature in a thermoneutral environment (GREENLEAF and CASTLE 1971; NIELSEN et al. 1971; NIELSEN 1974 h).

Therefore, it is likely that a perturbation in the systemic profile of the cations, at least within physiological limits, is probably not a factor in the normal regulation of one's resting body temperature. The two main reasons for this centre on (a) the blood–brain barrier, and (b) the remarkable buffering capacity of extracellular fluid within the brain-stem region containing neurones responsible for thermoregulatory control. However, in an animal subjected to temperature stress or to vigorous exercise, the blood–brain barrier may become leaky and thence, ion-penetrable (GREENLEAF 1978); an influx of Na^+ ions into the brain could perhaps account in part for the resultant change in body temperature. To illustrate, it is well known that the exposure of a rat to cold produces a marked change in the uptake and subsequent distribution of essential cations not only in the brain-stem but in the hypophysis as well (SABBOT and COSTIN 1974). In this connection, a rat acclimatized to severe cold for many days exhibits a sharp increase in the activity of the sodium pump in peripheral cell membranes. This activity could explain the mechanism for heat production by means of non-shivering thermogenesis, provided by skeletal muscle and liver (GUERNSEY and STEVENS 1977).

C. Action of Cations in the Cerebral Ventricles

During the course of studies in which the cerebral ventricles of the unrestrained cat were perfused, it was discovered that a solution containing only Na^+ ion evokes an intense rise in the cat's body temperature during the interval of perfusion (FELDBERG et al. 1970). In the same preparation, the addition of $CaCl_2$ to the perfusate, in a normal physiological concentration, prevents this hyperthermia. On the basis of these initial observations, the idea was proposed that "the correct level of calcium or its permeability in the hypothalamus" could serve as "the physiological basis of the set-point" for body temperature (FELDBERG et al. 1970). This early suggestion was made without the constraints of anatomical and functional considerations, which arose shortly thereafter.

In the unanaesthetized rhesus monkey, it was found initially that the perfusion of excess Ca^{2+} ions from the lateral to fourth cerebral ventricle produces a remarkably precise, concentration-dependent fall in the primate's body temperature (MYERS et al. 1971). This is illustrated in Fig. 1. The ventricular perfusion of solutions containing excess magnesium or potassium, in five or ten times their normal physiological concentration, failed to alter the core temperature of the monkey significantly. In the case of both Na^+ and Ca^{2+} ion perfusions, the respective hyper- and hypothermias were again dependent solely upon the interval of perfusion, the monkey's temperature returning to a normal baseline level as soon as the perfusion had been terminated.

In addition to the identical findings in the unanaesthetized rabbit, FELDBERG and SAXENA (1970) also showed that by increasing the Ca^{2+} ion concentration of

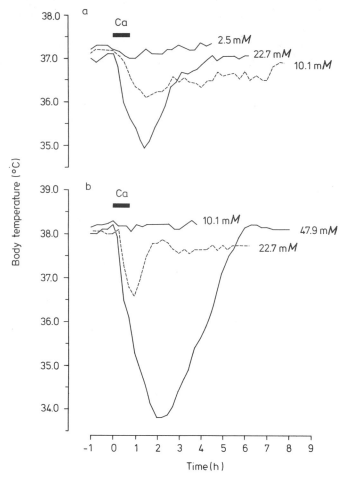

Fig. 1 a, b. Temperature records of two unanaesthetized monkeys in response to the 40 min perfusion (indicated by *heavy black lines*) from the lateral to the fourth ventricle at 100 μl/ min of a Krebs solution containing 2.5, 10.1, or 22.7 mM excess calcium **a**, and 10.1, 22.7, or 47.9 mM calcium **b**. (From Myers et al. 1971)

the perfusing fluid to 5.0 mM, the pyrexic response caused by the intravenous injection of 2.5 ml leucocyte pyrogen is prevented or nearly abolished. This Ca^{2+} concentration-dependent antagonism is illustrated in Fig. 2. From this result it was proposed that calcium could act as a kind of "brake," which would prevent Na^+ ions from exerting a temperature-elevating effect; and thus, if a pyrogen acted to remove the "calcium brake," it would bring about a sodium fever (Feldberg and Saxena 1970). It is of interest in relation to this idea, however, that an antipyretic such as Na^+ salicylate or acetaminophen fails to block the hyperthermic response caused by an intraventricular injection of disodium edetate (Na_2EDTA) in the un-anaesthetized cat (Clark 1971).

The universality of the involvement in central temperature control of Na^+ and Ca^{2+} ions soon became evident when different species were examined by use of the

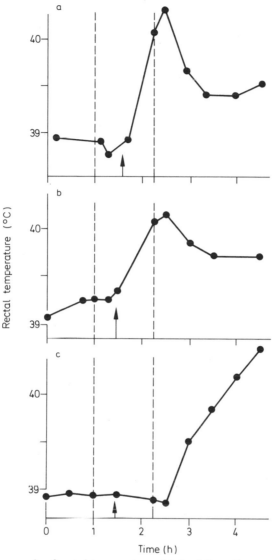

Fig. 2 a–c. Three records of rectal temperature obtained from the same rabbit on different days. The interval between the interrupted vertical lines indicates 75 min perfusion from left lateral ventricle to cisterna with artificial CSF containing different concentrations of calcium chloride. **a** perfusion with normal artificial CSF containing 1.25 mM calcium chloride; **b** perfusion with artificial CSF containing 3.75 mM; **c** containing 5 mM calcium chloride. The *arrow* in each of the records indicates an intravenous injection of 2.5 ml leucocyte pyrogen-containing plasma. (From FELDBERG and SAXENA 1970)

ventricular approach. In the unanaesthetized hibernator, the golden hamster, an increase in the ratio of Ca^{2+} to other ions in its CSF causes an immediate and deep hypothermia. When the hibernator is exposed to an ambient temperature of $+5\ °C$ or $-10\ °C$, excess calcium infused into the ventricle evokes a concentration-dependent decline in body temperature which averaged as much as 23.7 °C over an in-

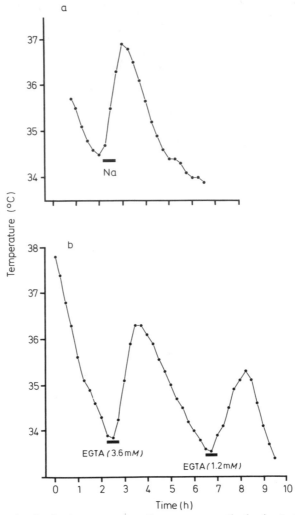

Fig. 3 a, b. Records of colonic temperature from two anaesthetized rats (1.5 g/kg urethane intraperitoneally) in response to 30 min ventricular perfusions of **a** a solution of 0.9% NaCl and **b** 3.6 mM EGTA and 1.2 mM EGTA. The perfusion intervals are indicated by *heavy black lines*. (From Myers and Brophy 1972)

terval of 4 h (Myers and Buckman 1972). Interestingly, the shift in the animal's temperature is accompanied by feeding, burrowing, and nesting behaviour, recapitulating the pattern of preparatory responses made by a normal hamster as it enters into a state of torpor. An artificial CSF solution infused intraventricularly and containing an excess in the ions of sodium, potassium, or magnesium did not affect the resting hamster's temperature at least in the concentrations which affect other species.

   In the anaesthetized or unanaesthetized rat, the perfusion of excess Ca^{2+} or Na^+ ions from the lateral ventricle to cisterna magna again evokes a similar hypo- or hyperthermia, respectively (Myers and Brophy 1972). Interestingly, the perfu-

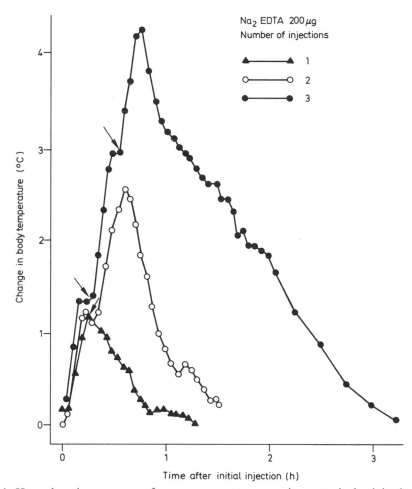

Fig. 4. Hyperthermic responses of one cat to one or more intraventricular injections of Na$_2$EDTA. *Arrows* indicate the time of successive injections in each series. (From CLARK 1971)

sion with ethyleneglycol tetra-acetic acid (EGTA), a relatively specific chelator of Ca^{2+} and having no mono- or divalent cation, evokes a sharp rise in temperature which is identical to that produced by excess sodium ions. The similarity of the pyrexic responses to the presence of Na$^+$ or absence of Ca^{2+} is portrayed in Fig. 3. In addition, sodium p-toluenesulphonate, used to control for the chloride ion, likewise elicits a hyperthermic response characteristic of sodium alone (MYERS and BROPHY 1972). The hyperthermic effect of Na$_2$EDTA has been shown recently in the rabbit; the similarity to the effect of a prostaglandin is quite remarkable (SASAKI and HORI 1977). The very intense hyperpyrexia due to repeated intraventricular infusions of Na$_2$EDTA in the cat (CLARK 1971) as shown in Fig. 4, underscores the significance of the ionic ratio in terms of the genesis of a hyperthermia.

Similarly, the infusion of other salts of sodium including palmitate, stearate, and oleate into the cerebral ventricle of the unanaesthetized cat also produces a concentration-dependent hyperthermia (BELESLIN et al. 1974). When Na_2EDTA is given in the ventricle of the conscious dog, an increase in temperature of 1.5 °C is accompanied by huddling, piloerection, vasoconstriction, shivering, and a drop in respiratory rate (SADOWSKI and SZCZEPAŃSKA-SADOWSKA 1974). Perfusion with physiological saline with an excess sodium concentration reportedly exerts no effect on the dog (SADOWSKI and SZCZEPAŃSKA-SADOWSKA 1974). In addition, DHU-MAL and GULATI (1974) report that a hyperthermic response could be produced with an inexplicable latency of as much as 40 min when a concentration of 47.8 mM Ca^{2+} was perfused in the dog's cerebral ventricle. However, a perfusion solution containing 105 mM Ca^{2+} ions in excess produced a hypothermia after which the dogs died within one to two hours. The reasons for the latter two results are not clear.

In avian species, the evolutionary consistency in the temperature response to an altered cation level in the brain has been further demonstrated. In the unanaesthetized pigeon kept at room temperature, excess Ca^{2+} ions infused into the cerebral ventricle evoke a fall in the bird's cloacal temperature (SAXENA 1976). NaCl solution by itself or Na_2EDTA both cause a rise in temperature, whereas potassium ions elicit hyperthermia when infused continuously. Only when the concentration of magnesium is elevated considerably is any hypothermic response in evidence. SAXENA has noted also that few if any changes are observed when the cations are infused intravenously in the pigeon. In the fowl, DENBOW and EDENS (1980) have observed essentially the same results: the infusion of normal NaCl solution into the lateral ventricle of the chicken, held at a thermoneutral environment, induces intense shivering, vasoconstriction, and a rise in the bird's body temperature. The hypothermia following intraventricular Ca^{2+} ions is directly related to the magnitude of vasodilatation, as reflected by an increase in the bird's foot temperature (DENBOW and EDENS 1980).

Although the body temperature of sheep increases after an infusion of Na^+ ions into the cerebral ventricle, it is essentially unchanged by a similar injection of excess Ca^{2+} ions (SEOANE and BAILE 1973). A cautionary note is necessary, however, since Ca^{2+} ions in the concentrations used elicited a strong feeding response, the activity of which may have tended to overcome the hypothermia observed in every other species. Within hypothalamic tissue, Ca^{2+}-sensitive sites which mediate feeding or evoke a fall in temperature are anatomically separate (MYERS et al. 1976a). The disparate actions of Ca^{2+} ions infused into the third ventricle of the rabbit are also documented: body temperature declines, intraocular pressure rises (KRUPIN et al. 1978). A pharmacological distinction is also evident in that systemic phenobarbitone blocks the Ca^{2+}-induced effect on intraocular fluid with no effect on temperature, whereas imidazole prevents Ca^{2+} hypothermia with no effect on the intraocular pressure response (KRUPIN et al. 1978).

D. Action of Cations on the Hypothalamus

By the late 1920s, the speculation had arisen that vegetative functions under the control of the central nervous system could be influenced or even regulated by the presence of cations which were transported from the bloodstream to the brain (e.g.

DEMOLE 1927). In this setting, HASAMA, a Japanese scientist working in Nagasaki, undertook an investigation of the direct effect of cations on the basal diencephalon, primarily the tuber cinerium. HASAMA (1930) proceeded to infuse solutions of different cations, each in a 50 µl volume, into the basal diencephalon of the cat while monitoring its body temperature. Although several cations produced a rather intense hyperthermia in the unanaesthetized cat, Na^+ and K^+ ions were particularly potent (HASAMA 1930). However, approximately three times the concentration of K^+ ions was required to produce the same elevation as that of sodium. When HASAMA injected excess calcium ions similarly into the tuberal region, a rapid fall in the animal's temperature occurred. These pioneering findings were among the first to demonstrate a clear-cut antagonistic action of two substances directly within the same region of the brain.

Using the same large 50 µl volume (because a microlitre syringe had not yet been invented), KYM (1934) then showed in the rabbit that Na^+ ions injected into the hypothalamus evoked a temperature rise that closely resembled the hyperthermia following intravenous ergotoxin (KYM 1934). This Na^+ hyperthermia could be prevented by an excess in Ca^{2+} ions, injected intrahypothalamically in the same volume, which provided the first evidence that calcium itself could serve as an antipyretic agent or a hypothalamic mediator of antipyresis. In addition, KYM (1934) found that K^+ ions infused in a very high concentration could also cause a rise in temperature in some animals, a finding confirmed later by COOPER et al. (1965), who instead infused excess K^+ directly into the rabbit's rostral hypothalamus. ROSENTHAL (1941) not only was able to verify KYM's results but also showed that Ca^{2+} ions intensify the decline in the rabbit's body temperature caused by a similar injection of picrotoxin into the hypothalamus. By taking this together with the earlier work of KYM, ROSENTHAL concluded that "injection of one mg of calcium chloride ($CaCl_2$) prevents all forms of experimental fever" (ROSENTHAL 1941).

I. Anatomical Localization of Ion-Induced Temperature Changes

Because of the large number of disparate anatomical structures reached and functions affected by a solution of excess cations infused intraventricularly, it was not possible to localize an effect of a specific cation to a circumscribed region of the diencephalon. Nor has it been possible on the basis of the earlier historical experiments to pinpoint the locus of action of a cation within the hypothalamus because of the large 50 µl volumes infused by the early investigators. In fact, from what is known today, a good portion of the 50 µl volume refluxed into the cerebral ventricle (e.g. MYERS 1974a).

In 1970, an attempt was made to identify the sites in the hypothalamus within which an imbalance in the Na^+:Ca^{2+} ion ratio could shift an animal's body temperature upward or downward. With respect to an anticipated localization of the ionic temperature phenomenon to the anterior hypothalamic preoptic area (AH/PO), all experimental efforts failed (see MYERS 1976a). Quite unexpectedly, however, MYERS and VEALE (1970) found that the cat's posterior hypothalamus, a region containing cells that are not thermally sensitive, was highly reactive to an imbalance in the ratio of Na^+ to Ca^{2+} ions. When the region dorsal to the mammillary bodies was perfused with excess Na^+ ions in a concentration less than

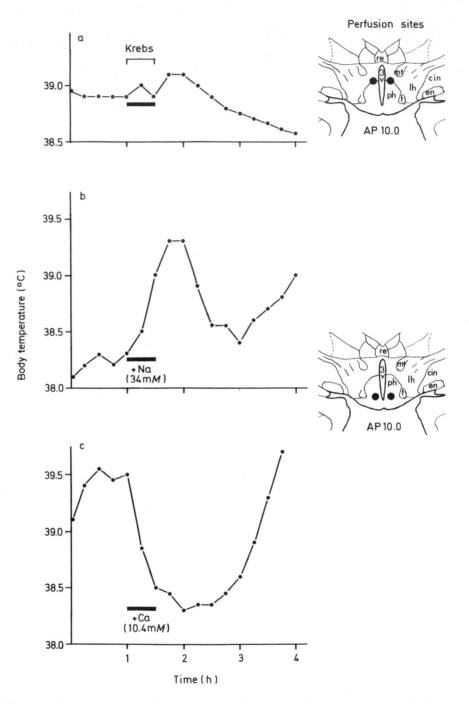

Fig. 5 a–c. Temperature records of an unanaesthetized cat in response to the local per-fusions for 30 min of **a**, Krebs solution alone; **b**, Krebs solution plus 34 m*M* excess sodium; **c**, Krebs solution plus 10.4 m*M* excess calcium. The sites of the bilateral perfusions are in-dicated by the *filled circles* in the *insets*. (From Myers and Veale 1971)

Table 1. Average maximal change from baseline temperature of unanaesthetized cats during the first 60 min of repeated push–pull perfusions of the anterior, posterior and other hypothalamic areas. (MYERS and VEALE 1971)

Ion	Concentration[a] (mM)	Number of perfusions	Mean change (°C) and standard error	
Posterior hypothalamic area				
Na	13.6	10	+0.55	±0.05
Na	34.0–68.0	8	+0.64	±0.10
Ca	2.6	4	−0.48	±0.02
Ca	10.4	11	−0.66	±0.11
K	4.7–47.0	9	−0.03	±0.08
Mg	1.2–12.0	4	0.00	±0.11
Controls[b]		10	+0.01	±0.01
Anterior hypothalamic area				
Na	13.6–68.0	8	−0.36	±0.19
Ca	2.6–10.4	6	+0.12	±0.23
K	4.7–23.5	3	−0.13	±0.30
Mg	1.2–6.0	3	−0.01	±0.33
Controls[b]		5	+0.18	±0.08
Other areas of the hypothalamus				
Na	13.6–68.0	35	−0.07	±0.06
Ca	2.6–10.4	17	−0.39	±0.09
K	4.7–47.0	5	−0.08	±0.07
Mg	1.2–12.0	3	0.00	±0.04
Controls[b]		11	−0.16	±0.07

[a] The millimolar values represent the ion concentrations above those in a standard Krebs solution

[b] The control perfusates consisted of isotonic sucrose; double isotonic sucrose; Krebs solution; Krebs solution with double the weight of each salt; and a solution containing Na, Ca, K, and Mg in physiological concentrations

10.0 mM in excess of normal CSF, by means of push–pull cannulae, the cat began to shiver, vasoconstrict, and exhibit an intense rise in body temperature. From 1.2 to 10.0 mM excess Ca^{2+} perfused within the same locus in the cat's posterior hypothalamus induced vasodilatation and a consequent and immediate hypothermia (MYERS and VEALE 1971).

In both instances, the changes in temperature depended solely upon (a) the aberrant ratio in the concentration of the ions and, (b) the anatomical sites of the push–pull perfusion as shown in Fig. 5. As long as the normal ratio of ions, one to the other, was constantly maintained, the temperature of the cat failed to change. When the p-toluenesulphonate salt of sodium was perfused as a control for possible chloride ion effects, a rise in temperature occurred of equal magnitude to that with Na^+ alone (MYERS and VEALE 1971). Perfusions at the same posterior hypothalamic sites of magnesium or potassium ions in a ratio increased proportionally to that of Na^+ or Ca^{2+} ions failed to alter the cat's body temperature. Table 1 presents the average changes in temperature caused by each of the afore-

mentioned cations together with the functional distinction between anatomical regions of perfusion.

Species continuity in terms of the cations' central action has been readily verified. A perturbation in the inherent balance between endogenous Na^+ and Ca^{2+}
ions within the hypothalamus also evokes changes in the body temperature of
the macaque monkey of the same magnitude and direction. The chelation of the
Ca^{2+} ions by EGTA, delivered to the caudal hypothalamus by push–pull cannulae,
results in a sharp increase in the primate's body temperature, following the shift
in the ratio of ions in favour of Na^+ (MYERS and YAKSH 1971).

By repetition of the push–pull perfusion of either Na^+ or Ca^{2+} ions at intervals
during the course of the day, a monkey's body temperature can also be re-set for
a prolonged period of time, even beyond 12 h. Thus, the cells of the posterior hypothalamus exhibit neither evidence of tachyphylaxis nor a decline in sensitivity to
an aberrant concentration of the two essential cations (MYERS and YAKSH 1971).
An important issue with respect to the conceptual distinction between a set-point
and regulatory mechanism has also been examined; that is, once the animal's body
temperature has been re-established at a high or low level by an excess in a respective ion species, will the animal nevertheless thermoregulate normally around the
new "set" level? In experiments with the monkey, the newly established temperature was stabilized by repeated perfusions of either Na^+ or Ca^{2+} ions. Then a thermal load in the form of hot or cold water was given by the intragastric route. The
effect of the thermal stimulus was entirely offset by normal thermoregulatory responses, which included shivering, piloerection, a change in respiratory rate, and
appropriate vasomotor responses (MYERS and YAKSH 1971). These responses were
in defence of the newly established level of body temperature and, in fact, following
a transient deflection due to the thermal load, the monkey's temperature returned
to its pre-load level.

One possible discrepancy has arisen with respect to the localization of an ion
imbalance. In the ground squirrel, excess Ca^{2+} ions reportedly exert a hypothermic
effect when perfused in the PO/AH (HANEGAN and WILLIAMS 1975). On close in-
spection of these data, particularly in comparison with those of the rat, it is clear
that the time of push–pull perfusion required to induce a 2.0 °C fall in the squirrel's
temperature due to excess Ca^{2+} ions is substantially greater than that when a perfusion is carried out in the caudal hypothalamus. Moreover, the concentration
required is twice as great. The facts suggest that because of the diminutive size of
the squirrel's diencephalon, the perfusate was, in fact, leaking or passing to the
caudal hypothalamus. Unfortunately, it is not known whether the caudal portion
of the hibernator's hypothalamus exhibits a greater sensitivity to the ions; hence,
the anatomical localization of this response has not yet been accomplished. To illustrate the clear-cut differences in the sensitivity of the posterior and anterior hypothalamic areas, VEALE et al. (1977) examined the hypothermic effects of Ca^{2+}
ions at two concentrations in the two regions of the rabbit. Their striking results
are presented in Fig. 6.

II. Specificity of Cation Actions

A non-specific depression of hypothalamic tissue caused by an imbalance of
cations has been ruled out for the most part by several different kinds of ex-

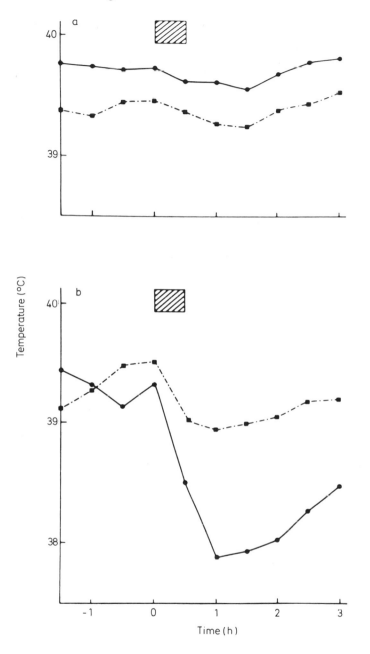

Fig. 6 a, b. Records of body temperature for rabbits during perfusion of the hypothalamus at an ambient temperature of 4.0 ± 2.0 °C. **a** perfusion of the anterior hypothalamic area with Ca^{2+} twice (5.2 mM) (*squares*) and five times (13.0 mM) (*circles*) in excess of the concentration found in extracellular fluid; **b** perfusion of the posterior hypothalamic area with Ca^{2+} twice (5.2 mM) (*squares*) and five times (13.0 mM) (*circles*) the concentration found in extracellular fluid. The duration of the perfusion is indicated by the *shaded box*. (From VEALE et al. 1977)

periments. First, the monkey consumes food in spite of significantly reduced body temperatures (e.g. 35 °C) caused by perfusion with excess Ca^{2+} ions (Myers and Yaksh 1972). Further, during deep Ca^{2+} hypothermia, the animal is nevertheless able to vasoconstrict, vasodilate, huddle, shiver, and/or piloerect when an externally given thermal load is imposed artificially. Interestingly, Borbély and his colleagues find that Ca^{2+} ions exert a very selective effect on the brain-stem mechanisms responsible for the differential states of sleep and arousal (Tószeghi et al. 1978; Borbély and Tobler 1979). As described earlier, excess Ca^{2+} ions also evoke vigorous eating behaviour in the rat, cat, and monkey without any sign of neuronal depression (e.g. Myers et al. 1976a).

In two other species, the powerful actions of Na^+ and Ca^{2+} ions have been morphologically isolated within the mammillary region of the hypothalamus. When excess Ca^{2+} ions are perfused within the posterior hypothalamus of the rat, a concentration-dependent fall in the animal's body temperature occurs. The exceptional sensitivity of this caudal region is documented by the fact that the amount of cation in the perfusate is well below that required for a similar sort of change in temperature following (a) a micro-injection of the cation at an homologous morphological site, or (b) after an infusion of Ca^{2+} ions into the animal's lateral cerebral ventricle (Myers et al. 1976a). A cholinergic–muscarinic link in the ion-induced change in temperature has also been postulated. Atropine but not mecamylamine, a nicotinic receptor blocker, accentuates even further the hypothermia caused by excess Ca^{2+} ions (Myers et al. 1976a).

Within the rabbit's posterior hypothalamus, the push–pull perfusion of excess Ca^{2+} or Na^+ ions produces the typical fall or rise in the rabbit's core temperature, respectively; the magnitude of the response is concentration- and site-dependent (Veale and Jones 1977; Veale et al. 1977). An important observation was made by Veale and his colleagues: the temperature-lowering effect caused by excess Ca^{2+} ions in the posterior hypothalamus is abolished by the addition of glucose to the push-pull perfusate. When a concentration of 53 mM glucose is present in the perfusate, the usual hypothermia evoked by excess Ca^{2+} ions is prevented, as indicated in Fig. 7. The availability of extra energy substrate within the hypothalamic tissue represents a logical explanation of this effect. The specificity of this utilizable energy substrate is underscored by the lack of effect of sucrose on calcium's action when the latter sugar is perfused in the hypothalamus in the same equimolar concentration as glucose (Jones et al. 1978).

E. Exercise, Cations, and Temperature Set-Point

Running, swimming or other forms of intense exercise typically cause a sharp rise in one's central body temperature. In humans, this elevation is entirely regulated in that the shift in temperature is independent of a wide range of ambient temperatures, hot or cold (Nielsen 1938; Greenleaf 1973).

Because of the suggestion that the set-point for body temperature is determined by the intrinsic ratio of Na^+ to Ca^{2+} in the caudal hypothalamus (Myers and Veale 1970), the physiological effects of altering the plasma concentration of these two cations was subsequently tested on the exercising human subject (Nielsen 1974b). It was found that Na^+ raises the equilibrium body temperature, whereas

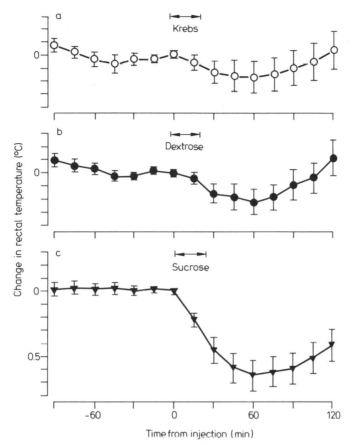

Fig. 7 a–c. Records of the mean changes in rectal temperatures of conscious cats from the temperatures recorded at the start of 20 min perfusions (indicated by double-headed arrows) with **a** control Krebs solution ($n=11$); **b** solutions in which (Ca^{2+}) was increased and simultaneously (Na^+) was reduced to produce a solution containing five times the normal Ca^{2+} : Na^+ ratio and brought to isomolarity with the addition of 53 mM dextrose ($n=11$); **c** solutions containing the same ionic constituents as above with 53 mM sucrose replacing the dextrose ($n=13$). *Vertical bars* represent the standard errors of the mean. The ordinate scale is the same on all three graphs. (From JONES et al. 1978)

excess Ca^{2+} ions reduce it. Before a 60 min period of strenuous exercise on a bicycle ergometer, the subjects drank 1.0–1.5 l of 2.0% NaCl or $CaCl_2$ solution. During the work interval, core temperature was higher but sweat rate was lower after the oral Na^+; both of these physiological responses were reversed following the ingestion of a Ca^{2+} solution before exercise was begun by the subject (NIELSEN 1974 b). Figure 8 depicts the differences in oesophageal temperature. Essentially the same results were obtained after the drinking of a Na^+ solution just before a period of exercise (GREENLEAF 1973). However, after a graded work load, the value of the actual plasma concentrations of Na^+ or Ca^{2+} shows that only the level of Na^+ ions correlates with the magnitude of displacement of the human subject's rectal temperature (GREENLEAF et al. 1977). STRÖMME et al. (1976), however, failed

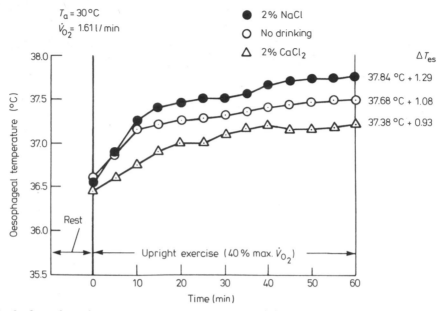

Fig. 8. Oesophageal temperature responses at rest and during 60 min of submaximal exercise after ingestion of hypertonic sodium and calcium solutions. [From Greenleaf (1979) re-drawn from Nielsen (1974b)]

to find any relationship whatsoever between serum cation concentration and the hyperthermia seen after cross-country skiing or treadmill exercise.

At either hot or cold ambient temperature, the oral intake of Na^+ elevates the rectal temperature of the human subject to the same extent as that observed at a thermoneutral temperature (Greenleaf et al. 1978). Following the ingestion of Ca^{2+} ions, the same sort of relationship is seen, albeit reversed; but ingested Ca^{2+} ions are not nearly as efficacious as Na^+ when the solutions are taken by this intragastric route.

Studies by Greenleaf and associates on the peripheral effects of plasma tonicity in the exercising dog tend to complement those on the human subject. An infusion of hypertonic NaCl solution into the hind-leg vein of a dog running on a treadmill evokes a slightly higher rise in rectal temperature than an isotonic or citrate solution given in the same way (Greenleaf et al. 1975). In addition, the rise in a dog's core temperature, accompanying treadmill exercise, correlates well with its plasma Na^+ concentration but not with plasma volume (Greenleaf et al 1976), an observation also confirmed in the human subject (Harrison et al. 1978). Interestingly, if the dog is permitted to drink water, the Na^+ ion, osmotic-induced, hyperthermia is attenuated.

I. Hypothalamic $Na^+ : Ca^{2+}$ Ratio and Exercise

Although the examination of changes in plasma ion dynamics is physiologically of great importance, the functional role played by the ionic milieu of the CNS in an exercise-induced shift in core temperature cannot be ascertained with this ex-

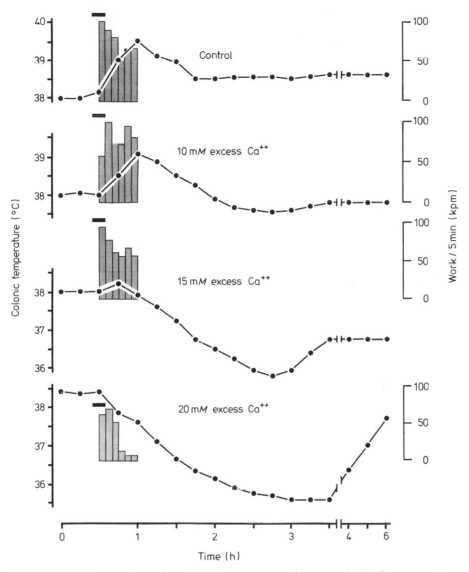

Fig. 9. Colonic temperature of a chaired macaque monkey recorded in four separate experiments, before, during, and after exercise on a "rowing machine." Work rate, recorded in kpm/5 min is denoted by vertical shaded bars. The 10 min interval of infusion of control CSF solution or of Ca^{2+} ions 10, 15, or 20 mM in excess of CSF, into the cerebral ventricle, is indicated by *black bar*. (From MYERS et al. 1977a)

perimental approach. One principal reason for this is the blood-brain barrier's delicate and effective maintenance of ionic stability within the brain's fluid compartments (otherwise the intake of salted peanuts, salt pork, and the like would play havoc with normal extracellular events such as a neurone's action potential, which is in major part governed by membrane Na^+ ions).

Table 2. Changes in colonic temperature from baseline control and total amount of work performed during exercise in neutral, cold, and hot environments. (Myers et al. 1977)

Neutral (22 °C db)	Solution	Temperature change (°C)	Total work (J per 30 min)
Monkey A	Control 5-ion	+1.45	2,018
	Ca^{2+} 2.5 mM	+0.40	1,258
	Ca^{2+} 10 mM	−0.45	1,018
Monkey B	Control 5-ion	+1.35	2,795
	Ca^{2+} 10 mM	+1.05	2,556
	Ca^{2+} 15 mM	+0.20	2,181
	Ca^{2+} 20 mM	−0.40	1,045
Hot (35 °C db)	Control 5-ion	+1.10	1,338
Monkey A	Ca^{2+} 2.5 mM	+0.45	1,192
Cold (0° C db)	Control 5-ion	+0.55	2,036
Monkey A	Ca^{2+} 2.5 mM	+0.05	1,367

[a] db = dry bulb

To determine if an exercising animal is affected in any way by a change in the ionic milieu of its hypothalamus, several sequential investigations were undertaken by Gisolfi and colleagues in the late 1970s. An important question was answered in 1976 when it was found that Ca^{2+} ions could, in fact, influence exercise-induced hyperthermia. When the posterior hypothalamus of a rat running steadily on a treadmill was perfused with a CSF solution containing excess Ca^{2+} ions for only 10 min, the already elevated temperatures suddenly declined (Gisolfi et al. 1976). In some cases the perfused rat continued to run uninterruptedly; however, in other animals a transient cessation in their motor activity occurred for several minutes.

Corresponding experiments with both Ca^{2+} ions and the calcium chelating agent, EGTA, have served to confirm this cation's involvement in the exercise-induced hyperthermia. The depletion of tissue calcium in the caudal hypothalamus by local push–pull perfusion with EGTA, carried out at the same time as the rat ran on the treadmill, augmented the exercise-related elevation in the rodent's core temperature (Wilson et al. 1978). Again the mechanism either for Ca^{2+}-stimulated heat dissipation or for Na^+ hyperthermia is mediated apparently through a coordinated vasomotor response. That is, the tail vein temperatures of the rat correlate inversely with the deflections in body temperature brought about by an excess or deficit in tissue calcium within the animal's posterior hypothalamus (Wilson et al. 1978).

In the macaque monkey trained to exercise on a specially devised "rowing machine" (Gisolfi et al. 1978), excess Ca^{2+} ions infused into its third cerebral ventricle reduce its body temperature significantly. As shown in Fig. 9, this decline was proportionately much greater than the reduction in the monkey's work output (Myers et al. 1977a). When the ambient temperature was raised to 35 °C or lowered to 3 °C, the pattern of the monkey's exercise was relatively unaffected by the injection of 2.5 mM. However, the colonic temperature remained stable or declined if the primate was exposed to an ambient temperature of 0°–3 °C (Myers

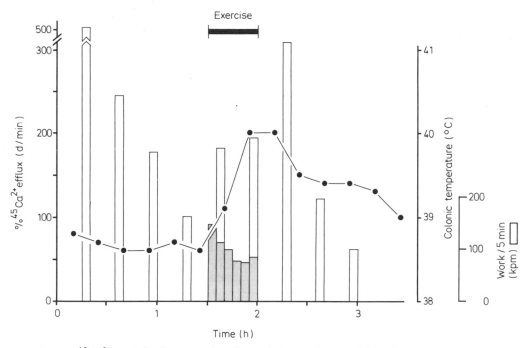

Fig. 10. $^{45}Ca^{2+}$ activity in successive diencephalic perfusates (left ordinate, open vertical bars). The d/min value in the perfusate collected just before exercise (*black bar*) served as the 100% baseline value for calculation of percentage changes in radioactivity. Colonic temperature (*solid circles*) of the monkey is in °C. Work output in N m/5 min (right ordinate, lower) is indicated by the *shaded vertical bars*. (From GISOLFI et al. 1977)

et al. 1977a, b). Table 2 presents a summary of changes in temperature and work output performed by two monkeys after Ca^{2+} infusions.

Thus, diencephalic Ca^{2+} ions seem to be involved in the steady-state regulated rise in core temperature ordinarily witnessed during vigorous exercise. SOBOCIŃSKA and GREENLEAF (1976) have found also that an infusion of excess Ca^{2+} ions into the lateral cerebral ventricle of the dog that was running on a treadmill significantly reduces the exercise-related hyperthermia. They conclude that the excess in Ca^{2+} ions in the CNS causes an increased loss of heat during physical exercise which is unrelated to the plasma concentration of Na^+ ions.

Physiological rather than pharmacological evidence of the involvement of central Ca^{2+} ions in the exercise-related set-point shift phenomenon has now been obtained. The kinetics of cation fluxes within the hypothalamus have been investigated following the pre-labelling with $^{45}Ca^{2+}$ of hypothalamic perfusion sites of a well-trained monkey exercising strenuously on a rowing machine. During the interval of exercise, the activity of $^{45}Ca^{2+}$ increases significantly at diencephalic sites in direct proportion to the concomitant rise in the primate's core temperature (GISOLFI et al. 1978). The enhanced efflux of $^{45}Ca^{2+}$ accompanying exercise-induced hyperthermia is shown in Fig. 10. As in the cat, cooling of the monkey's trunk evokes an immediate efflux of Ca^{2+} ions from the same diencephalic perfusion sites. Thus, the mechanism for heat production in the animal's hypothalamus, whether activated by cold or exercise, seems to be underpinned by the process of tissue transport, binding, or other cellular activity of Ca^{2+} ions within the caudal hypothalamus (Gisolfi et al. 1977).

F. Fever, Na$^+$:Ca^{2+} Ratio, and Set-Point Shift

A febrile reaction, which represents a major defence against bodily invasion by infectious bacteria, is considered to be an upward shift in the set-point for body temperature (Fox and MacPherson 1954; Hardy 1976). The rise is a regulated one and is amply defended by normal physiological responses against a hot or cold peripheral challenge (e.g. Cooper 1972). If, as was postulated, the set-point temperature is dependent upon the Na$^+$:Ca^{2+} ratio in the hypothalamus, then a distinct perturbation in ionic activity in this diencephalic structure should be demonstrable (Myers and Veale 1970, 1971). Since an endotoxin produces a fall in the serum concentration of Ca^{2+} ions (Skarnes 1968) and in brain-stem tissue (Veale 1971), a major issue has persistently revolved about the endogenous activity of the two vital cations in the brain during the induction and progress of a fever of bacterial origin.

I. In Vivo Cation Activity in the Diencephalon

In 1972, it was found that a bacterial pyrogen can act directly on brain tissue to disturb the cellular ratio of Na$^+$ to Ca^{2+} ions (Myers and Tytell 1972). The brain of the unrestrained cat was first labelled with either ^{22}Na$^+$ or ^{45}Ca^{2+} by an injection of the nuclide directly into the animal's lateral cerebral ventricle. Then the medial aspect of the diencephalon was perfused with CSF from one to the other lateral ventricle. Once the efflux of radioactivity had reached equilibrium, diluted *Salmonella typhosa* was infused into one lateral ventricle, and the perfusions were resumed. As the cat's body temperature began to rise, the efflux of ^{45}Ca^{2+} from the perfused diencephalon increased greatly. Alternatively, in the ^{22}Na$^+$-labelled cats, the efflux of Na$^+$ ions fell well below the control baseline level of radioactivity throughout the course of the pyrogen fever, with samples collected for up to seven hours after the typhoid infusion (Myers and Tytell 1972).

Table 3 illustrates the average percentage fluctuation, rise and decline, in ^{45}Ca^{2+} and ^{22}Na$^+$ efflux from brain-stem tissue, respectively, recorded temporally for the first five samples of perfusate. These findings provided the first direct evidence that bacteria, whether acting directly or indirectly on brain-stem cells, actually do disrupt the normal ratio of Na$^+$ to Ca^{2+} ions at least within CSF bathing the diencephalon. In human lumbar CSF no change in Na$^+$ or Ca^{2+} ions is detected in the febrile patient (Nielsen et al. 1973), which seems to correspond with the general lack of pharmacological effect of the two cations when ingested orally.

During the excitation of the nerve cells responsible for heat production, Ca^{2+} ions are apparently unbound from the neuronal membrane or extruded extracellularly. A reduction in cellular calcium would lead to an instability of the membrane, predominance of sodium, and presumably an enhanced rate of depolarization of

Table 3. Mean percentage change in radioactivity ($\pm$ standard error) in CSF samples collected at 30 min intervals beginning 15 min after the injection of the pyrogen. (MYERS and TYTELL 1972)

Time (min)	$^{45}Ca^{2+}$		$^{22}Na^+$	
	Increase (%)	ΔT (°C)	Decrease (%)	ΔT (°C)
Pyrogen injected				
15	91.2 ± 52.8^a	-0.09 ± 0.06	7.7 ± 24.0^b	0.08 ± 0.07
45	120.4 ± 63.7	0.28 ± 0.13	-28.5 ± 10.9	0.23 ± 0.13
75	96.5 ± 54.5	0.21 ± 0.18	-37.1 ± 11.5	0.30 ± 0.13
105	54.1 ± 40.4	0.44 ± 0.24	-36.0 ± 11.3	0.20 ± 0.05
135	83.3 ± 64.0	0.48 ± 0.13	-27.0 ± 10.9	0.26 ± 0.04
Mean	89.1 ± 10.71		-32.2 ± 3.0	
Control				
15	16.0^c	-0.03	24.6^c	-0.10
45	16.0	0.23	-1.6	0.00
75	0.0	0.08	8.2	$+0.10$
105	0.0	0.02	-16.4	-0.15
135	-36.0	0.00	6.6	$+0.15$
Mean	-0.8 ± 9.5		4.3 ± 6.7	

Nothing was injected into the controls. The increase in Ca^{2+} or the decrease in Na^+ for the animals that received the pyrogen was based on an average of three or four determinations for each sample and compared to the baseline concentration for each ion. For changes of the ions in control animals, one determination was made for each sample and compared with the baseline. Temperature change during each interval (ΔT) was also determined.
[a] $N=4$; [b] $N=3$; [c] $N=2$

hypothalamic neurones which are delegated to shivering, vasoconstriction, piloerection, and an increase in metabolism. When excess Ca^{2+} ions are applied to the selfsame cells, the opposite effect is produced, i.e. a reduction of neuronal firing and conceivably an enhanced release of transmitter subserving an inhibitory pathway which would lead to heat dissipation.

A direct test of these ideas was undertaken in the mid-1970s. The purpose was to identify precisely the anatomical site of cation efflux during thermogenesis due to a cold or pyrogen challenge. This is a particularly crucial question centred on the issue of the possible co-location of the region of sensitivity to a cation imbalance with the morphological site of cation efflux. In the cat, perfusion cannulae were lowered to the cation-reactive sites in the caudal hypothalamus after the site had been pre-labelled by a $^{45}Ca^{2+}$ micro-injection. Push–pull perfusions of the site were repeated until the egress of radioactivity began to equilibrate. The following observations were made (MYERS et al. 1976b).

First, exposure of the cat to an extremely cold ambient temperature of 0 °C causes shivering, vasoconstriction, piloerection, and a simultaneous and immediate efflux of $^{45}Ca^{2+}$ ions from the posterior hypothalamus. When the same cat is exposed to a high ambient temperature of 40 °C, the egress of Ca^{2+} ions from the

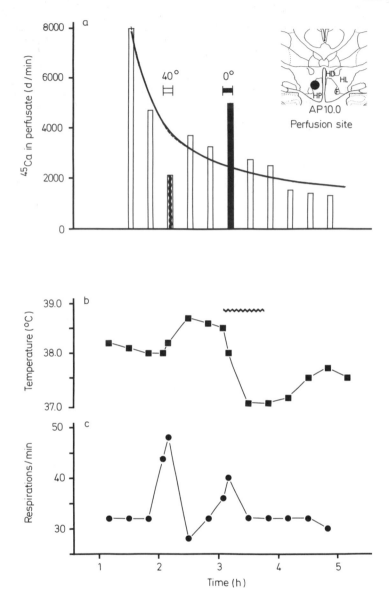

Fig. 11 a–c. Efflux (top) of $^{45}Ca^{2+}$ in successive push–pull perfusates collected at a rate of 50 µl/min from the perfusion site denoted by the dot in the histological *inset*. The site had been labelled with 1.0 µCi $^{45}Ca^{2+}$ 18 h earlier. The chamber temperature of the cat was raised to 40 °C or lowered to 0 °C just preceding and during the third and sixth perfusions, respectively, as denoted by the bars. Colonic temperature **b** and respiratory rate **c** were recorded continuously. Shivering is designated by the zigzag line **b**. The declining curve **a** denotes control washout of radioactivity. Anatomical abbreviations, here and in Figs. 12 and 13, are as follows: *C*, caudate nucleus; *CA*, anterior commissure; *CHO*, optic chiasm; *CM*, central medial nucleus; *CS*, subthalamic nucleus; *F*, fornix; *GP*, globus pallidus; *HD*, dorsal hypothalamic area; *HL*, lateral hypothalamus; *HP*, posterior hypothalamic area; *IC*, internal capsule; *MM*, mammillary bodies; *NPR*, prothalamic nucleus; *PP*, cerebral peduncle; *RPO* preoptic area; *S*, septum. From Myers et al. (1976 b)

same caudal site is inhibited. These changes are presented for a representative cat in Fig. 11. Second, when the thermosensitive neurones of the anterior hypothalamic preoptic area (AH/PO) are cooled by bilaterally positioned thermodes, at the same time that the posterior hypothalamus is perfused, again $^{45}Ca^{2+}$ activity is greatly enhanced. Alternatively, warming of the preoptic area similarly attenuates the efflux of Ca^{2+} ions. Third, the local anaesthesia of the cells in the PO/AH, with a procaine micro-injection blocks any change in $^{45}Ca^{2+}$ activity in the posterior hypothalamus when the cat is exposed to a cold or hot environmental temperature. Fourth, a bacterial pyrogen, S. typhosa, micro-injected into the PO/AH evokes a sharp efflux of $^{45}Ca^{2+}$ ions, again within the caudal part of the hypothalamus. This enhanced activity of Ca^{2+} ions coincides precisely with the pyrexic response, shivering, and vasoconstriction. Interestingly, prostaglandin E_1 (PGE_1) or serotonin (5-hydroxytryptamine, 5 HT) micro-injected in the same way as the typhoid organism exerts precisely the same action in augmenting Ca^{2+} efflux, which is accompanied by a profound hyperthermia. The initial efflux of $^{45}Ca^{2+}$ ions and subsequent extrusion into posterior hypothalamic perfusates following typhoid and PGE_1 micro-injections into the anterior hypothalamus are portrayed in Figs. 12 and 13. Since the posterior hypothalamus is not sensitive to a foreign lipopolysaccharide or other pyrogenic material, the change in temperature set-point occurring during a fever is apparently mediated by a change in calcium kinetics in the posterior hypothalamus. In fact, it is clear from the foregoing results that the Ca^{2+} ion mechanism, and perhaps Na^+ activity, operates whenever neuronal input from the periphery signals a severe thermal challenge to the rostral hypothalamus. When the local temperature of this anterior hypothalamic region is raised or lowered, the same Ca^{2+} response is generated (MYERS 1978). If thermogenesis is called for above and beyond that of a regulatory adjustment, i.e. a set-point shift upwards, as a consequence of a pyrogen's presence in the body, the Na^+ : Ca^{2+} ratio is displaced in favour of Na^+ by the relative depletion of Ca^{2+} ions from the cellular milieu of the caudal hypothalamus. In this instance, probably an exceedingly small number of Ca^{2+} ions are actually involved.

II. Antipyresis and Na^+ : Ca^{2+} Efflux

What happens to the Na^+ : Ca^{2+} ion ratio during defervescence following the administration of an antipyretic drug? Are the kinetics of Ca^{2+} flux now reversed?

In cats prepared with cerebral ventricular perfusion cannulae, the brain was pre-labelled with $^{45}Ca^{2+}$ or alternatively, $^{22}Na^+$ (MYERS 1976b). Following an injection of S. typhosa into the lateral ventricle, an intense fever developed. After Ca^{2+} or Na^+ extrusion from diencephalic tissue had achieved a steady state, paracetamol (acetaminophen) was administered parenterally (15–36 mg/kg). Even before the fever began to abate and the temperature began to decline, $^{45}Ca^{2+}$ efflux from the cat's diencephalon was reduced by as much as 40%. Conversely, in separate experiments, Na^+ ion activity was substantially elevated in the diencephalic perfusates as defervescence progressed. Of special note is the fact that the two divergent patterns of cation flux reversed themselves once the cat's body temperature started to rise again to fever level (MYERS 1976b).

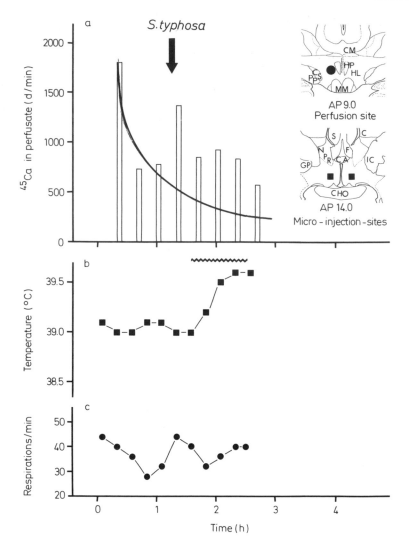

Fig. 12 a–c. Efflux **a** of $^{45}Ca^{2+}$ in successive push–pull perfusates collected at a rate of 50 μl/min from the perfusion site denoted by the *dot* in the histological *inset*. The site had been labelled with 1.0 μCi $^{45}Ca^{2+}$ 18 h earlier. A 1/10 dilution of *Salmonella typhosa* was micro-injected in a volume of 1.0 μl before the fourth perfusion, as indicated by the *arrow*, at the injection sites designated by the squares in the histological *inset*. Shivering indicated by the zigzag line, colonic temperature **b** and respiratory rate **c** are shown as in previous figures. The declining curve **a** denotes control washout of radioactivity. Anatomical abbreviations are the same as in Fig. 11. (From MYERS et al. 1976 b)

It is of interest here that in the afebrile cat prepared with both rostral and caudal hypothalamic cannulae, a fall in temperature affects the activity of the cation in the posterior hypothalamus. When noradrenaline (NA) is micro-injected into the PO/AH of a cat in which the $^{45}Ca^{2+}$-labelled hypothalamus is being perfused, the efflux of Ca^{2+} ions from the mammillary region declines transiently

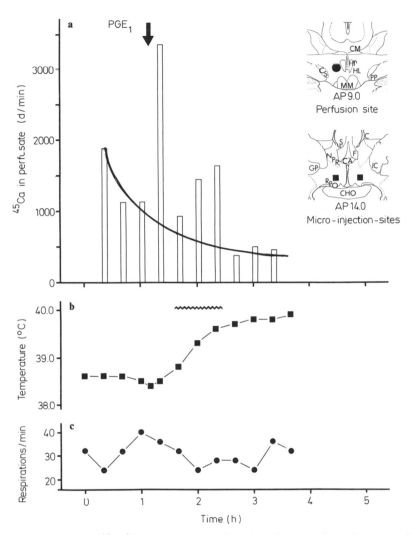

Fig. 13a–c. Efflux **a** of $^{45}Ca^{2+}$ in successive push–pull perfusates collected at a rate of 50 μl/min from the perfusion site denoted by the *dot* in the histological *inset*. The site had been labelled with 1.0 μCi $^{45}Ca^{2+}$, 18 h earlier. 100 ng of prostaglandin E_1 (PGE_1) were micro-injected in a volume of 1.0 μl before the fourth perfusion, as indicated by the *arrow*, at the injection sites designated by the squares in the histological *inset*. Shivering indicated by the zigzag line, colonic temperature **b** and respiratory rate **c** are shown as in previous figures. The declining curve **a** denotes control washout radioactivity. Anatomical abbreviations are the same as in Fig. 11. (From MYERS et al. 1976b)

(MYERS et al. 1976b). This physiological result corresponds with the previous finding which suggests that Ca^{2+} ions are retained in the posterior hypothalamus to bring about a lowering of the temperature set-point. Whether or not the concentration of Na^+ ions in the caudal hypothalamus is reduced concomitantly following the administration of an antipyretic or hypothermic agent is not yet known.

G. Critique of the Ionic Set-Point Mechanism for Body Temperature

Neither a precise definition nor the concept of the set-point for body temperature is agreed upon by the world community of physiologists (Boulant 1980). Generally speaking, the abundant number of physiological constants and reference values around which the bodily processes continually adjust, has provided a biological starting point for the elucidation of "set-point" theory.

From a functional standpoint, a set-point temperature itself would be derived from a cellular mechanism having a temperature-sensitive component as well as unique neurophysiological and morphological substrates (Benzinger 1969). One workable definition (Myers 1978) is that the set-point is established at birth as an intrinsic, built-in reference temperature of 37 °C in most mammals (at least domesticated). Regulatory adjustments are constantly made to defend and maintain the metabolically optimum and life-sustaining temperature. A basic set of assumptions which relates to the validity of this definition has been evolved as follows (e.g. Myers 1981):

First, the set-point mechanism should be universal across all species of mammals and possibly birds.

Second, because of this universality, a fundamental and inherent property of a select population of neurones should determine the body's set-point temperature.

Third, an intact and functional set-point should be present at birth, establishing the resting temperature at 37 °C, even though the animal's ability to defend this value against cold or heat challenges is not necessarily developed.

Fourth, although set-point neurones in the brain-stem should be in close anatomical proximity with and share neuronal connectivities with temperature-sensing cells, the site of the set-point mechanism in the brain would necessarily be anatomically separate from the neuronal locus involved in the thermoregulatory responses. Thus, neurones responsible for maintaining a set-point temperature would be distinct from those that alter their firing pattern to compensate for a warm or cold stimulus.

Fifth, when the set-point value is actually challenged, thermoregulatory responses around the set level of temperature defend this value by metabolic, vasomotor, pilomotor, sudomotor, respiratory, and other peripheral physiological responses.

Sixth, although normally an invariant reference value, the set-point temperature can be deflected upward or downward, without serious pathological consequences. Such a deflection occurs, however, only within certain upper and lower limits of body temperature, beyond which death would ensue.

I. Experimental Evidence for the Ionic Set-Point Theory

A summary analysis of the individual pieces of evidence, indirect, pharmacological and physiological, is presented in Table 4. Because of some potential discrepancies in the literature in this field and the interpretation of the findings obtained, a further elaboration of the salient points will be presented.

From a pharmacological point of view, at least three factors contribute to the specific action of a cation within the brain. For purposes of illustration, we will now consider calcium as an example. If a sufficiently high concentration of calcium ions is infused either into the cerebral ventricle or hypothalamus, a functional

Table 4. Summary evidence for the ionic theory of the temperature set-point, as taken from the text

Indirect Evidence

1) Evolution of a universal mechanism for maintenance of the ratio of cations in body tissue
2) Intrinsic stability of $Na^+:Ca^{2+}$ ratio in the extracellular fluid spaces under normal conditions
3) Universality across all species of effect on temperature of excess Na^+ and Ca^{2+} or reduction by chelating agent

Pharmacological evidence

1) Anatomical differences between the effects of cations on the posterior hypothalamus and the preoptic anterior hypothalamic area of thermosensitivity
2) Na^+ and Ca^{2+} ions act specifically in terms of the relative activity of other essential cations including K^+ and Mg^{2+}
3) Set-point temperatures can be reset by $Na^+:Ca^{2+}$ ratio shift for a prolonged period at high or low temperatures, within limits, without pathological sequelae
4) No tachyphylaxis to repeated level perfusions of excess cations; i.e., temperature set-point can be driven to the brink of death in either direction
5) Retention of the capacity to thermoregulate normally around a new temperature established by an altered ratio of Na^+ to Ca^{2+} ions; no evidence of non-specific depression or excitation of neurones
6) An exercise-induced rise in set-point temperature is overcome by elevating Ca^{2+} in the posterior hypothalamus while the animal continues to exercise
7) Peripheral cold or warm challenge blocks a typical Na^+-induced rise or Ca^{2+}-induced shift in set-point temperature
8) Behavioural responding to obtain heat during regulatory adjustments fails to occur during a change in temperature induced by cations perfused in the posterior hypothalamus
9) When the $Ca^{2+}:Na^+$ ratio is altered in other diencephalic structures, the cation-evoked response to feeding, arousal, sleep, drinking, etc. is functionally specific
10) Normality of EEG and the capacity to feed are retained after the set-point temperature is shifted artificially by excess Na^+ or Ca^{2+} in the posterior hypothalamus

Physiological (endogenous) evidence

1) Bacteria administered systemically or intracerebrally evoke a reciprocal shift in the ratio of endogenous Na^+ to Ca^{2+} ions in the diencephalon as a pyrogen fever develops
2) An antipyretic given systemically reverses reciprocally the induced shift in the endogenous diencephalic ratio of Na^+ to Ca^{2+} ions during defervescence
3) As the set-point temperature rises during exercise, the efflux of Ca^{2+} ions from the diencephalon is enhanced
4) A prostaglandin or bacterium injected into the anterior hypothalamus evokes a consequent efflux of Ca^{2+} ions within the posterior hypothalamus at the same time that the set-point temperature rises
5) A mild thermal stress of heat or cold, within a normal thermoregulatory bandwidth, fails to affect the endogenous ratio of Na^+ to Ca^{2+} ions in the posterior hypothalamus; i.e. cation ratio remains unchanged during thermoregulation
6) A severe peripheral challenge to the set-point temperature in terms of an intense cold or heat stressor causes an immediate compensatory shift in the activity of endogenous Ca^{2+} ions in the posterior hypothalamus
7) A sharp deflection of the preoptic anterior hypothalamic/area temperature sufficient to activate thermosensitive neurones augments the efflux or retention of endogenous Ca^{2+} ions within the posterior hypothalamus

According to this concept, the set-point is determined by a stable extracellular concentration of sodium and calcium in the posterior hypothalamus. This ionic milieu theoretically establishes a steady-state firing rate of efferent neurones in the caudal hypothalamic pathways for heat production and heat loss. (After MYERS 1981). For specific references see reviews of MYERS (1974a, b, 1976a, b, 1978)

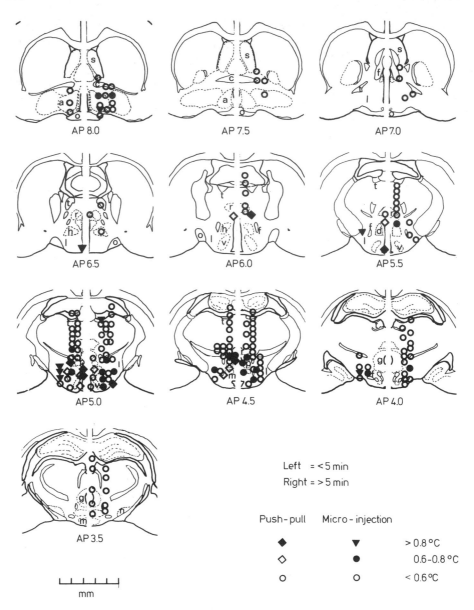

Fig. 14. Anatomical mapping of sites in the hypothalamus at which excess Ca^{2+} ions caused a fall in the rat's colonic temperature following push–pull perfusion or micro-injection of greater than 0.8 °C (*solid diamonds, solid triangles*), between 0.6 to 0.8 °C (*open diamonds, solid circles*) or less than 0.6 °C (*open circles*). Ca^{2+}-sensitive sites mediating hypothermia with a latency of less than 5 min are depicted on the left half of each map, and those with a latency greater than 5 min on the right half of each map. Anatomical abbreviations are: *a*, preoptic area; *c*, anterior commissure; *d*, dorsomedial nucleus of the hypothalamus; *f*, fornix, *g*, central gray; *h*, anterior hypothalamic area; *l*, lateral hypothalamic area; *m*, mammillary bodies; *n*, substantia nigra; *o*, optic tract; *p*, posterior area of the hypothalamus; *r*, nucleus reuniens of the thalamus; *s*, lateral septal nucleus; *t*, stria medullaris; *v*, ventromedial nucleus of the hypothalamus. (From Myers et al. 1976a)

depression of nerve cells will unquestionably occur. In fact, when a part of the brain is supersaturated with the cation, even the specificity of an anatomical region with its particular function is entirely overridden. By virtue of a given concentration gradient, many areas of the brain undoubtedly would be affected by a high calcium loading within CNS parenchyma. Therefore, which response could be considered as physiological and which is pharmacological are questions not easily answered without a careful concentration–response analysis.

Next, the route and/or site of administration of a cation such as Ca^{2+} – whether it be oral, intravenous, CSF, diencephalic, or directly into the hypothalamus – is crucial with respect to a given result. Clearly, the concentration of Ca^{2+} required to induce a shift in body temperature becomes less and less when the route of this cation's administration becomes more and more specific anatomically. Moreover, the brain's barriers to ionic penetration would tend to preclude an analysis of the systemic effects of an ionic imbalance in the physiological sense. In addition, the administration of a solution containing an aberrant cation concentration into the cerebrospinal fluid is subject to many more non-specific actions than that of a more direct anatomical approach. For example, as seen in the sheep, an intense behavioural response could indeed offset a temperature response.

Since the action of calcium is very selective anatomically, its excitation or suppression of certain neuronal systems would be expected. We have already seen that sleep states, intraocular pressure, feeding, and respiratory mechanisms are independently influenced by the unique attribute of the Ca^{2+} ion. VEALE and co-workers have clearly shown that the morphological distinctiveness, even within the hypothalamus between anterior and posterior areas, is unequivocal with respect to the cation's pharmacological actions. An analysis of the neuroanatomical specificity is presented in Fig. 14 for sites in the rat's hypothalamus within which an excess in Ca^{2+} ions lowered the rat's body temperature. Following histological evaluation and "mapping," the distribution of demarcated loci of reactivity to Ca^{2+} ions can be readily seen.

The means whereby a solution of an aberrant cation concentration is delivered to tissue can also contribute to a specific or non-specific change in the animal's physiological state. To illustrate, the perfusion of a cation via a push–pull cannula system is based on the principle of a tissue exchange of material present in the perfusate. In certain studies, it has been shown that there is as little as 5% exchange of the substances contained in the perfusion medium with the cerebral tissue surrounding the tips of the cannulae (MYERS 1974a). Thus, a so-called dose of cation in the perfusate is a misleading concept and cannot really be considered as such from a pharmacological standpoint. In reality, the concentration of Ca^{2+} ions which actually reaches the neuronal membranes, the synaptic junctions and other subcellular structures is the vital aspect and the sole determinant of the ultimate effect of the cation. On the other hand, a micro-injection into tissue of a Ca^{2+} ion solution leaves a bolus of concentrated cation which must diffuse away, equilibrate, or undergo transport from the site of micro-injection. In this instance, a dose–response analysis can be more easily generated, but the local action of the ion is not nearly so great as that witnessed during a constant exposure achieved by the perfusion procedure (MYERS et al. 1976a).

Finally, from all of the foregoing experiments, it is apparent that the ratio of one cation to another, principally sodium to calcium ions, constitutes the most important functional property of cations in hypothalamic tissue. As portrayed in Fig. 3, the nature of the hyperthermic response to Na^+ ions is identical to that seen when Ca^{2+} ions are locally depleted by a chelating agent, EGTA. In addition, the magnitude and duration of cation action are again precisely the same when the relative ion concentrations are identically matched. Thus, it is certain that an insufficiency of calcium is tantamount physiologically to an elevation of sodium. Greenleaf (1979) has quite rightly pointed out, however, that a proportional disturbance of the Na^+ ion concentration has a much greater functional impact than that of Ca^{2+}; by this is meant that only a very small percentage change in Na^+ ion concentration in diencephalic tissue will cause a rise in temperature, whereas a two-fold or four-fold increase in Ca^{2+} ions is required to produce a response of equal magnitude but in the opposite direction – hypothermia.

II. Primate Model of Temperature Control

How is the function of the cations in the posterior hypothalamus integrated with the proposed functions of putative neurotransmitters in the rostral and other parts of the hypothalamus? Figure 15 presents a schematic diagram of the neuronal pathways in the anterior (AH) and posterior (PH) hypothalamic areas which subserve the control of a primate's body temperature. Although many of the components of the model are derived from experiments with the monkey, studies of ion fluxes in the cat have been incorporated because of the identical anatomical and pharmacological results obtained with both species (Myers et al. 1976b).

The AH contains thermosensitive neurones which react to the local presence of 5HT (hyperthermia) and catecholamines (hypothermia). Cold exposure activates the release of 5HT from the AH, mediating heat production; heat stress evokes the release of noradrenaline (NA) and/or dopamine (DA) from the AH, mediating heat loss. Connecting cholinergic neurones (designated ACh to indicate the action of acetylcholine) in the mid-hypothalamus transmit signals for heat maintenance to the PH and through the PH. The steady-state ratio of Na^+ to Ca^{2+} ions within the cellular spaces of the PH stabilizes the firing rate of the PH neurones which are not thermosensitive, not pyrogen reactive, and not sensitive to monoamines. Thus these cells, by points of evidence presented in Table 3, could serve as neurones which establish the primate's set-point temperature of 37 °C.

From the accumulated physiological evidence, there are apparently two bandwidths for temperature control. The set-point bandwidth, as described previously (Myers et al. 1976b), is very broad. It can be shifted to a high or low temperature only within certain limits (hyperpyrexia or deep hypothermia) beyond which death occurs. The optimum set-point at euthermia for most primates is 37 °C. As indicated in Fig. 15, at euthermia, a balance in monoamine release between 5HT and catecholamine-containing neurones is extant in the AH, while the $Na^+ : Ca^{2+}$ ratio is in equilibrium within the PH. ACh neurones transmit impulses to the PH from AH monoaminergic neurones which signal the sensory state of thermoneutrality. Thus, functional responses for heat loss or gain are not activated.

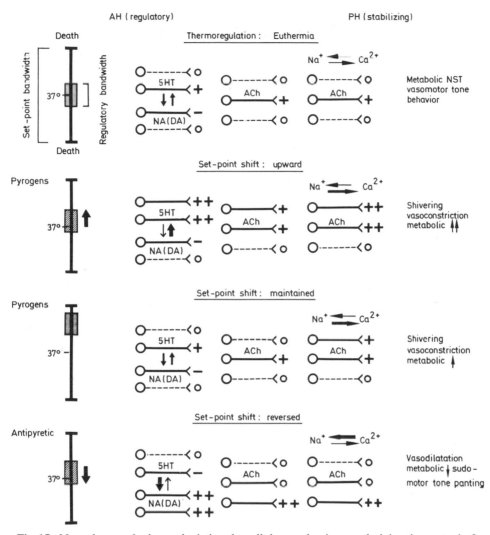

Fig. 15. Neurohumoral schema depicting the cellular mechanisms underlying the control of body temperature in the primate. The regulatory bandwidth around the optimal 37 °C set-point level is much more narrow than the set-point bandwidth which can be displaced upward or downward within the physiological limits of survival. As described in the text, monoaminergic neurones impinge upon cells whose ionic milieu is labile. Thus, a pyrogen challenge or treatment with an antipyretic during fever will bring about set-point changes by virtue of a coordinated set of cellular responses involving amines, Na^+ and Ca^{2+} ions

On exposure to endogenous pyrogen or other pyrexic material, 5 HT neurones are transiently excited, NA (and/or DA) neurones are inhibited and the cholinergic pathways for heat production set maximally in motion as indicated under the heading "Set-point shift-upward" in Fig. 15. The PH receives the physiologically significant signals that denote a maximal (indicated by $++$) challenge to body temperature, and the set-point mechanism is destabilized. The ion-ratio is shifted extracellularly toward the retention of Na^+ ions and the extrusion of Ca^{2+} from PH parenchyma. At the same time the more narrow regulatory bandwidth also shifts its position upward with the thermoregulatory capacity of AH cells still intact. Shivering, vasoconstriction, and intense metabolic heat production are stimulated through efferent impulses traversing cholinergic fibre systems.

The set-point shift, as portrayed in Fig. 15, is maintained by the steady efflux of Ca^{2+} ions and retention of Na^+ ions within the PH. This perturbation in the cation ratio serves to continue the heightened activity of the cholinergic heat production pathways. The regulatory bandwidth remains elevated with AH neurones ready to react to thermal stimuli (emanating from local vasculature or peripheral input). The respective motor and metabolic responses persist during the period when the set-point shift is maintained.

When the elevated set-point temperature is reduced by an antipyretic agent, the regulatory bandwidth returns to the 37 °C level. In this case, 5 HT release in the AH is transiently inhibited whereas NA (DA) release is greatly augmented, i.e. the balance in monoaminergic neurone activity favours the catecholamines. The maximal output (indicated in Fig. 15 by $++$) from AH to PH is carried by ACh neurones which signal the cells in the PH, as indicated in Fig. 15 by "Set-point shift-reversed." Here the ion ratio shifts to the retention of Ca^{2+} ions and the extrusion of Na^+ ions within the PH. The net effect of this is the maximal triggering of the cholinergic pathway for heat loss $(++)$. Sweating, vasodilatation, a decline in metabolic heat production, and an augmented respiratory rate are thereby activated. In this schema, crossed inhibitory pathways are not included since there is no direct anatomical or functional evidence of their existence at the level of the hypothalamus. Clearly, however, there must of necessity be a reciprocal inhibition of the firing of monoaminergic neurones delegated to temperature control (MYERS 1974 b), in order that an integrated regulatory response can take place (MYERS 1975).

In conclusion, the evidence now is almost unequivocal that the PH receives its input directly from the AH rather than from the periphery. Whether the physiologically significant signals arise from the thermosensitive neurones in the rostral hypothalamus or from the peripheral impulses that are transmitted by way of this rostral area, the net effect on the PH neurones is identical. If a severe cold or heat challenge exceeds the respective upper or lower threshold of the regulatory bandwidth, the activity of the ionic mechanism is altered immediately, as a result of transmission from the AH to the PH of the impulses reflecting the threshold information. The subsequent realignment of the molecular properties of the caudal aspect of the primate's hypothalamus results in the well-defined physiological responses that operate to establish a new set-point temperature.

References

Adey WR (1971) Evidence for cerebral membrane effects of calcium, derived from direct-current gradient, impedance, and intracellular records. Exp Neurol 30:78–102

Andersson K-E, Ekelund L-G, Johansson BW, Landmark K (1978) Calcium/antagonists (Ca-blockers). Acta Pharmacol Toxicol [Suppl 1] 43:5–14

Bawin SM, Adey WR, Sabbot IM (1978) Ionic factors in release of $^{45}Ca^{2+}$ from chicken cerebral tissue by electromagnetic fields. Proc Natl Acad Sci USA 75:6314–6318

Beleslin DB, Dimitrijević M, Samardžić R (1974) Hyperthermic effect of palmitate sodium, stearate sodium, and oleate sodium injected into the cerebral ventricles of conscious cats. Neuropharmacology 13:221–223

Benzinger TH (1969) Heat regulation: homeostasis of central temperature in man. Physiol Rev 49:671–795

Blaustein MP (1971) Preganglionic stimulation increases calcium uptake by sympathetic ganglia. Science 172:391–393

Blaustein MP (1977) Sodium ions, calcium ions, blood pressure regulation, and hypertension: a reassessment and a hypothesis. Am J Physiol 232:C 165–C 173

Borbély AA, Tobler I (1979) Cerebroventricular infusion in the rat: depression of motor activity and paradoxical sleep. Neurosci Lett 12:75–80

Boulant JA (1980) Hypothalamic control of thermoregulation. In: Morgane P, Panksepp J (eds) Handbook of the hypothalamus. Dekker, New York

Clark WG (1971) Hyperthermic effect of disodium edetate injected into the lateral cerebral ventricle of the unanaesthetized cat. Experientia 27:1452–1454

Colomo F, Rahamimoff R (1968) Interaction between sodium and calcium ions in the process of transmitter release at the neuromuscular junction. J Physiol (Lond) 198:203–218

Cooke WJ, Robinson JD (1971) Factors influencing ^{45}Ca metabolism in brain and other organs in vivo. Proc Soc Exp Biol Med 138:906–912

Cooper KE (1972) Central mechanisms for the control of body temperature in health and febrile states. Mod Trends Physiol 1:33 54

Cooper KE, Cranston WI, Honour AJ (1965) Effects of intraventricular and intrahypothalamic injection of noradrenaline and 5-HT on body temperature in conscious rabbits. J Physiol (Lond) 181:852–864

Demole V (1927) Pharmakologisch-anatomische Untersuchungen zum Problem des Schlafes. Arch Exp Pathol Pharmakol 120:229–258

Denbow DM, Edens FW (1978) Effects of cations on body temperature. Poult Sci 57:1133

Denbow DM, Edens FW (1980) Effects of intraventricular injections of sodium and calcium on body temperature in the chicken. Am J Physiol 239:62–65

Dhumal VR, Gulati OD (1974) Effect on body temperature in dogs of perfusion of cerebral ventricles with artificial CSF deficient in calcium or containing excess of sodium or calcium. Br J Pharmacol 49:699–701

Dreifuss JJ, Grau JD, Bianchi RE (1971) Antagonism between Ca and Na ions at neurohypophysial nerve terminals. Experientia 27:1295–1296

Edens FW (1976) Body temperature and blood chemistry responses in broiler cockerels given a single intravenous injection of Na$^+$ or Ca^{++} before an acute heating episode. Poult Sci 55:2248–2255

Feldberg W, Saxena PN (1970) Mechanism of action of pyrogen. J Physiol (Lond) 211:245–261

Feldberg W, Myers RD, Veale WL (1970) Perfusion from cerebral ventricle to cisterna magna in the unanaesthetized cat. Effect of calcium on body temperature. J Physiol (Lond) 207:403–416

Fox RH, MacPherson RK (1954) The regulation of body temperature during fever. J Physiol (Lond) 125:21 P–22 P

Freund H (1911) Über das Kochsalzfieber. Arch Exp Pathol Pharmakol 65:225–238

Gisolfi CV, Wilson NC, Myers RD, Phillips MI (1976) Exercise thermoregulation: Hypothalamic perfusion of excess calcium reduces elevated colonic temperature of rats. Brain Res 101:160–164

Gisolfi CV, Mora F, Myers RD (1977) Diencephalic efflux of calcium ions in the monkey during exercise, thermal stress and feeding. J Physiol (Lond) 273:617–630

Gisolfi CV, Mora F, Nattermann R, Myers RD (1978) New apparatus for exercising a monkey seated in a primate chair. J Appl Physiol 44:129–132

Graziani LJ, Kaplan RK, Escriva A, Katzman R (1967) Calcium flux into CSF during ventricular and ventriculocisternal perfusion. Am J Physiol 213:629–636

Greenleaf JE (1973) Blood electrolytes and exercise in relation to temperature regulation in man. In: Schönbaum E, Lomax P (eds) The pharmacology of thermoregulation. Karger, Basel, pp 72–84

Greenleaf JE (1978) Thresholds for Na^+ and Ca^{++} effects on thermoregulation. In: Girardier L, Seydoux J (eds) Effectors of thermogenesis. Birkhauser, Basel, pp 33–43

Greenleaf JE (1979) Hyperthermia and exercise. In: Robertshaw D (ed) Environmental physiology III. University Park Press, Baltimore, pp 157–208

Greenleaf JE, Castle BL (1971) Exercise temperature regulation in man during hypohydration and hyperhydration. J Appl Physiol 30:847–853

Greenleaf JE, Kozlowski S, Kacuiba-Uscilko H, Nazar K, Brzezinska Z (1975) Temperature responses to infusion of electrolytes during exercise. In: Lomax J, Schönbaum E, Jacob J (eds) Temperature regulation and drug action. Karger, Basel, pp 352–360

Greenleaf JE, Kolzowski S, Nazar K, Kacuiba-Uscilko H, Brzezinska Z, Ziemba A (1976) Ion-osmotic hyperthermia during exercise in dogs. Am J Physiol 230:74–79

Greenleaf JE, Convertino VA, Stremel RW, Bernauer EM, Adams WC, Vignau SR, Brock PJ (1977) Plasma $[Na^+]$, $[Ca^{2+}]$, and volume shifts and thermoregulation during exercise in man. J Appl Physiol 43:1026–1032

Greenleaf JE, Brock PJ, Morse JT, Van Beaumont W, Montgomery LD, Convertino VA, Mangseth GR (1978) Effect of sodium and calcium ingestion on thermoregulation during exercise in man. In: Houdas U, Guieu JD (eds) New trends in thermal physiology. Masson, Paris, pp 157–160

Guernsey DL, Stevens ED (1977) The cell membrane sodium pump as a mechanism for increasing thermogenesis during cold acclimation in rats. Science 196:908–910

Hanegan JL, Williams BA (1975) Ca^{2+} induced hypothermia in a hibernator (*Citellus Beechyi*). Comp Biochem Physiol 50 A:247–252

Hardy JD (1976) Fever and thermogenesis. Isr J Med Sci 12:942–950

Harrison MH, Edwards RJ, Fennessey PA (1978) Intravascular volume and tonicity as factors in the regulation of body temperature. J Appl Physiol 44:69–75

Hasama B (1930) Über den Einfluß der anorganischen Kationen auf Wärme- sowie Schweißzentrum im Zwischenhirn. Arch Exp Pathol Pharmakol 153:291–308

Hensel H, Schäfer K (1974) Effects of calcium on warm and cold receptors. Pflügers Arch 352:87–90

Itokawa Y, Tanaka C, Fujiwara M (1974) Changes in body temperature and blood pressure in rats with calcium and magnesium deficiencies. J Appl Physiol 37:835–839

Jones DL, Veale WL, Cooper KE (1978) Perfusions of the posterior hypothalamus of cats with various ions and saccharides; effects on body temperature. Can J Physiol Pharmacol 56:571–577

Jundt H, Prozig H, Reuter H, Stucki JW (1975) The effect of substances releasing intracellular calcium ions on sodium-dependent calcium efflux from guinea-pig auricles. J Physiol (Lond) 246:229–253

Kaczmarek L, Adey WR (1973) The efflux of $^{45}Ca^{2+}$ and $[^3H]\gamma$-aminobutyric acid from cat cerebral cortex. Brain Res 63:331–342

Krupin T, Grove JC, Gugenheim SM, Oestrich CJ, Podos SM, Becker B (1978) Increased intraocular pressure and hypothermia following injection of calcium into the rabbit third ventricle. Exp Eye Res 27:120–134

Kym O (1934) Die Beeinflussung des durch verschiedene fiebererzeugende Stoffe erregten Temperaturzentrums durch lokale Applikation von Ca, K und Na. Arch Exp Pathol Pharmakol 176:408–424

Lazarewicz JW, Haliamae H, Hamberger A (1974) Calcium metabolism in isolated brain cells and subcellular fractions. J Neurochem 22:33–45

Myers RD (1974a) Handbook of drug and chemical stimulation of the brain. Van Nostrand-Reinhold, New York, pp 237–301

Myers RD (1974b) Ionic concepts of the set-point for body temperature. In: Lederis K, Cooper KE (eds) Recent studies of hypothalamic function. Karger, Basel, pp 371–390

Myers RD (1975) An integrative model of monoamine and ionic mechanism in the hypothalamic control of body temperature. In: Lomax P, Schönbaum E, Jacob J (eds) Temperature regulation and drug action. Karger, Basel, pp 32–42

Myers RD (1976a) Chemical control of body temperature by the hypothalamus: A model and some mysteries. Proc Aust Physiol Pharmacol Soc 7:15–32

Myers RD (1976b) Diencephalic efflux of $^{22}Na^+$ and $^{45}Ca^{2+}$ ions in the febrile cat: effect of an antipyretic. Brain Res 103:412–417

Myers RD (1978) Hypothalamic mechanisms underlying physiological set-points. In: Lederis K, Veale WL (eds) Current studies of hypothalamic function. Karger, Basel, pp 17–28

Myers RD (1981) Hypothalamic control of thermoregulation: Neurochemical mechanisms. In: Morgane P, Panksepp J (eds) Handbook of the hypothalamus. Dekker, New York, pp 83–210

Myers RD, Brophy PD (1972) Temperature changes in the rat produced by altering the sodium-calcium ratio in the cerebral ventricles. Neuropharmacology 11:351–361

Myers RD, Buckman JE (1972) Deep hypothermia induced in the golden hamster by altering cerebral calcium levels. Am J Physiol 223:1313–1318

Myers RD, Tytell M (1972) Fever: Reciprocal shift in brain sodium to calcium ratio as the set-point temperature rises. Science 178:765–767

Myers RD, Veale WL (1970) Body temperature: Possible ionic mechanisms in the hypothalamus controlling the set point. Science 170:95–97

Myers RD, Veale WL (1971) The role of sodium and calcium ions in the hypothalamus in the control of body temperature of the unanaesthetized cat. J Physiol (Lond) 212:411–430

Myers RD, Yaksh TL (1971) Thermoregulation around a new 'set-point' established in the monkey by altering the ratio of sodium to calcium ions within the hypothalamus. J Physiol (Lond) 218:609–633

Myers RD, Yaksh TL (1972) The role of hypothalamic monoamines in hibernation and hypothermia. In: South FE, Hannon JP, Willis JR, Pengelley ET, Alpert NR (eds) Hibernation-hypothermia. Perspectives and challenges. Elsevier, Amsterdam, pp 551–575

Myers RD, Veale WL, Yaksh TL (1971) Changes in body temperature of the unanaesthetized monkey produced by sodium and calcium ions perfused through the cerebral ventricles. J Physiol (Lond) 217:381–392

Myers RD, Melchior CL, Gisolfi CV (1976a) Feeding and body temperature in the rat: diencephalic localization of changes produced by excess calcium ions. Brain Res Bull 1:33–46

Myers RD, Simpson CW, Higgins D, Nattermann RA, Rice JC, Redgrave P, Metcalf G (1976b) Hypothalamic Na^+ and Ca^{++} ions and temperature set-point: New mechanisms of action of a central or peripheral thermal challenge and intrahypothalamic 5-HT, NE, PGE_1, and pyrogen. Brain Res Bull 1:301–327

Myers RD, Gisolfi CV, Mora F (1977a) Role of brain Ca^{2+} in central control of body temperature during exercise in the monkey. J Appl Physiol 43:689–694

Myers RD, Gisolfi CV, Mora F (1977b) Calcium levels in the brain underlie temperature control during exercise in the primate. Nature 266:178–179

Nielsen B (1974a) Actions of intravenous Ca^{++} and Na^+ on body temperature in rabbits. Acta Physiol Scand 90:445–450

Nielsen B (1974b) Effect of changes in plasma Na^+ and Ca^{++} ion concentration on body temperature during exercise. Acta Physiol Scand 91:123–129

Nielsen B, Hansen G, Jørgensen O, Nielsen E (1971) Thermoregulation in exercising man during dehydration and hyperhydration with water and saline. Int J Biometerol 15:195–200

Nielsen B, Schwartz P, Alhede J (1973) Is fever in man reflected in changes in cerebrospinal fluid concentrations of sodium and calcium ions? J Clin Lab Invest 32:309–310

Nielsen M (1938) Die Regulation der Körpertemperatur bei Muskelarbeit. Scand Arch Physiol 79:193–230

Rosenthal FE (1941) Cooling drugs and cooling centres. J Pharm Exp Ther 71:305–314

Sabbot I, Costin A (1974) Effects of stress on the uptake of radiolabeled calcium in the pituitary gland and the brain of the rat. J Neurochem 22:731–734

Sadowski B, Szczepańska-Sadowska E (1974) The effect of calcium ions chelation and sodium ions excess in the cerebrospinal fluid on body temperature in conscious dogs. Pflügers Arch 352:61–68

Sasaki T, Hori T (1977) Temperature regulation and related problems in environmental physiology. Bull Inst Const Med Kumamoto Univ 27:1–85

Saxena PN (1976) Sodium and calcium ions in the control of temperature set-point in the pigeon. Br J Pharmacol 36:187–192

Schütz J (1916) Zur Kenntnis der Wirkung des Magnesiums auf die Körpertemperatur. Arch Exp Pathol Pharmakol 79:285–290

Seoane JR, Baile CA (1973) Ionic changes in cerebrospinal fluid and feeding, drinking, and temperature of sheep. Physiol Behav 10:915–923

Shea S, Sigafoos D, Scott D (1969) The effect of calcium and potassium on the thermal excitability of a model thermoreceptor. Comp Biochem Physiol 28:701–708

Skarnes RC (1968) *In vivo* interaction of endotoxin with a plasma lipoprotein having esterase activity. J Bacteriol 95:2031–2034

Snellen JW, Mitchell D, Busansky M (1972) Calorimetric analysis of the effect of drinking saline solution on whole-body sweating. I. An attempt to measure average body temperature. Pflügers Arch Ges Physiol 331:134–144

Sobocińska J, Greenleaf JE (1976) Cerebrospinal fluid $[Ca^{2+}]$ and rectal temperature response during exercise in dogs. Am J Physiol 230:1416–1419

Stahl WL, Swanson PD (1971) Movements of calcium and other cations in isolated cerebral tissues. J Neurochem 18:415–427

Strömme SB, Gullestad R, Meen HD, Refsum HE, Krog J (1976) Serum sodium and calcium and body temperature during prolonged exercise. J Sports Med 16:91–97

Tószeghi P, Tobler I, Borbély A (1978) Cerebral ventricular infusion of excess calcium in the rat: effects on sleep states, behavior and cortical EEG. Eur J Pharmacol 51:407–416

Veale WL (1971) Behavioral and physiological changes caused by the regional alteration of sodium and calcium ions in the hypothalamus of the unanaesthetized cat. PhD dissertation, Purdue University

Veale WL, Jones DL (1977) Alterations in hypothalamic ions: influence on limbic function. In: Deniker P, Radouco Thomas C, Villeneune A (eds) Proc Colloq Int Neuropsychopharmacol. Pergamon, Oxford, pp 407–413

Veale WL, Myers RD (1971) Emotional behavior, arousal, and sleep produced by sodium and calcium ions perfused within the hypothalamus of the cat. Physiol Behav 7:601–607

Veale WL, Benson MJ, Malkinson T (1977) Brain calcium in the rabbit: site of action for the alteration of body temperature. Brain Res Bull 2:67–69

Wilson NC, Gisolfi CV, Phillips MI (1978) Influence of EGTA on an exercise-induced elevation in the colonic temperature of the rat. Brain Res Bull 3:97–100

CHAPTER 8

Electrophysiology of the Anterior Hypothalamus: Thermoregulation and Fever

J. S. EISENMAN

A. Introduction

The neural control of body temperature has been studied using the various techniques available to neurobiologists, each of which contributes a particular body of data. Lesioning techniques delineate the central nervous system (CNS) areas whose integrity is important for proper thermoregulation; stimulation studies (physiological, electrical, or chemical) reveal the outputs generated by various CNS areas or sensitive neuronal populations functioning in thermoregulation. Electrophysiological techniques supply detailed information on the activities of neurones in the CNS which are presumed to act in thermoregulation, and to be acted upon by the physical (temperature) and chemical (hormones, transmitters, pyrogens) agents that drive or modify the function of the system.

In its capacity as a thermoregulator, the CNS serves two distinct, but overlapping, functions: an integrative one, generating appropriate regulatory effector output (vasomotor, sudomotor, somatomotor, respiratory, etc.) on the basis of a variety of inputs (skin and central temperatures, state of arousal, exercise); and a receptor function, monitoring brain temperature at several sites, thus providing some of the inputs to which the integrator responds. These two functions are in some instances subserved by the same anatomical regions (e.g. anterior hypothalamus and preoptic area). One of the goals of electrophysiological recording studies is to determine if these two functions can be mediated by the same neurone. The characterization of central neurones serving thermoregulatory functions into detectors and integrators (interneurones) has been a major thrust of such studies.

The integrative functions of the CNS in thermoregulation have been studied by lesioning techniques and electrical and chemical stimulations (HENSEL 1973). The presence of thermodetectors in the brain has been demonstrated by applying more-or-less localized thermal stimulation to CNS structures. That rostral brain-stem areas contained thermodetectors capable of generating appropriate regulatory outputs, when stimulated by local temperature changes, was demonstrated by the early work of KAHN (1904), BARBOUR (1912) and HAMMOUDA (1933). The sensitive area was localized to the preoptic anterior hypothalamic area (PO/AH) in anaesthetized cats by MAGOUN et al. (1938) and by HAMMEL et al. (1960) and FUSCO et al. (1961) in unanaesthetized dogs.

It has since been demonstrated that other CNS areas will respond to their own temperature; thermal stimulation of the medulla (LIPTON 1973) and of the spinal cord (SIMON 1974) will produce appropriate regulatory activity. Some reports indicate that the mid-brain is also sensitive to its own temperature (CABANAC and

HARDY 1969; CRONIN and BAKER 1977b) although this has been denied by others (ADAIR and STITT 1971; MURAKAMI et al. 1979).

While it is clear that several different CNS levels function as integrative and detector areas in thermoregulation, an extensive literature has evolved showing that pyrogens and antipyretics exert their actions primarily, if not exclusively, on neurones in the PO/AH. With one exception (NAKAYAMA and HORI 1973) electrophysiological studies of these effects have concentrated on the PO/AH neuronal population. This review will, therefore, be restricted to consideration of electrophysiological studies of neurones in the PO/AH presumed to be involved in thermoregulation, and to pyretic and antipyretic actions on these cells.

Recent reviews with somewhat different, but related, content include: HAYWARD (1977), which deals with the electrophysiology of hypothalamic cells, primarily with reference to neurosecretory systems; HENSEL (1973), on the neural mechanisms in thermoregulation; HELLON (1975) which reviews pharmacological aspects of thermoregulation and fever; and HELLON (1972b) and EISENMAN (1976) which review central thermoreceptor function.

B. Microelectrode Recording Techniques

I. Single-Unit Recordings

Electrophysiological recording of activity in the central nervous system is accomplished by positioning a fine, electrolyte-filled pipette (or insulated wire) electrode in the brain area being studied. The potentials recorded by such an extracellular electrode, representing neuronal action potentials or spike discharges, are amplified and displayed as a train of spikes (Fig. 1) and/or analysed in some way to quantitate the recorded activity (see Sect. B.IV). Recordings with intracellularly placed microelectrodes have not been obtained in the thermoregulatory system, as yet. In most instances, the electrode position is adjusted using a micromanipulator so as to bring the tip close to one of the active cells in the tissue. The spikes generated by this cell will be identifiable by their constant amplitude and waveform and by their larger size relative to the background activity generated by surrounding, but more distant, cells. In this way, single-unit or single-neurone activity can be studied.

Such recordings are most easily done in anaesthetized animals mounted in a stereotaxic instrument which incorporates the micromanipulator (NAKAYAMA et al. 1963) or in acutely prepared unanaesthetized animals similarly mounted (EISENMAN and JACKSON 1967; JELL and GLOOR 1972). Chronic preparations, in which the micromanipulator is surgically implanted on the animal's skull have also been used (HELLON 1967). The latter preparation has the advantage of avoiding the use of anaesthetics which could profoundly depress or alter the neuronal activity (MURAKAMI et al. 1967). The major problem encountered with use of the chronic preparation is difficulty in recording from a cell for a sufficiently long period of time to characterize its sensitivity or activity. Small movements of the animal can shift the position of the electrode relative to the neurone, either destroying the cell or reducing the size of the recorded potential to that of the background, unidentifiable noise.

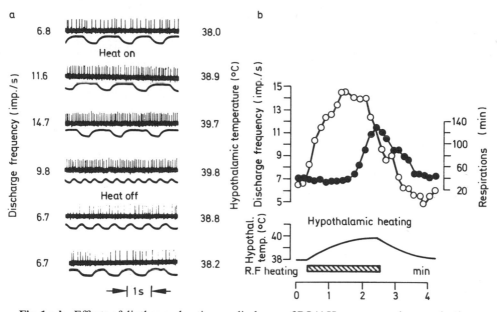

Fig. 1 a, b. Effects of diathermy heating on discharge of PO/AH neurone and on respiration. **a** spike trains and respiration at times indicated by arrows in right side of figure. **b** firing frequency of neurone (*open circles*) and respiratory rate (*solid circles*). (NAKAYAMA et al. 1963)

An alternative technique for recording neuronal activity in unanaesthetized animals involves positioning a semimicro wire in the tissue to be studied and permanently fixing its position by attaching it to the animal's skull. This system will record multiple-unit discharges, giving some indication of changes in the overall activity of the population of cells without allowing indentification of discharge patterns produced by any one cell in the population. Such recordings can be stable over long periods, even in a freely moving animal.

In all preparations, correlation of neuronal firing and regulatory effector activity can frequently be made (Fig. 1). This correlation will be poorest in the anaesthetized, or otherwise restricted, animal.

The microelectrode technique tends to select larger neurones rather than smaller ones since the best single-unit records will be derived from cells large enough to have an electrode positioned close to their surface without being destroyed or damaged (see Sect. B.V.1). This is a serious problem in the study of thermoregulation since most of the cells in the brain-stem core which functions in this system are quite small (15–20 µm) (BLEIER et al. 1966).

II. Functional Characterization of Neurones

In an area which mediates a variety of functions, like the hypothalamus, simply recording continuous neuronal activity provides little useful information. Functional characterization of the cell recorded from is essential, but is not easily accomplished. Ideally, it should be demonstrated that the cell under study: (1) has appro-

priate connections to thermoregulatory effector systems; (2) responds to inputs
from thermoreceptors which activate regulatory outputs; and, (3) is located in an
area which has been showed to function in thermoregulation by other experimental
techniques. For the most part, characterization of a recording as originating from
a thermoregulatory central neurone has been based on criteria (2) and (3): responsiveness to thermal input and location in thermoregulatory "centres." Except for
experiments on the thermosensitivity of spinal cord motoneurones (KLUSSMANN
1964; PIERAU et al. 1976), there have been no electrophysiological studies of effector neurones.

The responsiveness of central neurones can be studied by use of physiological,
electrical, and chemical or pharmacological stimuli. Each of these techniques has
been applied to the thermoregulatory system.

1. Physiological Stimuli

Physiological characterization of neuronal function in thermoregulation has been
attempted, for the most part, in terms of local thermosensitivity; i.e. responsiveness
to changes in the cell's own temperature. For this, diathermy wires (NAKAYAMA et
al. 1961) or water-perfused thermode tubes (NAKAYAMA et al. 1963) are implanted
around the area under study to allow variation of the temperature of the tissue containing the neurones recorded from by the microelectrode. A technical problem inherent in this system arises from the inability to record tissue temperature at the
electrophysiological recording site since a temperature probe (thermistor bead or
thermocouple junction) would destroy the cells in the area. Various symmetrical
arrangements of thermodes, temperature probes, and microelectrodes have been
used to minimize this problem. It is still not possible to prove that the cell under
study is, in fact, being affected by temperature changes recorded by the thermal
probe, rather than by some temperature in another part of the tissue block (CUN-
NINGHAM et al. 1967). All thermal response curves (correlations of neurone firing
rates and local temperature) may be in error, to some unknown degree, as a result
of this.

Central neurones lying outside the somatosensory projection pathways
(spinothalamic tracts) which respond to peripherally applied thermal stimuli, have
also been characterized as functioning in thermoregulation. Similarly, cells which
respond to thermal stimuli applied to some remote CNS area are considered to be
thermoregulatory in nature.

2. Electrical Stimuli

Another way of characterizing a neuron's role in CNS function is to study its responses to electrical stimulation applied in other areas of the brain. In contrast to
physiological stimulation, electrical currents will activate all cells affected by them,
regardless of function. Thus, these studies provide information about inputs to,
and outputs from, the area under study but not about the functional role of such
connections.

Stimuli applied in the mid-brain, pons, and hippocampus (EISENMAN 1974 b;
BOULANT and DEMIEVILLE 1977) have produced both excitation and inhibition of

PO/AH cells. In one instance (EISENMAN 1974b), antidromic activation of a PO/ AH neurone has demonstrated a direct, descending projection from the preoptic area to the mid-brain.

3. Pharmacological Stimuli

The actions of various pharmacological agents on PO/AH cells have been studied by parenteral administration, by intracerebroventricular (ICV) or intracerebral (IC) injection, and by micro-iontophoresis from multi-barrelled microelectrodes. The effects of anaesthetics (MURAKAMI et al. 1967), putative neurotransmitters (CUNNINGHAM et al. 1967), bacterial (exogenous) pyrogen (CABANAC et al. 1968; WIT and WANG 1968b; EISENMAN 1969), and leucocyte (endogenous) pyrogen (BE- LYAVSKII and ABRAMOVA 1975) have been examined following parenteral adminis- tration. More localized applications of pharmacological agents into the cere- broventricular system have been performed with neurotransmitters (CUNNINGHAM et al. 1967) and with prostaglandin E_2 (GORDON and HEATH 1979). Micro-injection into cerebral tissue, during single-unit recording has been done for acetylcholine and nicotine (KNOX et al. 1973a), for leucocyte pyrogen (SCHOENER and WANG 1975), and for prostaglandin E_1 (SCHOENER and WANG 1976).

The most localized form of application of chemical agents to neurones is by iontophoresis from a microelectrode (SALMOIRAGHI and WEIGHT 1967). In this technique, a multi-barrelled pipette is prepared by fusing several (3–7) glass tubes together before forming them into a microelectrode. One barrel is filled with elec- trolyte solution for recording unit activity, while the other barrels are filled with solutions of the salts of the agents to be tested. The drugs are discharged from the pipettes by application of a voltage of proper polarity. Once ejected into the tissue, the drugs will diffuse away to act on the cell, or cells, immediately adjacent to the electrode tip. The magnitude of the applied current is taken as a measure of the amount of drug applied.

It is difficult to quantitate drug application by this technique or to compare dif- ferent drug actions quantitatively. The actual drug transfer from the electrode will vary with the size and condition of the electrode (KRNJEVIĆ et al. 1963; BRADLEY and CANDY 1970). The current used to eject the agents (non-specific ion flow) may introduce an artifact, although in many cases this effect can be measured and cor- rected. Current leakage between barrels, and plugging or blocking of the electrode tip can introduce additional problems in the conduct and interpretation of these studies.

Iontophoretic studies on PO/AH neurones related to thermoregulatory func- tion include experiments using neurotransmitter agents by BECKMAN and EISEN- MAN (1970), HORI and NAKAYAMA (1973), MURAKAMI (1973), JELL (1974), STITT and HARDY (1975), and JELL and SWEATMAN (1977). Effects of iontophoretically applied prostaglandins (E_1, E_2, or $F_{2\alpha}$) were studied by FORD (1974), STITT and HARDY (1975), and JELL and SWEATMAN (1977).

III. In Vitro Recording

Single-unit recording techniques can be applied to neurones, in vitro. Recently, hy- pothalamic neurones maintained in cell cultures have been studied in this way,

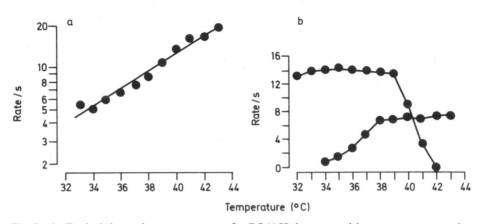

Fig. 2a, b. Typical thermal response curves for PO/AH thermosensitive neurones. **a** continuous function, detector-like response. **b** warm and cool interneurone-like responses. (EISENMAN 1970)

comparing their responses with those obtained in vivo. Both thermal and chemical stimulation of such cells has been accomplished (NAKAYAMA et al. 1978; MASON et al. 1978; H. M. GELLER, personal communication).

IV. Data Analysis

Data obtained from microelectrode studies consist of trains of spike discharges and the effects on these of various manipulations (Fig. 1). Several forms of quantitation or analysis are available.

1. Mean Firing Frequency and Thermosensitivity

The most commonly used quantitative measure of neuronal activity is mean firing frequency or rate. Since hypothalamic cells fire at comparatively slow and irregular rates, it is customary to average discharges over some short time interval (1–10 s) and to express this in terms of spikes/s. Thermosensitivity can be quantitated by plotting firing rate against local temperature and calculating the slope of the fitted line by least-squares regression (Fig. 2). Both linear (change in rate/°C) (NAKAYAMA et al. 1963) and semi-logarithmic (logarithm of firing rate versus °C) regressions have been used (EISENMAN and JACKSON 1967). The latter can also be expressed as Q_{10}; *i.e.* ratio of firing rates at temperatures 10 °C apart. Significant thermosensitivity has been variously defined as any regression coefficient greater than 0 or as a Q_{10} greater than 2. The latter criterion is based on the assumption that many biological processes will be temperature dependent and will double their rates with a 10 °C temperature rise.

Many PO/AH neurones do not exhibit a simple, direct relationship between firing rate and temperature. The responses of these cells will show some discontinuities in slope and so cannot be fitted by a single regression line (Fig. 2). Descriptions of this type of cell's activity range from simple designation as non-linear

(EISENMAN and JACKSON 1967; NAKAYAMA and HARDY 1969) to complex descriptions of the various segments of the response (GUIEU and HARDY 1970).

2. Patterns of Neuronal Discharge

Steady-state firing patterns have been analysed using interspike-interval histograms. In a steady-state record (i.e. at fixed temperature) the time intervals (in ms) between adjacent spikes is measured and the distribution of intervals displayed as a histogram (PERKEL et al. 1967). Statistical distribution functions can be fitted to such histogram data to quantitate the pattern. The effects of temperature on the interspike-interval distribution for PO/AH cells has been examined (EISENMAN 1972) and attempts have been made to correlate patterns of firing with thermoregulatory function (MURAKAMI 1974; REAVES and HEATH 1975).

A related form of analysis, the post-stimulus time histogram, has been used to describe the responses of PO/AH cells to electrical stimulation in other brain areas (EISENMAN 1974 b).

Periodicities in firing patterns and the effects of temperature on these have been examined by correlating a cell's discharge at different time intervals in a steady-state spike train (JAHNS and WERNER 1974 a, b). Some correlations between periodic discharge and thermosensitivity have been noted.

V. Critique of Microelectrophysiology

The utility of microelectrode recording techniques lies in enabling us to examine, in detail, the responses of individual neurones in the central nervous system, data essential for modelling of thermoregulatory neural mechanisms (HARDY 1972). The technique has limitations which should be recognized in interpreting data from such studies.

1. Non-Random Selection of Neuronal Population

The presence of a microelectrode close to the membrane of a CNS neurone can produce mechanical disruption of a membrane patch, leading to injury or death of the cell. This is most likely to occur in smaller neurones. It is common experience that CNS areas containing large cells are more easily recorded from than those with predominantly small cells. TOWE and HARDING (1970) studied this problem quantitatively in pyramidal tract cells of the pericruciate cortex in cats. They found significantly more large cells in their microelectrode-recorded population than in the histologically analysed total population of cortical cells. They compare microelectrode recording to "shooting fish in a barrel," in that, the larger the target (fish or cell) the more likely one is to "hit" it. The PO/AH region, as part of the older brain-stem core, is made up primarily of smaller diameter cells (BLEIER et al. 1966), making recording difficult, especially in the chronic preparation described earlier.

BOULANT and BIGNALL (1973 a), analysing the length of time that PO/AH cells could be recorded from, concluded that the thermosensitive cells lie at the smaller end of the general neuronal population range and that the reported percentage of sensitive cells is lower than the true percentages because of the size-selection bias introduced by this technique.

2. Lack of Positive Functional Characterization

As indicated earlier, cells recorded from in the PO/AH have been presumed to act in thermoregulation because: (a) they are responsive to local temperature changes, or (b) they respond to thermally generated inputs from other areas (e.g. skin, spinal cord), and (c) they are located in an area known to play an important role in the monitoring and/or regulation of body temperature. None of these criteria are absolute, and their validity has been questioned.

BARKER and CARPENTER (1970), for example, showed that the percentage of cells in the cerebral cortex of the cat, which are sensitive to local thermal changes (37%), is greater than that seen in the PO/AH. KOZYREVA (1972) found that 71% of the neurones in the sensorimotor cortex of rabbits were thermosensitive. A similar situation exists in the mid-brain, where as many as 72% of the cells studied were found to be thermosensitive (CRONIN and BAKER 1977a), yet local thermal stimulation of the mid-brain produces little (NAKAYAMA and HARDY 1969; CRONIN and BAKER 1977b) or no (ADAIR and STITT 1971; MURAKAMI et al. 1979) thermoregulatory effector output.

Clearly, thermosensitivity, per se, cannot be taken as proving a neurone's thermoregulatory function. The probability of such a classification being accurate is, however, considerably better when dealing with cells in known thermodetector or regulatory areas. An interesting, as yet unsolved, question is what function, if any, is mediated by thermosensitive cells located in brain areas apparently not related to thermoregulation.

The problems outlined above are not unique to the electrophysiological study of thermoregulation. KOEPCHEN et al. (1975) discuss the difficulties inherent in identification of neurones in the brain-stem subserving respiratory and cardiovascular functions. They raise the further question whether it is possible to distinguish brain-stem neurones acting in specific, autonomic mechanisms from non-specific, reticular neurones which might function in the ascending activating system. This latter question is relevant to the study of thermoregulation, as well, since the hypothalamus and preoptic area are rostral extensions of the brain-stem core. Further, thermal stimuli (peripheral or central) will influence cortical arousal and electroencephalogram (EEG) patterns (VON EULER and SODERBERG 1957; NAKAYAMA and HARDY 1969).

One conclusion drawn by KOEPCHEN et al. (1975) is that it may not be appropriate to attempt a precise classification of neuronal function, *in all instances.* In the context of thermoregulation, some neurones (e.g. thermodetectors) subserve specific and specialized functions; others may act in a more general way, mediating thermal, and non-thermal, information for overall, non-specific brain functioning which could include control of thermoregulatory effectors, as well. NAKAYAMA and HORI (1973) described neurones in the medullary reticular formation which were sensitive both to local temperature and to light mechanical stimulation of the skin. These cells also changed their firing rates after intravenous injection of bacterial pyrogen. Such cells may well belong to the second category of non-specific interneurones.

It is clear that microelectrode recording studies suffer from specific deficiencies which make their interpretation somewhat tentative. The data derived from such studies are, however, useful and necessary for analysis of the function of the body thermoregulator. Any dissection of CNS functions must include at its foundation some understanding of what the neurones are actually doing.

C. Thermosensitivity of PO/AH Neurones

Since the initial application of the microelectrode recording technique to the study of PO/AH thermosensitivity (NAKAYAMA et al. 1961), over 35 papers have appeared dealing with various aspects of the electrophysiology of this cell population. Table 1 summarizes, in chronological order, the results on thermoresponsiveness obtained in these studies. In almost all cases, some form of thermode was used to allow experimental manipulation of PO/AH temperature, which was recorded by a probe placed at a brain site symmetrical to that of the recording electrode. In order to make the results of these studies comparable, the table lists cells as warm-sensitive (increasing firing rates with increasing temperatures), cool-sensitive (increasing firing rates with decreasing temperatures), or insensitive, without regard to particular forms of the thermal responses or the various detailed classification schemes suggested by some authors.

An interesting technical point to emerge from this listing is that as the method was reapplied by different investigators, or even by the same worker, previously unobtainable responses were found. The earliest studies failed to find any central cool-sensitive cells in cats (NAKAYAMA et al. 1961, 1963), but later work described their presence in dogs (HARDY et al. 1964; CUNNINGHAM et al. 1967), cats (EISENMAN and JACKSON 1967), and rabbits (CABANAC et al. 1968). Similarly, earlier experiments could not demonstrate an effect of cutaneous thermoreceptors on PO/AH cells (HARDY et al. 1964; MURAKAMI et al. 1967), while later work did (WIT and WANG 1968a; HELLON 1970, 1972; KNOX et al. 1973b).

I. Thermoresponsiveness

The many studies on PO/AH thermosensitive cells agree on several broad points. There are cells in this area whose activity is related to local temperature; both warm-sensitive and cool-sensitive neurones are found. Most of the temperature-sensitive cells are located in the ventromedial portions of the septal area, and PO/AH. HELLON (1972a) has reported, however, that recordings made in the lateral PO/AH, in anaesthetized cats, gave a higher percentage of cool-sensitive cells than did more medial recordings.

1. Proportions of Thermosensitive Cells

The reported percentages of thermoresponsive cells (Table 1) ranges from 10% (HELLON 1967) to 76% (SIMON et al. 1977), the latter for a comparatively small cell population. In some instances, the reported population may not reflect the true distribution of sensitive versus insensitive cells, since the studies may have been intentionally biased to include more sensitive cells. Thus, studies of responses to iontophoretic drug application (BECKMAN and EISENMAN 1970; MURAKAMI 1973), pyrogens (WIT and WANG 1968b; EISENMAN 1969; STITT and HARDY 1975), or to stimuli applied elsewhere in the brain (EISENMAN 1974b; BOULANT and DEMIEVILLE 1977) may report higher proportions of thermosensitive cells. The actions of these agents or stimuli on responsive cells are of more interest and many non-sensitive cells may have been discarded without being tested and reported.

Table 1. Thermosensitive neurones in the PO/AH

Reference and Species	N^a	Warm-sensitive No. (%)	Cool-sensitive No. (%)	Non-sensitive No. (%)	W/C^b	Comment
Nakayama et al. (1963) Cat	?	(20)	0	(80)		
Hardy et al. (1964) Dog	88	28 (32)	7 (8)	53 (60)	4	No effect of face stimulation
Cunningham et al. (1967) Dog	114	44 (39)	7 (6)	63 (55)	6.3	Amine sensitivity studied
Eisenman and Jackson (1967) Cat	204	58 (28)	20 (10)	126 (62)	2.9	
Hellon (1967) Rabbit	227	17 (7)	6 (3)	204 (90)	2.9	Chronic recording
Murakami et al. (1967) Dog	270	156 (58)	0	114 (42)		Anaesthetic effects studied
Cabanac et al. (1968) Rabbit	?	50	27	?	1.9	Bacterial pyrogen
Wit and Wang (1968a) Cat	?	14	4	85	3.5	Ambient temperature effects. Pyrogen and antipyretic tested
Eisenman (1969) Cat	20	9 (45)	3 (15)	8 (40)	3	Pyrogen effect studied
Nakayama and Hardy (1969) Rabbit	51	27 (53)	3 (6)	21 (41)	9	Mid-brain units also
Beckman and Eisenman (1970) Cat, rat	52	33 (63)	5 (10)	14 (27)	6.6	Drug sensitivity studied
Guieu and Hardy (1970) Rabbit	102	25 (24)	6 (6)	71 (70)	4.2	Spinal cord stimulation
Hellon (1972a) Cat, rabbit	257	23 (9)	15 (6)	219 (85)	1.5	Ambient temperature effects
Jell and Gloor (1972) Cat	95	81 (85)	4 (4)	10 (11)	20	Decerebrated, anaesthetic study
Boulant and Bignall (1973a) Rat, squirrel	113	39 (35)	19 (17)	55 (48)	2.1	
Hori and Nakayama (1973) Rabbit	81	19 (23)	7 (9)	55 (68)	2.7	Drug sensitivity studied
Jell (1973) Cat	194	96 (49)	13 (7)	85 (44)	7.4	Drug sensitivity studied
Murakami (1973) Rat	73	40 (55)	15 (21)	18 (24)	2.7	Drug sensitivity studied
Beckman and Rozkowska-Ruttimann (1974) Rat	53	9 (17)	6 (11)	38 (72)	1.5	Drugs and salicylate studied
Boulant and Hardy (1974) Rabbit	204	51 (25)	27 (13)	126 (62)	1.9	Spinal cord and skin stimulation
Ford (1974) Cat	46	9 (19)	5 (11)	32 (70)	1.7	Decerebrated, PGE studied
Eisenman (1974b) Cat	156	56 (36)	3 (2)	97 (62)	19	Electrical stimulation of brain-stem
Jahns and Werner (1974a) Rat	52	12 (23)	7 (13)	33 (64)	1.7	Firing pattern analysis

Table 1. (continued)

Reference and Species	N^a	Warm-sensitive No. (%)	Cool-sensitive No. (%)	Non-sensitive No. (%)	W/C^b	Comment
JELL (1974) Cat	120	11 (9)	16 (13)	93 (78)	0.7	Peripheral thermo-sensitivity and drugs
BELYAVSKII and ABRAMOVA (1975) Rabbit	30	14 (47)	4 (13)	12 (40)	3.5	Pyrogen effects
SCHOENER and WANG (1975) Cat	?	21	9	?	2.3	Pyrogen and salicylate studied
STITT and HARDY (1975) Rabbit	138	63 (46)	10 (7)	65 (47)	6.3	PGE iontophoresis
SCHOENER and WANG (1976) Cat	?	12	4	?		PGE micro-injection
WÜNNENBERG et al. (1976) Hamster, guinea-pig	89	21 (24)	4 (5)	54 (61)	5.3	
JELL and SWEATMAN (1977) Cat	163	14 (8)	17 (11)	132 (81)	0.8	PGE ionto phoresis, peripheral stimulation
REAVES (1977) Rabbit	?	4	1	?	4	Ambient temperature effects
SIMON et al. (1977) Duck	21	11 (52)	5 (24)	5 (24)	2.2	Chronic recording
SPEULDA and WÜNNENBERG (1977) Hamster	73	20 (27)	0	53 (73)		Ambient temperature effects
BOULANT and DEMIEVILLE (1977) Rabbit	135	66 (49)	21 (16)	48 (35)	3.1	Electrical stimulation of brain stem and hippocampus
GORDON and HEATH (1979) Rabbit	15	5 (33)	5 (33)	5 (33)	1	PGE, chronic recording

JELL (1974) and JELL and SWEATMAN (1977) tested sensitivity to peripheral thermal stimuli only. All other data refer to local thermosensitivity
[a] N = total population
[b] W/C = ratio of warm- to cool-sensitive cells

For the most part, the data show that about 20%–40% of the neurones in the ventral septum, preoptic area, and anterior hypothalamus respond to changes in local temperature with significant changes in their firing rates. As indicated above, BOULANT and BIGNALL (1973a) suggest that the true proportion of thermosensitive cells in the PO/AH is considerably higher than this. Based on an analysis of firing rates and ability to continue recording from units for more than 90 min, they conclude that the small PO/AH cell population has 69% responsive cells and only 31% non-responsive. The greater difficulty in recording from the smaller cells is thought to account for the difference.

2. Ratio of Warm- to Cool-Sensitive Cells

The reports also agree that there are more warm-sensitive neurones than cool-sensitive in these areas, the ratio being about 3 or 4 to 1. The lack of cool-sensitive

cells in the large population of neurones studied by Nakayama et al. (1963) is puzzling, since a later study (Eisenman and Jackson 1967) in the same species (cat) using the same anaesthetic (urethane) and electrode type (metal) reported warm- to
cool-sensitive cells in a ratio of 2.9:1. Similarly, although Hardy et al. (1964) reported cool-sensitive cells in the anaesthetized dog (4:1 ratio), Murakami et al.
(1967) reported none in decerebrated or immobilized dogs. They did, however,
note that cells activated by cooling of the brain were occasionally encountered but
could not be studied long enough to be adequately characterized.

One possible explanation for these inconsistent results is that cool-sensitive
neurones are not only less common but are also smaller than warm-sensitive cells
and, therefore, harder to record from. The analysis of Boulant and Bignall
(1973a), of responses in small PO/AH cells, gave a ratio of warm- to cool-sensitive
cells of 3.4:1, which is in the range reported for PO/AH cells in general. Thus, it
appears that correcting for cell size does not change the proportion of cool-sensitive cells.

The warm- to cool-sensitive cell ratio may also depend on locus of recording.
Hellon (1972a) found that, of 19 thermosensitive cells isolated in the lateral PO/
AH of anaesthetized cats, 12 were cool-sensitive, giving ratio of 0.6:1. Most PO/
AH recording studies have concentrated on the medial zones since this is the area
most sensitive to thermal stimuli applied in chronic, thermoregulating animals
(Jessen 1976). At present, there are no *thermal* stimulation studies which suggest
that warm- and cool-sensitivity are localized in different areas of the PO/AH. It
is interesting that Metcalf and Myers (1978) localized the PO/AH area in which
noradrenaline micro-injection induces hypothermia to this same lateral zone. It
may be that the drug action is mediated by the cool-sensitive population located
in such high density there.

II. Detectors Versus Interneurones

Simple classification of PO/AH neurones as temperature-responsive or non-responsive does not provide sufficient information to characterize fully the functions
of the neurones studied. As discussed earlier, responsive cells could fall into two
categories: (1) thermodetectors; i.e. cells which are sensitive to local temperature
changes because of an inherent specialization, probably in their membranes; and,
(2) interneurones; i.e. cells which are not themselves thermosensitive but whose activities are modulated by synaptic inputs from thermodetector cells. When the thermal stimulus is applied to a block of brain tissue containing both types of cell, one
cannot distinguish these simply on the basis of responsiveness.

1. Thermal Response Form

One of the earliest attempts to make such a distinction, based on the form of the
thermal response, was that of Cunningham et al. (1967), who noted that the
changes in firing rates induced by rapid, local temperature shifts showed a time
phase shift or hysteresis for some cells. This indicated that the cells were responding
to temperature changes other than those recorded by the thermal probe. On the
assumption that the probe was recording the same temperature as that directly af-

Table 2. Classification of PO/AH neurones as detectors or interneurones by shape of thermal response curve

Reference	N [a]	Linear (detector) responses [b]		Non-linear (interneurone) responses	
		No.	(%)	Warm-sensitive No. (%)	Cool-sensitive No. (%)
EISENMAN and JACKSON (1967)	78	27 W	(35)	31 (40)	20 (25)
HELLON (1967)	13	4 W 1 C	(38)	4 (31)	4 (31)
NAKAYAMA and HARDY (1969)	30	6 W 3 C	(30)	21 (70)	
GUIEU and HARDY (1970)	31	9 W	(29)	16 (52)	6 (19)
BECKMAN and EISENMAN (1970)	38	24 W	(63)	9 (24)	5 (13)
HELLON (1972a)	38	17 W 9 C	(68)	6 (16)	6 (16)
Totals	228	100	(44)	87 (38)	41 (18)

[a] N = total thermosensitive population
[b] W = warm-sensitive; C = cool-sensitive

fecting the single neurone recorded from, cells showing such hysteresis in their responses were considered to be interneurones rather than primary detectors.

EISENMAN and JACKSON (1967) postulated that the activity of a detector cell should be a continuous function of the stimulus temperature and classified as detectors only those cells whose responses could be fitted to a single linear or semilogarithmic regression. Cells whose responses included threshold levels or discontinuities in slope were classified as interneurones (Fig. 2). In support of this hypothesis, they demonstrated that detector-like cells, with continuous or linear responses, were less sensitive to the depressant action of barbiturate anaesthetic than were the interneurone-like cells, with discontinuous or non-linear response forms. This analysis led to the conclusion that all cool-sensitive cells recorded from were of the interneurone type. GUIEU and HARDY (1970) and BECKMAN and EISENMAN (1970) likewise found no cool-sensitive cells with linear thermal responses to PO/AH heating or cooling. However, a few continuous function cool-sensitive cells were observed by HARDY et al. (1964), CUNNINGHAM et al. (1967), HELLON (1967), and NAKAYAMA and HARDY (1969).

Table 2 summarizes data from several studies in which cells were classified on the basis of these criteria. Most linearly responding cells in the PO/AH were warm-sensitive. Of 100 cells studied, 13 were cool-sensitive. Of these 9 were reported by HELLON (1972a), most of which were located lateral to the classical, medial thermosensitive preoptic zone. Overall, about 40% of the PO/AH thermosensitive cells were detector-like; in addition, warm-sensitive interneurones were twice as common as cool-sensitive.

It should be realized that many interneurones could show "detector-like" responses if their activity were dependent solely on inputs from the local detector cells. The interneurone-like response would be derived only from cells performing some integrative function, being acted upon by several different inputs.

These studies on the PO/AH, an area known to be an important thermodetector zone, can be compared with similar studies from less thermosensitive regions, such as mid-brain and posterior hypothalamus. Nakayama and Hardy (1969) reported on 62 thermosensitive cells in the mid-brain reticular formation: 28 (45%) were non-linear warm-sensitive; 22 (35%) were non-linear cool-sensitive; and 12 (19%) were linear cool-sensitive. This region produced no linear warm-sensitive recordings, the type of response associated with more than 40% of PO/AH cells. The mid-brain also contained many more cool-sensitive cells than did the PO/AH. Similarly, Edinger and Eisenman (1970), recording local thermoresponsiveness in the posterior hypothalamus, found only 21% linear warm-sensitive responses, 32% warm-sensitive interneurone and 47% cool-sensitive interneurone types. Wünnenberg and Hardy (1972) reported that only 3% of the cells in the posterior hypothalamus have linear warm-sensitive responses and received no inputs from other areas. Thus, areas of the brain concerned more with integration and less with thermodetection do have fewer cells with detector-like responses and more cool-sensitive cells.

These studies seem to support the concept that functionally different neurones have recognizably different response characteristics, although the separation into different categories appears to be less than perfect.

2. Extrahypothalamic Inputs

Another postulated distinction between detector and integrator neurones is that, by analogy with peripheral thermoreceptors, central detectors do not receive inputs from other neurones, but function as primary, or first-order, receptors (Eisenman and Jackson 1967; Guieu and Hardy 1970). Inputs to PO/AH cells have been studied with both thermal and electrical stimulation, and comparisons with thermal response forms have been made.

a) Thermal Inputs

Nakayama and Hardy (1969) correlated linearity of preoptic area thermal response and responsiveness to thermal stimulation of the mid-brain. Of 9 cells with linear preoptic thermal responses (detector-like), 2 (22%) responded to mid-brain temperatures, while 16 of 21 cells (76%) with non-linear response curves (interneurone-like) were affected by mid-brain stimulation. Guieu and Hardy (1970) extended these observations, correlating PO/AH sensitivity and responses to spinal cord thermal stimulation. None of the 9 PO/AH cells with linear responses were affected by spinal cord input, while about half (13 of 22) of the non-linear cells were.

Hellon (1970) found that 5 of 6 PO/AH cells responsive to ambient temperature changes in unanaesthetized rabbits were of the interneurone type; one such cell showed a detector-like, linear response. Hellon (1972a), however, found at least 4 (and perhaps 8) "linear" cells which were affected by ambient temperature changes.

Boulant and Bignall (1973b) and Boulant and Hardy (1974), in an extensive investigation of cutaneous and spinal cord thermal inputs to PO/AH neurones, found that the form of a unit's thermal response could be changed by changing the input to it from peripheral structures. This observation makes categorization of unit response very problematical under changing input conditions.

Overall, there does appear to be some correlation between responsiveness to extrahypothalamic thermal input and local thermal response form, but again, this is less than perfect.

b) Electrical Inputs

EISENMAN (1974b) studied responses of PO/AH cells to electrical stimulation of mid-brain and pontine areas known to project to the hypothalamus and found that of 19 linear thermosensitive cells, 11 (58%) responded to the evoked, ascending volley. Out of 40 non-linear thermosensitive cells 27 (68%) also responded, as did 58 of 97 insensitive cells (60%). Thus, inputs from the brain-stem are as prevalent on presumed detector cells as on other types. BOULANT and DEMIEVILLE (1977) reported that 43 out of 63 thermosensitive PO/AH cells (68%) responded to electrical stimulation in the brain-stem or hippocampus. Interestingly, only 6 out of 30 thermally insensitive cells (16%) responded to the electrically evoked inputs in their study.

The activity generated by electrical stimulation does not mimic thermally evoked inputs but more likely represents non-specific facilitatory and inhibitory modulation of PO/AH firing. The data show remarkably strong inputs to thermosensitive PO/AH cells, including presumed thermodetector-like cells.

3. Firing Pattern Analysis

Several reports have attempted to characterize thermosensitive PO/AH neurones by analysis of their steady-state firing patterns (see Sect. B.IV.2). EISENMAN (1972) illustrated some of the typical interspike-interval (ISI) histograms obtained from PO/AH cells, but found no correlation between histogram shape, or the effect of temperature on the ISI histogram, and other thermosensitivity characteristics. REAVES and HEATH (1975) noted that local temperature changes could produce changes in ISI histogram shape without affecting mean firing rate. This implies that thermal information could be coded by neurones in terms of firing *pattern* in addition to, or instead of, firing *rate*. Some apparently insensitive cells may actually be affected by temperature changes.

In an extensive analysis of the firing patterns of thermosensitive PO/AH cells, MURAKAMI (1974) found indications that firing pattern might reflect neuronal function, in some instances. Of 71 cells studied, the ISI histogram of 28 could be fitted with a specific distribution function: 17 were exponential and 11 were fitted with gamma functions of various orders. Following a suggestion of BRAITENBERG (1965), for analysis of excitability variations in frog cerebellar cells, MURAKAMI next noted that cells with ISI distributions fitted to gamma functions showed less variation in excitability when local temperature was changed than did cells with exponential ISI distributions. This was true even though cells in both groups were equally thermosensitive. The suggestion was made that the former distribution function derives from interneuronal cells and the latter from true thermodetectors. Unfortunately, most of the cells studied could not be specifically fitted with one of the two distribution functions. A large "grey area" existed in which this analysis

could not be applied. In addition, Murakami (1974) did not attempt to correlate
the results of this analysis with other forms of characterization, such as the shape
of the cell's thermal response curve.

In a recent paper, Murakami and Sakata (1979) comparing thermosensitive
medullary and PO/AH cells, found differences in the variability of firing exhibited
by neurones in the two groups. Again, the suggestion was made that thermosensitive cells of different function might be distinguished by analysis of patterns of responses.

Another aspect of the study of firing patterns in PO/AH cells relates to detection of periodic firing in a spike train. Bursting activity represents one, obvious
form of periodicity which has been noted (Eisenman 1972), but more subtle periodic or oscillatory behaviours have also been examined. Jahns and Werner
(1974b), studying PO/AH neurones in rats, found that more than half of the cells
showed periodicity in firing. Most warm-sensitive cells (10 of 12) had periodic discharges at one or more of the temperatures tested. In contrast, most non-sensitive
cells (31 of 32) had no periodic patterns at any temperature, or were periodic at
only one temperature. The few cool-sensitive cells studied did not reveal any periodic firing (3 of 4). No attempt was made to correlate these results with other
measures of cell characteristics, so that, for the present, it is not possible to decide
if determination of periodic behaviour could be a way of separating detectors from
interneurones.

III. In Vitro Recording of PO/AH Activity

Two reports have dealt with the activity of thermosensitive hypothalamic cells in
vitro. Nakayama et al. (1978) recorded from 38 thermosensitive cells in explants
of PO/AH from newborn mice; 33 warm-sensitive and 5 cool-sensitive cells were
studied. Responses obtained were very much like those seen with in vivo recordings, with respect to firing frequencies and temperature responsiveness. It is not
clear from this report if any thermally insensitive cells were found.

Mason et al. (1978), recording from cultured cells taken from 1-week-old rats,
found that about 80% of the cells (28 of 35) were temperature sensitive. In this
group, 6 cells were active only in a narrow, 2 °C temperature band centred at about
36 °C, and showed no activity at temperatures outside this band. This type of response has never been reported with in vivo recording. In cerebellar cells, studied
as controls, only 22% were thermosensitive (5 of 23), and the narrow-band type
of activity was not seen. Mason et al. suggest that this type of response might characterize an on–off trigger element in thermoregulation.

The in vitro recording technique is being applied to several problems in the
analysis of CNS functions: Yamamoto and Chujo (1978) in the hippocampus; Fukuda and Loeschke (1977) in the medulla; Hatton et al. (1978) and Geller and
Hoffer (1977) in the hypothalamus. It promises to become an increasingly potent
tool for such studies.

D. Pyrogenic and Antipyretic Actions

Fever generated by pyrogenic agents results from a coordinated shift in heat loss
and heat production levels leading to heat storage and a rise in body temperature.

This coordinated response makes it very likely that the pyrogen action is centrally mediated (STITT 1979). Several experimental studies have demonstrated that localized micro-injection of various pyrogens into the brain results in fevers only at PO/AH injection sites (VILLABLANCA and MYERS 1965; COOPER et al. 1967; JACKSON 1967; LIPTON et al. 1973; MYERS et al. 1974; WILLIAMS et al. 1977). The one exception to this is the report of ROSENDORFF and MOONEY (1971) that mid-brain injections also produced fevers. One possible explanation for this discordant observation is that the material injected at the mid-brain site may have leaked into the cerebroventricular system and acted at the sensitive PO/AH site.

Similarly, while the major site of antipyretic action is also the PO/AH, CRANSTON and RAWLINS (1972) found that mid-brain micro-injections of salicylate were antipyretic. The role of mid-brain neurones in thermoregulation, fever, and antipyresis is, thus, still unsettled. Electrophysiological studies of pyrogen and antipyretic actions have focused mainly on neurones in the PO/AH because of their demonstrated sensitivity to these agents.

I. Pyrogens and Antipyretics

1. Pyrogenic Agents

A variety of substances will induce an elevation of body temperature when administered to the intact animal (DINARELLO 1979). Those used in electrophysiological studies fall into three classes:

1) Bacterial pyrogens: whole killed bacterial cells or extracts of bacteria, such as vaccines of various types or Piromen, a crude lipopolysaccharide extracted from *Pseudomonas* bacteria. These substances are members of the group of exogenous pyrogens or endotoxins.

2) Leucocyte pyrogen: a small protein synthesized and released primarily by various bone-marrow derived phagocytic cells (DINARELLO 1979), also called endogenous pyrogen (ATKINS and WOOD 1955).

3) Prostaglandins: complex, unsaturated hydroxy-fatty acids derived from cell lipids. Prostaglandin synthesis and release in the brain can be stimulated by several factors including tissue trauma (RUDY et al. 1977), bacterial (PHILIPP-DORMSTON 1976) and leucocyte (ZIEL and KRUPP 1976) pyrogens.

2. Antipyretics

The antipyretics whose actions have been studied electrophysiologically all belong to the class of prostaglandin synthetase inhibitors (ROBINSON and VANE 1974). While it is clear that these substances will reduce the elevated body temperature found in fever, there is contradictory evidence on their effects in non-febrile states. Several studies have failed to demonstrate any action of salicylates in normothermic animals (CRANSTON and RAWLINS 1972; CRANSTON et al. 1970 a, b; MYERS et al. 1974), in animals hyperthermic because of PO/AH cooling (CRANSTON et al. 1970 b), or in hyperthermic, exercising humans (DOWNEY and DARLING 1962). However, hypothermic actions of salicylate were demonstrated in afebrile rats

Table 3. Action of bacterial and leucocyte pyrogen on PO/AH neurones

Neurone type	N^a	Facil[b] No. (%)	Inhib[c] No. (%)	No effect No. (%)
Warm-sensitive	65	2 (3)	61 (94)	2 (3)
Cool-sensitive	22	20 (91)	0	2 (9)
Non-sensitive	25	0	1 (4)	24 (96)

[a] N = number of units
[b] Facil = facilitation of firing
[c] Inhib = inhibition of firing

(SATINOFF 1972; POLK and LIPTON 1975; LIN 1978), rabbits (MURAKAMI and SAKATA 1975), and monkeys (LIN and CHAI 1975). No satisfactory explanation has been advanced for these contradictory results.

II. Electrophysiology of Pyrogen Action

The action of a pyrogen on CNS neurones should be appropriate to triggering the heat storage which results in an elevation of body temperature. Firing rates of cool-sensitive cells, presumed to drive heat production and conservation effectors, should be increased. Firing rates of warm-sensitive neurones, presumed to drive heat loss effectors, should be depressed. What effect might be noted on thermally insensitive units could not be predicted. On the assumption that such cells may serve as a thermostable firing reference for regulation (NAKAYAMA et al. 1963; CABANAC et al. 1968) they, too, might be affected by pyrogens.

An important technical problem that arises in performing pyrogen studies on single units is the need to record cell activity for fairly long times. Bacterial pyrogens act with latencies of 20–45 min and do not produce peak fevers for 1–3 h. Because of the long time course of this action comparatively few cells have been studied, some of these for as long as 5 h. The more rapid, and shorter duration, effect of prostaglandins can be studied more easily and several cells can be examined in a single animal.

1. Bacterial and Leucocyte Pyrogens

The action of intravascularly injected bacterial pyrogens (typhoid vaccine or Piromen) on PO/AH cells was studied by CABANAC et al. (1968), WIT and WANG (1968 b), EISENMAN (1969), and BELYAVSKII and ABRAMOVA (1975). SCHOENER and WANG (1975) and BELYAVSKII and ABRAMOVA (1975) have studied the actions of leucocyte pyrogen. The results of these various studies are highly consistent (Table 3).

In all, 112 neurones have been studied. Of these, 65 were warm-sensitive and 22 were cool-sensitive. Of the warm-sensitive group, 94% (61 of 65) were inhibited; 91% of the cool-sensitive cells (20 of 22) had their firing rates facilitated. These actions are those anticipated for increased heat storage leading to a rise in body tem-

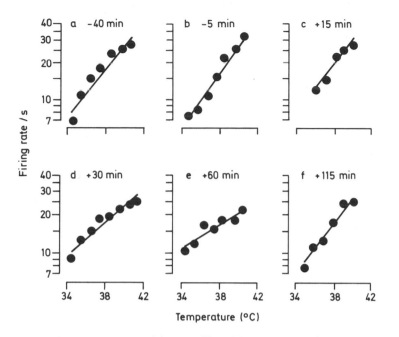

Fig. 3 a–f. Thermal response curves of detector-like PO/AH neurone taken at times indicated before (**a, b**) and after (**c–f**) injection of bacterial pyrogen. (EISENMAN 1969)

perature. Out of 25 thermally insensitive cells tested, only one (4%) responded to pyrogen with a depression of firing (CABANAC et al. 1968), suggesting that the pyrogenic action is specific to thermally sensitive, presumed thermoregulatory, PO/AH cells. It would, of course, be difficult to prove that no action occurs on any thermally insensitive cell, since this population is so large and heterogeneous in its function.

Another effect of pyrogen on PO/AH cells was noted in these studies which was not predictable on the basis of known febrile responses. By plotting unit firing rate against temperature before and after pyrogen treatment, both CABANAC et al. (1968) and EISENMAN (1969) demonstrated that the decrease in firing of warm-sensitive neurones was accompanied by a decrease in *thermosensitivity* (Figs. 3 and 4); the slope of the unit's thermal response curve was decreased after pyrogen treatment. Similar effects were noted, but not quantitated, by WIT and WANG (1968 b). For the linear, detector-like PO/AH neurone illustrated in Fig. 3, thermosensitivity in terms of Q_{10} was decreased from 9.5 to 3.1 by the pyrogen. Warm-sensitive, interneurone-like cells also showed a depression of thermosensitivity, but the effect seemed less pronounced in cool-sensitive cells (Fig. 5). The functional significance of this depressed thermosensitivity is still not clear since most studies on thermoregulation during fever do not indicate any decrease in regulatory precision or capacity (MACPHERSON 1959; COOPER et al. 1964; CRANSTON et al. 1976). EISENMAN (1974a), studying rabbits, and LIPTON and KENNEDY (1979), studying monkeys, both found a decrease in the animal's ability to respond to PO/AH thermal stimulation after bacterial pyrogen administration. They consider this to be a direct ef-

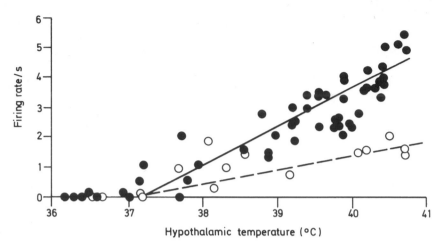

Fig. 4. Change in thermosensitivity of a warm-sensitive PO/AH neurone following bacterial pyrogen administration. *Solid circles* and *solid line* indicate data recorded before administration of vaccine; *open circles* and *broken line* are data recorded 18 min after administration of vaccine. (CABANAC et al. 1968)

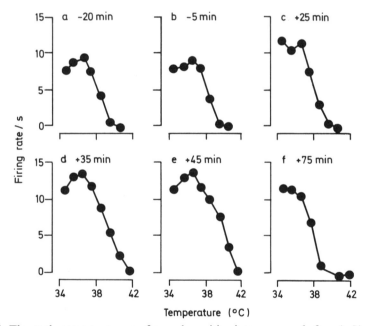

Fig. 5 a–f. Thermal response curves of a cool-sensitive interneurone before (**a, b**) and after (**c–f**) injection of bacterial pyrogen. (EISENMAN 1969)

fect on the central neurones. STITT et al. (1974), using prostaglandin E_1 as the pyrogen, consider the decreased central thermosensitivity during fever to be secondary to an induced change in peripheral thermal input to the central neurones. Such an action however would be minimal in the anaesthetized animals used for the electrophysiological experiments.

Analysis of the decrease in thermosensitivity (EISENMAN 1969) revealed that it resulted from an apparent rotation of the unit's thermal response curve around a point representing central temperatures of 37°–38 °C, close to the animal's normal body temperature (Fig. 3). CABANAC et al. (1968) also noted this phenomenon (Fig. 4). When PO/AH temperature was clamped at 38 °C, EISENMAN (1969) found that the firing rate of a detector-like neurone was not changed by pyrogen, even though the thermosensitivity was markedly depressed. This suggested that the actual drive to interneurones and effectors may originate from some cell population other than the central thermodetectors. It is possible that this observation was an artifact of the preparation since in a study of the intact, thermoregulating rabbit, EISENMAN (1974 a) found that the comparable "rotation point" was at central temperatures generally below normal body temperature, ranging from 34° to 38 °C for different animals.

The latencies for actions of bacterial pyrogen on PO/AH neurones ranged from 7 to 30 min. These values are somewhat shorter than the latency for fever development following pyrogen injection. This is to be expected since the neuronal drive should precede the effector response and the rise in body temperature should lag further due to the thermal inertia of the system. The duration of pyrogen action on the units was also comparable to the time to peak fever response. For the few neurones that were followed long enough, firing rates and thermosensitivities returned to control levels 100–150 min after pyrogen injection (EISENMAN 1969; WIT and WANG 1968 b), which precedes somewhat the latency to the peak of pyrogen-induced fever.

In the one electrophysiological study of pyrogen action outside the PO/AH, NAKAYAMA and HORI (1973) examined the effect of typhoid vaccine on mid-brain reticular formation cells. Following latencies of 6–15 min, these cells responded in a manner similar to the PO/AH neurones: 8 cool-sensitive cells were facilitated and 2 warm-sensitive were completely inhibited. It was found that 3 thermally insensitive neurones were not affected by the pyrogen. All of the cells tested were also sensitive to mechanical stimuli applied to the skin. The increased firing of cool-sensitive cells after pyrogen was not accompanied by a change in thermosensitivity, in agreement with the results obtained in the PO/AH. The thermosensitivities of the two warm-sensitive cells were not tested.

Studying the effects of a peripherally administered pyrogen cannot provide any insight into its site of action. Thus, the observations of NAKAYAMA and HORI (1973) do not necessarily show that the injected pyrogen acted on mid-brain neurones, just as the results on PO/AH cells do not prove a direct action at that site. SCHOENER and WANG (1975) micro-injected leucocyte pyrogen into the PO/AH close to their recording electrode and produced actions with a rapid onset, similar to those described above. This study demonstrates a localized action of the pyrogen on PO/AH cells, although not necessarily on the cells recorded from.

2. Prostaglandins

With the discovery by MILTON and WENDLANDT (1971) that prostaglandins of the E series (PGE_1 and PGE_2) produced hyperthermia when injected intracerebroventricularly, and with the work of VANE (1971) showing that aspirin-like antipyretics were inhibitors of prostaglandin synthesis, the concept developed that fevers resulted from synthesis and release of PGE at sensitive brain sites. Evidence has since been presented which casts doubt on this scheme, so that the relationship between pathological fevers and prostaglandins is still debatable (CRANSTON 1979). Whatever this relationship, it is clear that PGEs are among the most potent pyrogenic substances studied. Quantities as small as 100 pg will raise body temperature when injected into the sensitive PO/AH region (VEALE and WHISHAW 1976). The actions of several prostaglandins (PGE$_1$, PGE$_2$, and PGF$_{2\alpha}$) on PO/AH cells have been studied using localized forms of administration (micro-injection or iontophoresis). In contrast to the data obtained using bacterial or leucocyte pyrogen, these prostaglandin studies have not produced consistent or clearly interpretable results.

In an extensive study of 138 PO/AH cells in anaesthetized rabbits, STITT and HARDY (1975) found that 90%–92% of the cells were not affected by iontophoretically applied PGE$_1$, regardless of their local thermosensitivity. The few responses obtained (12 of 138) were all facilitatory, again not correlated to thermosensitivity.

JELL and SWEATMAN (1977) also studied a large population of 163 PO/AH cells, in cats, using iontophoresis of PGEs and PGF. They characterized thermosensitivity in terms of responsiveness of the neurone to peripheral thermal stimulation of the cat's face. Most (97%) of the thermally non-responsive cells were also not sensitive to PGE application, although several did respond to PGF$_{2\alpha}$. On the other hand, 28% of the warm-sensitive cells and 53% of the cool-sensitive cells responded to PGE, both primarily with increased firing. PGE$_2$ appeared slightly more effective than PGE$_1$; of cells tested with both prostaglandins, all PGE$_1$-responsive neurones were also sensitive to PGE$_2$, but the reverse was not true.

Data consistent with a direct pyrogenic action of PGE on thermosensitive PO/AH cells have been developed, but none of these studies is as extensive as the experiments of STITT and HARDY (1975) or JELL and SWEATMAN (1977). FORD (1974), using acutely decerebrated cats, examined the action of PGE$_1$ iontophoresis on 46 PO/AH cells whose local thermosensitivities were also determined. All 5 cool-sensitive neurones tested were facilitated by PGE, an effect consistent with the bacterial and leucocyte pyrogen data. However, only 2 of 9 warm-sensitive cells were inhibited. Most of the thermally insensitive cells (88%) were likewise not affected by PGE.

SCHOENER and WANG (1976) micro-injected PGE$_1$ intracerebrally while recording from PO/AH cells in cats. Peripheral and local thermosensitivities were determined and these were generally similar for any unit. The 12 warm-sensitive neurones studied were all depressed by PGE and the 4 cool-sensitive cells were excited.

Most recently, GORDON and HEATH (1979) recorded from PO/AH cells in chronically prepared unanaesthetized rabbits while infusing PGE$_2$ into the cerebral ventricles. They found that 5 cool-sensitive cells and 5 warm-sensitive cells all responded in the anticipated way: excitation of cool-sensitive cells and inhibition of warm-sensitive cells.

A comparison of the results obtained using bacterial and leucocyte pyrogens (Table 3) with those from PGE experiments (Table 4) shows the marked contrast in the two data sets. Predicted responses were seen in better than 90% of the units in the former series, but in only 20%–50% of the units in the latter. These data,

Table 4. Action of PGE_1 and PGE_2 on PO/AH neurones

Neurone type	N^a	Facil[b] No. (%)	Inhib[c] No. (%)	No effect No. (%)
Warm-sensitive	103	8 (8)	20 (19)	75 (73)
Cool-sensitive	41	21 (51)	3 (7)	17 (42)
Non-sensitive	234	8 (3)	6 (2)	220 (95)

[a] N = number of units
[b] Facil = facilitation of firing
[c] Inhib = inhibition of firing

in fact, have been taken as evidence that pyrogen fevers are not mediated by prostaglandins (VEALE et al. 1977). The two major iontophoretic studies have produced negative results. JELL and SWEATMAN (1977) could not correlate PGE action with responses to physiological thermal input. They did, however, find that PGE affected thermally responsive cells to a much greater extent than thermally insensitive ones, which suggests some form of specificity of action. Their finding that about 16% of PO/AH cells responded to PGE iontophoresis is a lower response rate than that reported by AVANZINO et al. (1966) for brain-stem neurones (30%–35%) or COCEANI and VITI (1975) for frog spinal cord cells (31%), although all agree that excitation is the primary action observed. POULAIN and CARETTE (1974) found that 84% of the hypothalamic cells tested (preoptic area and arcuate nucleus) responded to iontophoresis of PGE. As JELL and SWEATMAN (1977) point out, this latter study was done on barbiturate-anaesthetized animals, which may have distorted the results.

The very low yield of PGE-responsive neurones reported by STITT and HARDY (1975) is even more surprising in view of the higher degree of responsiveness reported by others. As a control for the effective iontophoretic ejection of PGE from their electrodes, STITT and HARDY tested their system on cerebellar Purkinje cells. These were found to respond as anticipated. Thus, the PGE was being applied, but did not appear to act on their cells as predicted for a pyrogenic effect, or as demonstrated by other iontophoretic studies. STITT and HARDY suggest that prostaglandins may not act on neurones directly, but rather may modulate the release of synaptic transmitters (HEDQVIST 1973), an action which might not produce changes in firing rates under the experimental conditions used. This does not explain the overall low response rate in this study compared with others.

It is possible that differences in the anaesthetic used could have caused the disparate results of the three iontophoretic studies. FORD (1974) worked on acutely prepared unanaesthetized cats; STITT and HARDY (1975) used urethane-anaesthetized rabbits, while JELL and SWEATMAN (1977) used the volatile anaesthetic methoxyflurane in cats, keeping the anaesthetic level as light as possible.

Another possible explanation may derive from the very localized application of substances in the iontophoretic technique. The ejected PGE may not have reached sensitive sites on the neurone studied or may not have been tested on PGE-sensitive neurones. It appears that the PO/AH region in which PGE acts is quite small, and is medially located (WILLIAMS et al. 1977); it may have been missed in some experiments. The grosser forms of application by micro-injection (Schoener and Wang 1976) or intraventricular injection (Gordon and Heath 1979) seem to produce results more consistent with predictions. Sorting out these discrepancies must await further experimentation.

3. Pyrogen Action on Peripheral Receptors

Evans et al. (1972) studied the action of bacterial pyrogen (intravenous typhoid vaccine) on activity of thermoreceptors in the tongue. No effects on these peripheral receptors were found. One conclusion derived from these results was that central thermosensitive cells, which are influenced by pyrogens, differ from peripheral receptors, which are not. However, if the action of the bacterial pyrogen on neural membranes requires some locally produced mediator (e.g. prostaglandin), the lack of effect on tongue thermoreceptors may have resulted from an inability of the peripheral tissue to respond to the injected pyrogen with production of the mediator. It would be interesting to re-study this problem using local injection of other, more directly acting pyrogens.

III. Electrophysiology of Antipyretic Action

Wit and Wang (1968b) first noted that intravenous or intracarotid injection of acetylsalicylate would counter the effects of previously administered bacterial pyrogen on PO/AH neurones. The latency for this effect was about 30 min. The study investigated 8 cells. In one additional neurone tested without prior pyrogen treatment, only a slight stimulatory effect was noted. Schoener and Wang (1975) micro-injected acetylsalicylate directly into the PO/AH during unit recording. In 6 thermosensitive cells without prior pyrogen treatment, no effect (3 cells) or a slight depression (3 cells) was noted. In addition, 5 warm-sensitive and 3 cool-sensitive cells were tested after leucocyte pyrogen administration, both substances being micro-injected into the same brain site. In all cases, the antipyretic reversed the effect produced by the pyrogen.

Localized iontophoretic application of salicylate to PO/AH cells was used in rats, without prior pyrogen treatment, by Beckman and Rozkowska-Ruttimann (1974). The antipyretic was found to excite 29% of the cells tested (30 of 104) and to depress 10 cells (10%). Of 53 cells tested, 15 were thermosensitive. Of 9 warm-sensitive cells examined, 8 were excited by salicylate; of 6 cool-sensitive neurones, only 1 responded and this was inhibited. Jell and Sweatman (1976) also studied the action of iontophoretically applied antipyretics on PO/AH cells in afebrile animals. Salicylate and fenoprofen were applied to 63 cells. Thermosensitivity was not determined. Both antipyretics produced depression of activity only; salicylate inhibited 5 cells (12% of the cells tested); fenoprofen, a more potent inhibitor of PG synthesis, depressed 12 cells (60% of those tested).

The results of Wit and Wang (1968b) and of Schoener and Wang (1975) support the view that antipyretics have no action in the absence of pyrogen fever, but do reverse the effects of pyrogens on neurones. The iontophoretic studies of Beckman and Rozkowska-Ruttimann (1974) and of Jell and Sweatman (1976), however, point to an action of antipyretics on neurones, even in the afebrile state.

JELL and SWEATMAN did not test thermosensitivity of their cells, so that it is not possible to correlate the observed antipyretic action with thermoregulatory function. The only effect noted in these experiments was a depression of firing (17 of 63 cells). Iontophoretic application of PGE_1 to 4 cells did not reverse the antipyretic depression of firing, suggesting that the depression was not related to inhibition of PG synthesis. Interestingly, cells which were depressed by the antipyretics were more likely to be sensitive to PGE than were cells not affected by the salicylate or fenoprofen. A direct action of salicylate on neuronal membranes, leading to hyperpolarization, has been described in molluscan ganglion cells (BARKER and LEVITAN 1971; LEVITAN and BARKER 1972). Such an action could account for the depression of firing rate reported by JELL and SWEATMAN (1976).

BECKMAN and ROZKOWSKA-RUTTIMANN (1974) reported a preponderance of excitatory effects on PO/AH neurones. In addition, they found some correlation between salicylate action and thermosensitivity in their cell population, in that warm-sensitive cells tended to be excited by the salicylate. Such effects would be in agreement with a hypothermic action of salicylate and could be evidence in support of the studies cited above on antipyretic actions in normothermic animals.

The interpretation of results from acute studies of antipyretic actions is complicated by the observations of RUDY et al. (1977) that traumatic injury to neural tissue in this area will cause fever ("puncture fever," ARONSOHN and SACHS 1884) which can be attenuated or blocked by the prostaglandin synthetase inhibitor, indomethacin. In acutely prepared animals, especially following implantation of thermode tubes and temperature probes, the surgical trauma may cause PG synthesis and release, even if the anaesthetic prevents manifestation of this by a rise in body temperature. Neurones examined in this state may be influenced by the locally produced PG and could, therefore, respond to antipyretics in an appropriate way. However, local application of salicylate by iontophoresis would not be expected to block PG synthesis at a distant, traumatized site. Further, if the antipyretics were acting by inhibition of this type of endogenous PG synthesis, the effect should have been most prominent in the experiments of SCHOENER and WANG (1975) where the injection cannula, through which the salicylate was administered, was in the immediate vicinity of the neurones studied. Yet, no effect of salicylate without prior pyrogen treatment was reported.

It appears that the antipyretics clearly reverse the effects of pyrogens on PO/AH neurones (WIT and WANG 1968b; SCHOENER and WANG 1975). There is also good evidence for actions of antipyretics on cells in the absence of exogenously administered pyrogen. On the question whether such actions are consistent with a hypothermic effect of antipyretics in afebrile animals, the data are inconclusive.

E. Summary

Application of electrophysiological techniques to the problems of pyrogenicity and antipyresis has produced data verifying previously known characteristics of thermoregulation during fever: latency and duration of action of bacterial pyrogen on PO/AH neurones are comparable to those seen in fever development and time to peak effect; changes in the firing rates of central thermosensitive neurones can be related to activation of appropriate heat loss and heat production–conservation effectors; antipyretics are seen to reverse the actions of pyrogens on central neurones.

The electrophysiological studies have also produced data which were not anticipated, some of which remain to be adequately explained. The observation that thermosensitivity of warm-sensitive cells in the PO/AH is depressed during fever has been confirmed in all microelectrode experiments in which this has been examined. Study of PO/AH thermosensitivity during fever in intact, thermoregulating animals has also demonstrated this effect. The nature of the effect (primary, central, or secondary to peripheral change), and its significance for thermoregulation during fever are by no means clear. The pyrogen-induced decrease in neuronal thermosensitivity appears to be absent or less prominent in cool-sensitive cells, presumed to drive heat production and conservation effectors. Yet, studies on regulation during fever have demonstrated a decrease in the regression of changes in metabolic rate on changes in preoptic area temperature. This is a striking instance of a lack of correlation between thermoregulatory and electrophysiological data that remains to be explained.

The decrease in sensitivity following pyrogen treatment appears to produce a rotation of thermal responsiveness around a point below, but close to, normal body temperature, suggesting that fever development would be depressed or even reversed during hypothermia. It is possible, at least theoretically, that in hypothermic states pyrogen would cause a further decrease in body temperature.

The nature of prostaglandin actions on PO/AH neurones is still unresolved. As potent pyrogens, PGs should act appropriately on central neurones, even if they are not the mediators of pathological fever. Some electrophysiological studies have substantiated this prediction; others have not.

Antipyretic effects have been demonstrated electrophysiologically, but the action of these agents on cells in the absence of pyrogen is still unsettled. This uncertainty at the neuronal level parallels the uncertainty at the level of the intact thermoregulating organism.

It is the nature of electrophysiological studies that data accumulate slowly. Experiments need to be repeated and confirmed independently, with each repetition improving our understanding of the system under study. Recent refinements in technique will improve data collection. Many of the problems, inconsistencies and uncertainties outlined are solvable and will undoubtedly be resolved in the near future.

References

Adair ER, Stitt JT (1971) Behavioral temperature regulation in the squirrel monkey: effects of midbrain temperature displacements. J Physiol (Paris) 63:191–194

Aronsohn E, Sachs J (1884) Ein Wärmezentrum in Grosshirn. Dtsch Med Wochenschr 10:823–825

Atkins E, Wood WB Jr (1955) Studies on the pathogenesis of fever: 1. the presence of transferable pyrogen in the blood stream following injection of typhoid vaccine. J Exp Med 101:519–528

Avanzino GL, Bradley PB, Wolstencroft JH (1966) Actions of prostaglandins E_1, E_2 and $F_{2\alpha}$ on brain stem neurons. Br J Pharmacol 27:157–163

Barbour H (1912) Die Wirkung unmittelbarer Erwärmung und Abkühlung der Wärmezentra auf Körpertemperatur. Arch Exp Pathol Pharmakol 70:1–26

Barker JL, Carpenter DO (1970) Thermosensitivity of neurons in the sensorimotor cortex of the cat. Science 169:597–598

Barker JL, Levitan H (1971) Salicylate: effect on membrane permeability of molluscan neurons. Science 172:1245–1247

Beckman AL, Eisenman JS (1970) Microelectrophoresis of biogenic amines on hypothalamic thermosensitive cells. Science 170:334–336

Beckman AL, Rozkowska-Ruttimann E (1974) Hypothalamic and septal neuronal responses to iontophoretic application of salicylate in rats. Neuropharmacology 13:393–398

Belyavskii EM, Abramova EL (1975) Effects of leucocyte pyrogen on thermosensitive neurons in the anterior hypothalamus. Bull Eksp Biol Med 80:17–20

Bleier R, Bard P, Woods JW (1966) Cytoarchitectonic appearance of the isolated hypothalamus of the cat. J Comp Neurol 128:255–311

Boulant JA, Bignall KE (1973a) Determinants of hypothalamic thermosensitivity in ground squirrels and rats. Am J Physiol 225:306–310

Boulant JA, Bignall KE (1973b) Hypothalamic neuronal responses to peripheral and deep-body temperatures. Am J Physiol 225:1371–1374

Boulant JA, Demieville HN (1977) Responses of thermosensitive preoptic and septal neurons to hippocampal and brain stem stimulation. J Neurophysiol 40:1356–1368

Boulant JA, Hardy JD (1974) The effect of spinal and skin temperatures on the firing rate and thermosensitivity of preoptic neurons. J Physiol (Lond) 240:639–660

Bradley PB, Candy JM (1970) Iontophoretic release of acetylcholine, noradrenaline and 5-hydroxytryptamine and D-lysergic acid diethylamide from micropipettes. Br J Pharmcol 40:194–201

Braitenberg V (1965) What can be learned from spike interval histograms about synaptic mechanisms. J Theor Biol 8:419–425

Cabanac M, Hardy JD (1969) Réponses unitaires et thermorégulatrices lors de réchauffements et refroidissments localisés de la region préoptique et du mésencéphale chez le lapin. J Physiol (Paris) 61:331–347

Cabanac M, Stolwijk JAJ, Hardy JD (1968) Effect of temperature and pyrogens on single-unit activity in the rabbit's brain stem. J Appl Physiol 24:645–652

Coceani F, Viti A (1975) Responses of spinal neurons to iontophoretically applied prostaglandin E_1 in the frog. Can J Physiol Pharmacol 53:273–284

Cooper KE, Cranston WI, Snell ES (1964) Temperature regulation during fever in man. Clin Sci 27:345–356

Cooper KE, Cranston WI, Honour AJ (1967) Observations on the site and mode of action of pyrogens in the rabbit brain. J Physiol (Lond) 191:325–337

Cranston WI (1979) Central mechanisms of fever. Fed Proc 38:49–51

Cranston WI, Rawlins MD (1972) Effects of intracerebral micro-injection of sodium salicylate on temperature regulation in the rabbit. J Physiol (Lond) 222:257–266

Cranston WI, Luff RH, Rawlins MD, Rosendorff C (1970a) The effects of salicylate on temperature regulation in the rabbit. J Physiol (Lond) 208:251–259

Cranston WI, Hellon RF, Rawlins MD, Rosendorff C (1970b) Observations on the mechanism of salicylate-induced antipyresis. J Physiol (Lond) 210:593–600

Cranston WI, Luff RH, Rawlins MD, Hellon RF, Mitchell D (1976) Thermoregulation in rabbits during fever. J Physiol (Lond) 257:767–777

Cronin MJ, Baker MA (1977a) Thermosensitive midbrain neurons in the cat. Br Res 128:461–472

Cronin MJ, Baker MB (1977b) Physiological responses to midbrain stimulation in the cat. Br Res 128:542–546

Cunningham DJ, Stolwijk JAJ, Murakami N, Hardy JD (1967) Responses of neurons in the preoptic area to temperature, serotonin, and epinephrine. Am J Physiol 213:1570–1581

Dinarello CA (1979) Production of endogenous pyrogen. Fed Proc 38:52–56

Downey JA, Darling RC (1962) Effect of salicylate on elevation of body temperature during exercise. J Appl Physiol 17:323–325

Edinger HM, Eisenman JS (1970) Thermosensitive neurons in tuberal and posterior hypothalamus of cats. Am J Physiol 219:1098–1103

Eisenman JS (1969) Pyrogen-induced changes in the thermosensitivity of septal and preoptic neurons. Am J Physiol 216:330–334

Eisenman JS (1972) Unit activity studies of thermoresponsive neurons. In: Bligh J, Moore RE (eds) Essays in temperature regulation. North-Holland, Amsterdam, pp 55–69

Eisenman JS (1974a) Depression of preoptic thermosensitivity by bacterial pyrogen in rabbits. Am J Physiol 227:1067–1073

Eisenman JS (1974b) Unit studies of brainstem projections to the preoptic area and hypothalamus. In: Lederis K, Cooper KE (eds) Recent studies of hypothalamic function. Karger, Basel, pp 328–340

Eisenman JS (1976) Sensory organs and thermogenesis. Isr J Med Sci 12:916–923

Eisenman JS, Jackson DC (1967) Thermal response patterns of septal and preoptic neurons in cats. Exp Neurol 19:33–45

Euler C von, Söderberg U (1957) The influence of hypothalamic thermoreceptive structures on the electroencephalogram and gamma motor activity. Electroencephalog Clin Neurophysiol 9:391–408

Evans MH, Frens J, Bligh J (1972) Unaltered activity of tongue temperature sensors after administration of pyrogen to rabbits. Eur J Pharmacol 18:333–337

Ford DM (1974) A selective action of prostaglandin E_1 on hypothalamic neurons in the cat which respond to brain cooling. J Physiol (Lond) 242:142P–143P

Fukuda Y, Loeschke HH (1977) Effect of H^+ on spontaneous neuronal activity in the surface layer of the rat medulla oblongata in vitro. Pfluegers Arch 371:125–134

Fusco MM, Hardy JD, Hammel HT (1961) Interaction of central and peripheral factors in physiological temperature regulation. Am J Physiol 200:572–580

Geller HM, Hoffer B (1977) Effect of calcium removal on monoamine-elicited depressions of cultured tuberal neurons. J Neurobiol 8:43–55

Gordon CJ, Heath JE (1979) The effect of prostaglandin E_2 on the firing rate of thermally sensitive and insensitive neurons in the preoptic/anterior hypothalamus of unanesthetized rabbits. Fed Proc 38:1295

Guieu JD, Hardy JD (1970) Effects of heating and cooling of the spinal cord on preoptic unit activity. J Appl Physiol 29:675–683

Hammel HT, Hardy JD, Fusco MM (1960) Thermoregulatory responses to hypothalamic cooling in unanesthetized dogs. Am J Physiol 198:481–486

Hammouda M (1933) The central and reflex mechanisms of panting. J Physiol (Lond) 77:319–336

Hardy JD (1972) Peripheral inputs to the central regulator for body temperature. In: Ito S, Ogata K, Yoshimura H (eds) Advances in climatic physiology. Igaku Shoin, Tokyo, pp 3–21

Hardy JD, Hellon RF, Sutherland K (1964) Temperature-sensitive neurons in the dog's hypothalamus. J Physiol (Lond) 175:242–253

Hatton GI, Armstrong WE, Gregory WA (1978) Spontaneous and osmotically-stimulated activity in slices of rat hypothalamus. Br Res Bull 3:497–508

Hayward JN (1977) Functional and morphological aspects of hypothalamic neurons. Physiol Rev 57:574–658

Hedqvist P (1973) Autonomic transmission. In: Ramwell PW (ed) The prostaglandins, vol 1. Plenum, New York, pp 101–131

Hellon RF (1967) Thermal stimulation of hypothalamic neurones in unanesthetized rabbits. J Physiol (Lond) 193:381–395

Hellon RF (1970) The stimulation of hypothalamic neurones by changes in ambient temperature. Pfluegers Arch 321:56–66

Hellon RF (1972a) Temperature-sensitive neurones in the brain stem: their responses to brain temperature at different ambient temperatures. Pfluegers Arch 335:323–334

Hellon RF (1972b) Central thermoreceptors and thermoregulation. In: Neil E (ed) Enteroreceptors. Handbook of sensory physiology, vol III/1. Springer, Berlin Heidelberg New York, pp 161–186

Hellon RF (1975) Monoamines, pyrogens and cations: their actions on central control of body temperature. Pharmacol Rev 26:289–321

Hensel H (1973) Neural processes in thermoregulation. Physiol Rev 53:948–1017

Hori T, Nakayama T (1973) Effect of biogenic amines on central thermoresponsive neurons in the rabbit. J Physiol (Lond) 232:71–85

Jackson DL (1967) A hypothalamic region responsive to localized injection of pyrogens. J Neurophysiol 30:586–602

Jahns R, Werner J (1974a) Special aspects of firing rates and thermosensitivity of preoptic neurons. Exp Brain Res 21:107–112

Jahns R, Werner J (1974b) Analysis of periodic components of hypothalamic spike-trains after central thermal stimulation. Pfluegers Arch 351:13–24

Jell RM (1973) Responses of hypothalamic neurones to local temperature and to acetylcholine, noradrenaline and 5-hydroxytryptamine. Brain Res 55:123–134

Jell RM (1974) Responses of rostral hypothalamic neurones to peripheral temperature and to amines. J Physiol (Lond) 240:295–307

Jell RM, Gloor P (1972) Distribution of thermosensitive and nonthermosensitive preoptic and anterior hypothalamic neurons in unanesthetized cats, and effects of some anesthetics. Can J Physiol Pharmacol 50:890–901

Jell RM, Sweatman P (1976) Actions of prostaglandin synthetase inhibitors on rostral hypothalamic neurones: thermoregulation and biogenic amines. Can J Physiol Pharmacol 54:161–166

Jell RM, Sweatman P (1977) Prostaglandin-sensitive neurones in cat hypothalamus: relation to thermoregulation and to biogenic amines. Can J Physiol Pharmacol 55:560–567

Jessen C (1976) Two dimensional determination of thermosensitive sites within the goat's hypothalamus. J Appl Physiol 40:514–520

Kahn RH (1904) Über die Erwärmung des Carotidenblutes. Arch Anat Physiol (Leipzig) [Suppl] 28:81–134

Klussman FW (1964) The influence of temperature on the activity of spinal α and γ motoneurones. Experientia 20:450

Knox GV, Campbell C, Lomax P (1973a) The effects of acetylcholine and nicotine on unit activity in the hypothalamic thermoregulatory centers of the rat. Brain Res 51:215–223

Knox GV, Campbell C, Lomax P (1973b) Cutaneous temperature and unit activity in the hypothalamic thermoregulatory centers. Exp Neurol 40:717–730

Koepchen HP, Langhorst P, Seller H (1975) The problem of identification of autonomic neurons in the lower brain stem. Brain Res 87:375–393

Kozyreva TV (1972) The influence of local fluctuations of brain temperature on unit activity in the sensorimotor cortex of rabbits. Fiziol Zh 58:1663–1668

Krnjević K, Laverty R, Sharman DF (1963) Iontophoretic release of adrenaline, noradrenaline and 5-hydroxytryptamine from micropipettes. Br J Pharmacol 20:491–496

Levitan H, Barker JC (1972) Membrane permeability: cation selectivity reversibly altered by salicylate. Science 178:63–64

Lin MT (1978) Effects of sodium acetylsalicylate on thermoregulatory responses of rats to different ambient temperatures. Pfluegers Arch 378:181–184

Lin MT, Chai CY (1975) Effect of sodium acetylsalicylate on body temperature of monkeys under heat exposure. J Pharmacol Exp Ther 194:165–170

Lipton JM (1973) Thermosensitivity of medulla oblongata in control of body temperature. Am J Physiol 224:890–897

Lipton JM, Kennedy JI (1979) Central thermosensitivity during fever produced by intra-PO/AH and intravenous injections of pyrogen. Brain Res Bull 4:23–34

Lipton JM, Welch JP, Clark WG (1973) Changes in body temperature produced by injecting prostaglandin E_1, EGTA and bacterial pyrogen into PO/AH region and the medulla oblongata of the rat. Experientia 29:806–808

MacPherson RK (1959) The effect of fever on temperature regulation in man. Clin Sci 18:281–287

Magoun HW, Harrison F, Brobeck JR, Ranson SW (1938) Activation of heat loss mechanisms by local heating of the brain. J Neurophysiol 1:101–114

Mason P, Hasan H, Valis M (1978) Spontaneous firing of hypothalamic neurones over a narrow temperature interval. Nature 273:242–243

Metcalf G, Myers RD (1978) Precise location within the preoptic area where noradrenaline produces hypothermia. Eur J Pharmacol 51:47–53

Milton AS, Wendlandt S (1971) Effect on body temperature of prostaglandins of the A, E and F series on injection into the third ventricle of unanesthetized cats and rabbits. J Physiol (Lond) 218:325–336

Murakami N (1973) Effect of iontophoretic application of 5-hydroxytryptamine, noradrenaline and acetylcholine upon hypothalamic temperature-sensitive neurones in rats. Jpn J Physiol 23:435–446

Murakami N (1974) A statistical analysis of spontaneous activity of the temperature-sensitive neurones in hypothalamus of rats. Bull Yamaguchi Med Sch 21:17–30

Murakami N, Sakata Y (1975) Effects of antipyretics on normothermic rabbits. Jpn J Physiol 28:29–40

Murakami N, Sakata Y (1979) Statistical analysis of the discharge patterns of medullary temperature-sensitive neurones in rabbits. Neurosci Lett 11:49–52

Murakami N, Stolwijk JAJ, Hardy JD (1967) Responses of preoptic neurons to anesthetics and peripheral stimulation. Am J Physiol 213:1015–1024

Murakami N, Uchimura H, Sakata Y (1979) Comparison of thermosensitivity of the preoptic/anterior hypothalamic area and the midbrain of the rabbit. Pfluegers Arch 379:113–116

Myers RD, Rudy TA, Yaksh TL (1974) Fever produced by endotoxin injected into the hypothalamus of the monkey and its antagonism by salicylate. J Physiol (Lond) 243:167–193

Nakayama T, Hardy JD (1969) Unit responses in the rabbit's brain stem to changes in brain and cutaneous temperature. J Appl Physiol 27:848–857

Nakayama T, Hori T (1973) Effects of anesthetic and pyrogen on thermally sensitive neurons in the brainstem. J Appl Physiol 34:351–355

Nakayama T, Eisenman JS, Hardy JD (1961) Single unit activity of anterior hypothalamus during local heating. Science 134:560–561

Nakayama T, Hammel HT, Hardy JD, Eisenman JS (1963) Thermal stimulation of electrical activity of single units of the preoptic region. Am J Physiol 204:1122–1126

Nakayama T, Hori T, Suzuki M, Yonezawa T, Yamamoto K (1978) Thermo-sensitive neurons in preoptic and anterior hypothalamic tissue cultures in vitro. Neurosci Lett 9:23–26

Perkel DH, Gerstein GL, Moore GP (1967) Neuronal spike trains and stochastic point processes: I. The single spike train. Biophys J 2:391–418

Phillip-Dormston WK (1976) Einfluß von Endotoxinen auf Temperaturregulation und Synthese von Transmittersubstanzen im Kaninchenhirn. Zentralbl Bakteriol [Orig A] 235:42–47

Pierau F-K, Klee MR, Klussman FW (1976) Effect of temperature on postsynaptic potentials of cat spinal motoneurones. Brain Res 114:21–34

Polk DL, Lipton JM (1975) Effects of sodium salicylate, aminopyrine and chlorpromazine on behavioral temperature regulation. Pharmacol Biochem Behav 3:167–172

Poulain P, Carette B (1974) Iontophoresis of prostaglandins on hypothalamic neurons. Brain Res 79:311–314

Reaves TA (1977) Gain of thermosensitive neurons in the preoptic area of the rabbit, Oryctolagus cuniculus. J Theor Biol 2:31–33

Reaves TA, Heath JE (1975) Interval coding of temperature by CNS neurones in thermoregulation. Nature 257:688–690

Robinson HJ, Vane JR (eds) (1974) Prostaglandin synthetase inhibitors – their effects on physiological function and pathological states. Raven, New York

Rosendorff C, Mooney JJ (1971) Central nervous system sites of action of a purified leucocyte pyrogen. Am J Physiol 220:597–603

Rudy TA, Williams JW, Yaksh TL (1977) Antagonism by indomethacin of neurogenic hyperthermia produced by unilateral puncture of the anterior hypothalamic/preoptic area. J Physiol (Lond) 272:721–736

Salmoiraghi GC, Weight F (1967) Micromethods in neuropharmacology; an approach to the study of anesthetics. Anesthesiology 28:54–64

Satinoff E (1972) Salicylate: action on normal body temperature in rats. Science 176:532–533

Schoener EP, Wang SC (1975) Leucocyte pyrogen and sodium acetylsalicylate on hypothalamic neurons in the cat. Am J Physiol 229:185–190

Schoener EP, Wang SC (1976) Effects of locally administered prostaglandin E_1 on anterior hypothalamic neurons. Brain Res 117:157–162

Simon E (1974) Temperature regulation: the spinal cord as a site of extrahypotalamic thermoregulatory functions. Rev Physiol Biochem Pharmacol 71:1–76

Simon E, Hammel HT, Oksche A (1977) Thermosensitivity of single units in the hypothalamus of the conscious Pekin duck. J Neurobiol 8:523–535

Speulda E, Wünnenberg W (1977) Thermosensitivity of preoptic neurons in a hibernator at high and low ambient temperatures. Pfluegers Arch 370:107–109

Stitt JT (1979) Fever versus hypothermia. Fed Proc 38:39–43

Stitt JT, Hardy JD (1975) Microelectrophoresis of PGE_1 onto single units in rabbit hypothalamus. Am J Physiol 229:240–245

Stitt JT, Hardy JD, Stolwijk JAJ (1974) PGE fever: its effect on thermoregulation at different low ambient temperatures. Am J Physiol 227:622–629

Towe AL, Harding GW (1970) Extracellular microelectrode sampling bias. Exp Neurol 29:366–381

Vane JR (1971) Inhibition of prostaglandin synthesis as a mechanism of action for action for aspirin-like drugs. Nature New Biol 231:232–235

Veale WL, Whishaw IQ (1976) Body temperature responses at different ambient temperatures following injection of prostaglandin E_1 and noradrenaline into the brain. Pharmacol Biochem Behav 4:143–150

Veale WL, Cooper KE, Pittman QJ (1977) Role of prostaglandins in fever and temperature regulation. In: Ramwell PW (ed) Prostaglandins, vol 3. Plenum, New York, pp 145–167

Villablanca J, Myers RD (1965) Fever produced by microinjection of typhoid vaccine into hypothalamus of cats. Am J Physiol 208:703–707

Williams JW, Rudy TA, Yaksh TL, Viswanathan CT (1977) An extensive exploration of the rat brain for sites mediating prostaglandin-induced hyperthermia. Brain Res 120:251–262

Wit A, Wang SC (1968a) Temperature-sensitive neurons in preoptic/anterior hypothalamic region: effect of increasing ambient temperature. Am J Physiol 215:1151–1159

Wit A, Wang SC (1968b) Temperature-sensitive neurons in preoptic/anterior hypothalamic region: actions of pyrogens and acetylsalicylate. Am J Physiol 215:1160–1169

Wünnenberg W, Hardy JD (1972) Responses of single units of the posterior hypothalamus to thermal stimulation. J Appl Physiol 33:547–552

Wünnenberg W, Merker G, Speulda E (1976) Thermosensitivity of preoptic neurones in hibernator (golden hamster) and a non-hibernator (guinea pig). Pfluegers Arch 363:119–123

Yamamoto C, Chujo T (1978) Long-term potentiation in thin hippocampal sections studied by intracellular and extracellular recordings. Exp Neurol 58:242–251

Ziel R, Krupp P (1976) Influence of endogenous pyrogen on the cerebral prostaglandin-synthetase system. Experientia 32:1451–1453

CHAPTER 9

Cyclic Nucleotides and Fever*

M. J. DASCOMBE

A. Introduction

The events taking place intracellularly within the central nervous system when pyrogens, putative neurotransmitters or other pharmacologically active substances raise body temperature during fever are poorly understood. Recognition of cyclic AMP as an intracellular mediator of adrenaline and glucagon-induced activation of hepatic glycolysis (SUTHERLAND and RALL 1960) may further the understanding of these central events. Cyclic AMP is at present thought to modulate metabolic activities in many tissue and cell types including those of the mammalian brain (see reviews by WEISS and KIDMAN 1969; GREENGARD and COSTA 1970; ROBISON et al. 1971; BLOOM 1975; DALY 1975a, b; DRUMMOND and MA 1975; KEBABIAN 1977; NATHANSON 1977).

Characterization of this so-called second messenger system has depended extensively on the use of biological systems reduced to the cellular or subcellular levels of organization. The physiological significance of the control mechanisms demonstrated in these simplified but not necessarily simple systems is not always readily apparent. In the case of the mammalian central nervous system, the apparent lack of significance may, as KEBABIAN (1977) suggested, reflect the inadequacy of our understanding of the physiology of the brain. Despite this ignorance and in an attempt to dispel it, the question arises as to whether the effects observed in vitro, as a consequence of perturbing the cyclic AMP system, also occur in the intact animal. It is of unquestionable benefit to the research worker attempting to substantiate in vivo the role (or roles) of cyclic AMP in the brain, to monitor a centrally mediated effect about which more rather than less is known. Few, if any such activities have been documented as extensively as the hyperthermia or fever associated with infection by micro-organisms. Determination of an involvement of cyclic AMP in the brain during the febrile response to pyrogens would serve not only to extend present knowledge of the pathogenesis of fever but could conceivably indicate the function of the cyclic nucleotide throughout the mammalian central nervous system.

---

* Abbreviations used in this chapter: AMP, adenosine 5'-monophosphate; ADP, adenosine 5'-diphosphate; ATP, adenosine 5'-triphosphate; cyclic AMP, adenosine 3',5'-monophosphate; cyclic GMP, guanosine 3',5'-monophosphate; Db-cAMP, N^6-2'-O-dibutyryl adenosine 3',5'-monophosphate; Db-cGMP, N^2-2'-O-dibutyryl guanosine 3',5'-monophosphate; GMP, guanosine 5'-monophosphate; GTP, guanosine 5'-triphosphate

B. Temperature Responses to Cyclic AMP in Different Species

Cyclic AMP does not readily penetrate cell membranes because of its phospory-lated nature (POSTERNAK 1971). In addition, the nucleotide is a substrate for cyclic nucleotide phosphodiesterase (SUTHERLAND and RALL 1958; DRUMMOND and PER-ROTT-YEE 1961; BUTCHER and SUTHERLAND 1962). These factors are thought to limit the efficacy of exogenous cyclic AMP in biological systems. In order to mimic the actions of endogenous intracellular cyclic AMP it is generally thought neces-sary to administer a derivative of the parent compound, for example Db-cAMP which may gain access more readily than cyclic AMP to the cell interior and is less susceptible to hydrolysis by cyclic nucleotide phosphodiesterase (POSTERNAK et al. 1962; HENION et al. 1967; CHEUNG 1970a; DRUMMOND and POWELL 1970; KAUKEL and HILZ 1972). Db-cAMP may serve as an intracellular source of cyclic AMP and/or biologically active metabolites such as N^6-monobutyryl cyclic AMP (HENION et al. 1967; KAUKEL and HILZ 1972; KAUKEL et al. 1972; NEELON and BIRCH 1973; SIGGINS and HENRIKSEN 1975) produced by N^6-butyryl aminohy-drolase and 2'-0-butyrylesterase activities present in tissues (BLECHER and HUNT 1972). There are reports, however, of Db-cAMP being less, not more, active than cyclic AMP in eliciting biological responses (KIM et al. 1968; RYAN and HEIDRICK 1968) and producing effects different from those of the parent nucleotide on vari-ous preparations including skeletal muscle (CHAMBAUT et al. 1969), melanophores (HADLEY and GOLDMAN 1969), intestinal smooth muscle (BOWMAN and HALL 1970), HeLa cells (HILZ and TARNOWSKI 1970), and isolated fat cells (SOLOMON et al. 1970). Divergent biological effects of cyclic AMP and Db-cAMP may be a con-sequence of different binding affinities of cyclic AMP and N^6-monobutyryl cyclic AMP to cyclic AMP-dependent protein kinase (NEELON and BIRCH 1973).

I. Mice

Db-cAMP (25 µg) injected intracerebroventricularly in a volume of 10 µl by the method of BRITTAIN and HANDLEY (1967) has been reported to produce no overt changes in either body temperature or behaviour over a period of 6 h in mice at an ambient temperature of $21° \pm 1$ °C (DOGGETT and SPENCER 1971). From the re-sults presented by DOGGETT and SPENCER, however, it appears that Db-cAMP may produce hypothermia in the mouse (Fig. 1). Paradoxically, the rate of recovery of body temperature from hypothermia induced by central injection of ouabain (DOGGETT and SPENCER 1971) or intraperitoneal injection of reserpine (DOGGETT and SPENCER 1973) is increased by Db-cAMP injected into the cerebral ventricles of mice although no thermogenic effect of the nucleotide was observed.

In contrast with the latter observations on behaviour, reduced locomotor activ-ity for up to 10 min after intracerebroventricular injection of Db-cAMP (10 µg) in-to mice was observed by LEONARD (1972) associated with a concomitant increase in brain glycolysis. HERMAN and SZKILNIK (1977) found Db-cAMP (10 µg or 20 µg) injected intracerebroventricularly produced a stuporous state with convulsive episodes in mice, with an onset 30 min after injection and lasting up to approxi-mately 2 h. Neither LEONARD (1972) nor HERMAN and SZKILNIK (1977) report the effects, if any, of Db-cAMP on body temperature concomitant with the observed

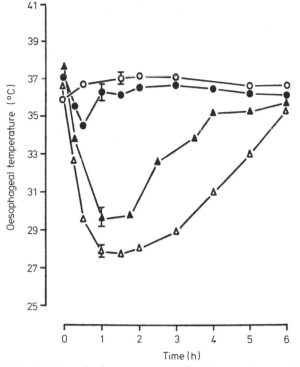

Fig. 1. Effect of Db-cAMP on body temperature after intracerebroventricular injection in mice at time *zero*. Vertical lines define standard error of the mean. 10 µl saline (*open circles*); Db-cAMP 25 µg (*solid circles*); Db-cAMP 25 µg + ouabain 0.3 µg (*solid triangles*); ouabain 0.3 µg (*open triangles*). (After DOGGETT and SPENCER 1971)

changes in locomotor activity. The observation by WATANABE and PASSONNEAU (1974, 1975) that stab wound damage to brain tissue causes an increase in brain tissue levels of cyclic AMP in mice makes estimation of the effective concentration of cyclic AMP at the site of injection difficult.

Intraperitoneal injection of Db-cAMP into mice maintained at an ambient temperature of 22° ± 1 °C induces a dose-related (10–75 mg/kg) decrease in spontaneous locomotor activity and exploratory activity in addition to eliciting mild diarrhoea and urination (WEINER and OLSON 1973). Behavioural effects of Db-cAMP administered intraperitoneally were not observed if mice were treated 24 h earlier with the compound. Although WEINER and OLSON (1973) do not report on the temperature effects of Db-cAMP in mice, their data indicate that peripheral injection of Db-cAMP can induce behavioural responses which may be of central origin and to which tolerance rapidly develops.

II. Rats

Implantation of solid Db-cAMP (500 µg) into the anterior hypothalamus or the arcuate nucleus produces hyperthermia in rats (BRECKENRIDGE and LISK 1969). In this study cyclic AMP had a similar but less potent effect on body temperature to that of Db-cAMP, whereas AMP was without effect. Various non-thermoregulatory responses to Db-cAMP were also induced including lengthening of the oestrous cycle, pseudopregnancy, aggression, hyperphagia, and increased locomotor activity. Increased locomotor activity together with convulsions, salivation, and vocalization lasting up to 4 h have been reported by HERMAN (1973) in response to Db-cAMP dissolved in artificial cerebrospinal fluid. Solutions (20 μl) of Db-cAMP were injected into a lateral cerebral ventricle in rats and doses of 100 μg or 200 μg were effective but not 50 μg Db-cAMP. In this study, cyclic AMP (100–400 μg) was without effect on behaviour unless rats were pre-treated with the cyclic nucleotide phosphodiesterase inhibitor, theophylline (100 mg/kg intraperitoneally) and/or dimethylsulphoxide (100 μg intracerebroventricularly) where upon cyclic AMP induced behavioural effects in some rats similar to those produced by Db-cAMP. HERMAN (1973) makes no report on the effects, if any, of cyclic AMP or Db-cAMP on body temperature in rats. The effect of intrahypothalamic injection of Db-cAMP on food intake by rats, reported to be hyperphagia by BRECKENRIDGE and LISK (1969) appears to be a variable response and may be an enlargement or a diminution of meal size (BOOTH 1972). Water intake may be increased by injection of Db-cAMP into the lateral hypothalamus in the rat (RINDI et al. 1972). It is not clear, therefore, whether the hyperthermic response to cyclic AMP and Db-cAMP in the rat (BRECKENRIDGE and LISK 1969) is thermoregulatory or a non-specific effect secondary to other centrally evoked responses. Administration of Db-cAMP into a lateral cerebral ventricle attentuates pentobarbitone-induced narcosis but not barbiturate-induced hypothermia (ISOM et al. 1978).

III. Rabbits

Cyclic AMP or Db-cAMP (20–500 μg) injected into a lateral cerebral ventricle produces a fall in rectal temperature in rabbits, the response to 500 μg cyclic AMP being comparable to that produced by 20 μg Db-cAMP (DUFF et al. 1972). With higher doses, hypothermia is followed by a rise in body temperature beginning not less than 90 min after central injection. PHILIPP-DORMSTON and SIEGERT (1975a) report the effect of Db-cAMP on body temperature after injection into a lateral cerebral ventricle to be dose dependent in rabbits. Doses of Db-cAMP up to 15 μg/kg were without effect but 25 μg/kg or 50 μg/kg produced a slight decrease in rectal temperature lasting about 20 min, which was followed by a rise in temperature up to 2 °C above control values. Changes in body temperature were associated with increased pulmonary ventilation and increased locomotor activity. Two hours after injection of Db-cAMP (25 or 50 μg/kg) body temperature and behaviour began to return towards normal values. PHILIPP-DORMSTON and SIEGERT (1975a) found that higher doses of Db-cAMP (75–200 μg/kg) elicit a rapid rise in rectal temperature associated with recurrent episodes of locomotor hyperactivity, catatonia, and convulsions culminating in death for some rabbits. In contrast with the hypothermic effect of cyclic AMP reported by DUFF et al. (1972), PHILIPP-DORMSTON and SIEGERT (1975a) found administration of cyclic AMP in doses up to 100 μg/kg into a lateral cerebral ventricle to be without effect on body temperature as was intravenous injection of cyclic AMP or Db-cAMP in doses up to 1.5 mg/kg.

LABURN et al. (1974) localized a dose-dependent hyperthermic effect of Db-cAMP in the preoptic/anterior hypothalamic area in rabbits. A maximum rise in body temperature of over 1.8 °C was produced by 2.5 µg Db-cAMP injected unilaterally at this site. In subsequent studies by these workers (WILLIES et al. 1976a; WOOLF et al. 1976) 3 µg Db-cAMP injected similarly into rabbits evoked a smaller rise in temperature, approximately 0.5 °C. Bilateral injection of Db-cAMP into the hypothalamus produces hyperthermia which is dose dependent over the range 0.25–10 µg (WOOLF et al. 1975). Doses of 5 µg and 10 µg Db-cAMP induce prolonged febrile responses but these are not as great in amplitude as the response to 2.5 µg Db-cAMP. Hyperthermia was associated with marked vasoconstriction and some shivering. Hyperexcitability was apparent in about one-third of the rabbits used and culminated in death for some animals. Hyperthermia in response to intrahypothalamic administration of Db-cAMP is not preceded by hypothermia in the rabbit (WOOLF et al. 1975; WILLIES et al. 1976a) and is apparently resistant to the antipyretic action of sodium salicylate (WILLIES et al. 1976b).

IV. Cats

In a study of the behavioural effects produced by seemingly non-sterile injections of Db-cAMP (50–500 µg) into the anterior hypothalamus of the cat, GESSA et al. (1970) reported the incidence of hyperthermia associated with piloerection and panting together with non-thermoregulatory behavioural and autonomic activities including increased locomotor activity, convulsions, mydriasis, salivation, micturition, and defecation. VARAGIĆ and BELESLIN (1973) and CLARK et al. (1974) reported a dose-dependent hyperthermic response to Db-cAMP (20–1,000 µg) injected into a lateral cerebral ventricle in cats. The rise in body temperature was sustained for 12 h or more and was associated with sedation. CLARK et al. (1974) found the onset of hyperthermia to be about 3 h after intracerebroventricular injection of Db-cAMP and the hyperthermia to be attenuated by indomethacin or paracetamol (Fig. 2). In some experiments prolonged hyperthermia in response to Db-cAMP was preceded by a fall in rectal temperature (VARAGIĆ and BELESLIN 1973; CLARK et al. 1974). Hypothermia had an onset within 30 min and a duration of 1–3 h, a maximal fall in body temperature of 1.9 °C being observed by CLARK and his colleagues. A transient rise in body temperature lasting 30–60 min and accompanied by increased locomotor activity and other evidence of psychomotor stimulation was seen by CLARK et al. (1974) in some cats before the onset of the aforementioned sustained hyperthermia. These workers concluded that the transient rise was secondary to general central nervous system stimulation. Four of the ten cats used in this study died within 1 h of administration of Db-cAMP (750–1,000 µg), death being associated with a rapid increase in body temperature and convulsions. On the basis that Db-cAMP caused many hyperthermic responses without hypothermia or observable excitement, but never caused hypothermia or excitement without the subsequent development of hyperthermia, CLARK et al. (1974) favoured the sustained hyperthermia as the principal effect of Db-cAMP. In contrast with this conclusion, VARAGIĆ and BELESLIN (1973) found that injection of ATP or butyrate (unspecified metal) into a lateral cerebral ventricle also produced a long-lasting hyperthermia in cats and concluded it to be possible that the sustained rise in body

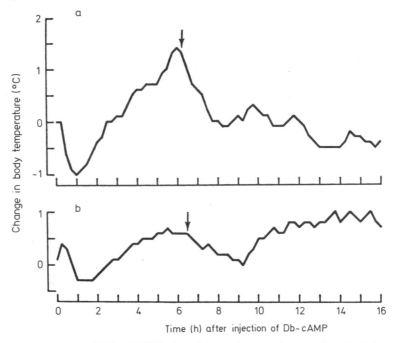

Fig. 2 a, b. Reduction of Db-cAMP-induced hyperthermia in cats by (**a**) indomethacin 40 µg/kg and (**b**) paracetamol 20 mg/kg injected intravenously at the times indicated by the *arrows*. Individual responses. (After CLARK et al. 1974)

temperature produced by Db-cAMP could be produced by an action not related specifically to the cyclic nucleotide. VARAGIĆ and BELESLIN (1973) considered the biphasic effect consisting of hypothermia followed by hyperthermia to represent a genuine response to Db-cAMP despite being seen in only one-third of their experiments.

Db-cAMP injected into the preoptic/anterior hypothalamic area in cats at an ambient temperture of $22° \pm 2 °C$ produces a fall in rectal temperature which is dose dependent over the range 50–500 µg (DASCOMBE and MILTON 1975 a). Hypothermia had an onset within 20 min and was maximal, as much as 1 °C below control values, 60–90 min after injection. The fall in body temperature in response to Db-cAMP was associated with ear skin vasodilatation, polypnoea, panting, and occasionally sweating from the paw pads. After this period, body temperature returned to pre-injection values 2–3 h after injection accompanied by peripheral vasoconstriction and shivering. Db-cAMP, particularly higher doses in the range 50–500 µg injected into the preoptic/anterior hypothalamic area, induced non-thermoregulatory behavioural and autonomic activities similar to those described by GESSA et al. (1970), following intrahypothalamic administration, and by MCKEAN et al. (1969), after intracerebroventricular injection. In the study of DASCOMBE and MILTON (1975 a) behavioural and autonomic responses to Db-cAMP lasted less than 3 h whereas GESSA et al. (1970) reported a duration of many hours. A sustained hyperthermia accompanied by sedation, cutaneous vasoconstriction and shivering was observed by DASCOMBE and MILTON in some, but not all, cats after the consistent hypothermic response to Db-cAMP injected into the preoptic/anterior hypothalamic area. Long-lasting hyperthermia in response to Db-cAMP was seen only in those cats responding to intrahypothalamic injections of vehicle, with or without the addition of sodium chloride or sodium *n*-butyrate, with a similar rise in body temperature and was attenuated or abolished by paracetamol. It appears, therefore, that central injections (VARAGIĆ and BELESLIN 1973; DASCOMBE and MILTON 1975a) or intracerebroventricular perfusions (FELDBERG et al. 1970) can produce a non-specific and long-lasting rise in body temperature in cats, possibly as a result of tissue damage and prostaglandin release about the site of injection (DEY et al. 1974). It is not possible to determine from these micro-injection studies to what extent increased synthesis of prostaglandins may be a direct consequence of the substance injected. A transient rise in body temperature seen first after intrahypothalamic injection of Db-cAMP was seen in some cats by DASCOMBE and MILTON (1975a), and may have been due to general stimulation of the central nervous system made manifest as increased locomotor activity, as suggested by CLARK et al. (1974). In some of the experiments in this study, however, the apparent hyperthermia of brief duration may have been the consequence of the hypothermic response to Db-cAMP having onset after the initiation of a tissue-damage fever. Cyclic AMP injected into the preoptic/anterior hypothalamic area has a similar but less potent hypothermic effect in the cat to that produced by Db-cAMP (DASCOMBE and MILTON 1975a). The fall in body temperature was associated with slight cutaneous vasodilatation only, the extreme hyperactivity and agitation produced by the dibutyryl derivative of the nucleotide were not elicited by the parent compound. Sustained hyperthermia was apparent after hypothermia induced by cyclic AMP only in those cats responding to intrahypothalamic injections of vehicle with a similar sustained rise in body temperature. DASCOMBE and MILTON concluded the predominant effect of cyclic AMP and Db-cAMP injected into the preoptic/anterior hypothalamic area to be hypothermia, and consequently considered it unlikely that cyclic AMP in this region of the brain mediates fever in cats.

Localized application of ATP, ADP, and AMP to the preoptic/anterior hypothalamic area, in quantities equimolar with 250 µg and 500 µg Db-cAMP, produce qualitatively similar effects on body temperature in the cat to those of Db-cAMP (DASCOMBE and MILTON 1975a). Hypothermia and associated heat loss activity, primarily cutaneous vasodilatation, appear to be common effects of the adenine nucleotides in the cat (Fig. 3), effects which may be independent of the cyclic structure of cyclic AMP. A localized increase in free Ca^{2+} ions was suggested by DASCOMBE and MILTON (1975a) as a possible common basis of hypothermia in response to adenine nucleotides since DUFFY and SCHWARZ (1974) have reported a non-specific displacement of Ca^{2+} ions from isolated erythrocyte membranes in response to cyclic AMP and ATP. This hypothesis is supported by the observation that when DASCOMBE and MILTON (1975a) injected Ca^{2+} ions, in quantities equimolar with the doses of adenine nucleotides used, into the preoptic/anterior hypothalamic area, hypothermia was produced in cats. It is possible, however, that administration of non-cyclic nucleotides may increase levels of endogenous cyclic AMP in brain tissue (SATTIN and RALL 1970).

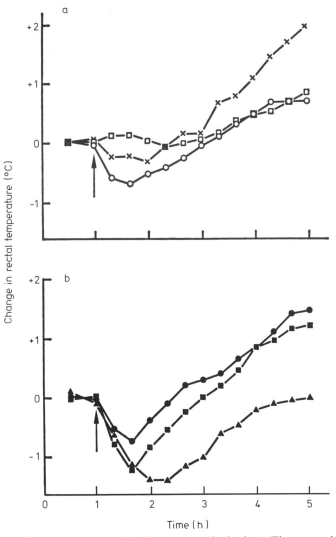

Fig. 3 a, b. Rectal temperature records of an unanaesthetized cat. The *arrows* indicate injection of 2.5 μl drug solution into the optic chiasma, 1 mm ventral to the preoptic/anterior hypothalamic area. **a** 0.9% NaCl (*open squares*); cyclic AMP 0.48 μmol (*crosses*); AMP 0.48 μmol (*open circles*). **b** ADP 0.48 μmol (*solid circles*); ATP 0.48 μmol (*solid squares*); Db-cAMP 0.48 μmol (*solid triangles*). (After DASCOMBE and MILTON 1975 a)

Cyclic AMP (5 and 10 mg/kg) injected intravenously evokes hypothermia in cats at an ambient temperature of $22° \pm 2$ °C (DASCOMBE and MILTON 1975 b, 1976). Cyclic AMP in doses of 0.1 mg/kg and 1 mg/kg was without effect on body temperature after intravenous administration. Hypothermia had an onset in 2–3 min and was associated with ear skin vasodilatation. In one cat, in response to cyclic AMP 10 mg/kg, polypnoea and sweating from the paw pads were also seen. Maximum falls in rectal temperature, 0.3°–0.5 °C below control values, were produced by intravenous cyclic AMP (5 or 10 mg/kg) within 30 min. Body tempera-

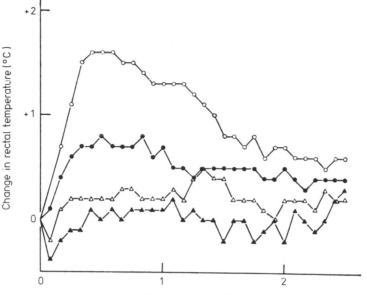

Fig. 4. Effects on rectal temperature in the squirrel monkey of bilateral intracerebral injections of Db-cAMP and prostaglandin E_1 into the same brain sites. Injection sites were previously shown to be sensitive to *S. typhosa* endotoxin. PGE_1 500 ng (*solid circles*); PGE_1 750 ng (*open circles*); Db-cAMP 500 ng (*solid triangles*); Db-cAMP 750 ng (*open triangles*). (After LIPTON and FOSSLER 1974)

ture returned to pre-injection values 3–4 h after injection of cyclic AMP. Hypothermia in response to cyclic AMP administered intravenously may be a centrally mediated effect, because it has been shown that the cyclic nucleotide can enter the cerebrospinal fluid from the blood (DASCOMBE and MILTON 1975c, 1976). However, heat loss consequent to a direct vasodilatory effect of cyclic AMP cannot be discounted (PETTINGER et al. 1970).

V. Dogs

ONO et al. (1976) found Db-cAMP (10–100 mg/kg) injected into a cephalic vein had no significant effect on body temperature in dogs despite production of decreased locomotor activity, vomiting, and diarrhoea. In one experiment, Db-cAMP 300 mg/kg induced tonic convulsions culminating in death. Cyclic AMP (100 mg/kg), sodium butyrate, and butyric acid injected intravenously into dogs in this study were without significant behavioural or vegetative effect.

VI. Primates

Db-cAMP (500–750 ng) injected bilaterally into the preoptic/anterior hypothalamic area is reported to have no consistent effect on body temperature in the squirrel monkey at an ambient temperature of $23° \pm 0.5$ °C (LIPTON and FOSSLER 1974). Although results presented by LIPTON and FOSSLER indicate a slight hypothermic effect to 500 ng and 750 ng Db-cAMP (Fig. 4), the lack of a marked effect on body temperature in the primate could be due to insufficient nucleotide being administered since microgram quantities of Db-cAMP are found necessary to alter body temperature in other species (Table 1). In one monkey, however, Lipton and Fossler (1974) found bilateral application of 75 µg Db-cAMP to be without effect on body temperature.

VII. Birds

Db-cAMP injected into the hypothalamus (0.1–0.2 µmol, approximately 49–98 µg) or into the third cerebral ventricle (1 µmol, equivalent to about 491 µg) of adult fowls maintained at an ambient temperature of 20°–25 °C produces a rise in body temperature (Marley and Nistico 1972). Hyperthermia began within 30 min of injection and was in excess of 2 °C above control values for body temperature after 4 h. Rises in body temperature were associated with behavioural changes in the fowl, having onset within 5 min and including increased locomotor activity, contralateral head movement, escape behaviour, vocalization, and polypnoea. Convulsions and death occured in some birds treated with Db-cAMP. Injection of cyclic AMP into the hypothalamus (0.1–0.4 µmol, approximately 35–139 µg) or into the third cerebral ventricle (0.3 or 0.4 µmol, approximately 104 µg and 139 µg) had no effect on either body temperature or behaviour in the fowl, unless the bird was pre-treated intramuscularly with the cyclic nucleotide phosphodiesterase inhibitor, aminophylline (110 µmole/kg, approximately 28.4 mg/kg) (Marley and Nistico 1972). Cyclic AMP injected centrally into aminophylline-treated fowls evoked behavioural and electrocortical sleep in contrast with the arousal elicited by Db-cAMP but had no significant effect on body temperature.

The effects of central injection of Db-cAMP on body temperature in several species are summarized in Table 1. Both hypothermia and hyperthermia have been reported for the rabbit and the cat, the two species most commonly employed in studies on fever. Hypothermia when present is a relatively transient effect seen first after administration of the nucleotide whereas hyperthermia when present is generally of later onset and of longer duration than the fall in body temperature. Penetration of Db-cAMP to more that one site in the central nervous system after central injection may be responsible for the multiple components of the temperature response. The specific thermoregulatory nature of the hyperthermia is often difficult to assess owing to the concomitant increase in locomotor activity seen commonly in most species after central injection of Db-cAMP. In experiments where dissociation between hyperthermia and increased locomotor activity is apparent, non-specific effects, such as brain tissue damage in cats, may explain in part the sustained rise in body temperature. Central injection of cyclic AMP has either no effect or a similar, but less potent, effect on body temperature to that of Db-cAMP in species so far tested. These findings are in agreement with the proposal that cyclic AMP does not readily penetrate cell membranes (Posternak 1971) and is readily hydrolysed (Sutherland and Rall 1958; Drummond and Perrott-Yee 1961; Butcher and Sutherland 1962). The possibility exists that injection of cyclic AMP and its derivatives may initiate responses including effects on body temperature, by extracellular rather than intracellular interactions. Responses

Table 1. Summary of effects of Db-cAMP on body temperature after central administration in different species

Species	Route of administration	Dose (μg)	Response	Comments	Reference
Mouse	ICV	25	0 (↓?)	See Fig. 1	DOGGETT and SPENCER (1971)
Rat	AH	500	↑	Solid implant. Db-cAMP also increases locomotor activity	BRECKENRIDGE and LISK (1969)
Rabbit	LV	20–500	↓↑	Hyperthermia in all rabbits. Hyperthermia onset more than 90 min after injection of higher doses	DUFF et al. (1972)
	PO/AH	0.25–10 (bilateral)	↑	Hyperthermia prolonged and associated with hyperexcitability in some rabbits	WOOLF et al. (1975)
	LV	25–50/kg	↓↑	Higher doses (75–200 μg/kg) produce rapid rise in temperature associated with increased locomotor activity	PHILIPP-DORMSTON and SIEGERT (1975a)
Cat	AH	50–500	↑	Non-sterile injections? Db-cAMP increases locomotor activity	GESSA et al. (1970)
	LV	50–150	↓↑	Hyperthermia in all cats whereas hypothermia in 5 of 17 animals. ATP and butyrate raise temperature	VARAGIC and BELESLIN (1973)
	LV	250–1,000	↓↑	Sustained hyperthermia reduced by indomethacin and paracetamol. See Fig. 2	CLARK et al. (1974)
	PO/AH	50–500	↓↑	Hypothermia in all cats with subsequent hyperthermia in animals developing fever after injections of vehicle	DASCOMBE and MILTON (1975a)
Monkey	PO/AH	0.5–75	0 (↓?)	A single monkey received Db-cAMP above the dose-level 0.75 μg. See Fig. 4	LIPTON and FOSSLER (1974)
Fowl	H	49–98 (approx.)	↑	Db-cAMP also increases locomotor activity	MARLEY and NISTICO (1972)
	III	491 (approx.)	↑	Db-cAMP also increases locomotor activity	MARLEY and NISTICO (1972)

Db-cAMP injected into the anterior hypothalamus (AH), the preoptic anterior hypothalamic area (PO/AH) or the third cerebral ventricle (III). Arrows denote the direction and the chronological order but not the magnitude or the duration of the change in temperature. (↓?) signifies a hypothermic response apparent from published data, which may or may not be significant and does not represent a conclusion of the original authors the cerebroventricular system (ICV), the hypothalamus (H), a lateral cerebral ventricle (LV),

evoked by exogenous cyclic AMP administered into the brain by micro-injection techniques may not, therefore, mimic the function of endogenous intracellular nucleotide.

C. Enzymes Related to Cyclic AMP

The intracellular concentration of endogenous cyclic AMP in the brain, as in other tissues, appears to be a balance between the rate of synthesis of the nucleotide by adenylate cyclase from the substrate ATP (RALL and SUTHERLAND 1958, 1962; SUTHERLAND et al. 1962) and its rate of hydrolysis by cyclic nucleotide phosphodiesterase to AMP (SUTHERLAND and RALL 1958; DRUMMOND and PERROTT-YEE 1961; BUTCHER and SUTHERLAND 1962).

I. Adenylate Cyclase

The presence, distribution, and properties of adenylate cyclase in the brain indicate the possible importance of the enzyme in brain function. Highest specific activities of adenylate cyclase in mammalian tissues are found in the brain (SUTHERLAND et al. 1962), these levels being exceeded only by those in fractions of dark-adapted frog retina (BITENSKY et al. 1971a). The distribution of the enzyme varies throughout the brain in several species but appears not to correlate with the presence of cyclic nucleotide phosphodiesterase activity or certain putative neurotransmitter substances (VOIGT and KRISHNA 1967; WEISS and COSTA 1968; WILLIAMS et al. 1969). CRAMER et al. (1971) suggested that the occurrence of cyclic AMP in the brain may be related to the turnover of noradrenaline, as documented by IVERSEN and GLOWINSKI (1966), rather than to absolute concentrations of the catecholamine. Brain adenylate cyclase activity is associated mainly with particulate subcellular fractions (RALL and SUTHERLAND 1958; SUTHERLAND et al. 1962; DE ROBERTIS et al. 1967; WEISS and COSTA 1968) being most concentrated in factions rich in synaptic membrane (DE ROBERTIS et al. 1967; ISAAC and GRAHAME-SMITH 1972). Adenylate cyclase in the rat pineal gland appears to be situated both postsynaptically (WEISS and COSTA 1967) and presynaptically (DUBOCOVICH et al. 1978).

Adenylate cyclase activity is assayed by the rate of accumulation of cyclic AMP by preparations of tissue in vitro (KRISHNA et al. 1968), although it is conceivable this parameter may be influenced independently by changes in the rate of degradation of the nucleotide. A consideration of possibly greater importance is that studies on adenylate cyclase in brain tissue may not monitor enzyme activity present solely in neurones since neurohumoral sensitive adenylate cyclase is present in glial cells (CLARK and PERKINS 1971; GILMAN and NIRENBERG 1971; GILMAN and SCHRIER 1972; SCHULTZ et al. 1972; PALMER 1973).

1. Activators of Adenylate Cyclase
a) Microbial Toxins

Escherichia coli lipopolysaccharide increases the response of hepatic and splenic adenylate cyclase to adrenaline after administration of endotoxin either in vitro or in vivo in mice (BITENSKY et al. 1971b). Endotoxin was without effect on basal adenylate cyclase activity and had no discernible influence on glucagon-activated enzyme in the liver. In contrast with these findings, *E. coli* endotoxin has been found to stimulate adenylate cyclase activity in the liver of the guinea-pig following administration of the lipopolysaccharide either in vivo or in vitro (GIMPEL et al. 1971). DONLON and WALKER (1976) reported that *Salmonella typhosa* lipopolysaccharide increases the basal activity of adenylate cyclase in homogenates of mouse liver but reduces adrenaline-stimulated activity. The mechanism of action of bacterial lipopolysaccharides in stimulating adenylate cyclase activity is not known. The affinity of these compounds for phospholipids in cell membranes (ROTHFIELD and HORNE 1967; SHANDS 1973) can result in disruption of cell membranes at high concentrations (ČIŽNÁR and SHANDS 1971). Membrane effects such as this may alter the activity of membrane-bound adenylate cyclase although ČŽNÁR and SHANDS (1971) thought it unlikely membrane effects contribute to the toxicity of lipopolysaccharides, because the concentrations necessary to produce membrane disruption in vitro exceed levels found in vivo. The possibility exists that stimulation of adenylate cyclase activity is not a property of lipopolysaccharides. Enterotoxins of *E. coli* have been shown to stimulate adenylate cyclase activity in several tissues in vitro including adipocytes (EVANS et al. 1972), intestine (EVANS et al. 1972; HYNIE et al. 1974; KANTOR et al. 1974), thyroid (MASHITER et al. 1973), ovaries (GUERRANT et al. 1974), liver (HYNIE et al. 1974), thymocytes (ZENSER and METZGER 1974), myocardium (DORNER and MAYER 1975), and kidney cells (STAVRIC et al. 1978). Unlike the endotoxin activity associated with lipopolysaccharides, the enterotoxicity of *E. coli* resides in a heat-labile, protein-like fraction (EVANS et al. 1973; JACKS et al. 1973). Attempts by JACKS et al. (1973) to dissociate enterotoxicity from endotoxicity were unsuccessful and led these workers to propose that the same macromolecule or complex may be responsible for both activities, with a glycolipid fraction conferring classical endotoxicity (NOWOTNY 1971) and a protein-like fraction responsible for enterotoxic activity. Preparations of toxins from enteropathogenic bacteria such as *E. coli* presumably contain both endotoxin and enterotoxin and it is undetermined whether stimulation of adenylate cyclase activity by such preparations is an expression of endotoxicity and/or enterotoxicity.

An apparently pure protein enterotoxin, choleragen, has been prepared from *Vibrio cholerae* (FINKELSTEIN and LOSPALLUTO 1969, 1970, 1972). Choleragen, or culture filtrates of *V. cholerae* containing the enterotoxin stimulate adenylate cyclase activity in a variety of tissues including the small intestine (KIMBERG et al. 1971; EVANS et al. 1972; GUERRANT et al. 1972; GRAND et al. 1973; HYNIE et al. 1974), liver (GORMAN and BITENSKY 1972; BECKMAN et al. 1974; HYNIE et al. 1974), thyroid (MASHITER et al. 1973), leucocytes (BOURNE 1973; BOURNE et al. 1973; LICHTENSTEIN et al. 1973), thymocytes (BOYLE and GARDINER 1974; ZENSER and METZGER 1974), gall bladder (MERTENS et al. 1974), nucleus accumbens (MILLER and KELLY 1975), pineal gland (MINNEMAN and IVERSEN 1976a), substantia nigra (QUENZER et al. 1977), hypothalamus (NISTICO et al. 1978), and kidney cells (STAVRIC et al. 1978). The possible involvement of cyclic AMP in the pathogenesis of cholera has been reviewed (ADAMS 1973; GILL 1977). Cholera toxin causes a characteristically delayed accumulation of cyclic AMP which is long lasting and persists after removal of the toxin from the incubation medium. The effect of choleragen

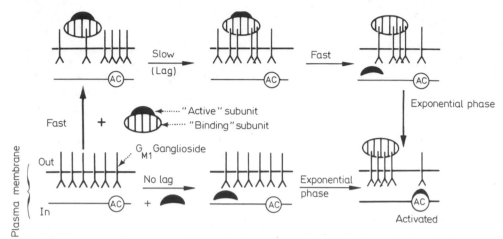

Fig. 5. Diagrammatic summary of postulated sequence of events in the activation of adenylate cyclase (*AC*) by native choleragen and by the "active" subunit (subunit A, see text). The specific mechanism by which the active subunit modifies the cyclase complex is unknown and is therefore unspecified. Although the "binding" subunit is fundamentally not an essential component, it serves to give specificity and orientation, to enhance the affinity for the toxin, and to provide a specialized water-soluble vehicle for direct delivery of the active molecular species. (After SAHYOUN and CUATRECASAS 1975)

on adenylate cyclase contrasts with the rapid, reversible response of the enzyme to isoprenaline and prostaglandin E_1 (BOURNE et al. 1973; KIMBERG et al. 1974). Stimulation of adenylate cyclase by choleragen is subsequent to the toxin binding to the cell membrane, probably at gangliosides like G_{M1}, a monosialoganglioside (G_M) with four neutral sugar residues (CUATRECASAS 1973; BOYLE and GARDINER 1974; VAN HEYNINGEN 1974). The action of choleragen on adenylate cyclase is thought to be effected by a particular component, subunit A, of the enterotoxin (FINKELSTEIN et al. 1974; SAHYOUN and CUATRECASAS 1975; VAN HEYNINGEN and KING 1975) and appears to be directly on the enzyme (Fig. 5) because solubilization of cell membranes does not inhibit the response (BECKMAN et al. 1974). Several groups of workers have found the effects of *E. coli* toxin on adenylate cyclase similar to those of cholera toxin (EVANS et al. 1972; MASHITER et al. 1973; GUERRANT et al. 1974; HYNIE et al. 1974; KANTOR et al. 1974; ZENSER and METZGER 1974; STAVRIC et al. 1978).

GTP is a prerequisite for adenylate cyclase activity in several tissue preparations (RODBELL et al. 1971; BOCKAERT et al. 1972; GOLDFINE et al. 1972; KRISHNA and HARWOOD 1972; LERAY et al. 1972; WOLFF and COOK 1973). Guanyl imidodiphosphate, an analogue of GTP containing a metabolically stable P–N–P linkage (YOUNT et al. 1971), activates adenylate cyclase by a process apparently similar to that of GTP (LONDOS et al. 1974; SPIEGEL and AURBACH 1974; LEFKOWITZ 1975; PFEUFFER and HELMREICH 1975; SCHRAMM and RODBELL 1975). Activation of adenylate cyclase by guanyl imidodiphosphate is sustained, resistant to dilution, and is not inhibited by sonication or solubilization of the membrane-bound enzyme (SCHRAMM and RODBELL 1975). As pointed out by FLORES and SHARP (1975), these features are not unlike those of choleragen-induced activation of the enzyme and these workers suggested that choleragen and guanyl imidodiphosphate may share a common site of action in the adenylate cyclase complex, presumably the guanyl nucleotide binding site described by RODBELL et al. (1971).

The effects of activators of adenylate cyclase, such as choleragen and guanyl imidodiphosphate, on body temperature are clearly of interest. Purified cholera enterotoxin injected into a lateral cerebral ventricle induces hyperthermia in cats after a latency period of 2–3 h (CLARK et al. 1974). Febrile responses to 1 μg cholera enterotoxin were maximal and persisted for more than 32 h but were attenuated by intraperitoneal injection of paracetamol, indomethacin, or sodium salicylate. Indomethacin and paracetamol were shown by CLARK et al. (1974) to reduce the febrile response to Db-cAMP injected into a lateral cerebral ventricle in the cat (Fig. 2) indicating a similar mechanism for the production of hyperthermia by both cholera enterotoxin and Db-cAMP. Cholera toxin did not mimic the general stimulation of the central nervous system or the periods of hypothermia induced in cats by Db-cAMP, even when supramaximal doses of toxin, up to 100 μg were administered. CLARK and his co-workers favour the explanation that excitation and hypothermia are characteristic of concentrations of cyclic AMP higher than those that can be induced by cholera enterotoxin.

b) Putative Neurotransmitters of Fever

The ability of many neurotransmitter and modulator substances to increase adenylate cyclase activity in brain tissue has been extensively documented and reviewed (WEISS and KIDMAN 1969; GREENGARD and COSTA 1970; BLOOM 1975; DALY 1975 a, b; DRUMMOND and MA 1975; KEBABIAN 1977, NATHANSON 1977). Suffice it here to say that the substances generally accepted as stimulating adenylate cyclase activity in brain tissue in vitro include many of the endogenous compounds at present thought to be involved in central neuronal pathways during the genesis of fever, for example, noradrenaline, dopamine, 5-hydroxytryptamine, and prostaglandins of the E series. There are contradictory reports of some of these substances having little or no effect on adenylate cyclase activity in vitro (KLAINER et al. 1962; VOIGT and KRISHNA 1967; WILLIAMS et al. 1969; ISAAC and GRAHAME-SMITH 1972). These studies were based on preparations of homogenized brain tissue, however, and may indicate that homogenization can cause sufficient damage to the adenylate cyclase system to render it less sensitive, or even insensitive, to the presence of neurohormones. Additions to assay systems utilizing homogenized brain tissue may be necessary before neurohormone-induced changes in adenylate cyclase activity are demonstrable, for example, the presence of GTP markedly potentiates the response of the brain enzyme to histamine (HEGSTRAND et al. 1976). Noradrenaline, 5-hydroxytryptamine, and histamine, but not acetylcholine, injected intracisternally in rats increase adenylate cyclase activity in the cerebral cortex (CHO et al. 1971). The involvement of central neurotransmitter substances in the pathogenesis of fever is discussed in Chap. 4 of this volume.

2. Inhibitors of Adenylate Cyclase

An exotoxin from *Bacillus thuringiensis* has been found to inhibit adenylate cyclase activity in pigeon erythrocytes and in the adrenals and the brain of the rat (GRA-

Hame-Smith et al. 1975). The exotoxin, a phosphoallomucyl glycoside of adenine (Šebesta and Horská 1968, Bond et al. 1969), appears to inhibit adenylate cyclase by competition with the enzyme substrate ATP (Grahame-Smith et al. 1975). Unilateral intrahypothalamic injection of *B. thuringiensis* toxin (10 µg) attenuates fever induced by intrahypothalamic administration of bacterial pyrogen (65 ng) and prostaglandin E_1 (0.5 µg) in rabbits (Willies et al. 1976a). These workers showed that the effect of the exotoxin is not a non-specific inhibition of heat production since hyperthermia induced by intrahypothalamic injections of Db-cAMP (3 µg) in rabbits was unaffected by the toxin. *B. thuringiensis* toxin itself has a slight hyperthermic effect following intrahypothalamic injection in rabbits at an ambient temperature of 21°–22 °C (Willies et al. 1976a). The effect of the exotoxin may not, however, be specific for adenylate cyclase as the bacterial product inhibits RNA polymerase also (Beebee and Korner 1972; Beebee and Bond 1973).

In summary, it appears that bacterial toxins and putative neurohormones of fever can, in addition to inducing hyperthermia after injection in vivo, also stimulate adenylate cyclase activity in vitro. Furthermore, an exotoxin from *B. thuringiensis* can both attenuate the febrile response to centrally administered bacterial pyrogen and prostaglandin E_1 but not that to Db-cAMP in the rabbit, and inhibit adenylate cyclase activity in vitro. These observations are circumstantial evidence that adenylate cyclase in the brain may be stimulated during the febrile response to bacterial pyrogens or neurohormones injected centrally. An obvious lack of information exists as to whether adenylate cyclase activity is actually increased in the central neuronal pathways involved in the genesis of hyperthermia, particularly during fever associated with peripheral infection.

The possibility exists that adenylate cyclase activity may be diminished not increased in some brain cells during fever. Hypothalamic warm-sensitive neurones may be such cells for their stimulation by capsaicin results in a fall in body temperature (Jancsó and Jancsó-Gábor 1965; Jancsó-Gábor et al. 1970a, b) which is associated with increased adenylate cyclase activity in the preoptic area in the rat (Jancsó and Wolleman 1977).

II. Cyclic Nucleotide Phosphodiesterase

High levels of cyclic nucleotide phosphodiesterase activity are found in the mammalian brain (Sutherland and Rall 1958; Drummond and Perrott-Yee 1961; Butcher and Sutherland 1962) with regional variations in specific activity (Voigt and Krishna 1967; Weiss and Costa 1968; Williams et al. 1969). Cyclic nucleotide phosphodiesterase is associated primarily with mitochondrial and microsomal fractions (Cheung 1967; Cheung and Salganicoff 1967; De Robertis et al. 1967; Weiss and Costa 1968) with most activity in the rat brain in the immediate vicinity of the postsynaptic membrane (Florendo et al. 1971). Cyclic nucleotide phosphodiesterase activity in many tissues including the mammalian brain can be resolved by several techniques into multiple forms or isoenzymes (Brooker et al. 1968; Beavo et al. 1970a; Cheung 1970a; Jard and Bernard 1970; Kakiuchi et al. 1971; Thompson and Appleman 1971a, b; Monn and Christiansen 1971; Campbell and Oliver 1972; Uzunov and Weiss 1972; Pledger et al. 1974). Some single cell types namely human blood platelets (Amer and Mayol

1973; PICHARD et al. 1973) and cloned astrocytoma and neuroblastoma cells (UZUNOV et al. 1973, 1974) also contain multiple forms of cyclic nucleotide phosphodiesterase. The isoenzymes differ in their molecular weights, kinetic characteristics, tissue distributions, stabilities, and ionic requirements. Although most forms of the enzyme hydrolyse several cyclic nucleotides in addition to cyclic AMP, for example, and perhaps most significantly, cyclic GMP, kinetic analyses indicate each isoenzyme exhibits a relative selectivity for a particular substrate.

1. Activators of Cyclic Nucleotide Phosphodiesterase

Cyclic nucleotide phosphodiesterase separated from brain tissue loses activity upon purification (CHEUNG 1969) apparently as a result of the loss of an endogenous activator of the enzyme (CHEUNG 1970b). The endogenous activator of cyclic nucleotide phosphodiesterase has been characterized as a heat-stable protein with a molecular weight of 19,200–27,000 daltons and an absolute requirement for Ca^{2+} ions (CHEUNG 1970b, 1971; GOREN and ROSEN 1971; KAKIUCHI et al. 1973; TEO et al. 1973; LIN et al. 1974; WOLFF and BROSTROM 1974). The calcium-dependent protein does not increase the activity of all phosphodiesterase isoenzymes equally, but selectively activates one of the major forms found primarily in brain tissue (UZUNOV and WEISS 1972; UZUNOV et al. 1974). This isoenzyme has a high Michaelis constant (K_m) for cyclic AMP and a low K_m for cyclic GMP (GOREN and ROSEN 1972) and although hydrolysis of both nucleotides is increased by the activator of phosphodiesterase, the relatively greater effect on the degradation of cyclic GMP may be of greater physiological importance (KAKIUCHI et al. 1973). The same calcium-dependent protein appears to activate adenylate cyclase (BROSTROM et al. 1975; CHEUNG et al. 1975) and Ca^{2+}/Mg^{2+} ATPase (GOPINATH and VINCENZI 1977; JARRETT and PENNISTON 1977). An involvement of this calcium-dependent protein in fever has not been established although bacterial pyrogens may act by reducing the effective concentration of calcium in the hypothalamus (FELDBERG and SAXENA 1970).

Nicotinic acid increases cyclic nucleotide phosphodiesterase activity (KRISHNA et al. 1966). Injected unilaterally into the hypothalamus nicotinic acid (50 µg) attenuates the febrile response to prostaglandin E_1 (0.5 µg) administered simultaneously in rabbits (WOOLF et al. 1975). Intrahypothalamic injection of nicotinic acid alone produces a slight rise in rectal temperature ($0.23° \pm 0.03$ °C standard error of mean) in rabbits at an ambient temperature of $21°–23$ °C. WOOLF et al. (1975) acknowledge that the dose (50 µg) of nicotinic acid used in these experiments is possibly cytotoxic and suggest their results must be interpreted with caution in view of the possible non-specific effects of the compound.

2. Inhibitors of Cyclic Nucleotide Phosphodiesterase

The rate of hydrolysis of cyclic AMP by cyclic nucleotide phosphodiesterase in vitro can be reduced by other purine and pyrimidine derivatives particularly by nucleotides such as cyclic GMP with purine as a base (BEAVO et al. 1970a; ROSEN 1970; FRANKS and MACMANUS 1971; GOREN and ROSEN 1971, 1972; HARRIS et al. 1971; RUSSELL et al. 1973; SCHRÖDER and RICKENBERG 1973). These observations indicate the ratio of different nucleotides to be an important determinant of their individual endogenous concentrations. Db-cAMP inhibits the hydrolysis of cyclic AMP in cat heart (HARRIS et al. 1971, 1973) but not in rat liver (MENAHAN et al. 1969) or bovine brain (CHEUNG 1970 a). It is conceivable, therefore, that administration of Db-cAMP may increase intracellular levels of cyclic AMP in tissues like the cat heart by inhibition of phosphodiesterase activity. Cyclic nucleotide phosphodiesterase activity in vitro is inhibited by the substrate and a product of the adenylate cyclase reaction, ATP and inorganic pyrophosphate (CHEUNG 1966). CHEUNG proposed that during synthesis of cyclic AMP in vivo the inhibition of phosphodiesterase activity by ATP and pyrophosphate produced conditions unfavourable for the degradation of the intracellular mediator. The mechanism of inhibition of cyclic nucleotide phosphodiesterase by nucleotide triphosphates and inorganic polyphosphates may be chelation of divalent metal ions essential for phosphodiesterase activity (CHEUNG 1967), a property attributed to bacterial pyrogens (FELDBERG and SAXENA 1970).

Cyclic nucleotide phosphodiesterase activity in vitro can be inhibited by numerous drugs including caffeine (1,3,7-trimethylxanthine) and theophylline (1,3-dimethylxanthine) (SUTHERLAND and RALL 1958; BUTCHER and SUTHERLAND 1962), diazoxide (SCHULTZ et al. 1966), some benzodiazepines and phenothiazines (HONDA and IMAMURA 1968; YAMAMOTO and MASSEY 1969; UZUNOV and WEISS 1971; BEER et al. 1972), papaverine (TRINER et al. 1970), apomorphine (SHEPPARD and WIGGAN 1971 a; SHEPPARD et al. 1971), some tricyclic antidepressant drugs (MUSCHEK and MCNEILL 1971), and some ergot derivatives (IWANGOFF and ENZ 1973). CHASIN and HARRIS (1976) have reviewed the literature on agents inhibiting or stimulating cyclic nucleotide phosphodiesterase activity. Potentiation of a biological response by an inhibitor of phosphodiesterase may be accepted as presumptive evidence that the response is mediated by a cyclic nucleotide. The mechanism of inhibition and the particular isoenzyme (or isoenzymes) of phosphodiesterase affected differ with the drug used and may confer a degree of selectivity as to the form of the enzyme affected (WEISS et al. 1974).

The methylxanthines caffeine and theophylline have been used by several workers to investigate the possible involvement of cyclic AMP in fever. DASCOMBE and MILTON (1972) reported that caffeine (13.3 mg/kg) injected intraperitoneally in rabbits potentiated the febrile response to intravenous bacterial pyrogen. Some control animals in this study, however, exhibited a rise in rectal temperature ($0.63° \pm 0.45$ °C standard deviation) which, upon comparison with paired caffeine-treated rabbits, appears to have masked a hyperthermic response to caffeine (DASCOMBE 1977). Hyperthermia induced by caffeine (13.3 mg/kg) injected intraperitoneally in rabbits adds to but does not potentiate submaximal febrile responses to bacterial pyrogen (Fig. 6) and endogenous pyrogen (DASCOMBE 1977). The origin of caffeine-induced thermogenesis in the restrained rabbit is uncertain but in the unrestrained cat, caffeine (15 mg/kg) induces a low-grade hyperthermia, similar to that seen in rabbits, and is associated with increased locomotor activity (DASCOMBE 1977). In this study, caffeine (5 or 15 mg/kg) injected intraperitoneally had no effect on the temperature or behavioural response to bacterial pyrogen in the cat, the increased locomotor activity evoked by the drug being suppressed by the onset of fever and associated sedation.

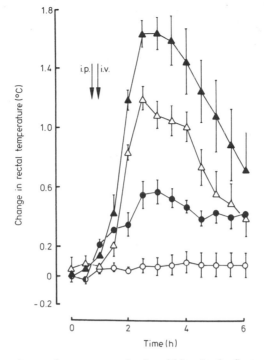

Fig. 6. Mean change in rectal temperature in six rabbits. At the first *arrow* (*IP*) 0.9% NaCl or caffeine 13.3 mg/kg was injected intraperitoneally. After 15 min, at the second *arrow* (*IV*) 0.9% NaCl or *Shigella dysenteriae* 1 µg/kg was injected intravenously. Vertical lines define standard error of the mean. 0.9% NaCl+0.9% NaCl (*open circles*); caffeine+0.9% NaCl (*solid circles*); 0.9% NaCl+*S. dysenteriae* (*open triangles*); caffeine+*S. dysenteriae* (*solid triangles*). (After DASCOMBE 1977)

Irradiation of the hypothalamic region in cats and rabbits with X-rays causes a rise in rectal temperature of about 1 °C after a latent period of 60–90 min, which is enhanced by intravenous injection of theophylline (2 mg/kg) (VENINGA 1972). Exposure of the body trunk to X-rays also causes an increase in body temperature in rabbits maintained at an ambient temperature of 23 °C but this response is not potentiated by theophylline (VENINGA and DIEKEMA 1974). The pathology of these hyperthermic responses to X-rays is undetermined but conceivably involves endogenous pyrogens, although, as the authors pointed out, the possibility that other biochemical mediators are involved has to be considered. PHILIPP-DORMSTON (1975, 1976) reported intravenous injection of theophylline (5 mg/kg) to have no effect on body temperature in afebrile rabbits but to potentiate fever induced by intravenous bacterial pyrogen. Theophylline enhanced the raised concentrations of cyclic AMP but not those of prostaglandin E_2 found in the anterior hypothalamus (PHILIPP-DORMSTON 1975) and in cerebrospinal fluid (PHILIPP-DORMSTON 1976) during fever. In contrast with the latter observations, DASCOMBE (1977) found intraperitoneal injection of theophylline (13.3 mg/kg) to have no effect on body temperature in either afebrile or febrile rabbits.

The absence of potentiation of fever following systemic administration of phosphodiesterase inhibitors could be due to the drugs not being in the brain in sufficient concentration to inhibit enzyme activity. Injection of drugs directly into the brain reduces this possibility and also introduces some degree of selectivity as to the tissue affected. WOOLF et al. (1975) reported hyperthermia produced by bacterial pyrogen injected intravenously in rabbits to be potentiated by multiple injections of theophylline directly into the hypothalamus. These workers also showed that simultaneous administration of prostaglandin E_1 (0.5 µg) and theophylline (50 µg) induced a significantly greater fever than that produced by prostaglandin E_1 alone, and concluded that central cyclic AMP may mediate pyrexia. Aminophylline (theophylline with ethylenediamine), equivalent to 1 mg of theophylline, injected into the third cerebral ventricle is without effect on body temperature in both afebrile and febrile cats (DASCOMBE 1977). Caffeine injected into the third cerebral ventricle (1 mg) or into the anterior hypothalamus (25 µg or 50 µg) is also without effect on body temperature or behaviour in afebrile or pyrogen-treated cats when compared with responses to control injections of vehicle (0.9 %w/v NaCl in water). There appears to be a difference, therefore, between the effects of centrally applied methylxanthines on fever in the rabbit and the cat. Theophylline and caffeine are not potent inhibitors of cyclic nucleotide phosphodiesterase activity and the absence of potentiation of fever in the cat may be attributable to a lack of enzyme inhibition following a single application of the drug, despite the use of concentrated drug solutions. The use of more potent inhibitors of phosphodiesterase activity such as 1-methyl-3-isobutylxanthine (BEAVO et al. 1970b), SQ 20,009 (etazolate hydrochloride; 1-ethyl-4-(isopropylidenehydrazine)-1 H-pyrazole-(3,4-b)-pyridine-5-carboxylic acid, ethyl ester, hydrocholoride) (CHASIN 1971) or Ro 20-1724(4-(3-butoxy-4-methoxybenzyl)-2-imidazolidinone) (SHEPPARD and WIGGAN 1971 b; SHEPPARD et al. 1971) may help resolve the apparent difference between the rabbit and the cat.

An alternative explanation for the difference between species is afforded by the observation of DASCOMBE (1977) that hyperthermia, resulting from damage to brain tissue caused by central injections, summates with the febrile response to bacterial pyrogen injected intravenously in cats. The occurrence of non-specific febrile responses to central injections has been documented most extensively for the cat (FELDBERG et al. 1970; VARAGIĆ and BELESLIN 1973; DEY et al. 1974; DASCOMBE and MILTON 1975a) but may be seen in rabbits after perfusion of the cerebral ventricles (FELDBERG and SAXENA 1970). Gradual development of tissue damage and associated fever (DASCOMBE and MILTON 1975a) may render interpretation of differences between responses, obtained in the same animal but at different times, difficult. As suggested by DASCOMBE (1977), summation of tissue-damage hyperthermia with the febrile response to pyrogens could be interpreted erroneously as potentiation of fever by phosphodiesterase inhibitors in the absence of control injections. WOOLF et al. (1975) compared the febrile responses to bacterial pyrogen in theophylline-treated rabbits with fevers in animals which apparently did not receive multiple control injections of vehicle bilaterally into the hypothalamus.

Potentiation of a response by inhibitors of cyclic nucleotide phosphodiesterase activity can be accepted as presumptive evidence that the response is mediated by cyclic AMP; this represents an important criterion in determining involvement of the nucleotide (BUTCHER 1968; ROBISON et al. 1971). It is not, however, conclusive evidence owing to possible changes in the hydrolysis of cyclic GMP in addition to other effects of the compounds which may be unrelated to a cyclic nucleotide system. The results of such studies must, as WOOLF et al. (1975) indicated, be interpreted with caution.

D. Endogenous Cyclic AMP in Fever

I. Cyclic AMP in Brain Tissue

The apparent concentration of cyclic AMP in brain tissue varies with the method of preparation of the tissue for assay. The amount of cyclic AMP in brain tissue increases rapidly post mortem, apparently as a result of ischaemia (BRECKENRIDGE 1964; KAKIUCHI and RALL 1968; SCHMIDT et al. 1971; UZUNOV and WEISS 1971; STEINER et al. 1972). Attempts to minimize if not abolish post-mortem rises in cyclic AMP concentrations have centred on the development of methods arresting enzyme activities by freezing or microwave irradiation (SCHMIDT et al. 1971; LUST et al. 1973; JONES et al. 1974; DELAPAZ et al. 1975). Both methods of preparation give levels of cyclic AMP lower than those in brain tissue prepared from decapitated animals. Lowest values for cyclic AMP content are presently given by methods emphasizing rapid fixation of tissue by freezing (NAHORSKI and ROGERS 1973) or microwave irradiation (JONES and STAVINOHA 1977). Low levels of cyclic AMP are interpreted by some workers as indicating rapid fixation of tissue with minimal anoxia but LUST et al. (1973) report microwave-irradiated brain tissue to be anoxic as indicated by changes in phosphocreatinine, ATP, lactate, and phosphorylase levels, despite low concentrations of cyclic AMP. Fixation of brain tissue by freezing was found by these workers to give samples more closely resembling the metabolic state in vivo. In addition, non-uniform microwave irradiation can result in the development of "hot spots" in the brain which may facilitate diffusion of substances from one brain region to another (LENOX et al. 1977) or across the blood-brain barrier (MERRITT et al. 1978). Dissection of frozen tissue is difficult, however, and microwave irradiation as a means of tissue fixation may be preferable for the comparative ease of dissection of discrete brain areas.

Most studies on brain tissue levels of cyclic AMP have been with the rat. Results tend to be contradictory, for example, after intracerebroventricular injection in vivo of noradrenaline, increased cyclic AMP concentrations are found in the whole brain when tissue is prepared for assay by freezing (BURKARD 1972) but not after microwave irradiation (SCHMIDT et al. 1972). This discrepancy may be attributable in part to the different methods of tissue fixation.

Concentrations of cyclic AMP in the anterior hypothalamus of the rabbit are increased about three-fold during fever induced by intravenous endotoxin when compared with samples from afebrile animals (PHILIPP-DORMSTON 1975). Cyclic AMP levels in all other brain areas remained unchanged during fever. Theophylline administered intravenously enhanced both the febrile response to pyrogen and the levels of cyclic AMP in the anterior hypothalamus, whereas paracetamol reduced both fever and cyclic AMP. Fever induced in rabbits by prostaglandin E_2 injected into a lateral cerebral ventricle was also found by PHILIPP-DORMSTON

(1975) to be associated with raised levels of cyclic AMP in the anterior hypothalamus. Prostaglandin E_2 which may enter the brain from the blood (Dascombe and Milton 1979) produces sedation and stupor together with increased concentrations of cyclic AMP in the brain, including the hypothalamus, after intravenous injection in mice and rats (Wellman and Schwabe 1973). Increases in the hypothalamic content of cyclic AMP are also produced in rats exposed to an ambient temperature of 36 °C for up to 30 min (Siegel et al. 1976; Kornbluth et al. 1977) but not in rats exposed to 4 °C (Mao et al. 1974a). Siegel et al. (1976) and Kornbluth et al. (1977) did not find a rise in cyclic AMP in the cerebral cortex of rats maintained at 36 °C and proposed that their data indicate that acute heat exposure affects cyclic AMP in central thermoregulatory areas. These workers suggested also that the elevated nucleotide levels could be a result of changes in the capacity of these brain regions to synthesize or catabolize cyclic AMP in the short but finite time that elapses between death and tissue fixation.

II. Cyclic AMP in Cerebrospinal Fluid

Indications are that levels of pyrogens or their endogenous mediators increase in cerebrospinal fluid during fever (Cooper and Veale 1972a, b; Feldberg and Gupta 1973; Feldberg et al. 1973). Cyclic AMP is found in mammalian cerebrospinal fluid in concentrations of approximately 2×10^{-8} M (Henion and Sutherland 1971). The functional significance of cyclic AMP in extracellular fluid is uncertain. Davoren and Sutherland (1963) found avian erythrocytes able to extrude cyclic AMP against an apparent concentration gradient and this may be a means whereby intracellular concentrations of the nucleotide are regulated.

Raised levels of cyclic AMP are found in the cisternal cerebrospinal fluid of cats (Dascombe and Milton 1975b, 1976) and rabbits (Philipp-Dormston and Siegert 1975b; Philipp-Dormston 1976; Siegert et al. 1976) during the febrile response to pyrogens injected intravenously. An approximately two-fold increase in basal levels of cyclic AMP occurs in both species. A smaller increase has been reported for a child suffering meningococcal meningitis (Myllylä et al. 1975). The rise in cerebrospinal fluid levels of cyclic AMP is dependent on the dose of bacterial lipopolysaccharide (2 or 20 µg/kg) injected intravenously in cats and is prevented by prior administration of paracetamol (75 mg/kg intraperitoneally) which suppresses fever (Dascombe and Milton 1975b, 1976). In the rabbit also both the febrile response and the rise in cerebrospinal cyclic AMP are inhibited by intraperitoneal injection of paracetamol (50 mg/kg) whilst theophylline (5 mg/kg intravenous) enhances both responses to pyrogen (Philipp-Dormston 1976). Philipp-Dormston (1976) showed the nature of the pyrogen not to be crucial in eliciting an increase in cerebrospinal fluid cyclic AMP since pyrogens from bacterial, viral, and endogenous sources were all effective in the rabbit. The increase in cerebrospinal fluid cyclic AMP appears to be associated with the pathogenicity of pyrogens and not to be a consequence of heat production and/or heat conservation activities or a rise in body temperature (Dascombe and Milton 1975c, 1976; Siegert et al. 1976). Philipp-Dormston and Siegert (1975b) and Philipp-Dormston (1976) propose that as cyclic AMP does not cross the blood-brain barrier (Gessa et al. 1970), concentrations of cyclic AMP in cerebrospinal fluid represent biosynthesis

in brain regions adjoining the cerebral ventricles and that raised levels of the nucleotide during fever imply cyclic AMP to be a central mediator of fever in the rabbit. However, SIEGERT et al. (1975, 1976) have reported an apparent dissociation
between raised cerebrospinal fluid levels of cyclic AMP and fever in the rabbit.
Cycloheximide injected intravenously in rabbits prevents the febrile response to
Newcastle disease virus but not the increase in cyclic AMP. Apparent dissociation
of pyrexia and raised cerebrospinal fluid levels of cyclic AMP in the cat have been
observed by DASCOMBE and MILTON (1976) on two occasions. First, paracetamol
at doses (50 and 100 mg/kg intraperitoneally) shown to be antipyretic, injected after the onset of the febrile response to bacterial pyrogen, had no significant effect
on raised concentrations of cyclic AMP during a period of nearly 3 h. Secondly,
a single cat responded to bacterial pyrogen with collapse and hypothermia as described for rabbits by JONA (1916). Concentrations of cyclic AMP in cerebrospinal
fluid from this cat during and after collapse and hypothermia were similar to those
for cats with marked pyrexia, although fever was attenuated in this animal. Dissociation of fever and raised levels of cyclic AMP in cisternal cerebrospinal fluid
could be due to the fluid content in the cisterna magna not reflecting accurately
concentrations of the nucleotide in brain areas involved with the genesis of fever.
Assay of cyclic AMP in samples obtained closer to such sites may give an unequivocal indication of cyclic AMP involvement in fever.

Cyclic AMP in cerebrospinal fluid may not, as proposed by PHILIPP-DORMSTON
and SIEGERT (1975 b) and PHILIPP-DORMSTON (1976), represent only changes in nucleotide biosynthesis in brain regions neighbouring on the cerebroventricular system. GESSA et al. (1970) cited unpublished work, the nature of which was not revealed, that cyclic AMP does not cross the blood–brain barrier. This observation
does not exclude the possibility that the nucleotide enters the cerebrospinal fluid
from the blood. Both tritiated and non-radioactive cyclic AMP enter cisternal cerebrospinal fluid after intravenous injection in cats (DASCOMBE and MILTON 1975 c,
1976). Cyclic AMP (0.1–10 mg/kg) administered intravenously in cats produces a
dose-related increase in the concentration of the nucleotide in cerebrospinal fluid
which is not mimicked by adenosine. DASCOMBE and MILTON (1976) proposed that
whilst it is unlikely that a large and rapid increase in plasma cyclic AMP, such as
that produced by intravenous injection of the nucleotide would occur naturally, the
concentration of cyclic AMP in cerebrospinal fluid may be affected by or be in
equilibrium with that in the plasma. In contrast with these findings, SEBENS and
KORF (1975) found no consistent increase in cerebrospinal fluid cyclic AMP after
intravenous injection of the nucleotide (1.5×10^5 pmol, approximately 60 µg/rab-
bit) into two rabbits weighing 3.0–4.5 kg. These workers assumed a total blood volume of about 300 ml for the distribution of exogenous cyclic AMP in their rabbits,
but rapid hepatic metabolism (LEVINE et al. 1969) and renal excretion (BROADUS
et al. 1970) of the nucleotide would presumably result in a greater apparent volume
of distribution. The absence of cyclic AMP from rabbit cerebrospinal fluid following intravenous injection of cyclic AMP (SEBENS and KORF 1975) may be a consequence of rapid clearance of the nucleotide (1.5×10^5 pmol) from the blood. JOÓ
et al. (1975) report intravenous Db-cAMP to increase the permeability of brain
capillaries in rats to passage of ferritin and propose cyclic AMP may regulate brain
capillary permeability. Increases in cerebrospinal fluid cyclic AMP equivalent to

those found in cats during lipopolysaccharide-induced fever (about 25–30 pmol/ml) but in response to intravenous injection of the nucleotide are without effect on body temperature in cats (Dascombe and Milton 1975c, 1976). Furthermore, levels of cerebrospinal fluid cyclic AMP greater than those during fever, in excess of 100 pmol/ml, are associated with autonomic heat loss activity and hypothermia. Indications are, therefore, that raised concentrations of cyclic AMP in cerebrospinal fluid in response to bacterial pyrogen do not elicit hyperthermia in the cat but are possibly a consequence of altered peripheral metabolism. Cyclic AMP levels in plasma are increased during fever in cats (Dascombe and Milton 1976), possibly as a consequence of altered carbohydrate metabolism induced in peripheral tissues by bacterial pyrogens (Berry et al. 1959; Berry and Smythe 1959; Spitzer et al. 1973). Raised hepatic concentrations of cyclic AMP are associated with hyperinsulinaemia and hyperglucagonaemia induced in rats by pneumococcal sepsis (Zenser et al. 1974; Curnow et al. 1976) although *Serratia marcescens* endotoxin injected in vivo is reported to have no effect on hepatic cyclic AMP in the rat (Gartner 1975). A rise in cerebrospinal fluid cyclic AMP may also result from decreased active transport of the nucleotide from the cerebral ventricular system (Cramer et al. 1972a, b).

E. Cyclic GMP in Fever

A second cyclic nucleotide, cyclic GMP is present in the mammalian brain in concentrations approximately 47 times less (68 pmol/g wet weight) than those of cyclic AMP (Goldberg et al. 1969; Ishikawa et al. 1969). Cyclic GMP is formed from the substrate GTP under the influence of guanylate cyclase, an enzyme distinct from adenylate cyclase (Hardman and Sutherland 1969; Ishikawa et al. 1969; White and Aurbach 1969; White et al. 1969; Schultz et al. 1969; Kimura and Murad 1974, 1975). The mode of action of cyclic GMP in the brain appears to be similar to that of cyclic AMP, involving activation of protein kinases specific for the nucleotide (Miyamoto et al. 1969a, b; Greengard and Kuo 1970; Kuo and Greengard 1970). As with cyclic AMP, cyclic GMP is hydrolysed at the 3′-phosphate linkage to yield GMP by cyclic nucleotide phosphodiesterase (Beavo et al. 1970a). The existence of multiple molecular forms of cyclic nucleotide phosphodiesterase with varying capacities to hydrolyse cyclic GMP and/or cyclic AMP has been reviewed (Sect. C.II). Work by Hardman et al. (1969) first indicated cyclic GMP to be regulated by factors distinct from those influencing accumulation of cyclic AMP. Levels of cyclic GMP in the perfused rat heart (George et al. 1970) and thyroid slices (Yamashita and Field 1972) are raised independently of cyclic AMP by acetylcholine, indicating an involvement of cyclic GMP in cholinergic responses. Cholinomimetics increase cyclic GMP concentrations in brain tissue (Ferrendelli et al. 1970; Kuo et al. 1972) apparently via muscarinic receptors (Lee et al. 1972; Kebabian et al. 1975; Palmer and Duszynski 1975). Glycine, glutamate, and γ-aminobutyric acid (Ferrendelli et al. 1974; Mao et al. 1974b), opiates (Gullis et al. 1975; Bonnet 1975; Minneman and Iversen 1976b), sodium azide, and hydroxylamine (Kimura et al. 1975) have also been found to influence concentrations of cyclic GMP in brain tissues or cells.

A possible involvement of cyclic GMP in central thermoregulatory pathways is indicated by the observation that levels of the nucleotide are raised in the cerebellum but not in the striatum of rats exposed to an ambient temperature of 4 °C (MAO et al. 1973). MAO et al. (1974a) confirmed that cold-exposure raised cyclic GMP concentrations in the rat cerebellum and found levels of the nucleotide to be increased also in the hypothalamus and brain stem within 5–15 min of cold-exposure. Cyclic AMP levels in these brain areas were not affected by an ambient temperature of 4 °C (MAO et al. 1973, 1974a). In contrast with observations in the rat, LUST and PASSONNEAU (1973) found cerebellar cyclic GMP to be unchanged in mice rendered hypothermic but raised up to three-fold in hyperthermic mice. The cerebellum content of cyclic AMP in the hypothermic mice was decreased by 60%, whilst that of the hyperthermic mice remained unchanged.

Db-cGMP (2 mg) injected into the third cerebral ventricle of the cat produces hypothermia, as much as 2.2 °C below control retroperitoneal temperature, associated with tachypnoea and lasting about 2 h (CLARK 1978). Hypothermia induced by Db-cGMP was followed after 2 h by a rise in body temperature, about 0.6 °C above control values, with a duration of approximately 12 h. Db-cGMP (1 mg) injected into the third cerebral ventricle had a similar but less marked effect on body temperature to that produced by 2 mg Db-cGMP, in only some of the cats tested, whereas 0.5 mg Db-cGMP was ineffectual. Cyclic GMP (5 mg) injected intracerebroventricularly produced initial hypothermia in four of six cats and hyperthermia in all animals (CLARK 1978). Defecation, vocalization, and vomiting were elicited by Db-cGMP and cyclic GMP in cats. CLARK (1978) likened the thermoregulatory effects of cyclic GMP and Db-cGMP to those of Db-cAMP introduced into the third cerebral ventricle in cats but emphasized that high concentrations of exogenous cyclic GMP can mimic cyclic AMP in several systems and may not necessarily mimic the effects of elevated concentrations of endogenous cyclic GMP, a caution expounded by GOLDBERG et al. (1973).

F. Summary

It is apparent that the information pertaining to a role for cyclic GMP in the brain during fever is less than that for cyclic AMP. Despite the greater volume of information relating to cyclic AMP, however, the evidence for an involvement of this nucleotide in the brain during fever is equivocal at present. This lack of consensus is due in part to the comparatively gross nature of methods used to study brain function in vivo. Present methods can generate data which may or may not be related to the central events associated with fever. Such data can be interpreted in various ways, one of these being that cyclic AMP does mediate pyrexia, but any interpretation requires verification by experiments with more discrimination than most conducted to date.

References

Adams MME (1973) Cholera: new aids in treatment and prevention. Science 179:552–555
Amer MS, Mayol RF (1973) Studies with phosphodiesterase. III. Two forms of the enzyme from human blood platelets. Biochim Biophys Acta 309:149–156

Beavo JA, Hardman JG, Sutherland EW (1970a) Hydrolysis of cyclic guanosine and adenosine 3′,5′-monophosphates by rat and bovine tissues. J Biol Chem 245:5649–5655

Beavo JA, Rogers NL, Crofford OB, Hardman JG, Sutherland EW, Newman EV (1970b) Effects of xanthine derivatives on lipolysis and on adenosine 3′,5′-monophosphate phosphodiesterase activity. Mol Pharmacol 6:597–603

Beckman B, Flores J, Witkum PA, Sharp GWG (1974) Studies on the mode of action of cholera toxin. Effects on solubilized adenylate cyclase. J Clin Invest 53:1202–1205

Beebee TJC, Bond RPM (1973) Effect of the exotoxin of *Bacillus thuringiensis* on normal and ecdysone-stimulated ribonucleic acid polymerase activity in intact nuclei from the fat-body of *Sarcophaga bullata* larvae. Biochem J 136:1–7

Beebee T, Korner A (1972) Differential inhibition of mammalian ribonucleic acid polymerases by an exotoxin from *Bacillus thuringiensis*. The direct observation of nucleoplasmic ribonucleic acid polymerase activity in intact nuclei. Biochem J 127:619–624

Beer B, Chasin M, Clody DE, Vogel JR, Horovitz ZP (1972) Cyclic adenosine monophosphate phosphodiesterase in brain: effect of anxiety. Science 176:428–430

Berry LJ, Smythe DS (1959) Effects of bacterial endotoxin on metabolism. II. Protein-carbohydrate balance following cortisone. Inhibition of intestinal absorption and adrenal response to ACTH. J Exp Med 110:407–418

Berry LJ, Smythe DS, Young LG (1959) Effects of bacterial endotoxin on metabolism. I. Carbohydrate depletion and the protective role of cortisone. J Exp Med 110:389–405

Bitensky M, Gorman RE, Miller WH (1971a) Adenyl cyclase as a link between photon capture and changes in membrane permeability of frog photoreceptors. Proc Nat Acad Sci USA 68:561–562

Bitensky MW, Gorman RE, Thomas L (1971b) Selective stimulation of epinephrine-responsive adenyl cyclase in mice by endotoxin. Proc Soc Exp Biol Med 138:773–775

Blecher M, Hunt NH (1972) Enzymatic deacylation of mono- and dibutyryl derivatives of cyclic adenosine 3′,5′-monophosphate by extracts of rat tissues. J Biol Chem 247:7479–7484

Bloom FE (1975) The role of cyclic nucleotides in central synaptic function. Rev Physiol Biochem Pharmacol 74:1–103

Bockaert J, Roy C, Jard S (1972) Oxytocin-sensitive adenylate cyclase in frog bladder epithelial cells: role of calcium, nucleotides, and other factors in hormonal stimulation. J Biol Chem 247:7073–7081

Bond RPM, Boyce CBC, Brown VK, Tipton JD (1969) Some chemical and biological studies on an exotoxin from *Bacillus thuringiensis* var. *thuringiensis* Berliner. Biochem J 114:1p

Bonnet KA (1975) Regional alterations in cyclic nucleotide levels with acute and chronic morphine treatment. Life Sci 16:1877–1882

Booth DA (1972) Unlearned and learned effects of intrahypothalamic cyclic AMP injection on feeding. Nature New Biol 237:222–224

Bourne HR (1973) Cholera enterotoxin: failure of anti-inflammatory agents to prevent cyclic AMP accumulation. Nature 241:399

Bourne HR, Lehrer RI, Lichtenstein LM, Weissmann G, Zurier R (1973) Effects of cholera enterotoxin on adenosine 3′,5′-monophosphate and neutrophil function. Comparison with other compounds which stimulate leukocyte adenyl cyclase. J Clin Invest 52:698–708

Bowman WC, Hall MT (1970) Inhibition of rabbit intestine mediated by α- and β-adrenoceptors. Br J Pharmacol 38:399–415

Boyle JM, Gardiner JD (1974) Sequence of events mediating the effect of cholera toxin on rat thymocytes. J Clin Invest 53:1149–1158

Breckenridge BMcL (1964) The measurement of cyclic adenylate in tissues. Proc Nat Acad Sci USA 52:1580–1586

Breckenridge BMcL, Lisk RD (1969) Cyclic adenylate and hypothalamic regulatory functions. Proc Soc Exp Biol Med 131:934–935

Brittain RJ, Handley SL (1967) Temperature changes produced by the injection of catecholamines and 5-hydroxytryptamine into the cerebral ventricles of the conscious mouse. J Physiol (Lond) 192:805–813

Broadus AE, Kaminsky NI, Hardman JG, Sutherland EW, Liddle GW (1970) Kinetic parameters and renal clearances of plasma adenosine 3',5'-monophosphate and guanosine 3',5'-monophosphate in man. J Clin Invest 49:2222–2236

Brooker G, Thomas LJ Jr, Appleman MM (1968) The assay of adenosine 3',5'-cyclic monophosphate in biological materials by enzymatic radioisotopic displacement. Biochemistry 7:4177–4181

Brostrom CO, Huang YC, Breckenridge BMcL, Wolff DJ (1975) Identification of a calcium-binding protein as a calcium-dependent regulator of brain adenylate cyclase. Proc Nat Acad Sci USA 72:64–68

Burkard WP (1972) Catecholamine induced increase of cyclic adenosine 3',5'-monophosphate in rat brain in vivo. J Neurochem 19:2615–2619

Butcher RW (1968) Role of cyclic AMP in hormone actions. N Engl J Med 279:1378–1384

Butcher RW, Sutherland EW (1962) Adenosine 3',5'-phosphate in biological materials. I. Purification and properties of cyclic 3',5'-nucleotide phosphodiesterase and use of this enzyme to characterize adenosine 3',5'-phosphate in human urine. J Biol Chem 237:1244–1250

Campbell MT, Oliver IT (1972) 3':5'-Cyclic nucleotide phosphodiesterase in rat tissues. Eur J Biochem 28:30–37

Chambaut AM, Eboué-Bonis D, Hanoune J, Clauser H (1969) Antagonistic actions between dibutyryl adenosine-3',5'-cyclic monophosphate and insulin on the metabolism of the surviving rat diaphragm. Biochem Biophys Res Commun 34:283–290

Chasin M (1971) A potent new cyclic nucleotide phosphodiesterase (PDE) inhibitor. Fed Proc 30:1268

Chasin M, Harris DN (1976) Inhibitors and activators of cyclic nucleotide phosphodiesterase. Adv Cyclic Nucleotide Res 7:225–264

Cheung WY (1966) Inhibition of cyclic nucleotide phosphodiesterase by adenosine 5'-triphosphate and inorganic pyrophosphate. Biochem Biophys Res Commun 23:214–219

Cheung WY (1967) Properties of cyclic 3',5'-nucleotide phosphodiesterase from rat brain. Biochemistry 6:1079–1087

Cheung WY (1969) Cyclic 3',5'-nucleotide phosphodiesterase. Preparation of a partially inactive enzyme and its subsequent stimulation by snake venom. Biochim Biophys Acta 191:303–315

Cheung WY (1970a) Cyclic nucleotide phosphodiesterase. Adv Biochem Psychopharmacol 3:51–65

Cheung WY (1970b) Cyclic 3',5'-nucleotide phosphodiesterase. Demonstration of an activator. Biochem Biophys Res Commun 38:533–538

Cheung WY (1971) Cyclic 3',5'-nucleotide phosphodiesterase. Evidence for and properties of a protein activator. J Biol Chem 246:2859–2869

Cheung WY, Salganicoff L (1967) Cyclic 3',5'-nucleotide phosphodiesterase: localization and latent activity in rat brain. Nature 214:90–91

Cheung WY, Bradham LS, Lynch TJ, Lin YM, Tallant EA (1975) Protein activator of cyclic 3',5'-nucleotide phosphodiesterase of bovine or rat brain also activates its adenylate cyclase. Biochem Biophys Res Commun 66:1055–1062

Cho WS, Ho AKS, Loh HH (1971) Neurohormones on brain adenyl cyclase activity in vivo. Nature New Biol 233:280–281

Čižnár I, Shands JW Jr (1971) Effect of alkali-treated lipopolysaccharide on erythrocyte membrane stability. Infect Immun 4:362–367

Clark RB, Perkins JP (1971) Regulation of adenosine 3':5'-cyclic monophosphate concentration in cultured human astrocytoma cells by catecholamines and histamine. Proc Nat Acad Sci USA 68:2757–2760

Clark WG (1978) Effects of third cerebral ventricular injections of cyclic guanosine nucleotides on body temperature of cats. Proc Soc Exp Biol Med 158:655–657

Clark WG, Cumby HR, Davis HE IV (1974) The hyperthermic effect of intracerebroventricular cholera enterotoxin in the unanaesthetized cat. J Physiol (Lond) 240:493–504

Cooper KE, Veale WL (1972a) Potentiation of fever, produced by intravenous leucocyte pyrogen, following the injection of paraffin oil in the cerebral ventricles of the unanaesthetized rabbit. Experientia 28:917–918

Cooper KE, Veale WL (1972 b) The effect of injecting an inert oil into the cerebral ventricular system upon fever produced by intravenous leucocyte pyrogen. Can J Physiol Pharmacol 50:1066–1071

Cramer H, Paul MI, Silbergeld S, Forn J (1971) Determination of regional distribution of adenosine 3',5'-monophosphate in rat brain. J Neurochem 18:1605–1608

Cramer H, Goodwin FK, Post RM, Bunney WE Jr (1972 a) Effects of probenecid and exercise on cerebrospinal-fluid cyclic A.M.P. in affective illness. Lancet 1:1346–1347

Cramer H, Ng LKY, Chase TN (1972 b) Effect of probenecid on levels of cyclic A.M.P. in human cerebrospinal fluid. J Neurochem 19:1601–1602

Cuatrecasas P (1973) Gangliosides and membrane receptors for cholera toxin. Biochemistry 12:3558–3566

Curnow RT, Rayfield EJ, George DT, Zenser TV, DeRubertis FR (1976) Altered hepatic glycogen metabolism and glucoregulatory hormones during sepsis. Am J Physiol 230:1296–1301

Daly J (1975 a) Role of cyclic nucleotides in the nervous system. In: Iversen LL, Iversen SD, Snyder SH (eds) Handbook of psychopharmacology, vol 5. Plenum, New York London, pp 47–130

Daly JW (1975 b) Cyclic adenosine 3',5'-monophosphate role in the physiology and pharmacology of the central nervous system. Biochem Pharmacol 24:159–164

Dascombe MJ (1977) Effects of methylxanthine drugs on pyrogen-induced hyperthermia. Eur J Pharmacol 45:389–392

Dascombe MJ, Milton AS (1972) The effect of caffeine on the antipyretic action of aspirin administered during endotoxin induced fever. Br J Pharmacol 46:548–549 P

Dascombe MJ, Milton AS (1975 a) The effects of cyclic 3',5'-adenosine monophosphate and other adenine nucleotides on body temperature. J Physiol (Lond) 250:143–160

Dascombe MJ, Milton AS (1975 b) Cyclic adenosine-3',5'-monophosphate in cerebrospinal fluid during fever and antipyresis. J Physiol (Lond) 247:29–31 P

Dascombe MJ, Milton AS (1975 c) Cyclic adenosine 3',5'-monophosphate in cerebrospinal fluid. Br J Pharmacol 54:254–255 P

Dascombe MJ, Milton AS (1976) Cyclic adenosine 3',5'-monophosphate in cerebrospinal fluid during thermoregulation and fever. J Physiol (Lond) 263:441–463

Dascombe MJ, Milton AS (1979) Study on the possible entry of bacterial endotoxin and prostaglandin E_2 into the central nervous system from the blood. Br J Pharmacol 66:565–572

Davoren PR, Sutherland EW (1963) The effect of 1-epinephrine and other agents on the synthesis and release of adenosine 3',5'-phosphate by whole pigeon erythrocytes. J Biol Chem 238:3009–3015

Delapaz RL, Dickman SR, Grosser BI (1975) Effects of stress on rat brain adenosine 3',5'-monophosphate in vivo. Brain Res 85:171–175

De Robertis E, Arnaiz R de LG, Alberici M, Butcher RW, Sutherland EW (1967) Subcellular distribution of adenyl cyclase and cyclic phosphodiesterase in rat brain cortex. J Biol Chem 242:3487–3493

Dey PK, Feldberg W, Gupta KP, Milton AS, Wendlandt S (1974) Further studies on the rôle of prostaglandin in fever. J Physiol (Lond) 241:629–646

Doggett NS, Spencer PSJ (1971) Pharmacological properties of centrally administered ouabain and their modification by other drugs. Br J Pharmacol 42:242–253

Doggett NS, Spencer PS (1973) Pharmacological properties of centrally administered agents which interfere with neurotransmitter function: a comparison with the central depressant effects of ouabain. Br J Pharmacol 47:26–38

Donlon MA, Walker RI (1976) Adenyl cyclase activity of mouse liver membranes after incubation with endotoxin and epinephrine. Experientia 32:179–181

Dorner F, Mayer P (1975) Escherichia coli enterotoxin: stimulation of adenylate cyclase in broken-cell preparations. Infect Immun 11:429–435

Drummond GI, Ma Y (1975) Metabolism and functions of cyclic AMP in nerve. Prog Neurobiol 2:119–176

Drummond GI, Perrott-Yee S (1961) Enzymatic hydrolysis of adenosine 3',5'-phosphoric acid. J Biol Chem 236:1126–1129

Drummond GI, Powell AC (1970) Analogues of adenosine 3',5'-cyclic phosphate as activators of phosphorylase b kinase and as substrates for cyclic 3',5'-nucleotide phosphodiesterase. Mol Pharmacol 6:24–30

Dubocovich ML, Langer SZ, Pelayo F (1978) Effect of cyclic nucleotides on [³H] – neuro transmitter release induced by potassium stimulation in the rat pineal gland. Br J Pharmacol 62:383–384P

Duff GW, Cranston WI, Luff RH (1972) Cyclic 3',5' adenosine monophosphate in central control of body temperature. Proc Fifth Int Congr Pharmacol Abstr 360. Karger, Basel, p 60

Duffy MJ, Schwarz V (1974) The effects of adenosine 3':5'-cyclic monophosphate and adenosine triphosphate on calcium ion binding in erythrocyte membranes. Biochem Soc Trans 2:406–407

Evans DG, Evans DJ, Pierce NF (1973) Differences in the response of rabbit small intestine to heat-labile and heat-stable enterotoxins of *Escherichia coli*. Infect Immun 7:873–880

Evans DJ, Chen LC, Curlin GT, Evans DG (1972) Stimulation of adenyl cyclase by *Escherichia coli* enterotoxin. Nature New Biol 236:137–138

Feldberg W, Gupta KP (1973) Pyrogen fever and prostaglandin-like activity in cerebrospinal fluid. J Physiol (Lond) 228:41–53

Feldberg W, Saxena PN (1970) Mechanism of action of pyrogen. J Physiol (Lond) 211:245–261

Feldberg W, Myers RD, Veale WL (1970) Perfusion from cerebral ventricle to cisterna magna in unanaesthetized cat. Effect of calcium on body temperature. J Physiol (Lond) 207:403–416

Feldberg W, Gupta KP, Milton AS, Wendlandt S (1973) Effect of pyrogen and antipyretics on prostaglandin activity in cisternal c.s.f. of unanaesthetized cats. J Physiol (Lond) 234:279–303

Ferrendelli JA, Chang MM, Kinscherf DA (1974) Elevation of cyclic GMP levels in central nervous system by excitatory and inhibitory amino acids. J Neurochem 22:535–540

Ferrendelli JA, Steiner AL, McDougal DB Jr, Kipnis DM (1970) The effect of oxotremorine and atropine on cGMP and cAMP levels in mouse cerebral cortex and cerebellum. Biochem Biophys Res Commun 41:1061–1067

Finkelstein RA, LoSpalluto JJ (1969) Pathogenesis of experimental cholera. Preparation and isolation of choleragen and choleragenoid. J Exp Med 130:185–202

Finkelstein RA, LoSpalluto JJ (1970) Production of highly purified choleragen and choleragenoid. J Infect Dis 121:S63–S72

Finkelstein RA, LoSpalluto JJ (1972) Crystalline cholera toxin and toxoid. Science 175:529–530

Finkelstein RA, Boesman M, Neoh SH, Larve MK, Delaney R (1974) Dissociation and recombination of the subunits of the cholera enterotoxin (choleragen). J Immunol 113:145–150

Florendo NT, Barnnett RJ, Greengard P (1971) Cyclic 3',5'-nucleotide phosphodiesterase: cytochemical localization in cerebral cortex. Science 173:745–747

Flores J, Sharp GWG (1975) Effects of cholera toxin on adenylate cyclase: studies with guanylylimidodiphosphate. J Clin Invest 56:1345–1349

Franks DJ, Macmanus JP (1971) Cyclic GMP stimulation and inhibition of cyclic AMP phosphodiesterase from thymic lymphocytes. Biochem Biophys Res Commun 42:844–849

Gartner SL (1975) Hepatic levels of cyclic AMP in normal and lead-sensitized rats after treatment with bacterial endotoxin. Experientia 31:566–567

George WJ, Polson JB, O'Toole AG, Goldberg ND (1970) Elevation of guanosine 3',5'-cyclic phosphate in rat heart after perfusion with acetylcholine. Proc Nat Acad Sci USA 66:398–403

Gessa GL, Krishna G, Forn J, Tagliamonte A, Brodie BB (1970) Behavioral and vegetative effects produced by dibutyryl cyclic AMP injected into different areas of the brain. In: Greengard P, Costa E (eds) Role of cyclic AMP in cell function. Raven, New York, pp 371–381

Gill DM (1977) Mechanism of action of cholera toxin. Adv Cyclic Nucleotide Res 8:85–118

Gilman AG, Nirenberg M (1971) Effects of catecholamines on adenosine 3′,5′-monophosphate concentrations of clonal satellite cells of neurons. Proc Nat Acad Sci USA 68:2165–2168

Gilman AG, Schrier BK (1972) Adenosine cyclic 3′,5′-monophosphate in fetal rat brain cell cultures. I. Effect of catecholamines. Mol Pharmacol 8:410–416

Gimpel LP, Hodgins DS, Jacobson ED (1971) Effect of endotoxin on liver adenyl cyclase. Clin Res 19:475

Goldberg ND, Dietz SB, O'Toole AG (1969) Cyclic guanosine 3′,5′-monophosphate in mammalian tissues and urine. J Biol Chem 244:4458–4466

Goldberg ND, O'Dea RF, Haddox MK (1973) Cyclic GMP. Adv Cyclic Nucleotide Res 3:155–223

Goldfine ID, Roth J, Birnbaumer L (1972) Glucagon receptors in β-cells. Binding of ^{125}I-glucagon and activation of adenylate cyclase. J Biol Chem 247:1211–1218

Gopinath RM, Vincenzi FF (1977) Phosphodiesterase protein activator mimics red blood cell cytoplasmic activator of (Ca^{2+}–Mg^{2+}) ATPase. Biochem Biophys Res Commun 77:1203–1209

Goren EN, Rosen OM (1971) The effect of nucleotides and a nondialyzable factor on the hydrolysis of cyclic AMP by a cyclic nucleotide phosphodiesterase from beef heart. Arch Biochem Biophys 142:720–723

Goren EN, Rosen OM (1972) Purification and properties of a cyclic nucleotide phosphodiesterase from bovine heart. Arch Biochem Biophys 153:384–397

Gorman RE, Bitensky MW (1972) Selective effects of cholera toxin on the adrenaline responsive component of hepatic adenyl cyclase. Nature 235:439–440

Grahame-Smith DG, Isaac P, Heal DJ (1975) Inhibition of adenyl cyclase by an exotoxin of *Bacillus thuringiensis*. Nature 253:58–60

Grand RJ, Torti FM, Jaksina S (1973) Development of intestinal adenyl cyclase and its response to cholera enterotoxin. J Clin Invest 52:2053–2059

Greengard P, Costa E (eds) (1970) Role of cyclic AMP in cell function. Raven, New York

Greengard P, Kuo JF (1970) On the mechanism of action of cyclic AMP. In: Greengard P, Costa E (eds) Role of cyclic AMP in cell function. Raven, New York, pp 287–306

Guerrant RL, Chen LC, Sharp GWG (1972) Intestinal adenyl-cyclase activity in canine cholera: correlation with fluid accumulation. J Infect Dis 125:377–381

Guerrant RL, Brunton LL, Schnaitman TC, Rebhun LI, Gilman AG (1974) Cyclic adenosine monophosphate and alteration of Chinese hamster ovary cell morphology: a rapid, sensitive *in vitro* assay for the enterotoxins of *Vibrio cholerae* and *Escherichia coli*. Infect Immun 10:320–327

Gullis R, Traber J, Hamprecht B (1975) Morphine elevates levels of cyclic GMP in a neuroblastoma × glioma hybrid cell line. Nature 256:57–59

Hadley ME, Goldman JM (1969) Effects of cyclic 3′,5′-AMP and other adenine nucleotides on the melanophores of the lizard (*Anolis carolinensis*). Br J Pharmacol 37:650–658

Hardman JG, Sutherland EW (1969) Guanyl cyclase, an enzyme catalyzing the formation of guanosine 3′,5′-monophosphate from guanosine triphosphate. J Biol Chem 244:6363–6370

Hardman JG, Davis JW, Sutherland EW (1969) Effects of some hormonal and other factors on the excretion of guanosine 3′,5′-monophosphate and adenosine 3′,5′-monophosphate in rat urine. J Biol Chem 244:6354–6362

Harris DN, Phillips MB, Goldenberg HJ (1971) Interaction of cyclic nucleotides with cyclic nucleotide phosphodiesterases of the cat heart. Fed Proc 30:219

Harris DN, Chasin M, Phillips MB, Goldenberg H, Samaniego S, Hess SM (1973) Effect of cyclic nucleotides on activity of cyclic 3′,5′-adenosine monophosphate phosphodiesterase. Biochem Pharmacol 22:221–228

Hegstrand LR, Kanof PD, Greengard P (1976) Histamine-sensitive adenylate cyclase in mammalian brain. Nature 260:163–165

Henion WF, Sutherland EW (1971) Cyclic AMP and hormone action. In: Robison GA, Butcher RW, Sutherland EW (eds) Cyclic AMP. Academic Press, New York London, pp 17–47

Henion WF, Sutherland EW, Posternak T (1967) Effects of derivatives of adenosine 3',5'-phosphate on liver slices and intact animals. Biochim Biophys Acta 148:106–113

Herman ZS (1973) Behavioural effects of dibutyryl cyclic 3',5' AMP, noradrenaline and cyclic 3',5' AMP in rats. Neuropharmacology 12:705–709

Herman ZS, Szkilnik R (1977) Central effects of dibutyryl cyclic 3',5' AMP and dibutyryl cyclic 3',5' GMP in mice. Acta Med Pol 18:1–6

Hilz H, Tarnowski W (1970) Opposite effects of cyclic AMP and its dibutyryl derivative on glycogen levels in HeLa cells. Biochem Biophys Res Commun 40:973–981

Honda F, Imamura H (1968) Inhibition of cyclic 3',5'-nucleotide phosphodiesterase by phenothiazine and reserpine derivatives. Biochim Biophys Acta 161:267–269

Hynie S, Rašková H, Sechser T et al. (1974) Stimulation of intestinal and liver adenyl cyclase by enterotoxin from strains of *Escherichia coli* enteropathogenic for calves. Toxicon 12:173–179

Isaac P, Grahame-Smith DG (1972) Adenosine 3':5'-cyclic monophosphate and adenyl cyclase in subcellular fractions of rat brain. Biochem J 126:14P

Ishikawa E, Ishikawa S, Davis JW, Sutherland EW (1969) Determination of guanosine 3',5'-monophosphate in tissues and of guanyl cyclase in rat intestine. J Biol Chem 244:6371–6376

Isom GE, McCarthy TA, Eells JT, Wimer ER (1978) Influence of intracerebroventricular injections of $N^6,O^{2'}$-dibutyryl adenosine 3':5'-cyclic monophosphate on sodium pentobarbital-induced narcosis in rats. Neuropharmacology 17:53–58

Iversen LL, Glowinski J (1966) Regional studies of catecholamines in the rat brain. II. Rate of turnover of catecholamines in various brain regions. J Neurochem 13:671–682

Iwangoff P, Enz A (1973) Inhibition of phoshodiesterase by dihydroergotamine and hydergine in various organs of the cat in vitro. Experientia 29:1067–1069

Jacks TM, Wu BJ, Braemer AC, Bidlack DE (1973) Properties of the enterotoxic component in *Escherichia coli* enteropathogenic for swine. Infect Immun 7:178–189

Jancsó G, Wollemann M (1977) The effect of capsaicin on the adenylate cyclase activity of rat brain. Brain Res 123:323–329

Jancsó VN, Jancsó-Gábor A (1965) Die Wirkungen des Capsaicins auf die hypothalamischen Thermoreceptoren. Naunyn-Schmiedeberg Arch Exp Pathol Pharmakol 251:136–137

Jancsó-Gábor A, Szolcsányi J, Janscó N (1970a) Irreversible impairment of thermoregulation induced by capsaicin and similar pungent substances in rats. J Physiol (Lond) 206:495–507

Jancsó-Gábor A, Szolcsányi J, Jancsó N (1970b) Stimulation and desensitization of the hypothalamic heat-sensitive structures by capsaicin in rats. J Physiol (Lond) 208:449–459

Jard S, Bernard M (1970) Presence of two 3'-5'-cyclic AMP phosphodiesterases in rat kidney and frog bladder epithelial cells extracts. Biochem Biophys Res Commun 41:781–788

Jarrett HW, Penniston JT (1977) Partial purification of the Ca^{2+}–Mg^{2+} ATPase activator from human erythrocytes: its similarity to the activator of 3':5'-cyclic nucleotide phosphodiesterase. Biochem Biophys Res Commun 77:1210–1216

Jona JL (1916) A contribution to the experimental study of fever. J Hyg (Lond) 15:169–194

Jones DJ, Stavinoha WB (1977) Levels of cyclic nucleotides in mouse regional brain following 300 ms microwave inactivation. J Neurochem 28:759–763

Jones DJ, Medina MA, Ross DH, Stavinoha WB (1974) Rate of inactivation of adenyl cyclase and phosphodiesterase: determinants of brain cAMP. Life Sci 14:1577–1585

Joó F, Rakonczay Z, Wollemann M (1975) cAMP-mediated regulation of the permeability in the brain capillaries. Experientia 31:582–584

Kakiuchi S, Rall TW (1968) Studies on adenosine 3',5'-phosphate in rabbit cerebral cortex. Mol Pharmacol 4:379–388

Kakiuchi S, Yamazaki R, Teshima Y (1971) Cyclic 3',5'-nucleotide phosphodiesterase. IV. Two enzymes with different properties from brain. Biochem Biophys Res Commun 42:968–974

Kakiuchi S, Yamazaki R, Teshima Y, Uenishi K (1973) Regulation of nucleoside cyclic 3',5'-monophosphate phosphodiesterase activity from rat brain by a modulator and Ca^{2+}. Proc Nat Acad Sci USA 70:3526–3530

Kantor HS, Tao P, Wisdom C (1974) Action of *Escherichia coli* enterotoxin: adenylate cyclase behaviour of intestinal epithelial cells in culture. Infect Immun 9:1003–1010

Kaukel E, Hilz H (1972) Permeation of dibutyryl cAMP into HeLa cells and its conversion to monobutyryl cAMP. Biochem Biophys Res Commun 46:1011–1018

Kaukel E, Mundhenk K, Hilz H (1972) N^6-Monobutyryladenosine 3′:5′-monophosphate as the biologically active derivative of dibutyryladenosine 3′:5′-monophosphate in HeLa S3 cells. Eur J Biochem 27:197–200

Kebabian JW (1977) Biochemical regulation and physiological significance of cyclic nucleotides in the nervous system. Adv Cyclic Nucleotide Res 8:421–508

Kebabian JW, Bloom FE, Steiner AL, Greengard P (1975) Neurotransmitters increase cyclic nucleotides in postganglionic neurones: immunocytochemical demonstration. Science 190:157–159

Kim TS, Shulman J, Levine RA (1968) Relaxant effect of cyclic adenosine 3′,5′-monophosphate on the isolated rabbit ileum. J Pharmacol Exp Ther 163:36–42

Kimberg DV, Field M, Johnson J, Henderson A, Gershon E (1971) Stimulation of intestinal mucosal adenyl cyclase by cholera enterotoxin and prostaglandins. J Clin Invest 50:1218–1230

Kimberg DV, Field M, Gershon E, Henderson A (1974) Effects of prostaglandins and cholera enterotoxin on intestinal mucosal cyclic AMP accumulation. Evidence against an essential role for prostaglandins in the action of toxin. J Clin Invest 53:941–949

Kimura H, Murad F (1974) Evidence for two different forms of guanylate cyclase in rat heart. J Biol Chem 249:6910–6916

Kimura H, Murad F (1975) Localization of particulate guanylate cyclase in plasma membranes and microsomes of rat liver. J Biol Chem 250:4810–4817

Kimura H, Mittal CK, Murad F (1975) Increases in cyclic GMP levels in brain and liver with sodium azide an activator of guanylate cyclase. Nature 257:700–702

Klainer LM, Chi YM, Freidberg SL, Rall TW, Sutherland EW (1962) Adenyl cyclase: the effects of neurohormones on the formation of adenosine 3′,5′-phosphate by preparations from brain and other tissues. J Biol Chem 237:1239–1243

Kornbluth I, Siegel RA, Conforti N, Chowers I (1977) cAMP in temperature- and ADH-regulating centers after thermal stress. J Appl Physiol 42:257–261

Krishna G, Harwood JP (1972) Requirement for guanosine triphosphate in the prostaglandin activation of adenylate cyclase of platelet membranes. J Biol Chem 247:2253–2254

Krishna G, Weiss B, Davies JI, Hynie S (1966) Mechanism of nicotinic acid inhibition of hormone-induced lipolysis. Fed Proc 25:719

Krishna G, Weiss B, Brodie BB (1968) A simple sensitive method for the assay of adenyl cyclase. J Pharmacol Exp Ther 163:379–385

Kuo JF, Greengard P (1970) Cyclic nucleotide-dependent protein kinases. Isolation and partial purification of a protein kinase activated by guanosine 3′,5′-monophosphate. J Biol Chem 245:2493–2498

Kuo JF, Lee TP, Reyes PL, Walton KG, Donnelly TE Jr, Greengard P (1972) Cyclic nucleotide-dependent kinases. X. An assay method for measurement of guanosine 3′,5′-monophosphate in various biological materials and a study of agents regulating its levels in heart and brain. J Biol Chem 247:16–22

Laburn H, Rosendorff C, Willies G, Woolf C (1974) A role for noradrenaline and cyclic AMP in prostaglandin E_1 fever. J Physiol (Lond) 240:49–50P

Lee TP, Kuo JF, Greengard P (1972) Role of muscarinic cholinergic receptors in regulation of guanosine 3′:5′-cyclic monophosphate content in mammalian brain, heart muscle, and intestinal smooth muscle. Proc Nat Acad Sci USA 69:3287–3291

Lefkowitz RJ (1975) Guanosine triphosphate binding sites in solubilized myocardium. Relation to adenylate cyclase activity. J Biol Chem 250:1006–1011

Lenox RH, Meyerhoff JL, Gandhi OP, Wray HL (1977) Regional levels of cyclic AMP in rat brain: pitfalls of microwave inactivation. J Cyclic Nucleotide Res 3:367–379

Leonard BE (1972) Effect of phentolamine on the increase in brain glycolysis following the intraventricular administration of dibutyryl-3,5-cyclic adenosine monophosphate and sodium fluoride to mice. Biochem Pharmacol 21:115–117

Leray FA, Chambaut AM, Hanoune J (1972) Role of GTP in epinephrine and glucagon activation of adenyl cyclase of liver plasma membrane. Biochem Biophys Res Commun 48:1385–1391

Levine RA, Lewis SE, Shulman J, Washington A (1969) Metabolism of cyclic adenosine 3',5'-monophosphate-8-^{14}C by isolated perfused rat liver. J Biol Chem 244:4017–4022

Lichtenstein LM, Henney CS, Bourne HR, Greenough WB III (1973) Effects of cholera toxin on in vitro models of immediate and delayed hypersensitivity. Further evidence for the role of cyclic adenosine 3',5'-monophosphate. J Clin Invest 52:691–697

Lin YM, Liu YP, Cheung WY (1974) Cyclic 3':5'-nucleotide phosphodiesterase. Purification, characterization, and active form of the protein activator from bovine brain. J Biol Chem 249:4943–4954

Lipton JM, Fossler DE (1974) Fever produced in the squirrel monkey by intravenous and intracerebral endotoxin. Am J Physiol 226:1022–1027

Londos C, Salomon Y, Lin MC, Harwood JP, Schramm M, Wolff J, Rodbell M (1974) 5'-Guanylylimidodiphosphate, a potent activator of adenylate cyclase systems in eukaryotic cells. Proc Nat Acad Sci USA 71:3087–3090

Lust WD, Passonneau JV (1973) Influence of certain drugs on cyclic nucleotide levels in mouse brain following electroconvulsive shock. Trans Am Soc Neurochem 4:115

Lust WD, Passonneau JV, Veech RL (1973) Cyclic adenosine monophosphate, metabolites, and phoshorylase in neural tissue: a comparison of methods of fixation. Science 181:280–282

Mao CC, Guidotti A, Lehne R, Costa E (1973) Effect of cold exposure on adenosine 3', 5'-monophosphate (cyclic AMP) and guanosine 3', 5'-monophosphate (cyclic GMP) concentrations of rat cerebellum and striatum. Trans Am Soc Neurochem 4:116

Mao CC, Guidotti A, Costa E (1974a) Interactions between γ-aminobutyric acid and guanosine cyclic 3',5'-monophosphate in rat cerebellum. Mol Pharmacol 10:736–745

Mao CC, Guidotti A, Costa E (1974b) The regulation of cyclic guanosine monophosphate in rat cerebellum: possible involvement of putative amino acid neurotransmitters. Brain Res 79:510–514

Marley E, Nistico G (1972) Effects of catecholamines and adenosine derivatives given into the brain of fowls. Br J Pharmacol 46:619–636

Mashiter K, Mashiter GD, Hauger RL, Field JB (1973) Effects of cholera and E. coli enterotoxins on cyclic adenosine 3',5'-monophosphate levels and intermediary metabolism in the thyroid. Endocrinology 92:541–549

McKean CM, Peterson NA, Raghupathy E (1969) Effects of N[6]-2'-O-dibutyryladenosine-3',5'phosphate introduced into the cerebral ventricles of cats. Fed Proc 28:776

Menahan LA, Hepp KD, Wieland O (1969) Liver 3':5'-nucleotide phosphodiesterase and its activity in rat livers perfused with insulin. Eur J Biochem 8:435–443

Merritt JH, Chamness AF, Allen SJ (1978) Studies on blood-brain barrier permeability after microwave – radiation. Radiat Environ Biophys 15:367–377

Mertens RB, Wheeler HO, Mayer SE (1974) Effects of cholera toxin and phosphodiesterase inhibitors on fluid transport and cyclic adenosine 3',5'-monophosphate concentrations in rabbit gall bladder. Gastroenterology 67:898–906

Miller RJ, Kelly PH (1975) Dopamine-like effects of cholera toxin in the central nervous system. Nature 255:163–166

Minneman KP, Iversen LL (1976a) Cholera toxin induces pineal enzymes in culture. Science 192:803–805

Minneman KP, Iversen LL (1976b) Enkephalin and opiate narcotics increase cGMP accumulation in slices of rat neostriatum. Nature 262:313–314

Miyamoto E, Kuo JF, Greengard P (1969a) Adenosine 3',5'-monophosphate-dependent protein kinase from brain. Science 165:63–65

Miyamoto E, Kuo JF, Greengard P (1969b) Cyclic nucleotide-dependent protein kinases. III. Purification and properties of adenosine 3',5'-monophosphate-dependent protein kinase from bovine brain. J Biol Chem 244:6395–6402

Monn E, Christiansen RO (1971) Adenosine 3',5'-monophosphate phosphodiesterase: multiple molecular forms. Science 173:540–542

Muschek LD, McNeill JH (1971) The effect of tricyclic antidepressants and promethazine on 3′,5′-cyclic AMP phosphodiesterase from rat brain. Fed Proc 30:330

Myllylä VV, Eeikkinen ER, Similä S, Hokkanen E, Vapaatalo H (1975) Cerebrospinal fluid concentration and urinary excretion of cyclic adenosine-3′,5′-monophosphate in various diseases in children. Z Kinderheilkd 118:259–264

Nahorski SR, Rogers KJ (1973) The adenosine 3′,5′-monophosphate content of brain tissue obtained by an ultra-rapid freezing technique. Brain Res 51:332–336

Nathanson JA (1977) Cyclic nucleotides and nervous system function. Physiol Rev 57:157–256

Neelon FA, Birch BM (1973) Cyclic adenosine 3′:5′-monophosphate-dependent protein kinase. Interaction with butyrylated analogues of cyclic adenosine 3′:5′-monophosphate. J Biol Chem 248:8361–8365

Nistico G, Macchia V, Mandato E (1978) Molecular mechanisms of motor effects of dopamine and cholera toxin in chicks. J Pharm Pharmacol 30:49–50

Nowotny N (1971) Chemical and biological heterogeneity of endotoxins. In: Weinbaum G, Kadis S, Ajl SJ (eds) Microbial toxins, vol 4. Academic Press, New York, pp 309–329

Ono H, Taira N, Hashimoto K (1976) Behavioural and vegetative effects of dibutyryl cyclic AMP on conscious dogs. Neuropharmacology 15:571–575

Palmer GC (1973) Adenyl cyclase in neuronal and glial-enriched fractions from rat and rabbit brain. Res Commun Chem Pathol Pharmacol 5:603–613

Palmer GC, Duszynski CR (1975) Regional cyclic GMP content in incubated tissue slices of rat brain. Eur J Pharmacol 32:375–379

Pettinger WA, Bautz GT, Wiggan GA, Sheppard H (1970) Cyclic AMP as a mediator of vasodilation: indirect evidence. Pharmacologist 12:291

Pfeuffer T, Helmreich EJM (1975) Activation of pigeon erythrocyte membrane adenylate cyclase by guanylnucleotide analogues and separation of a nucleotide binding protein. J Biol Chem 250:867–876

Philipp-Dormston WK (1975) Cyclic AMP synthesis in rabbit brain during experimental fever. Proc Tenth Meet Eur Biochem Soc, Paris Abstr 1330. Soc de Chimic Biologique, Paris

Philipp-Dormston WK (1976) Evidence for the involvement of adenosine 3′,5′-cyclic monophosphate in fever genesis. Pfluegers Arch 362:223–227

Philipp-Dormston WK, Siegert R (1975a) Fever produced in rabbits by N^6,O2-dibutyryl adenosine 3′,5′-cyclic monophosphate. Experientia 31:471–472

Philipp-Dormston WK, Siegert R (1975b) Adenosine 3′,5′-cyclic monophosphate in rabbit cerebrospinal fluid during fever induced by E. coli-endotoxin. Med Microbiol Immunol 161:11–13

Pichard AL, Hanoune J, Kaplan JC (1973) Multiple forms of cyclic adenosine 3′,5′-monophosphate phosphodiesterase from human blood platelets. Biochim Biophys Acta 315:370–377

Pledger WJ, Stancel GM, Thompson WJ, Strada SJ (1974) Separation of multiple forms of cyclic nucleotide phosphodiesterases from rat brain by isoelectrofocusing. Biochim Biophys Acta 370:242–248

Posternak T (1971) Chemistry of cyclic nucleoside phosphates and synthesis of analogs. In: Robison GA, Butcher RW, Sutherland EW (eds) Cyclic AMP. Academic Press, New York London, pp 48–68

Posternak T, Sutherland EW, Henion WF (1962) Derivatives of cyclic 3′,5′-adenosine monophosphate. Biochim Biophys Acta 65:558–560

Quenzer LF, Galli CL, Neff NH (1977) Activation of the nigrostriatal dopaminergic pathway by injection of cholera enterotoxin into the substantia nigra. Science 195:78–80

Rall TW, Sutherland EW (1958) Formation of a cyclic adenine ribonucleotide by tissue particles. J Biol Chem 232:1065–1076

Rall TW, Sutherland EW (1962) Adenyl cyclase. II. The enzymatically catalyzed formation of adenosine 3′,5′-phosphate and inorganic pyrophosphate from adenosine triphosphate. J Biol Chem 237:1228–1232

Rindi G, Sciorelli G, Poloni M, Acanfora F (1972) Induction of ingestive responses by cAMP applied into the rat hypothalamus. Experientia 28:1047–1049

Robison GA, Butcher RW, Sutherland EW (eds) (1971) Cyclic AMP. Academic Press, New York London

Rodbell M, Birnbaumer L, Pohl SL, Krans HMJ (1971) The glucagon-sensitive adenyl cyclase system in plasma membranes of rat liver. V. An obligatory role of guanyl nucleotides in glucagon action. J Biol Chem 246:1877–1882

Rosen OM (1970) Interaction of cyclic GMP and cyclic AMP with a cyclic nucleotide phosphodiesterase of the frog erythrocyte. Arch Biochem Biophys 139:447–449

Rothfield L, Horne RW (1967) Reassociation of purified lipopolysaccharide and phospholipid of the bacterial cell envelope: electron microscopic and monolayer studies. J Bacteriol 93:1705–1721

Russell TR, Terasaki WL, Appleman MM (1973) Separate phosphodiesterases for the hydrolysis of cyclic adenosine 3',5'-monophosphate and cyclic guanosine 3',5'-monophosphate in rat liver. J Biol Chem 248:1334–1340

Ryan WL, Heidrick ML (1968) Inhibition of cell growth in vitro by adenosine 3',5'-monophosphate. Science 162:1484–1485

Sahyoun N, Cuatrecasas P (1975) Mechanism of activation of adenylate cyclase by cholera toxin. Proc Nat Acad Sci USA 72:3438–3442

Sattin A, Rall TW (1970) The effects of adenosine and adenine nucleotides on the cyclic adenosine 3',5'-phosphate content of guinea pig cerebral cortex slices. Mol Pharmacol 6:13–23

Schmidt MJ, Schmidt DE, Robison GA (1971) Cyclic adenosine monophosphate in brain areas: microwave irradiation as a means of tissue fixation. Science 173:1142–1143

Schmidt MJ, Schmidt DE, Robison GA (1972) Cyclic AMP in the rat brain: microwave irradiation as a means of tissue fixation. Adv Cyclic Nucleotide Res 1:425–434

Schramm M, Rodbell M (1975) A persistent active state of the adenylate cyclase system produced by the combined actions of isoproterenol and guanyl imidodiphosphate in frog erythrocyte membranes. J Biol Chem 250:2232–2237

Schröder J, Rickenberg HV (1973) Partial purification and properties of the cyclic AMP and the cyclic GMP phosphodiesterase of bovine liver. Biochem Biophys Acta 302:50–63

Schultz G, Senft G, Losert W, Sitt R (1966) Biochemische Grundlagen der Diazoxid-Hyperglykämie. Naunyn-Schmiedeberg Arch Exp Pathol Pharmakol 253:372–387

Schultz G, Böhme E, Munske K (1969) Guanyl cyclase. Determination of enzyme activity. Life Sci 8:1323–1332

Schultz J, Hamprecht B, Daly JW (1972) Accumulation of adenosine 3':5'-cyclic monophosphate in clonal glial cells: labeling of intracellular adenine nucleotides with radioactive adenine. Proc Nat Acad Sci USA 69:1266–1270

Sebens JB, Korf J (1975) Cyclic AMP in cerebrospinal fluid: accumulation following probenecid and biogenic amines. Exp Neurol 46:333–344

Šebesta K, Horská K (1968) Inhibition of DNA-dependent RNA polymerase by the exotoxin of Bacillus thuringiensis var. gelechiae. Biochim Biophys Acta 169:281–282

Shands JW Jr (1973) Affinity of endotoxin for membranes. J Infect Dis 128:S197–S201

Sheppard H, Wiggan G (1971a) Different sensitivities of the phosphodiesterases (adenosine-3',5'-cyclic phosphate 3'-phosphohydrolase) of dog cerebral cortex and erythrocytes to inhibition by synthetic agents and cold. Biochem Pharmacol 20:2128–2130

Sheppard H, Wiggan G (1971b) Analogues of 4-(3,4-dimethoxybenzyl)-2-imidazolidinone as potent inhibitors of rat erythrocyte adenosine cyclic 3',5'-phosphate phosphodiesterase. Mol Pharmacol 7:111–115

Sheppard H, Wiggan G, Tsien WH (1971) The differential inhibition of the phosphodiesterase (PD) preparations from canine cerebral cortex and erythrocytes by chemical agents and cold. Fed Proc 30:330

Siegel RA Kornbluth I, Conforti N, Chowers I (1976) The effect of acute heat exposure on cyclic adenosine-3',5'-monophosphate concentrations in the preoptic area, posterior medial hypothalamus, supraoptic-paraventricular nuclei and neurohypophysis of the rat. Isr J Med Sci 12:1060–1062

Siegert R, Philipp-Dormston WK, Radsak K, Menzel H (1975) Inhibition of Newcastle disease virus-induced fever in rabbits by cycloheximide. Arch Virol 48:367–373

Siegert R, Philipp-Dormston WK, Radsak K, Menzel H (1976) Mechanism of fever induction in rabbits. Infect Immun 14:1130–1137

Siggins GR, Henriksen SJ (1975) Analogs of cyclic adenosine monophosphate: correlation of inhibition of Purkinje neurons with protein kinase activation. Science 189:559–561

Solomon SS, Brush JS, Kitabchi AE (1970) Divergent biological effects of adenosine and dibutyryl adenosine 3′,5′-monophosphate on the isolated fat cell. Science 169:387–388

Spiegel AM, Aurbach GD (1974) Binding of 5′-guanylyl-imidodiphosphate to turkey erythrocyte membranes and effects on β-adrenergic-activated adenylate cyclase. J Biol Chem 249:7630–7636

Spitzer JA, Kovách AGB, Sándor P, Spitzer JJ, Storck R (1973) Adipose tissue and endotoxin shock. Acta Physiol Acad Sci Hung 44:183–194

Stavric S, Speirs JI, Konowalchuk J, Jeffrey D (1978) Stimulation of cyclic AMP secretion in Vero cells by enterotoxins of *Escherichia coli* and *Vibrio cholerae*. Infect Immun 21:514–517

Steiner AL, Ferrendelli JA, Kipnis DM (1972) Radioimmunoassay for cyclic nucleotides. III. Effect of ischemia, changes during development and regional distribution of adenosine 3′,5′-monophosphate and guanosine 3′,5′-monophosphate in mouse brain. J Biol Chem 247:1121–1124

Sutherland EW, Rall TW (1958) Fractionation and characterization of a cyclic adenine ribonucleotide formed by tissue particles. J Biol Chem 232:1077–1091

Sutherland EW, Rall TW (1960) The relation of adenosine-3′,5′-phosphate and phosphorylase to the actions of catecholamines and other hormones. Pharmacol Rev 12:265–299

Sutherland EW, Rall TW, Menon T (1962) Adenyl cyclase. I. Distribution, preparation, and properties. J Biol Chem 237:1220–1227

Teo TS, Wang TH, Wang JH (1973) Purification and properties of the protein activator of bovine heart cyclic adenosine 3′,5′-monophosphate phosphodiesterase. J Biol Chem 248:588–595

Thompson WJ, Appleman MM (1971a) Multiple cyclic nucleotide phosphodiesterase activities from rat brain. Biochemistry 10:311–316

Thompson WJ, Appleman MM (1971b) Characterization of cyclic nucleotide phosphodiesterases of rat tissues. J Biol Chem 246:3145–3150

Triner L, Vulliemoz Y, Schwartz I, Nahas GG (1970) Cyclic phosphodiesterase activity and the action of papaverine. Biochem Biophys Res Commun 40:64–69

Uzunov P, Weiss B (1971) Inhibition by phenothiazine tranquilizers of the cyclic 3′,5′-AMP system of rat brain. Fed Proc 30:330

Uzunov P, Weiss B (1972) Separation of multiple molecular forms of cyclic adenosine-3′,5′-monophosphate phosphodiesterase in rat cerebellum by polyacrylamide gel electrophoresis. Biochim Biophys Acta 284:220–226

Uzunov P, Shein HM, Weiss B (1973) Cyclic AMP phosphodiesterase in cloned astrocytoma cells: norepinephrine induces a specific enzyme form. Science 180:304–306

Uzunov P, Shein HM, Weiss B (1974) Multiple forms of cyclic 3′,5′-AMP phosphodiesterase of rat cerebrum and cloned astrocytoma and neuroblastoma cells. Neuropharmacology 13:377–391

Van Heyningen S (1974) Cholera toxin: interaction of subunits with ganglioside G_{M1}. Science 183:656–657

Van Heyningen S, King CA (1975) Subunit A from cholera toxin is an activator of adenylate cyclase in pigeon erythrocytes. Biochem J 146:269–271

Varagić VM, Beleslin DB (1973) The effect of cyclic N-2-O-dibutyryl-adenosine-3′,5′-monophosphate, adenosine triphosphate and butyrate on the body temperature of conscious cats. Brain Res 57:252–254

Veninga TS (1972) The role of monoamines in the hyperthermia produced in cats and rabbits by irradiation of the hypothalamic area. Br J Pharmacol 45:163–164P

Veninga T, Diekema A (1974) Elevation of body temperature in rabbits by X-irradiation of the trunk. Life Sci 14:1777–1784

Voigt KM, Krishna G (1967) Correlation between the distribution of adenyl cyclase (AC), cyclic 3′,5′-AMP phosphodiesterase (PD) and various biological amines in various areas of brain. Pharmacologist 9:239

Watanabe H, Passonneau JV (1974) The effect of trauma on cerebral glycogen and related metabolites and enzymes. Brain Res 66:147–159

Watanabe H, Passonneau JV (1975) Cyclic adenosine monophosphate in cerebral cortex. Alterations following trauma. Arch Neurol 32:181–185

Weiner M, Olson JW (1973) The behavioral effects of dibutyryl cyclic AMP in mice. Life Sci 12:345–356

Weiss B, Costa E (1967) Adenyl cyclase activity in rat pineal gland: effects of chronic denervation and norepinephrine. Science 156:1750–1752

Weiss B, Costa E (1968) Regional and subcellular distribution of adenyl cyclase and 3′,5′-cyclic nucleotide phosphodiesterase in brain and pineal gland. Biochem Pharmacol 17:2107–2116

Weiss B, Kidman AD (1969) Neurobiological significance of cyclic 3′,5′-adenosine monophosphate. Adv Biochem Psychopharmacol 1:131–164

Weiss B, Fertel R, Figlin R, Uzunov P (1974) Selective alteration of the activity of the multiple forms of adenosine 3′,5′-monophosphate phosphodiesterase of rat cerebrum. Mol Pharmacol 10:615–625

Wellmann W, Schwabe U (1973) Effects of prostaglandins E_1, E_2 and $F_{2\alpha}$ on cyclic AMP levels in brain in vivo. Brain Res 59:371–378

White AA, Aurbach GD (1969) Detection of guanyl cyclase in mammalian tissues. Biochim Biophys Acta 191:686–697

White AA, Aurbach GD, Carlson SJ (1969) Identification of guanyl cyclase in mammalian tissues. Fed Proc 28:473

Williams RH, Little SA, Ensinck JW (1969) Adenyl cyclase and phosphodiesterase activities in brain areas of man, monkey and rat. Am J Med Sci 258:190–202

Willies GH, Woolf CJ, Rosendorff C (1976a) The effect of an inhibitor of adenylate cyclase on the development of pyrogen, prostaglandin and cyclic AMP fevers in the rabbit. Pfluegers Arch 367:177–181

Willies GH, Woolf CJ, Rosendorff C (1976b) The effect of sodium salicylate on dibutyryl cyclic AMP fever in the conscious rabbit. Neuropharmacology 15:9–10

Wolff DJ, Brostrom CO (1974) Calcium-binding phosphoprotein from pig brain: identification as a calcium-dependent regulator of brain cyclic nucleotide phosphodiesterase. Arch Biochem Biophys 163:349–358

Wolff J, Cook GH (1973) Activation of thyroid membrane adenylate cyclase by purine nucleotides. J Biol Chem 248:350–355

Woolf CJ, Willies GH, Laburn H, Rosendorff C (1975) Pyrogen and prostaglandin fever in the rabbit. I. Effects of salicylate and the role of cyclic AMP. Neuropharmacology 14:397–403

Woolf CJ, Willies GH, Rosendorff C (1976) Does cyclic AMP have a role in the pathogencsis of fever in the rabbit? Naturwissenschaften 63:94–95

Yamamoto M, Massey KL (1969) Cyclic 3′,5′-nucleotide phosphodiesterase of fish (Salmo gairdnerii) brain. Comp Biochem Physiol 30:941–954

Yamashita K, Field JB (1972) Elevation of cyclic guanosine 3′,5′-monophosphate levels in dog thyroid slices caused by acetylcholine and sodium fluoride. J Biol Chem 247:7062–7066

Yount RG, Babcock D, Ballantyne W, Ojala D (1971) Adenylyl imidodiphosphate, an adenosine triphosphate analog containing a P-N-P linkage. Biochemistry 10:2484–2489

Zenser TV, Metzger JF (1974) Comparison of the action of Escherichia coli enterotoxin on the thymocyte adenylate cyclase-cyclic adenosine monophosphate system to that of cholera toxin and prostaglandin E_1. Infect Immun 10:503–509

Zenser TV, DeRubertis FR, George DT, Rayfield EJ (1974) Infection-induced hyperglucagonemia and altered hepatic response to glucagon in the rat. Am J Physiol 227:1299–1305

CHAPTER 10

Prostaglandins in Fever and the Mode of Action of Antipyretic Drugs

A. S. MILTON

A. Introduction

It was in the year 1763 that the REVEREND EDWARD STONE of Chipping Norton in Oxfordshire, England presented to the Royal Society in London the results of his observations on the use of the bark of the willow tree in the treatment of ague (Fig. 1). This is the first scientific account published on the use of an antipyretic drug. Just over 200 years later we are beginning to understand the mechanisms of action of antipyretic drugs. This chapter will be concerned with the developments from the beginning of the last decade, when the word "prostaglandin" was intro-

[195]

XXXII. *An Account of the Succeſs of the Bark of the Willow in the Cure of Agues. In a Letter to the Right Honourable* George *Earl of* Macclesfield, *Preſident of R. S. from the Rev. Mr.* Edmund Stone, *of* Chipping-Norton *in* Oxfordſhire.

My Lord,

Read June 2d, 1763.

AMong the many uſeful diſcoveries, which this age hath made, there are very few which, better deſerve the attention of the public than what I am going to lay before your Lordſhip.

There is a bark of an Engliſh tree, which I have found by experience to be a powerful aſtringent, and very efficacious in curing aguiſh and intermitting diſorders.

About ſix years ago, I accidentally taſted it, and was ſurpriſed at its extraordinary bitterneſs; which immediately raiſed me a ſuspicion of its having the properties of the Peruvian bark. As this tree delights in a moiſt or wet ſoil, where agues chiefly abound, the general maxim, that many natural maladies carry their cures along with them, or that their remedies lie not far from their cauſes, was ſo very appoſite to this particular caſe, that I could not help applying it; and that this might be the intention of Providence here, I muſt own had ſome little weight with me.

The exceſſive plenty of this bark furniſhed me, in my ſpeculative diſquiſitions upon it, with an

D d 2   argument

[200]

cinnamon or lateritious colour, which I believe is the caſe with the Peruvian bark and powders.

I have no other motives for publiſhing this valuable ſpecific, than that it may have a fair and full trial in all its variety of circumſtances and ſituations, and that the world may reap the benefits accruing from it. For theſe purpoſes I have given this long and minute account of it, and which I would not have troubled your Lordſhip with, was I not fully perſuaded of the wonderful efficacy of this Cortex Salignus in agues and intermitting caſes, and did I not think, that this perſuaſion was ſufficiently ſupported by the manifold experience, which I have had of it.

I am, my Lord,

with the profoundeſt ſubmiſſion and reſpect,

Chipping-Norton, Oxfordſhire, April 25, 1763.

your Lordſhip's moſt obedient humble Servant

Edward Stone.

XXXIII. *An*

Fig. 1. An account of the success of the bark of the willow in the cure of agues. First and last pages of the paper presented to the Royal Society of London on 2 June 1763 by the REVEREND EDWARD STONE. (Note the error in the title, where his name is incorrectly printed as *Edmund* Stone)

duced into our thermoregulatory repertoire by MILTON and WENDLANDT, to the present day. From the year 1763 until the beginning of the 1970s our understanding was confused and illogical. In particular there was the apparently puzzling relationship between the three dissimilar actions of the salicylates and related drugs, namely their antipyretic, analgesic, and anti-inflammatory properties. To many pharmacologists it seemed surprising that such simple drugs, for example aspirin, should have these three entirely separate actions, all mediated differently. It seemed far more logical that there should be one simple mechanism of action to explain all three properties.

In order to relate the recent history of the studies on their antipyretic action one must go back to the 1960s, when FELDBERG and MYERS proposed that the amines noradrenaline (NA) and 5-hydroxytryptamine (5-HT) were the neurotransmitters present in the hypothalamus involved in the central control of body temperature. For example, they had shown that the intracerebroventricular injection of 5-HT into the hypothalamus of the cat produced a rise in deep body temperature and NA a fall (FELDBERG and MYERS 1964). In their paper they postulated that fever might result from an imbalance in these two neurotransmitters, though they also admitted in the same paper that fever might result from some entirely different mechanism. It was as a result of reading this paper that the author of this chapter decided to determine whether any changes in central amine release could be found during fever and also, if any changes were observed, whether they could be modified by antipyretic drugs. At that time several sites of action had been proposed for the antipyretics (see COOPER et al. 1968; RAWLINS et al. 1971). In order to ascertain whether a central action was involved, MILTON and WENDLANDT (1968) injected endotoxin centrally into the lateral ventricles of the conscious cat and found that the resulting fever could either be prevented or abolished by the peripheral or central administration of the antipyretic drug 4-acetamidophenol (4-Ac) (paracetamol, acetaminophen) at the appropriate times. Attempts were then made to obtain CSF from a cat during fever and assay it for biological activity. If the ideas of FELDBERG and MYERS were correct then one might expect an elevated level of 5-HT. Experiments showed that biological activity as measured using the rat fundus strip preparation of VANE (1957) was present; however, since the response of the tissue to the extract remained after treatment with 5-HT blocking drugs, the biological activity could not be attributed to 5-HT. Insufficient material was obtained in these first experiments to make any identification of the active principle present (MILTON and WENDLANDT 1970). However, since the rat fundus strip was known to be sensitive to certain of the prostaglandins it was decided to inject prostaglandin E_1 (PGE_1) into the ventricular system and measure body temperature. The very first experiment showed that PGE_1 in microgram quantities produced a marked rise in deep body temperature accompanied by shivering and vasoconstriction and with the animal adopting a "curled up" position, symptoms very similar to those observed following the central administration of endotoxin.

A report of this first observation was published by MILTON and WENDLANDT in 1970. One of the most exciting findings of this early work was the observation that 4-Ac had no effect on the febrile response to PGE_1, in contrast to its action in suppressing fever produced by endotoxin as reported previously (MILTON and WENDLANDT 1968). From their observations with PGE_1 and 4-Ac MILTON and

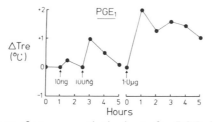

Fig. 2. Rectal temperature of an unanaesthetized cat after PGE₁ injection. *Arrows* indicate the times at which the various doses were administered. (MILTON and WENDLANDT 1971 a)

WENDLANDT put forward the proposal that "PGE₁ may be acting as a modulator in temperature regulation and that the action of antipyretics may be to interfere with the release of PGE₁ by pyrogen". At that time there was no experimental evidence to indicate how antipyretic drugs might affect the release of prostaglandins; however, the answer was to come a few months later when VANE (1971) showed that the non-steroidal anti-inflammatory drugs, including aspirin, inhibited the synthesis of prostaglandins from arachidonic acid by lung homogenates. From his observations VANE proposed that since fever could be mimicked by prostaglandins, as mentioned above, and because of the proposed involvement of prostaglandins in inflammation and pain, the prostaglandins were mediators in all these three pathological conditions, and the non-steroidal anti-inflammatory drugs produced their antipyretic, anti-inflammatory and analgesic actions by inhibition of the synthesis of the prostaglandins. This proposal of VANE provided an answer to the question already posed as to why aspirin-like drugs should have these three apparently dissimilar therapeutic effects.

Since the original proposal of MILTON and WENDLANDT many published papers have dealt with the actions of the prostaglandins in thermoregulation and fever. As with all new theories there is evidence both for and against, and the final words are yet to come.

B. Temperature Responses to Prostaglandins

I. Cats

1. Prostaglandins E₁ and E₂

The first species in which a prostaglandin was injected into the cerebroventricular system and temperature changes observed, was the cat (MILTON and WENDLANDT 1970). The authors observed that doses of between 1.0 ng and 1.0 µg injected into the third ventricle produced dose-dependent rises in deep body temperture (see Fig. 2). The hyperthermia was accompanied by vigorous shivering and skin vasoconstriction with the animals curling up in a ball; with the larger doses piloerection, sedation and stupor were observed (see also MILTON and WENDLANDT 1971 a; WENDLANDT 1972). The most important observation was that the threshold dose required to produce an effect corresponded to 3×10^{-11} mol, making PGE₁ very much more active in producing thermoregulatory changes than any other substance previously injected into the ventricular system with the possible exception

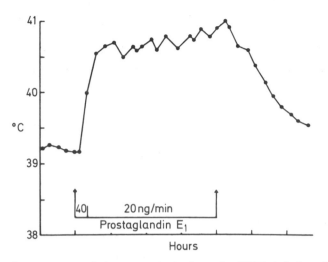

Fig. 3. Rectal temperature of an unanaesthetized cat after PGE$_1$ infusion. At the *first arrow* 40 ng/min was infused; after 20 min the infusion rate was reduced to 20 ng/min. (Feldberg and Saxena 1971 a)

of endogenous pyrogen itself. Milton and Wendlandt also observed that the latency of onset of hyperthermia following the injection of PGE$_1$ was only a few minutes and the response was also short lasting.

Feldberg and Saxena (1971 a) infused PGE$_1$ into a lateral ventricle of the conscious cat and found that if 40 ng/min was infused for 20 min the temperature rose rapidly; at that time the infusion rate was lowered to 20 ng/min and the elevated temperature remained steady for as long as infusion was continued. After cessation of infusion the temperature fell to the pre-infusion level (Fig. 3). Shivering, vasoconstriction and sedation were observed, as previously described by Milton and Wendlandt.

In a subsequent paper Feldberg and Saxena (1971 b) observed that PGE$_1$ in doses of between 2 and 100 ng produced a dose-depenent rise in body temperature when injected directly into the pre-optic area of the anterior hypothalamus (PO/AH); no effect on temperature was seen when PGE$_1$ was injected into the posterior hypothalamus. This observation is of importance in localising the hyperthermic action of the prostaglandin to the thermoregulatory centre of the brain. Milton and Wendlandt (1971 a) showed that the intracerebroventricular injection of PGE$_2$ produced exactly the same responses in the cat as PGE$_1$, and also that PGE$_1$ and PGE$_2$ were equally potent.

2. Prostaglandins F$_{1\alpha}$ and F$_{2\alpha}$

Milton and Wendlandt (1970, 1971 a) injected PGF$_{1\alpha}$ into the third ventricle of the cat. In doses of 1 or 10 μg there was no immediate effect on temperature in some cats, in others a small rise was observed and in a very few, rises of nearly 1 °C occurred. These rises differed from those produced by PGE$_1$ or PGE$_2$ in that they were not associated with shivering and vasoconstriction; however, restlessness and diarrhoea were seen.

PGF$_{2\alpha}$ in doses from 100 ng to 10 μg produced small rises (0.2–0.5 °C); however, the authors were not convinced that the effects they saw were significant. Subsequently, EWEN et al. (1976) re-investigated the effects of PGF$_{2\alpha}$ and obtained significant hyperthermia, but PGF$_{2\alpha}$ was far less potent than PGE$_2$, the ratio of equiactive doses being approximately 27:1. Since prostaglandins of both the F and the E series have been extracted from cat brain (HORTON and MAIN 1967), the authors state that PGF$_{2\alpha}$ could be involved in pyrogen-induced fever and normal thermoregulation.

3. Prostaglandin A$_1$

Intraventricular injections of PGA$_1$ 1–10 μg have no immediate effect on body temperature (MILTON and WENDLANDT 1970, 1971 a), though in some cats a rise developed after a latency of 30 min and lasted for another 12 h. If 4-Ac was administered prior to the PGA the hyperthermic response was abolished or inhibited for several hours. This long-lasting fever is probably another example of the non-specific fever (see Sect. O).

4. Prostaglandin D$_2$

Prostaglandin D$_2$ is a stereo-isomer of PGE$_2$. In doses of from 400 ng to 64 μg it elicited a small hyperthermic response, which was not dose dependent (EWEN et al. 1976) and was sufficiently indeterminate to conclude that PGD$_2$ is not hyperthermic. The results are important in that they illustrate the specificity of PGEs and the importance of the double bond oxygen atom in the 9 position of the pentane ring.

5. Environmental Temperature and PGE$_1$ Response

MILTON and WENDLANDT (1971 b) subjected cats to different environmental temperatures. At 1 °C, at which temperature the animals were thermoregulating normally, 100 ng PGE$_1$ injected into the third ventricle produced a rise in deep body temperature associated with vigorous shivering. The response was variable and less than that observed at room temperature (20°–22 °C). When the temperature of the environment was raised to 44 °C the cats had considerable difficulty in thermoregulating and body temperature rose passively; however even under these extreme conditions PGE$_1$ was still able to raise the deep body temperature, though shivering was less pronounced than at lower temperatures.

II. Rabbits

Injection of PGE$_1$ into a lateral ventricle or into the third ventricle of conscious rabbits produces a dose-dependent rise in deep body temperature (FELDBERG and SAXENA 1971 a; MILTON and WENDLANDT 1971 c). In doses of between 20 ng and 2.5 μg the effects on body temperature appeared to be mediated primarily through ear skin vasoconstriction. There was also an increase in muscle tone but shivering was only occasionally observed. PGE$_2$ was subsequently found to produce similar effects to PGE$_1$ and in similar dose ranges (HORI and HARADA 1974; CRAWFORD et al. 1979; MILTON et al. 1980; MILTON and SAWHNEY 1981).

Stitt (1973) confirmed that in the rabbit, as in the cat, the site of action of PGE$_1$ for producing hyperthermia was the anterior hypothalamus. Micro-injections of doses of PGE$_1$ between 20 ng and 1 µg produced dose-dependent hyperthermias, whereas similar injections into the posterior hypothalamus or into the midbrain reticular formation were without effect on body temperature. Upon injection into the PO/AH, decrease in heat loss and increase in heat production were observed within 1–2 min, and temperature began to rise within 2–4 min. Interestingly, there was no difference in the magnitude of the response whether the injections were made unilaterally or bilaterally. Stitt et al. (1974) measured the thermosensititivy of the PO/AH in rabbits prior to and during fever produced by intrahypothalamic injections of PGE$_1$ at ambient temperatures of $+17$, $+5$, and -5 °C. Administration of 500 ng PGE$_1$ did not alter the thermosensitivity during the chill phase of the fever but resulted in an upward displacement by 1.8 °C of the PO/AH temperature threshold for increased metabolic rate. The authors conclude that fever is produced by an upward displacement of a central reference point rather than a change in central thermosensitivity.

In their paper on the effects of PGE$_1$ and PGE$_2$, Hori and Harada (1974) showed that the hyperthermic responses to PGE$_1$ were approximately equal in magnitude and time-course irrespective of the ambient temperature. However, the ambient temperature affected the mechanisms by which the temperature rose in a very similar way to that previously reported for the sheep by Bligh and Milton (1973). For example, in the cold the effect was brought about mainly by heat production whereas in a warm environment it was brought about by suppression of heat loss with very little change in heat production. Hori and Harada also found that the PGE hyperthermia was attenuated by warming and enhanced by cooling the hypothalamus. These effects were different from those seen with NA, and the authors argue that the PGE hyperthermia is not mediated through NA and that their results support the theory that prostaglandins are involved in fever.

III. Sheep

1. Adult Sheep

Bligh and Milton (1973) studied the effects of intracerebroventricular infusions of PGE$_1$ in the Welsh mountain sheep. The sheep was chosen as an experimental animal because it is able to maintain a constant deep body temperature when exposed to a wide range of ambient air temperatures. It does this by regulating both heat loss and heat gain mechanisms and the responses can be readily monitored. Bligh and Milton recorded deep body temperature, ear skin temperature, respiratory rate and shivering.

When the ambient air temperature was 10 °C the respiratory rate was low and the ear skin temperature was the same as the air temperature, indicating vasoconstriction; an occasional burst of activity observed from electrical recordings of the thigh muscle indicated shivering. These measurements showed that the animal was maintaining deep body temperature by minimising heat loss and occasionally increasing heat production. When PGE$_1$ was infused intracerebroventricularly at the rate of 1 µg per min, the respiratory rate dropped slightly. There was no change in ear skin temperature but violent shivering was observed and deep body temperature began to rise immediately. As soon as the infusion was stopped, shivering ceased and the animals began to pant and continued to do so until deep body temperature had returned to normal. In contrast, when the ambient air temperature was 45 °C, well above deep body temperature, the animals panted vigorously, the ear vessels were dilated and no shivering was seen at all, indicating that the animals were actively preventing body temperature from rising, primarily through increased evaporative heat loss. When the PGE_1 infusion was started the respiratory rate dropped dramatically but there was no effect on the ear skin temperature and no shivering was observed. As a result of the decrease in respiratory rate, evaporative heat loss by panting was suppressed and deep body temperature rose rapidly. When the PGE_1 infusion was stopped, panting resumed and the respiratory rate rose well above the pre-infusion level. This elevated level was maintained until deep body temperature had returned to normal. When the animals were maintained at room temperature (18 °C), the ear skin temperature was between ambient temperature and deep body temperature and the animals did not shiver. At this ambient temperature PGE_1 infusion produced a fall in respiratory rate, a decrease in ear skin temperature (indicating vasoconstriction) and occasional bursts of shivering. When the PGE_1 infusion was stopped, shivering ceased, ear temperature increased and the respiratory rate rose. The deep body temperature quickly fell to normal.

These experiments on the Welsh mountain sheep showed that PGE_1 increased deep body temperature by inhibiting heat loss mechanisms, including evaporative heat loss (panting) and surface heat loss (vasomotor), and by stimulating heat gain mechanisms such as shivering (metabolic heat production). The predominant pattern of thermo-effector activity depended on the ambient air temperature and therefore on the thermoregulatory pathways being driven at the time. Of particular interest was the observation that as soon as the PGE_1 infusion was stopped, the animals rapidly lost the heat they had gained during the infusion and deep body temperature was quickly restored to normal. This is reminiscent of the effects of antipyretic drugs in reducing fever produced by bacterial pyrogens.

HALES et al. (1973) examined the response of the adult Merino sheep not only to PGE_1 but also to PGE_2, $PGF_{1\alpha}$, and $PGF_{2\alpha}$. They found that in a cool environment all the prostaglandins caused the very faint shivering normally present to increase when injected into a lateral ventricle; in addition peripheral vasoconstriction became maximal. In a thermoneutral environment shivering and vasoconstriction were produced whereas in a warm environment panting was markedly reduced and there was slight vasoconstriction. PGE_1 and PGE_2 were most effective in producing hyperthermia, $PGF_{2\alpha}$ was less effective, and $PGF_{1\alpha}$ considerably less active. HALES et al. concluded that the prostaglandins may be involved in transmission along neural pathways concerned with (a) the stimulation of heat production and increased peripheral vasomotor tone and (b) the inhibition of heat loss mechanisms.

In contrast to the work of BLIGH and MILTON, and HALES et al., PITTMAN et al. (1977b) injected PGE_1 and PGE_2 (0.2–2.0 µg) into 92 sites within the hypothalamus of the sheep and found a complete absence of fever on all occasions. Injection of 100 µg of PGE_1 into a lateral ventricle caused fever which reached a peak after about 1 h. When they injected endotoxin into the same sites as the PGE_1, fever was produced on some but not all occasions. The authors concluded that sheep may be able to develop fever without the central involvement of prostaglandins, or if prostaglandins do play a role they may act within the brain at a site other than the PO/AH.

2. New-born Lambs

PITTMAN et al. (1975) injected PGE_1 in doses of 2–200 µg into the lateral ventricle of conscious new-born lambs (aged from 4 to 168 h). Of the 40 injections, 15 were followed by rises in deep body temperature; in the remaining animals there was no change or a fall in temperature. There was no relationship between effect on deep body temperature and age or dose. Some of the lambs which did not develop fever to PGE_1 did so to intravenous endotoxin. Intracerebroventricular pyrogen (3 µg) produced no changes in body temperature in four animals tested whereas 300 µg produced a fever in three out of the four. On the basis of these results the authors suggested that the new-born lamb may be able to develop fever independent of central PGE_1. Alternatively, they considered that the intracerebroventricular approach may not be relevant to new-born lambs. Subsequently, KASTING et al. (1979), investigating the response of new-born lambs to endotoxin and to endogenous pyrogens, found that at 5 h of age lambs do not become febrile to relatively large doses of endotoxin or to endogenous pyrogen but rather become hypothermic. At 32 h and all subsequent times fever could be elicited. Onset time of fevers in lambs was initially short and gradually lengthened over the first 9 days of life; by the end of this period it was similar to the onset time in adult sheep. COOPER et al. (1979) suggested that the lack of febrile response to endotoxin in the new-born lamb occurs beyond the stage of production of endogenous pyrogen and may represent either an immmaturity of the brain mechanisms for heat production and heat conservation which are stimulated by endogenous pyrogen or the presence of an endogenous antipyretic substance in the circulation. KASTING et al. (1978 a, b) had previously shown that in the pregnant ewe febrile response to both bacterial endotoxin and endogenous pyrogen was reduced from about 4 days before until at least 5 h after parturition. They showed that this effect was due to a circulating vasopressin-like substance which had antipyretic activity, and it is therefore possible that in the new-born lamb a similar substance is present.

IV. Rats

The response of the rat to endotoxin differs depending upon whether the route of administration is central or peripheral. Upon intravenous injection the usual response is hypothermia, although hyperthermic responses have been reported, especially if live yeast is used as the pyrogenic agent (see VAN MIERT and FRENS 1968; KIM et al. this volume, Chap. 12). In contrast, as was demonstrated by MILTON and WENDLANDT (1971 a) and FELDBERG and SAXENA (1975), endotoxin regularly produces fever when injected into the cerebral ventricles of the rat.

In the unanaesthetized rat kept at an ambient temperature of 20°–25 °C injections of 5 ng to 5 µg of PGE_1 into a lateral cerebral ventricle were found to produce sharp rises in rectal temperature in restrained rats (FELDBERG and SAXENA 1971 c). Similar results were obtained by MILTON and WENDLANDT (1971 b) in unrestrained rats. Hyperthermia was also obtained with PGE_2 on injection into a lateral cerebral ventricle of restrained rats (POTTS and EAST 1972). It was later shown (FELD-BERG and SAXENA 1975) that the hyperthermia associated with sedation was produced not only by the E but also by the F prostaglandins when injected into a lateral cerebral ventricle of restrained rats. When comparing their potencies PGE_2 was found to be the most potent hyperthermic prostaglandin, followed in descending order by PGE_1, $PGF_{2\alpha}$, and $PGF_{1\alpha}$. A dose of 20 ng, which was sub-threshold for the F prostaglandins, produced hyperthermia with the E prostaglandins. The temperature effect of the E prostaglandins differed further from that of the F prostaglandins in being followed by a fall to below the pre-injection level. As in other species, the hyperthermia appears to result from an action on the PO/AH region; LIPTON et al. (1973) obtained large rises in rectal temperature upon injection of 1 µg of PGE_1 into this region, the effect being maximal when injections were made within 0.9 mm of the midline. RUDY and VISWANATHAN (1975) obtained a mean rise in temperature of 1.3 °C following unilateral injections of 100 ng of PGE_1 into the PO/AH region. Subsequently, WILLIAMS et al. (1977) carried out an extensive exploration of the rat brain for sites mediating prostaglandin-induced hyperthermia. They tested 272 sites, forming a matrix encompassing much of the subcortical tissue rostral to the medulla. Injections of PGE into a sensitive site typically produced a rapidly developing short-lasting monophasic rise in body temperature. Almost all of the active sites were within the PO/AH region, the sites of greatest activity being in the ventricular aspect of the tissue lying between the anterior commissure and the optic chiasma. The authors indicate that the PO/AH is probably the only supramedullary site of action of PGE_1 in the rat brain. VEALE and WISHAW (1976) also obtained hyperthermias in the unrestrained rat with micro-injections of 5 ng into the region of the PO/AH whereas injections into the lateral posterior hypothalamus did not affect temperature.

LIPTON et al. (1973) found that the same doses of PGE_1 that produced hyperthermia upon injection into the PO/AH region caused a pronounced fall in rectal temperature when injected into the medulla oblongata in a region below the fourth ventricle, although cooling or heating of this region had the same effect on rectal temperature as cooling and heating the PO/AH region. It is possible that the hypothermia following the hyperthermia produced by large doses of E prostaglandins injected into a lateral cerebral ventricle (FELDBERG and SAXENA 1975) results from an action on this region.

SPLAWINSKI (1977) and SPLAWINSKI et al. (1978) have also shown that when PGE_2 is injected into the hypothalamus of the rat it produces a rise in deep body temperature. VEALE and WISHAW (1976) studied the effects of PGE_1 in unanaesthetized rats at different ambient temperatures. The responses to PGE_1 were unaffected by the ambient temperature whereas the responses to NA were affected. They suggested that this is further support for the theory that pyrogens act in the hypothalamus by releasing prostaglandin. They found that PGE_1 produced a dose-dependent rise when injected into the hypothalamus but had no significant effect in the lateral ventricle, midbrain or hippocampus.

V. Mice

The response of the mouse to bacterial pyrogen appears to depend not only on the strain of mouse used but also on the experimental conditions. MILTON et al. (1982)

injected PGE_2 into the PO/AH of MF1 mice. The experiments were carried out at an ambient temperature of 32 °C. PGE_2 produced an increase in oxygen consumption and skin vasoconstriction followed by an increase in deep body temperature. The effects of PGE_2 on body temperature were dose dependent, the threshold dose required to produce an effect being 100 ng. The response was unaffected by 4-Ac. This strain of mouse was found to be unresponsive both to hypothalamic and intravenous injection of endotoxin. No pyrogenic activity was found in neutrophils prepared from peritoneal exudates of this strain of mouse. WILLIS et al. (1972) injected both PGE_1 and PGE_2 directly through the skull into the cerebroventricular spaces of the mouse at a dose of 0.6 µg. They reported that both prostaglandins produced an increase in deep body temperature.

VI. Guinea-pigs

SZÉKELY and KOMÁROMI (1978) reported that PGE_1 produced hyperthermia in 0–3 day old guinea-pigs and from their results they concluded that a prostaglandin of the E series was involved in endotoxin fever. In contrast, BLATTEIS (1980) reported that he had been unable to see any response to intra-pre-optic administration of PGE_2 in the new-born guinea-pig. It is interesting to note that, like the new-born lamb, the new-born guinea-pig is refractory to bacterial pyrogen (COOPER et al. 1979). The problems of fever development in the new-born are dealt with by SZÉKELY and SZELÉNYI (this volume, Chap. 15).

VII. Monkeys

LIPTON and FOSSLER (1974) compared the action of PGE_1 and endotoxin on temperature responses in the conscious squirrel monkey. They observed a rise in deep body temperature when PGE_1 was injected into the PO/AH, the threshold dose being 10 ng; however, very much larger doses (500–750 ng) were required to obtain consistent fevers. As with other species, the latency of the response was short (5–10 min), much less than when endotoxin was injected into the same site. Other sites in the diencephalon were found to be insensitive to both PGE_1 and endotoxin. CRAWSHAW and STITT (1975) also investigated the effect of PGE_1 in the squirrel monkey and found dose-dependent hyperthermias following injections of between 20 and 500 ng into the PO/AH. Their experiments were carried out at 21 °C, which is below the thermoneutral temperature of the squirrel monkey, and CRAWSHAW and STITT found that all the heat gained by the monkeys was from an increase in metabolic rate. Similar rises in body temperature following the injections of PGE_1 into the PO/AH were seen by WALLER and MYERS (1973) in the rhesus monkey and by HORI and HARADA (1974) in the crab-eating macaque following injection into the cerebral ventricles.

Both WALLER and MYERS (1973) and CRAWSHAW and STITT (1975) reported that in behavioural experiments in which the monkeys were able to vary ambient temperature by switching on and off heat lamps, the time of heating was increased following injection of PGE_1 into the PO/AH. The authors of both these papers indicated that this is evidence for an upward shift of the set point by PGE_1.

It is interesting to note that many primates, such as the rhesus monkey, baboon, and chimpanzee, are relatively intensitive to endotoxin when it is injected intravenously. In many cases only hypothermia is observed, with fever occurring with very high doses of the endotoxin. Other monkeys, such as the squirrel monkey, do however respond normally with a fever to intravenous injections of small doses of endotoxin. These differences in response to endotoxin between the species of monkeys are not seen when the endotoxins are injected directly into the cerebral ventricles or into the PO/AH region.

VIII. Man

The author has been unable to learn of any experiments in which prostaglandins have been administered directly into the CNS of man. However, they are used routinely for the induction of labour and the production of abortion in women. They may be given either by intravenous drip or directly into the uterus. The side-effects most frequently reported are diarrhoea and vomiting, with hyperpyrexia a common occurrence. It has been assumed that these febrile episodes are due to the prostaglandin concerned entering the CNS and acting on the PO/AH. The doses given in labour and for abortion are in the milligram range and it is therefore possible that sufficient amounts may pass into the CNS. On a dose basis, prostaglandins of the E series are more potent that those of the F series (see KARIM 1979).

IX. Monotremes

BAIRD et al. (1974) injected PGE_1 and PGE_2 into the lateral cerebral ventricles of the common echidna *(Tachyglossus aculeatus)*. Both prostaglandins produced the same effects, with PGE_1 being more active than PGE_2. In the cool (14 °C) 2 µg PGE_1 produced a marked fall in deep body temperature, with a marked rise in foot temperature indicating vasodilatation. The metabolic rate decreased slightly and shivering which only occurred at this low temperature was inhibited. At thermoneutrality (22 °C) the effects were similar but far less marked than at 14 °C, and at a high ambient temperature (26 °C) there was a slight fall in deep body temperature accompanied by a slight rise in foot temperature. There was no effect on body metabolism. At none of the ambient temperatures used did PGE_1 or PGE_2 affect respiration.

Interestingly, the authors also injected 5-HT, NA, and acetylcholine into the cerebral ventricles of this species and all three neurotransmitter substances produced falls in deep body temperature. The differences in the responses of this species of non-placental mammal from those of other mammalian species have not yet been fully explained (see discussion, Sect. Q).

X. Birds

1. Adult Chickens

When PGE_1 is infused in doses between 1 and 10 µg into the third cerebroventricle or into the hypothalamus of adult chickens, it produces an increase in deep body temperature (NISTICO and MARLEY 1973). These authors' experiments were carried out at an environmental temperature of between 20° and 25 °C, within the thermoneutral range for the chicken. The chickens exhibited changed behavioural responses, with abduction of the wings and extension of the tail and body feathers. Shivering was occasionally observed and the birds were either sedated or asleep. The effects of the PGE_1 on temperature were dose dependent. Injections into other areas of the brain, such as the palaeostriatum augmentatum, right telencephalon and mesencephalon, were without effect on cortical activity and body temperature. NISTICO and MARLEY (1976) later demonstrated that PGE_2, when infused intracerebroventricularly over 4 min in doses of 2.8–42 nmol, induced behavioural and cortical sleep which lasted between 40 and 80 min. During this time body temperature rose. The effects seen were dose dependent; as sleep abated, heat production occurred with visible muscle tremor, heat loss mechanisms such as wing abduction and tachypnoea also being involved. The activity of PGE_2 was less than that of PGE_1 (NISTICO and MARLEY 1973). In addition to PGE_1 the authors also examined the effects of PGA_1 and $PGF_{2\alpha}$. PGA_1 was similar to PGE_2 but less potent, whereas $PGF_{2\alpha}$ produced no behavioural or cortical changes but lowered body temperature. Intrahypothalamic injections of all three prostaglandins resulted in similar responses. No effect on body temperature or behaviour was seen when the prostaglandins were injected into other areas of the brain. NISTICO and MARLEY stated that the central effects of the prostaglandins would appear to depend on their chemical structure, reduction of the oxy substituent on the cyclopentane ring to form $PGF_{2\alpha}$ abolishing the ability to produce fever and sleep.

PITTMAN et al. (1976) compared the actions of bacterial pyrogen and PGE_1 in adult chickens. Single doses of the endotoxin from *Salmonella abortus equi* (0.05–0.5 µg) injected into a wing vein produced no effect on temperature, whereas 2–10 µg caused a fall of up to 1.1 °C accompanied by increased respiratory rate and flushing of the comb. These effects were not abolished by aspirin (1 g p.o.). Injection of 0.1 µg of the endotoxin into the anterior hypothalamus (AH) produced fever (1.24 °C) which was abolished by aspirin; endotoxin was without effect when injected into other brain stem areas. Injection of 0.1 µg PGE_1 into the AH also produced fever of about 1 °C. The author states that this work is supportive evidence that prostaglandins are involved in pyrogen fever but that in the chicken the action of endotoxin when given intravenously differs from that when it is administered into the hypothalamus.

NISTICO and ROTIROTI (1978) found that when the endotoxin from *S. dysenteriae* was injected into the third ventricle or hypothalamus in adult fowls at ambient temperatures of either 21°–24 °C or − 5 °C it elevated body temperature. The antipyretic agents indomethacin, aspirin, and ibuprofen given intravenously, intramuscularly or into the third ventricle abolished or delayed the fever but had no effect if administered before the endotoxin. PGE_1 and PGE_2 also produced fever which was not attenuated by the same antipyretic agents. The authors suggest that the differences seen when giving the antipyretic before fever development (no antiypresis) and after development (antipyresis) is evidence that pyrogen fever and PGE fever are dissimilar.

2. Chicks

In the chick ARTUNKAL and MARLEY (1974) found that PGE_1, when infused into the hypothalamus, elevated body temperature when the ambient temperature was thermoneutral but lowered body temperature when it was below thermoneutrality. At both temperatures PGE elevated the temperature of the exposed lower limbs, and behavioural and electrocortical sleep were also observed. Indomethacin potentiated the hyperthermia both at thermoneutrality and at ambient temperatures below thermoneutrality. Very similar results were obtained when PGE_1 was given intravenously or intra-arterially.

A potentiation of prostaglandin effects by antipyretic drugs was reported by MILTON and WENDLANDT (1971 a) when they found that injection of PGE_1 into the third ventricle of the cat could be potentiated by 4-Ac. Since it became known that indomethacin can inhibit the dehydrogenase enzyme responsible for the breakdown of prostaglandins (FLOWER 1974), ARTUNKAL et al. (1975) and NISTICO and MARLEY (1976) used 5,8,11,14-eicosatetraynoic acid (TYA), which is said to inhibit the cyclo-oxygenase without inhibiting the dehydrogenase. This substance was also found to potentiate PGE fever. These authors also observed that whereas at an ambient temperature of 16 °C *S. dysenteriae* produced fever, PGE_1 produced hypothermia. These authors maintained from these experiments that there was a dissociation between the effects of PGE_1, which produces both hyper- and hypothermia, and bacterial pyrogen, which produces hyperthermia alone. From the observations that PGE_1 produces sedation, sleep and vasodilatation of peripheral vessels in the leg it is obvious that the prostaglandin is inducing heat loss at the same time as it is producing heat gain. The overall effect will depend upon the magnitude of each of these parameters and obviously at temperatures below thermoneutral heat loss may predominate, resulting in a fall in body temperature. Why prostaglandins are more effective in promoting heat loss and bacterial pyrogen needs further investigation. At present there is no explanation as to why TYA should potentiate prostaglandin fever. It could be that it is inhibiting the removal of prostaglandins from CSF since it is known that the CSF can rapidly clear prostaglandins (HOLMES and HORTON 1968).

XI. Miscellaneous Species

Other mammalian species which have been shown to respond by hyperthermia to prostaglandins of the E series include the alpaca (BAUMANN et al. 1975).

Various non-mammalian vertebrates and also invertebrates have been shown to select warm environments following injection of prostaglandins of the E series and therefore to raise their deep body temperatures (see reviews by CASTERLIN and REYNOLDS and by REYNOLDS and CASTERLIN this volume, Chaps. 19 and 20).

C. Prostacyclin

Prostacyclin (PGI_2), a cyclic derivative of arachidonic acid, was discovered by MONCADA ct al. in 1976 and is the major metabolite of arachidonic acid in certain arterial walls as well as being present in other tissue, including the CNS. Its immediate precursors are the endoperoxides: mainly PGH_2, to some extent PGG_2. PGI_2 is extremely labile at physiological pH and is rapidly degraded to the stable metabolite 6-oxo-$PGF_{1\alpha}$.

Milton et al. (1980) injected PGI_2 and 6-oxo-$PGF_{1\alpha}$ into the third ventricle of conscious cats and rabbits and compared their actions on body temperature with that of PGE_2. In cats injection of 100 and 200 µg PGI_2 into the third ventricle produced a rise in deep body temperature within a few minutes, associated with vigorous shivering, ear skin vasoconstriction and pilo-erection. Some shivering was also observed after a lower dose (50 µg) although no effect on body temperature was observed. Sedation was a consistent feature of all three doses. No significant differences were observed between the responses to 100 and 200 µg PGI_2, both producing less hyperthermia than 1 µg PGE_2. The hyperthermic response to PGI_2 lasted several hours – considerably longer than that produced by PGE_2. 6-oxo-$PGF_{1\alpha}$ (50, 100, and 200 µg) was also injected in the third ventricle of cats. The lower dose had no effect on body temperature or on the behaviour of the animal. Both 100 and 200 µg produced temperature responses very similar to those produced by PGI_2, but the behavioural effects were different: restlessness and an increase in the frequency of respiration often accompanied the rise in deep body temperature but vigorous shivering and vasoconstriction did not appear to be associated with the rise in temperature.

PGI_2, when injected in doses of 10, 50, and 100 µg into the third ventricle of rabbits, produced a dose-related hyperthermia. The maximum increase in temperature following 100 µg PGI_2 was similar to that occurring after 5 µg PGE_2; however the duration of the response to PGI_2 was greater than that to PGE_2. The behavioural effects produced by PGI_2 also differed from those produced by PGE_2 in that rabbits became very active immediately after the injection of PGI_2 whereas PGE_2 produced sedation. 6-oxo-$PGF_{1\alpha}$ (100 µg) produced effects on temperature and behaviour in rabbits very similar to those observed after the same dose of PGI_2.

Clark and Lipton (1979) treated six cats with 100 µg PGI_2; five rapidly developed fever, in the sixth the temperature declined by 1.2 °C. Larger doses (1 mg) produced marked hyperthermia in four of the initial responders, the increases being somewhat delayed, with a transient decrease seen in three cats. The development of the hyperthermia was associated with shivering. All six cats responded normally to PGE_1. Indomethacin (2 mg/kg i.v.) was without effect on the recovery phase to PGI_2.

Milton et al. and Clark and Lipton are in agreement that PGI_2 is less potent but that the response is more sustained than with either PGE_1 or PGE_2. They also discuss the problems related to the lability of PGI_2. Milton et al. point out that PGI_2 and its degradation product 6-oxo-$PGF_{1\alpha}$ are more potent hyperthermic agents in rabbits than in cats whereas PGE_2 is more potent in cats than in rabbits. They conclude that these results provide no evidence for a role for PGI_2 in pyrogen fever.

D. Prostaglandin Endoperoxide Analogues

The two prostaglandin endoperoxides PGG_2 and PGH_2, which are intermediates in the biosynthesis of PGE_2 and $PGF_{2\alpha}$ as well as PGI_2 and the thromboxanes (see Fig. 4), are extremely labile and impractical to work with in vivo on thermoregulatory studies. Two stable endoperoxide analogues are available (Bundy 1975) in

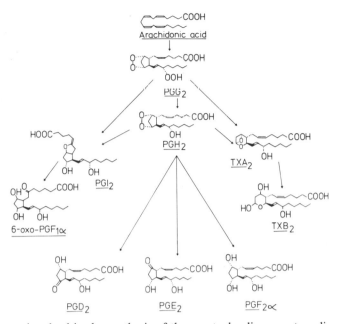

Fig. 4. Pathways involved in the synthesis of the prostaglandins, prostacyclin and thromboxanes

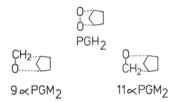

Fig. 5. Ring structures of 9_α and 11_α PGM_2 compared with the endoperoxide PGH_2

which one of the oxygen atoms bridging the cyclopentane ring has bccn replaced by a methano group. These two compounds are, respectively, (15 S)-hydroxy-9_α,11_α-(epoxymethano)prosta-5 Z,13 E-dienoic acid (Upjohn, U-46619), in which the oxygen group in the 9 position has been replaced by a methano group, and (15 S)-hydroxy-11_α,9_α-(epoxymethano)prosta-5 Z,13 E-dienoic acid (Upjohn, U-44069), in which the oxygen group in the 11 position has been replaced by a methano group (Fig. 5).

CREMADES-CAMPOS and MILTON (1978) and MILTON et al. (1980) examined the thermoregulatory responses of these two compounds, which they refer to respectively as 9_α PGM_2 and 11_α PGM_2, in conscious cats and rabbits.

Injected into the third ventricle of conscious cats in doses of 5–20 µg, 11_α PGM_2 produced a rise in deep body temperature accompanied by shivering, ear vasoconstriction and sedation. The effects were similar to those observed following the intraventricular injection of either PGE_2 or bacterial pyrogen. 11_α PGM_2 was less active than PGE_2, 20 µg of the former corresponding to 1 µg of the latter. The effects came on quickly and lasted 2–3 h; in some experiments a secondary rise in deep body temperature was observed. The antipyretic agent 4-Ac had no effect on the initial hyperthermia but completely suppressed the secondary rise. The secondary rise was considered by the authors to be a "non-specific" fever (see Sect. O) associated with disturbances of the ventricular system and resulting in prostaglandin release.

By contrast, in all experiments with cats 9_α PGM$_2$ in the same dose range produced a very marked fall in deep body temperature accompanied by panting, vasodilatation, sweating from paw pads and sedation. In some experiments a secondary fever developed; this fever was suppressed by 4-Ac, which, however, had no effect on the fall in deep body temperature produced by 9_α PGM$_2$.

In 16 rabbits used in a total of 63 experiments doses of between 5 and 20 μg of either 11_α or 9_α PGM$_2$ injected into the cerebral ventricles were without effect on deep body temperature. Other effects, such as ear skin vasodilatation, increased frequency of respiration and sedation, were frequently observed regardless of the doses tested. A dose of 20 μg of either 9_α or 11_α PGM$_2$ was fatal in over 60% of the animals, death occurring by cardiac arrest within a few minutes. This is thought to be subsequent to thrombus formation in the pulmonary veins.

The hypothermic effect of 9_α PGM$_2$ is of considerable interest as this is the only known example of a prostaglandin which produces a fall in deep body temperature in placental mammals at thermoneutrality. There is some evidence that 9_α PGM$_2$ resembles thromboxane A$_2$ in its pharmacological properties (Malmsten et al. 1975; Gorman et al. 1978). The hypothermic action of a 9_α PGM$_2$ in cats could be explained if this analogue were to cause a localised increase of free calcium ions, as hypothermia may result from infusion of calcium ions into the cerebral ventricles (Myers and Veale 1971; see also this volume, Chap. 7). Thromboxane A$_2$ has been reported to cause displacement of Ca^{2+} from the bound to the free state, which would fit in with the suggestion that 9_α PGM$_2$ resembles thromboxane A$_2$ in its actions.

In 11_α PGM$_2$ the position of the single bonded oxygen atom is the same as the double bonded oxygen atom present in PGE$_1$ and PGE$_2$, namely the 9 position, and both of these are potent hyperthermic agents. In contrast, PGD$_2$, which is without hyperthermic activity, has the double bonded oxygen in the 11 position with a single bonded hydroxyl group in the 9 position. PGF$_{1\alpha}$, PGF$_{2\alpha}$, and 6-oxo PGF$_{1\alpha}$, all of which have very little hyperthermic activity, have single bonded constituents in the 9 position. The structure-activity relationship of the prostaglandins in producing hyperthermia is therefore complex and needs further investigation. The experiments with the two endoperoxide analogues do not provide any evidence as to whether the naturally occurring endoperoxides have any role in pyrogen fever. The peculiar differences between the actions of these two analogues in the cat and the rabbit are also of interest.

E. Brain Trauma and Prostaglandin Synthesis

Damage to brain tissue may result in hyperpyrexia: it has been observed in man following head injury and neurosurgical procedures and in a variety of animal species following lesions to the pre-optic area of the anterior hypothalamus. The underlying mechanisms are not understood, however. RUDY et al. (1977) investigated the problem by producing unilateral lesions in the PO/AH of rats by acute mechanical puncture and observing the temperature changes produced following recovery from surgery. They observed a neurogenic hyperthermia which began immediately and reached a maximum (mean, $+2.3\ °C$) within 60–90 min. The hyperthermia persisted for 8–16 h, after which temperature fell to close to that observed before making the lesions. If indomethacin, a prostaglandin synthetase inhibitor, was administered intraperitoneally in doses of 5 and 15 mg/kg 1 h before puncture of the PO/AH region the febrile response was attenuated. The higher dose reduced the maximum temperature rise by 80% and the 6-h fever index by 88%.

In addition, if indomethacin (10–15 mg/kg i.p.) was administered after making the lesion then the temperature fell to near the pre-lesion value. This occurred both when the indomethacin was administered whilst the temperature was rising and when it was administered during the plateau phase of the fever.

RUDY et al. suggest that the neurogenic hyperthermia produced by the unilateral lesions of the PO/AH resulted from a prostaglandin being released from damaged tissue and possibly from blood. They give evidence to suggest that the most likely sites of action of the released prostaglandins are the remaining part of the PO/AH region in the punctured side and on the intact contralateral PO/AH region. From their results the authors feel that certain neurogenic hyperthermias may be true febrile responses involving the synthesis and release of prostaglandin.

F. Endogenous Pyrogen and Prostaglandin Synthesis In Vitro

ZIEL and KRUPP (1976) prepared endogenous pyrogen (EP) from rabbit peritoneal exudate cells, and a prostaglandin synthetase system from both bovine cerebral cortex (grey matter only) and bovine seminal vesicles. They used a micro-assay system for measuring prostaglandin synthesis using both ^{14}C labelled and unlabelled arachidonic acid. The prostaglandin formed was isolated by column chromatography and the amount synthesised determined radiometrically. They did not characterise the prostaglandin synthesised.

The authors of this paper found that the biotransformation of arachidonic acid to prostaglandin in vitro was specifically augmented by EP, the augmentation depending upon (a) the concentration of EP applied and (b) the fact that the prostaglandin synthesising system was derived from the microsomal fraction of the cerebral cortex. No potentiation of prostaglandin synthesis was observed in the seminal vesicle microsomal preparation. Neither lipopolysaccharide nor ovalbumin had any effect on prostaglandin synthesis by cerebral cortex microsomes. This potentiating effect on prostaglandin synthesis by endogenous pyrogen was inhibited by non-steroidal anti-inflammatory agents.

The differences between cerebral cortex and seminal vesicle may be due to differences in the synthesising ability of the tissue, which is low in cortex and high in seminal vesicles. The authors wonder whether different iso-enyzmes are present in the different tissues and also whether the differences could be due to the isolation procedure used in the two different tissues. However, they conclude that their results are compatible with the hypothesis that prostaglandins act as mediators of the febrile reaction induced by endogenous pyrogen.

G. Release of Prostaglandins by Pyrogens

I. Release of Prostaglandin in the CNS by Bacterial Pyrogen

If a prostaglandin of the E series is to be considered a neuromediator for fever then evidence should be available showing release of PGE in the CNS following the administration of bacterial or endogenous pyrogen. For technical reasons it is very difficult to measure PGE release in brain tissue in vivo, and to attempt to assay brain tissue post-mortem is fraught with danger, especially considering the ability of most tissues to synthesise prostaglandin following trauma or damage. This would almost certainly happen if attempts were made to remove brain tissue and assay it for prostaglandin levels. For this reason most of the attempts to correlate fever and prostaglandins have been carried out by measuring the levels of prostaglandins in CSF collected from living animals.

1. Prostaglandins in Cat Cerebrospinal Fluid

In 1970 Milton and Wendlandt found a biologically active substance present in the CSF of the conscious cat when collected from the cisterna magna during endotoxin fever. The biological activity as assayed on the rat fundus strip suggested that the substance was a prostaglandin; however, insufficient material was present for a definitive characterisation. Feldberg and Gupta (1972, 1973) collected CSF from the third ventricle of conscious cats and also measured the biological activity using the rat fundus strip preparation. They found that the CSF in afebrile cats contained small amounts of biological activity, which was greatly increased at the peak fever following administration of the endotoxin from *S. dysenteriae* into the third ventricle. The biological activity of the CSF was not abolished by treating the rat fundus strip with 2-bromolysergic acid diethylamide (BOL). The authors concluded that the biological activity was due to a prostaglandin of the E series. Their conclusion was based on the fact that of the four prostaglandins which were known at that time to contract the rat fundus strip – namely PGE_1, PGE_2, $PGF_{1\alpha}$, and $PGF_{2\alpha}$ – only PGE_1 and PGE_2 had been shown to produce fever.

When Feldberg et al. (1972, 1973) collected CSF from the cisterna magna of the conscious cat they found that the levels of biological activity in control animals or animals receiving intravenous saline were normally below those detectable by the rat fundus strip preparation treated with BOL and made more sensitive to prostaglandins by inhibiting endogenous release of prostaglandins with indomethacin (<1 ng/ml PGE). When the endotoxin from *S. dysenteriae* was administered to these cats either directly into the third ventricle or the cisterna magna or intravenously, there was always a rise in PGE levels paralleling the rise in deep body temperature (see Fig. 6). Subsequently, samples of the CSF were prepared for thin-layer chromatography and all the biologically measurable activity was found to correspond to prostaglandins of the E series. When material collected either from control (afebrile) animals or from animals during fever was radio-immunoassayed for PGEs, the prostaglandin present was found to be PGE_2. As previously reported by Milton and Wendlandt (1971 a), in the cat PGE_2 is equipotent to PGE_1 in producing hyperthermia. It was therefore concluded by Feldberg et al. (1973) that the prostaglandin released during pyrogen fever and responsible for the hyperpyrexia was PGE_2.

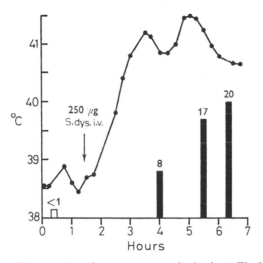

Fig. 6. Record of rectal temperature from an unanaesthetized cat. The length of the columns and the values above them refer to PGE$_1$-like activity of cisternal CSF in ng/ml. The position of the columns refers to the time but not to the duration of the CSF collection. At the *arrow*, 250 μg of the O-somatic antigen of *S. dysenteriae* was injected intravenously. (FELD-BERG and et al. 1973)

It is generally assumed that the pyrogenic activity of the endotoxins are present in the lipid A part of the lypopolysaccharide structure (see Chap. 4) and that this lipid A is similar in all gram-negative bacteria. DEY et al. (1974 b) and DEY et al. (1975) reported that lipid A injected into the conscious cat either intravenously or into the cerebral ventricles produced a fever which was accompanied by a rise in the PGE$_2$ content of the CSF collected from the cisterna magna. Lipid A was found to be more potent than endotoxin. DEY et al. reasoned that since lipid A is similar in all endotoxins, the endotoxin should act in the same way and produce fever by stimulating prostaglandin synthesis.

PGF$_{1\alpha}$ or PGF$_{2\alpha}$ occur in cat brain (HORTON and MAIN 1967); however, as previously mentioned, FELDBERG et al. (1973), using bio-assay, failed to detect any PGF in cat CSF. Since PGF$_{2\alpha}$ is pyrogenic in cats (EWEN et al. 1976), albeit in higher doses than PGE$_2$, MILTON et al. (1977) assayed for PGF in cat CSF using the more sensitive technique of radio-immunoassay. Two distinct types of febrile responses to the endotoxin of *S. dysenteriae* were observed. In some animals which had not previously received pyrogen the fever developed after a long latency (approximately 90 min), whereas in other animals which had received pyrogen previously the fever developed after a short latency (approximately 30 min). In all animals both PGE and PGF were detected in the CSF. In afebrile animals PGE levels were in the order of 140 pg/ml and PGF levels 100 pg/ml. In the short latency fevers significant increases of both PGE and PGF which paralleled the increase in deep body temperature were seen; however, during the long latency fevers no significant increases in either PGE or PGF levels were shown during the febrile response to endotoxin. An explanation for these two dissimilar responses has not been forthcoming.

2. Prostaglandins in Rabbit Cerebrospinal Fluid

Prostaglandins have been found in the CSF of rabbits during pyrogen fever. PHIL-IP-DORMSTON and SIEGERT (1974 a, b) collected CSF from the cisterna magna and assayed the samples by radio-immunoassay for prostaglandins of both the E and F series. However, no differentiation was made between PGE_1 and PGE_2, nor between $PGF_{1\alpha}$ and $PGF_{2\alpha}$. The animals were lightly anaesthetized by pentobarbitone just prior to the collection of the CSF. In control animals which had not received pyrogen, small amounts of prostaglandins of both the E and F series were found. When the samples were collected following the production of fever with the endotoxin of *E. coli* (10 µg/kg i.v.), the concentration of PGE was more than double that found in animals not receiving endotoxin. The CSF of control animals contained between 0.24 and 2.8 ng/ml PGE, with a mean of 1.87 ng/ml, whereas the samples from febrile animals contained between 2.01 and 4.98 ng/ml, with a mean of 4.11 ng/ml. There were no changes in the concentration of PGF during endotoxin fever. PHILIPP-DORMSTON and SIEGERT (1974 b) administered Newcastle disease virus in addition to *E. coli* endotoxin to rabbits and found that the virus also increased the level of PGE in the CSF by approximately twofold, but again there was no increase in PGF levels.

In 1975 HARVEY et al. measurd PGE_2 levels in rabbit CSF using the rat fundus strip preparation for their assay. They also used a different collection procedure from that of PHILIPP-DORMSTON and SIEGERT, the samples of CSF being collected from the cisterna magna immediately after killing the rabbit by injection of air into the heart. In the samples which were collected from rabbits which were afebrile after receiving intravenous injection of sterile saline the PGE content of the CSF was less than 1 ng/ml. In those animals which had received the endotoxin from *S. dysenteriae*, the CSF collected at the height of the ensuing pyrogen fever contained between 31 and 85 ng/ml PGE_2, while in the animals that received the endotoxin from *Proteus vulgaris* it contained between 41 and 60 ng/ml. If the collection of CSF from endotoxin-treated rabbits was delayed until the fever had subsided, the levels of PGE_2 in the CSF were found to be less than 1 ng/ml.

3. Prostaglandins in Human Cerebrospinal Fluid

SAXENA et al. (1979) measured the prostaglandin-like activity of human CSF obtained from pyrexic patients with bacterial or viral infections. The CSF was obtained by lumbar puncture and tested for biological activity on the rat fundus strip preparation. Several samples showed activity which was antagonised by the 5-HT receptor blocking drug methysergide, and it was concluded that the activity might be due to 5-HT. However, in some samples contractile activity was still manifest in the presence of methysergide. The authors concluded that the methysergide-resistant contractile response indicated the presence of prostaglandin. They assayed their response in comparison with a known solution of PGE_1. PGE_1-like activity was found in the CSF of patients suffering from high fever (39 °C or greater) of short duration (less than 3 days). From their experimental records it would appear that a 1-ml sample of CSF obtained from a patient with tubercular meningitis contained approximately 1 ng PGE_1, and a sample from another patient with typhoid fever, 3 ng PGE_1/ml. Prostaglandin-like activity was found in patients suffering from viral encephalitis or pyrogenic meningitis, and also in cases of undiagnosed fever. Prostaglandin-like activity was only occasionally detectable when the fever was of a lower magnitude (less than 39 °C) or of longer duration (5 days or more). No activity was present in the CSF of afebrile patients. The authors suggest that prostaglandins may play some role in the initial stages of pyrexia in man.

II. Release of Prostaglandins by Endogenous Pyrogen

Endotoxins, tissue damage and other stimuli which produce fever are thought to do so by stimulating the synthesis and release of endogenous pyrogen (EP), a low molecular weight protein, from various cells within the body (see ATKINS and BODEL 1974). Assuming that this is so and that fever results from stimulation of the release of prostaglandin in the region of the PO/AH, then EP fever should also be associated with increased acticity of PGE in the CSF.

1. Cats

HARVEY and MILTON (1975) prepared EP from cat peritoneal exudate cells and injected it either intravenously in a single dose or infused it intravenously into conscious cats. CSF was collected using the method of FELDBERG et al. (1973) and assayed for PGE_2. Doses of EP prepared from 5×10^6 cells produced a mean rise of 1.5 °C, and the PGE_2 levels increased from <1 ng/ml to a mean of 3.2 ng/ml at the height of the febrile response. If the EP (4×10^6 cell exudate/ml) was infused at a rate of 0.5 ml/min for 5 min followed by 0.05 ml/min, a rapid rise in deep body temperature was produced and sustained for as long as the infusion was continued, and PGE_2 levels rose from <1 ng/ml to between 2.7 and 5.1 ng/ml and remained elevated until the infusion was stopped. HARVEY and MILTON also obtained plasma from cats during fever produced by the administration of the O-somatic antigen of S. dysenteriae, injected either intravenously or into the cerebral ventricular system. The plasma was infused into the jugular veins of conscious cats previously made tolerant to S. dysenteriae. This was to prevent any possibility of a febrile response to S. dysenteriae endotoxin which might have been still circulating in the donor animal, though this was unlikely as endotoxin is very rapidly removed from the circulation by body tissues. When the plasma taken from cats receiving endotoxin intravenously was infused into recipient cats, an increase in deep body temperature was observed and this was associated with an increase in CSF PGE_2 levels. Plasma obtained from donors which had received no endotoxin but 0.9% sodium chloride instead was found to be non-pyrogenic when infused into the recipient cats, and no increases in CSF PGE_2 levels were found.

In a cat which developed a postoperative fever the deep body temperature was found to be 40.05 °C. A sample of CSF was taken and found to contain 7.8 ng/ml PGE_2. Plasma taken from the animal was infused into a recipient cat and produced a sustained fever, the temperature rising by 1.55 °C, and the PGE content of the CSF of the recipient increased from <1 to 3.8 ng/ml (Fig. 7).

A particularly important observation which HARVEY and MILTON made was that plasma collected from a cat in which fever had been produced by the injection of endotoxin into the cerebral ventricles produced neither an increase in body tem-

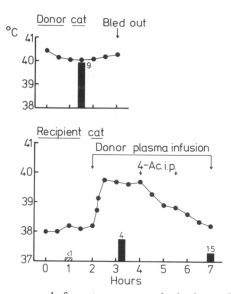

Fig. 7. Rectal temperature records from two unanaesthetized cats. The length of the columns and the values above them refer to PGE$_2$-like, activity of cisternal CSF expressed as ng/ml. The *top trace* is from a cat with a postoperative fever. The *lower trace* is from an endotoxin-resistant cat. Between the *large arrows* the plasma from the febrile cat was injected i.v. (5 ml/kg), followed by an infusion of 0.1 ml/min. At the *small arrows* 4-Ac 50 mg/kg was injected i.p. (Figure previously unpublished, for text see HARVEY and MILTON 1975)

perature in the recipient nor an increase in the PGE$_2$ levels in the CSF of the recipient, although the CSF and PGE$_2$ levels of the donor animal were increased. Endotoxin injected into the ventricular system is thought to act directly on the brain (to stimulate prostaglandin release) and not by the peripheral activation of EP synthesis and release. This experiment confirmed this and also confirmed that the pyrogenic circulating material shown to be present following intravenous administration of endotoxin was not produced subsequent to the development of fever.

2. Rabbits

PHILIPP-DORMSTON and SIEGERT (1974 b) obtained serum from rabbits by cardiac puncture at the height of fever produced by *Newcastle disease* virus. They assumed that the serum contained the EP which should be circulating in the rabbit during the virus-induced fever. When the serum was injected intravenously into afebrile rabbits it produced a fever which was associated with an increase in CSF levels of PGE but not PGF; these results were similar to those which they had obtained with Newcastle disease virus itself.

Further experiments with rabbits and EP were carried out by CRANSTON et al. (1975 a, b). They initiated steady state fever by continuous infusion of EP prepared from rabbit blood incubated with purified *Proteus* endotoxin. Samples of CSF were collected from the cisterna magna at hourly intervals and bioassayed for PGE$_2$. During the fever the PGE content of the CSF increased from undetectable levels (<1 ng/ml) to 3.6 ng/ml.

BERNHEIM et al. (1980) also produced fever in rabbits by intravenous injection of EP. They collected CSF from the third ventricle, which is nearer the PO/AH than the cisterna magna, and found an increase in PGE levels which they measured by radio-immunoassay. The PGE content was found to rise from 2–3 ng/ml to 11–12 ng/ml. Of particular interest were their observations that heating or cooling the hypothalamus which affected the animal's thermoregulation was without effect on the levels of PGE in the CSF.

III. Peripheral Actions of Antipyretics

It is the basic premise of this chapter that EP synthesized and released peripherally activates the synthesis and release of a prostaglandin which is the final modulator of fever; however, there are those who do not accept this and would suggest that pyrogens can act directly on neurones within the hypothalamus. Similarly, it is accepted that the predominant action of antipyretic drugs is within the CNS, either by inhibiting prostaglandin synthesis, as maintained here, or by acting directly on cells within the hypothalamus or by blocking the action of pyrogens on similar cells (see RAWLINS et al. 1971). However, antipyretics may also be able to exert an antipyretic action at the level of the neutrophil or other EP synthesising cell within the body to prevent the synthesis and/or release of EP. GANDER et al. (1967) found that antipyretic drugs such as aspirin, inhibited endotoxin fever in rabbits but not endogenous pyrogen fever. They suggested that the antipyretics were acting between the endotoxin and the circulating EP. They also showed that if neutrophils prepared from buffy coat were incubated with endotoxin then EP was released and this effect could be inhibited by the antipyretic drugs under investigation. These same authors subsequently obtained similar results using indomethacin and phenylbutazone (unpublished work). The drugs which they used were all good anti-inflammatory agents as well as being antipyretic; however, when experiments were repeated by GANDER et al. (1972) using 4-Ac, which has little anti-inflammatory action, no inhibition of EP release from neutrophils could be measured despite the finding that 4-Ac is antipyretic in the rabbit. In fact GANDER et al. (1972) showed that during antipyresis induced by 4-Ac circulating endogenous pyrogenic material was still present in the plasma of the rabbit. Subsequently, HARVEY (1976) showed that in the rabbit 4-Ac was antipyretic to the fevers produced both by intravenous injection of endotoxin and EP.

In summary, certain antipyretic agents, particularly those with anti-inflammatory properties, can block the synthesis or release of EP and may possibly exert part of their antipyretic action by this mechanism. However, I consider that the major site of action of antipyretic agents which have little anti-inflammatory action and which do not exert an effect at the neutrophil level is within the CNS.

H. Antipyretics and Prostaglandin Synthesis

I. Action on Prostaglandin Fever

In their first publication on the "fever"-producing effects of PGE$_1$ when injected into the third cerebral ventricle of the conscious cat, MILTON and WENDLANDT

(1970) showed that the hyperthermic action of PGE_1, in contrast to the fever produced by endotoxin (MILTON and WENDLANDT 1968), was not prevented or abolished by 4-Ac. This observation led to the proposal that prostaglandins are modulators of fever and that antipyretics act by inhibiting prostaglandin release in some way. As a result of the work of VANE (1971) we now know that it is not the release of prostaglandin which is inhibited by antipyretics but their synthesis. However, as PIPER and VANE (1971) pointed out, "prostaglandin release can often be equated with prostaglandin synthesis; for many tissues can be provoked to release more prostaglandins than they contain." These early observations on the resistance of prostaglandin fever to the action of antipyretics have been confirmed and extended to other species, to prostaglandins other than PGE_1, particularly PGE_2, and to antipyretics other than 4-Ac [see MILTON and WENDLANDT 1971 b; MILTON 1972; SCHOENER and WANG 1974; CLARK and CUMBY 1975 b; (cats) – MILTON and WENDLANDT 1971 b; KANDASAMY et al. 1975; WOOLF et al. 1975; (rabbits) – MILTON and WENDLANDT (1971 b) (rats) – WILLIS et al. 1972 (mice) – ARTUNKAL and MARLEY 1974; ARTUNKAL et al. 1975; (chicks)]. There are reports that the effects of the prostaglandins may in fact be potentiated by antipyretics. There are two possible explanations for the enhancement of the prostaglandin fever. Firstly, the inhibition of prostaglandin synthesis, and secondly, retardation of the breakdown of the prostaglandin (because certain antipyretics such as indomethacin also inhibit prostaglandin dehydrogenase). However, other explanations may also have to be considered (see p. 297).

II. Action on Prostaglandin Release During Endotoxin and Endogenous Pyrogen Fever

In the experiments described by FELDBERG and GUPTA (1972, 1973) in which they measured prostaglandin-like activity in CSF collected from the third ventricle of the conscious cat, they found that intraperitoneal injection of 4-Ac not only lowered the fever but also reduced the prostaglandin-like activity to below detectable levels. FELDBERG et al. (1972) developed a method for collecting CSF from the cisterna magna of the conscious cat. Using this technique they studied the effects of 4-Ac and indomethacin on the febrile response and CSF prostaglandin levels following injections of the endotoxin of *S. dysenteriae* not only into the cerebral ventricles but also into the cisterna magna and intravenously. In all cases the elevated levels of PGE (identified as PGE_2) found during fever were reduced during antipyresis (Fig. 8).

Similar results were obtained by HARVEY et al. (1975), who also collected CSF from the cisterna magna of the rabbit (see p. 276), where the elevated levels of PGE in the CSF during endotoxin fever were lowered not only by 4-Ac and indomethacin but also by aspirin.

As mentioned earlier (p. 275) the lipid A part of the endotoxin molecule is considered to be either the same or similar in all gram-negative bacterial endotoxins, and also to be responsible for the pyrogenic activity of the molecule. DEY et al. (1974 b, 1975), using lipid A, found that both the fever and the elevated PGE_2 activity in the CSF produced by the lipid A injected intravenously or into the cerebral

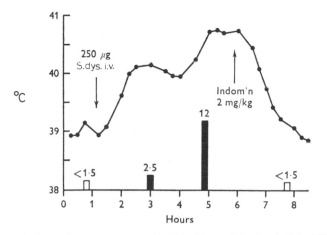

Fig. 8. Record of rectal temperature and PGE_1-like activity (mg/ml) in CSF from an unanaesthetized cat. Description as for Fig. 6. At the *first arrow* 250 μg of the endotoxin from *S. dsenteriae* was injected intravenously; at the *second arrow* 2 mg/kg indomethacin was injected intraperitoneally. (FELDBERG et al. 1973)

ventricles were lowered or prevented by intraperitoneal injections of aspirin, 4-Ac and indomethacin.

Since EP is thought to be the circulating mediator for all peripherally induced fevers, HARVEY and MILTON (1975) and HARVEY (1976) prepared EP from cat peritoneal exudate and injected it intravenously and centrally into the conscious cat (see p. 277). In these experiments they found that 4-Ac not only reduced the fever and lowered the elevated prostaglandin levels following central administration of EP but also did so during intravenous infusion of EP. When the antipyretic agent was given whilst the EP infusion was maintained, antipyresis occurred in the presence of circulating EP.

Similar results were obtained by HARVEY and MILTON (1975) when plasma from a febrile cat suffering from a postoperative infection was infused into an afebrile recipient cat. Again, the febrile response was associated with elevated prostaglandin levels in the CSF of the recipient, in which both the fever and prostaglandin levels were rapidly lowered following the intraperitoneal injection of 4-Ac (Fig. 7).

Experiments with EP were also carried out by CRANSTON et al. (1975a, b), who produced a steady state fever by continuous infusion of EP prepared from rabbit blood. During the steady state fever produced by the pyrogen the PGE concentrations rose from undetectable levels to 3.6 ng/ml. When the infusion was preceded by a continuous infusion of sodium salicylate, a weak antipyretic in the rabbit, the PGE concentrations were below detectable levels though the increase in body temperature still occurred. (The significance of these results is discussed on p. 294.)

III. Antagonism of Sodium Arachidonate Hyperthermia by Antipyretics

In 1976 CLARK and CUMBY infused arachidonic acid, the precursor of the E_2 prostaglandins, into the lateral cerebral ventricle of the conscious cat and obtained hyperthermias. These effects are similar to those reported in the rat by Splawinski et al. (1978). When antipyretic agents were administered at the height of the arachidonic hyperthermia Clark and Cumby found differences in effects between the different antipyretics. For example, sodium salicylate (40 and 160 mg/kg i.p.) inhibited the hyperthermia after a delay of approximately 4 h, with a small but significant hyperthermia occurring in the first hour after administration. 4-Ac (10 and 40 mg/kg) likewise inhibited the hyperthermic response, though the initial hyperthermia was not seen. In contrast, 10 µg indomethacin was without effect, though larger doses (40 µg/kg) produced antipyresis. However, the hypothermic effect of indomethacin was said to be not much less than the hypothermia produced indomethacin alone. When the authors compared the inhibition of arachidonic acid fever with that of endotoxin fever they found that the endotoxin fever was antagonised to a considerably greater degree and that inhibition occurred immediately, in contrast to the 3–4 h delay with arachidonate fever. This occurred using both 4-Ac and indomethacin. The authors conclude by saying that comparison of the relative effectiveness of the antipyretics in blocking hyperthermic responses to pyrogens and to sodium arachidonate indicates that if prostaglandins do mediate pyrogen-induced fever these antipyretics exert their prime reaction at a step before prostaglandin synthesis and not by inhibiting prostaglandin synthesis itself (for discussion of these results see p. 297).

J. Interactions Between Prostaglandins and Endotoxins

I. Hypothalamic Destruction

Veale and Cooper (1975), in studying the sites of action of pyrogen and prostaglandin, destroyed the entire PO/AH region of the rabbit. They found that PGE_1 and EP no longer induced fever when injected into this area, which is what would be expected; however, when they administered the same agents into the cerebral ventricles, PGE_1 still did not produce an effect but intravenous EP did. In both these latter cases though the temperature rose more gradually than in control animals it still reached the same maximum. These results suggest that besides the PO/AH region there is some other site within the brain responsive to EP to promote fever (the significance of these observations is discussed on p. 295).

II. Inhibition of Prostaglandin Breakdown

Splawinski (1977) reported that in rat hypothalamus PGE_2, unlike $PGF_{2\alpha}$ or arachidonic acid, shared the site of hyperthermic action with E. coli endotoxin. Splawinski also found that the in vitro catabolism of PGE_2 in the hypothalamus of endotoxin-treated rats was significantly suppressed. He therefore proposed that endotoxin fever in rats was due to the inhibition of PGE breakdown in the hypothalamus. He also showed that rat hypothalami homogenates transformed arachidonic acid mainly to prostaglandins, with barely detectable formation of thromboxane A_2. In a subsequent paper Splawinski et al. (1978) intimated that PGE_2 produces fever (not hyperthermia) by acting on the PO/AH. Conversely, $PGF_{2\alpha}$ and arachidonic acid produced virtually similar hyperthermias with no correlation between the micro-injection sites in the diencephalon and the observed hyperthermia. Additional evidence was provided by these authors to suggest that thromboxane A_2 and PGI_2 were unlikely to be involved. Arachidonic acid increased the levels of both $PGF_{2\alpha}$ and a mixture of $PGF_{2\alpha}$ and PGE_2 with $PGF_{2\alpha}$ predominating. SPLAWINSKI et al. say that it is unlikely that endotoxin produces fever either through increased availability of arachidonic acid or through activation of prostaglandin endoperoxide synthesis in the hypothalamus; therefore the mechanisms remain unknown.

In another paper SPLAWINSKI et al. (1979) continued their studies on PGE_2 breakdown and found that in the rat PGE_2 accumulated in the hypothalamus following administration of endotoxin and that this accumulation was due to inhibition of the 15-hydroxyprostaglandin dehydrogenase by the endotoxin. This conclusion was based on experiments in which the enzyme was inhibited by polyphloretin phosphate (PPP) a substance said to be a competitive inhibitor. Inhibition resulted in a prolongation of both endotoxin fever and PGE_2 fever. In addition, in normal afebrile rats inhibition of the enzyme with PPP led to an increase in body temperature whereas systemic administration of aspirin produced a fall. Degradation of PGE_2 by the hydrogenase enzyme from the hypothalami of rats with endotoxin-induced fever was significantly slower than degradation by the enzyme prepared from afebrile animals.

K. Effects of Prostaglandins on Neuronal Activity in the PO/AH

Conflicting and confusing results have been obtained from studies comparing the effects of prostaglandins and pyrogens on neuronal activity in the PO/AH (see EISENMANN, this volume, Chap. 8). In addition, the effects observed with the prostaglandins are difficult to interpret. For example FORD (1974), using an isolated diencephalic preparation, studied the effects of PGE_1 applied iontophoretically from multilabelled pipettes onto 46 excitable hypothalamic neurones. Of the 32 neurones which were not affected by either local warming or cooling, 1 was excited, 3 were suppressed and 28 did not respond to PGE_1. Of the 9 excited by warming 2 were suppressed and 7 did not respond to PGE_1, whereas all 5 that were excited by cooling were excited by PGE_1. With just a few neurones which were responding to temperature changes the main effect of PGE_1 was therefore to excite cold-sensitive ones which are presumed to drive heat production and heat conservation. Using anaesthetized rabbits, STITT and HARDY (1975) made an extensive study of the effects of micro-electrophoretic application of PGE_1 onto single units in the PO/AH region. The firing rates of all but 12 of the 138 units tested were not affected by PGE_1 regardless of their local thermosensitivity. Of the 17 that responded, the effects were facilitatory, indicating to the authors no correlation with thermosensitivity.

JELL and SWEATMAN (1977) studied the effects of both PGEs and PGFs in the cat. Twenty-eight percent of the warm-sensitive cells and 53% of the cold-sensitive cells responded to PGE, both types predominantly with increased firing rates. PGE_2 was a little more active than PGE_1. Interestingly, all cells which responded to PGE_1 also responded to PGE_2; however there were cells which responded to

PGE_2 without responding to PGE_1. Of the non-thermosensitive cells, 97% were also unaffected by either PGE_1 or PGE_2. A few of these cells responded to $PGF_{2\alpha}$.

Schoener and Wang (1976) recorded from PO/AH cells and micro-injected PGE_1 intracerebrally. Of 12 warm-sensitive neurones examined, all were depressed by PGE_1, whereas 4 cool-sensitive neurones were excited.

In order to eliminate the depressant effects of anaesthetics on neuronal activity, Gordon and Heath (1980) recorded the single unit activity of thermoregulatory neurones in the PO/AH of unanaesthetized rabbits. Intracerebroventricular injections of PGE_2 induced consistent excitatory effects (up to 190% increase in firing rate) on cold-sensitive cells and inhibitory effects (up to 50%) on warm-sensitive cells. Single units that were insensitive or had changes in firing rate that could not be correlated with PO/AH temperature were either facilitated or inhibited by PGE_2. The authors state that the consistent effect of PGE_2 on the thermoregulatory neurones supports the proposal of PGE modulation of thermoregulatory neurones during the development of fever.

L. Prostaglandin Antagonists

An obvious way to investigate the role of prostaglandins in fever would be to attempt to block the hyperthermic effects of both PGE and pyrogens with prostaglandin receptor blocking drugs. Unfortunately, to the present day there are no highly specific active compounds available. Three compounds have been studied, polyphloretin phosphate (PPP), 1-acetyl-2(8-chloro-10,11-dihydrodibenz-(b,f)-(1,4)-oxazepine-10-carbonul) hydrazine (Searle, SC-19220) and the prostaglandin analogue 8-ethoxycarbonyl-10,11-dihydro-A-prostaglandin (Hoechst, HR-546).

When injected into the cerebroventricular system of the conscious cat PPP produced marked restlessness and increased motor activity, with the animals eventually going into sustained convulsions. Body temperature rose almost certainly as a result of the increased motor activity. Because of these undesirable effects the experiments were abandoned (Milton unpublished work). PPP also inhibits the prostaglandin degradation enzyme 15-hydroxyprostaglandin dehydrogenase, and recently Splawinski et al. have shown that systemic administration of PPP significantly prolongs the duration of PGE and endotoxin fever. SC-19220 has been investigated by Sanner (1974), Clark and Cumby (1975a), Cranston et al. (1976a, b), and Laburn et al. (1977). Sanner reported that when SC-19220 was administered to rats intraperitoneally it inhibited the hyperthermia produced by the intracerebroventricular injection of PGE_1. He also stated that it produced a hypothermia in its own right but that it did not reduce pyrogen-induced fever. In his paper he gives no details of how his results were obtained. Clarke and Cumby reported that SC-19220 in doses of between 3 and 9 ml/kg i.v. produced in the conscious cat a dose-related hypothermia; other effects included emesis, mydriasis, tachypnoea, and occasional panting. Repeated administration of SC-19220 resulted in tolerance to the effects with no hypothermia. When these authors obtained a steady state hypothermia with a continuous intravenous infusion of SC-19220, the ability of intraventricular PGE_1 to produce hyperthermia was abolished and that of EP given intravenously either abolished or markedly attenuated. PGE_1 and EP were effective in producing hyperthermia when administered after the hypothermic effect of the SC-19220 had subsided or if the dose of SC-19220 was insufficient to produce hypothermia. CLARK and CUMBY suggested that if SC-19220 is acting as a prostaglandin antagonist the resulting hypothermia might indicate (a) a role for prostaglandins in normal thermoregulation and (b) that the blockade of the hyperthermic responses to PGE$_1$ and EP is evidence for the role of prostaglandins in fever. However, they mention the possibility that the hypothermic actions of SC-19220, a relatively non-specific agent, is entirely unrelated to the prostaglandin blockade.

CRANSTON et al. (1976a, b) in experiments designed to disprove the prostaglandin fever theory injected SC-1900 directly into the lateral ventricles of conscious rabbits. Administration of 15 μmol SC-19220 dissolved in 20 μl dimethylsulphoxide (DMSO) produced a rise in deep body temperature of 0.6 °C over a period of 3 h. However, a similar rise in temperature was produced by DSMO alone or after a similar dose of artificial CSF. When they injected 2.5 nmol PGE$_2$ together with the SC-19220 a slow rise in rectal temperature took place which was indistinguishable from the rise following the administration of SC-19220 alone. In contrast, PGE$_2$ administered with DMSO exerted its normal hyperthermic action superimposed on the slow rise produced by DMSO alone. Administration of 2.4 nmol PGE$_2$ produced a rise of 0.8 °C. Injection of 15 μl of 0.9% NaCl solution containing rabbit EP resulted in a rapid rise in deep body temperature of the same magnitude as that produced by PGE$_2$. When SC-19220 was administered together with the EP the response was unaltered. The authors conclude by saying that the prostaglandin antagonist SC-19220 injected intracerebroventricularly blocked the hyperthermic effect to PGE$_2$ but not the fever produced by EP, and that this is not consistent with the theory that pyrogen fever is mediated by a prostaglandin. One fundamental criticism of their results concerns the dose of SC-19220 used, which is extremely large and on a molar basis 6×10^3 times that of the dose of prostaglandin used. In most pharmacological situations the affinity of the antagonist to receptors is considerably greater than that of the agonist. In addition the solution of SC-19220 is extremely concentrated and is hypertonic (0.75 M) and therefore hyperosmotic. CRANSTON et al. (1976a, b) carried out similar experiments with the antagonist HR-546. The effects which they observed similar to those obtained with SC-19220. The hyperthermic response to PGE$_2$ was considerably attenuated during the first hour following injection of HR-546, whereas the substance had no effect on EP fever. The dose ratio of HR-546 to PGE$_2$ was 176:1, and similar criticisms can therefore be levelled at these experiments as at those involving SC-19200. The authors conclude from their results that they can find no evidence to support the theory that EP produces fever by releasing a prostaglandin and suggest that EP acts directly on the anterior hypothalamus (see also p. 293).

LABURN et al. (1977) investigated the effects of SC-19220 and HR-546 on arachidonate fever in the rabbit. They studied the effects of these two compounds on the hyperthermia produced by intracerebral injections of PGE$_1$ and on the hyperthermia resulting from the intraventricular administration of arachidonic acid, the precursor of PGE$_2$ and PGF$_{2\alpha}$. They found that sodium arachidonate injected into a lateral cerebral ventricle in a dose of 60–320 nmol produced dose-dependent hyperthermias which lasted in excess of 6 h, with a peak response occurring after about 3 h.

When indomethacin (280 nmol) was injected into a lateral ventricle together with 250 nmol sodium arachidonate the resulting hyperthermia was significantly less for the first 140 min than that produced by sodium arachidonate alone. Injection of PGE_1 (4 nmol) into a lateral ventricle produced marked hyperthermia similar to that produced by 250 nmol sodium arachidonate; the hyperthermia lasted several hours. When SC-19220 (15 µmol) was administered simultaneously with PGE_1 it abolished the hyperthermic response, and HR-546 (440 nmol) also reduced this response, though to a lesser degree. In contrast, both SC-19220 and HR-546 attenuated the fever produced by sodium arachidonate for only the first 30–40 min; thereafter a normal hyperthermia developed.

The authors suggest that their results indicate that the hyperthermic actions of arachidonate are due to its derivatives and not to the parent substance itself, the evidence for this being the inhibition of the response by indomethacin. Indomethacin is a fatty acid cyclo-oxygenase inhibitor which inhibits the enzyme responsible for the conversion of arachidonic acid into its metabolites. Since the PGE_1 effect was blocked by the two inhibitors after the first few minutes, the authors conclude that PGE is not the only pyrogenic derivative of arachidonic acid and suggest that either on endoperoxide or a thromboxane is responsible. Inhibition of the cyclo-oxygenase by indomethacin would, of course, inhibit the formation of all these compounds (see Fig. 4). The main criticism of this paper is similar to that of the papers by Cranston et al. (1976 a, b), namely that very high doses of inhibitor were used; also it is not clear why the authors used PGE_1 when arachidonic acid is the precursor of the prostaglandin 2 series, i.e. PGE_2 and $PGF_{2\alpha}$.

In summary, the use of low specificity and low activity prostaglandin antagonists has provided interesting observations; however, the results need to be repeated when highly active and highly specific prostaglandin antagonists are available. Until then no definite statements can be made that antagonist drugs provide evidence to show that prostaglandins are not involved in pyrogen fever.

M. Prostaglandins and Thermoregulation

Experiments to date provide no evidence that prostaglandins are involved in normal physiological thermoregulation. Cammock et al. (1976) subjected conscious cats to various different environmental temperatures (45 °C, 25 °C, and 0 °C), collected CSF from the cisterna magna and assayed it for PGE activity using radioimmunoassay. During a period of cold stress (110 min) the animals assumed a crouched position. Vigorous, continuous shivering, vasoconstriction and some pilo-erection were observed. Deep body temperature was maintained but PGE levels remained the same as during the 90-min period prior to the cold stress and as after the cessation of the cold stress; at both these times the animals were at room temperature (25 °C). In contrast to the thermoregulatory responses to cold, when the animals were subjected to heat stress they lay stretched out. Sweating from the foot pads and panting occurred and rectal temperature rose passively. However, as under cold stress, no changes in the cisternal PGE levels could be detected. Observations by Myers and Sharpe (1968) had previously shown that both heat and cold stress can alter the release of transmitter substances from the PO/AH. The observations reported by Cammock et al. indicate that prostaglandins are not amongst these transmitter substances. However, the authors do stress the point that the CSF was collected from the cisterna magna and that it may be preferable to assay perfusates from the PO/AH region itself to establish whether in fact the prostaglandins have a function in normal thermoregulation.

Subsequently, in 1980 BERNHEIM et al. subjected rabbits to cold and heat exposure and to heating and cooling of the hypothalamus. They collected CSF from the third ventricle and assayed the fluid for PGE activity by radio-immunoassay. Neither environmental nor hypothalamic temperature changes produced any changes in PGE levels, in contrast to the administration of EP, which produced a marked increase in PGE levels in the CSF. The resting and febrile levels of PGE found by BERNHEIM et al. were considerably greater than those reported to be present in cisternal CSF, and they stress in the discussion to their paper the importance of collecting CSF from the third ventricle, which they consider reflects a truer picture of what is happening in the region of the PO/AH.

N. Prostaglandins and Cyclic Nucleotides

Many of the neurotransmitters which are thought to be involved in thermoregulation or fever, including the E prostaglandins, have been shown to stimulate cyclic adenosine $3'5'$-monophosphate (cAMP) in brain tissue (ZOR et al. 1969), and it is also thought that some of the muscarinic actions of acetylcholine may be mediated by cyclic guanosine $3'5'$-monophosphate (cGMP) (KEBABIAN et al. 1975).

I. Cyclic GMP

DASCOMBE and MILTON (1980, 1981) injected cGMP and its dibutyryl derivative db-cAMP into the third cerebral ventricle of the conscious cat and compared the thermoregulatory behavioural effects seen with those produced by acetylcholine and physostigmine. cGMP and db-cGMP (10–1,250 nmol) had no effect on body temperature in cats exposed to an ambient temperature of 20°–24 °C; in contrast, acetylcholine (100 nmol) plus physostigmine (100 nmol) injected together intracerebroventricularly produced a rise in deep body temperature which was abolished by pretreatment with atropine (200 nmol i.c.v.).

At an environmental temperature of 9°–11 °C both cGMP and db-cGMP in doses of 1,250 nmol produced hypothermia. Administration of the O-somatic antigen of *S. dysenteriae* (20 mg/kg i.v.) resulted in fever in cats which was not potentiated by the phosphodiesterase inhibitor caffeine (25 mg/kg i.p.). Levels of endogenous cGMP in CSF taken from the cisterna magna during bacterial pyrogen fever in the presence or absence of the antipyretic drug 4-Ac and/or caffeine were similar to the values obtained in CSF from afebrile animals. The authors conclude that exogenously applied cGMP and db-cGMP can inhibit central events mediating autonomic and behavioural thermoregulation in cats exposed to cold environments – however there was no evidence to suggest that cGMP is involved in pyrogen fever in the cat.

DASCOMBE (1981) observed a fall in the deep body temperature of rabbits when they were exposed to an environmental temperature of 21°–23 °C and 10–200 µg db-GMP was administered into the PO/AH region.

II. Cyclic AMP

The effects on body temperature of cAMP and its more lipid soluble dibutyryl derivative db-cAMP as well as other adenosine nucleotides have been examined in
a number of species when injected into the ventricular system, into the PO/AH region and parenterally.

1. Mice

In mice, DASCOMBE et al. (1980) observed that db-cAMP (4, 16, and 32 µg) injected
intracerebroventricularly produced hypothermia which was associated with a fall
in oxygen consumption together with behavioural and autonomic heat loss activities, but with no cutaneous vasodilatation. The effects on rectal temperature
and oxygen consumption were dose dependent. The falls in rectal temperature and
oxygen consumption following db-cAMP administration were decreased by elevation of the environmental temperature from 22 °C to 32 °C, and abolished at
36 °C. It was concluded that in the mouse db-cAMP may inhibit central events mediating the rise in metabolic heat production upon exposure to cold environments.

2. Rats

In rats BRECKENRIDGE and LISK (1969) found that implants of db-cAMP, cAMP,
and AMP into the anterior hypothalamus produced a rise in deep body temperature which was associated with hyperactivity and aggressive behaviour. In contrast, DASCOMBE (1980) injected db-cAMP into the PO/AH of the rat and observed
a fall in deep body temperature which was occasionally followed by hyperthermia
secondary to the increased motor activity.

3. Monkeys

In squirrel monkeys in which PGE_1 and endotoxin injected into the PO/AH had
produced the expected rises in deep body temperature, LIPTON and FOSSLER (1974)
found that doses of db-cAMP in the order of 500–750 ng were without hyperthermic activity.

4. Cats

In cats VARAGIC and BELESLIN (1973) examined the effect on body temperature of
injections of cAMP, ATP, db-cAMP and butyrate itself into a lateral cerebral ventricle. Long-lasting hyperthermias of more than 12 h were produced by all of these
substances; however, the hyperthermia produced by db-cAMP was sometimes preceded by transient hypothermia. A biphasic effect on body temperature was obtained by CLARK et al. (1974) when db-cAMP was injected into the lateral cerebral
ventricles. CLARK et al. particularly noted the long duration of the hyperthermia
and also the long latency, the temperature beginning to rise only about 3 h after
the injection. They also showed that the hyperthermia was reduced by the antipyretic drugs indomethacin and 4-Ac. They concluded that cAMP could not me-

diate prostaglandin fever but that it might induce prostaglandin synthesis. DASCOMBE and MILTON (1975) found that not only db-cAMP and cAMP but also ATP, ADP, and AMP applied by micro-injection into the PO/AH region of the cat regularly produced hypothermia which was dose dependent. A secondary long-lasting fever was occasionally produced and it was found that this effect was abolished by 4-Ac. DASCOMBE and MILTON concluded that this secondary hyperthermia was a non-specific fever (see p. 290), as was the fever seen by CLARK et al. They also concluded that the genuine or specific effect of cAMP and db-cAMP acting on the PO/AH of the cat was a fall in temperature and therefore "that it is unlikely that endogenous cAMP in this region mediates the hyperthermic response to pyrogens or to prostaglandins."

Subsequently, DASCOMBE and MILTON (1976) measured cAMP levels in the CSF of unanaesthetized cats during active thermoregulation and during pyrogen fever. Even though appropriate thermoregulatory responses were elicited in the cat at high and low ambient temperature exposure, no changes in the concentrations of cAMP and cisternal CSF were detected. This suggested that cAMP was not involved in normal central thermoregulatory pathways in the cat. In contrast, they found that intravenous injection of the endotoxin of *S. dysenteriae* was associated with a dose-related increase in both body temperature and the concentration of cAMP in the cisternal CSF. Intraperitoneal administration of 4-Ac before injection of pyrogen was found to suppress not only the rise in body temperature but also the increase in cerebrospinal cAMP. However, they also observed an apparent dissociation between fever and increased cAMP in the CSF. For example, 4-Ac injected after the onset of fever in cats in doses shown to be antipyretic had no apparent effect on the raised concentrations of the cAMP. Therefore, although injection of 4-Ac before pyrogen prevented the increase in cAMP, the sustained increase in cAMP concentration following the administration of the drug after the onset of fever indicated that either the change in biosynthesis of the nucleotide in response to pyrogen is not affected by 4-Ac once the change has been initiated and/or that the nucleotide is slowly cleared from the CSF. Secondly, they observed a single incident of a cat responding to intravenous pyrogen with a collapsed hypothermia. The concentrations of cAMP in CSF from this animal following collapse were similar to the values in the cats with marked pyrexia. The finding of apparent dissociation between increased concentration of cAMP in the CSF and the occurrence of fever indicates that raised concentrations of the nucleotide in the CSF do not directly mediate fever in cats. This hypothesis was supported by the finding that when the nucleotide was injected intravenously increases in cerebrospinal cAMP equivalent to those found during fever (25–35 pmol/ml) were found, but there was no effect on temperature. Furthermore, increases greater than those during fever (> 100 pmol/ml) are associated with heat loss and a fall in body temperature.

That cAMP rapidly entered the CSF from the blood in the cat led DASCOMBE and MILTON (1976) to investigate the effect of fever on the concentration of the nucleotide in the blood. Fever induced by *S. dysenteriae* was associated with an increase in the concentrations of cAMP in plasma which was similar to that observed in the CSF for the same cats. It therefore appeared that the rise in cerebrospinal cAMP in response to bacterial pyrogen may be due to a change in the biosynthesis of the nucleotide in the periphery.

5. Rabbits

An injection of cAMP or db-cAMP (20–500 µg) into a lateral cerebral ventricle of rabbits was reported by DUFF et al. (1972) to produce a significant fall in body temperature; when a rise occurred after large doses it did not appear until 90 min after the injection and the authors considered that this represented an unspecific rise in body temperature. DASCOMBE (1981) has also reported a fall in body temperature in the rabbit following intracerebral injection of db-cAMP. In contrast to these findings, LABURN et al. (1974) and WOOLF et al. (1975, 1976) obtained dose-dependent rises with db-cAMP with a mean latency of approximately 3.5 min after injection into the PO/AH. Since in the rabbit noradrenaline produces a rise in deep body temperature when injected into the cerebral ventricles, WOOLF et al. (1977) proposed that in the rabbit during fever prostaglandins mediate their hyperthermic response by activating the release of noradrenaline, which in turn activates adenyl cyclase, leading to the production of cAMP. They suggested that cAMP was responsible for the increase in heat gain and decrease in heat loss. In a further investigation of the rabbit, CREMADES-CAMPOS and MILTON (1982) studied the inter-relationship between PGE_2 and db-cAMP and the antipyretic drug 4-Ac. They found that PGE_2 in doses of 100 ng to 10 µg produces a dose-related rise in deep body temperature associated with ear skin vasoconstriction and occasional shivering and that this hyperthermic response was unaffected by the administration of the antipyretic drug ketoprofen (6 mg/kg s.c.). In contrast to the action of PGE_2, db-cAMP in doses of 50, 100, and 200 µg produced immediate hypothermia. This response was coupled with vasodilatation and an increase in respiratory rate. The hypothermic response lasted for approximately 60 min, after which secondary hyperthermia was produced. The initial hypothermia was unaffected by ketoprofen, whereas the secondary hyperthermia was blocked. A large dose of db-cAMP (400 µg) produced recurrent episodes of locomotor hyperactivity followed by catatonia and eventually convulsions culminating in death. These responses were associated with a rise in deep body temperature. This rise in deep body temperature was unaffected by ketoprofen. Since the immediate effect of db-cAMP is hypothermia whereas the immediate effect of PGE_1 hyperthermia, it is unlikely that PGE_1 can be producing its effect by the production of cAMP. Even if the secondary hyperthermia produced by db-cAMP is a true response to the db-cAMP itself and not an unspecific fever, the fact that it is abolished by ketoprofen, a prostaglandin synthetase inhibitor, indicates that it is due to PGE release and therefore that it is the db-cAMP which is causing the release of PGE and not vice versa. (For a complete discussion on the role of cyclic nucleotides in thermoregulation and fever, see DASCOMBE, this volume, Chap. 9.)

O. Non-specific Febrile Response

It has been observed on many occasions that injections of non-pyrogenic solutions of apparently innocuous substances such as artificial CSF or 0.9% NaCl may produce a long-lasting febrile response, generally after a delay of varying length (sometimes as long as several hours) (FELDBERG et al. 1970; FELDBERG and SAXENA 1970, 1971 b; MILTON and WENDLANDT 1971 a). DEY et al. (1974a) showed that in the cat this febrile response was associated with an increase in the levels of PGE_2 in the cisternal CSF and that antipyretic drugs not only blocked the febrile response but at the same time reduced the levels of PGE_2 in the CSF to those found in the afebrile state. In 1975 DASCOMBE and MILTON saw a similar febrile response following micro-injections into the region of the PO/AH and showed that this fever was also inhibited by 4-Ac. Interestingly, they observed that the latency of the rise in temperature was dependent upon the exact placement of the injection cannula, being shorter when the injections were made into sites nearer to the PO/AH. These results suggested that the response was initiated in this region of the brain; it should therefore be considered a prostaglandin fever. This fever may be explained by the assumption that injections or perfusions produce a disturbance in the ventricular walls or in the surface structures of the brain-stem, resulting in increased synthesis and release of PGE. In other words this is a local inflammatory response. What is important is that apparently innocuous stimuli can trigger off this response. Therefore long-lasting fever produced when investigating the thermoregulatory responses of drugs injected into the cerebral ventricles or into brain tissue is very likely to be a "non-specific" fever, particularly if it is not consistent or suddenly occurs in animals in which it has not occurred previously. Routinely, if such a response is seen, non-steroidal anti-inflammatory agents should immediately be administered. Abolition of the response by these drugs indicates that it is due to prostaglandin release. If a drug were to stimulate prostaglandin synthesis in its own right and not by producing local tissue damage or irritation, difficulties would be apparent: One would obtain a long-lasting fever indistinguishable from the "non-specific" response. For example, in 1964 FELDBERG and MYERS showed that 5-HT injected into the cerebral ventricles of the conscious cat produced a long-lasting biphasic hyperthermia; subsequently, MILTON and WENDLANDT (1968) showed that this response could be inhibited or abolished by 4-Ac. Does 5-HT therefore activate prostaglandin synthesis directly or is this another example of the "non-specific" fever?

Now that we are aware of this response we must be very careful in making claims for thermoregulatory responses occurring after the injection of substances directly into the CNS; we must also critically examine all work already published, particularly before 1974.

P. Sodium Fever

In 1970 *Feldberg* et al. perfused the ventricular system of the conscious cat with solutions in which the calcium and sodium ion concentrations were altered. If the ventricles were perfused with 0.9% sodium chloride or artificial CSF lacking in calcium, the animals began to shiver vigorously and body temperature rose; if calcium ions were then added to the solutions the body temperature returned to normal. FELDBERG et al. referred to this hyperthermia as a "sodium fever" and maintained that under normal physiological conditions the hyperthermic effect of the sodium ions was held in check by the calcium ions. These observations are particularly important when considering the effects on temperature of drugs which may interfere with calcium ions (see MYERS, this volume, Chap. 7).

Dey et al. (1974a) showed that prostaglandins were not involved in the sodium fever. The antipyretic drugs 4-Ac and indomethacin did not block the hyperthermia produced by perfusing the cerebroventricles of the cat from the lateral ventricle to the cisterna magna with artificial CSF containing no calcium ions, nor were there any changes seen in the PGE_2 content of perfusate collected from the cisterna magna.

In the same series of experiments Dey et al. showed that the fevers produced by intracerebroventricular injections of endotoxin, PGE_1 and PGE_2 could be suppressed by perfusing the ventricles with CSF containing a high calcium ion concentration. The reversal of pyrogen and PGE fevers can be fully accounted for by the fact that the hypothalamus has become insensitive to the hyperthermic action of the PGE, although the possibility cannot be excluded that with the pyrogen fever inhibition of prostaglandin synthesis is involved as well.

Q. Discussion

It is undeniable that when prostaglandins of the E series are injected into the cerebroventricular system or the PO/AH area they produce a rise in body temperature in all the placental mammals so far studied. The action is specific to the PO/AH area, for when they are injected into other areas of the brain thermoregulatory responses are not initiated, though other responses may be seen. Of all the prostaglandins, prostaglandin precursors and derivatives so far examined, PGE_1 and PGE_2 are by far the most active in producing hyperthermia when applied to the PO/AH. The hyperthermia results from a co-ordinated activation of heat gain mechanisms and inhibition of heat loss mechanisms. It is therefore reasonable to postulate that there is a specific PGE receptor in the PO/AH. Assuming the existence of this receptor, what is its function? Three possibilities come to mind: (a) that it is involved in some way in the processes concerned with the normal physiological control of body temperature, (b) that it is involved in some way with the processes concerned with pathophysiological thermoregulatory situations, e.g. fever, and (c) that it is simply a "pharmacological curiosity."

There is no convincing evidence to suggest that prostaglandins are involved in normal physiological thermoregulation (see p. 286); therefore until such evidence is obtained, this role for prostaglandins and the prostaglandin receptor must be discounted.

The weight of evidence is for a role in fever: that fever produced by pyrogens is mediated by a prostaglandin of the E series, probably PGE_2. The evidence for this is based on the following findings:

1. PGE_2, a natural constituent of hypothalamic tissue, produces fever "when injected in minute amounts into the PO/AH."
2. The PGE_2 content of CSF, which is normally extremely low, increases markedly during fever produced by either bacterial endotoxin or endogenous pyrogen.
3. Antipyretic drugs which inhibit the synthesis of PGE_2 in brain tissue (and elsewhere) prevent or abolish pyrogen fever but do not inhibit PGE_2 "fever."
4. During antipyresis brought about by the non-steroidal anti-inflammatory drugs the raised levels of PGE_2 present in the CSF decrease markedly as temperature falls, even though endotoxin or EP may still be present in the body.

This last finding is further strengthened by the work initiated by VANE (1971) showing that the anti-inflammatory and analgesic actions of the non-steroidal aspirin-like drugs are mediated through the inhibition of prostaglandin synthesis. We therefore have three pathological conditions all of which are relieved by aspirin-like drugs, all of which can be mimicked by exogenous prostaglandins and all of which involve the release of prostaglandins. Is it conceivable that in all three cases the presence of prostaglandins is irrelevant to the disease and that inhibition of the prostaglandin synthesis by aspirin-like drugs is irrelevant to relief of the symptoms? Or, although it is admittedly less likely, is it conceivable that prostaglandins are involved in inflammation and pain but not in fever and that the aspirin-like drugs act as prostaglandin synthesis inhibitors in inflammation and pain but inhibit fever by some entirely different mechanism?

Further support for the theory that prostaglandins are involved in fever is provided by the observation of ZIEL and KRUPP (1976), who showed that EP can stimulate the synthesis of prostaglandin by brain tissue but not by seminal vesicle tissue. Also, as has been pointed out by KIM et al. (this volume, Chap. 12), there is general correspondence between the antipyretic potency and the anti-inflammatory potency of the aspirin-like drugs, with the more potent anti-inflammatory drugs being better antipyretics. In addition, there is a correlation between cyclooxygenase inhibitory activity and anti-inflammatory activity of these same drugs (FLOWER 1972). Other evidence in support of the prostaglandin theory is contained in this chapter and has previously been extensively discussed by FELDBERG and MILTON (1978).

Obviously there are those who do not accept the prostaglandin theory of fever and antipyresis, and experimental evidence has been published to support their views. These publications are dealt with in the main body of this chapter but for convenience are reiterated here. The arguments are almost all entirely based on results obtained where the actions of pyrogens and of prostaglandins are divorced from each other, e.g. the experiments of CRANSTON et al. (1976a, b) and LABURN et al. (1977), where they showed that the hyperthermic responses to PGE_1 or PGE_2 could be blocked by prostaglandin receptor blocking drugs whereas the fever resulting from EP or arachidonic acid was not affected. Unfortunately, as discussed earlier (p. 286), the inhibitors used were non-specific and very weak and the concentrations applied were extremely high. It is well known that it is considerably more difficult to inhibit endogenously produced modulators or transmitters than to inhibit the same substances exogenously applied. The number of receptors and the concentration at the receptors of the agonist may be very different if the agonist comes from an endogenous as opposed to an exogenous source. Similarly because of tissue penetration antagonists may be less effective in blocking endogenous agonist than exogenously applied agonist. Until such time as a potent, specific, centrally active prostaglandin antagonist is available, no conclusions can be reached from such research.

Another example also comes from the research of CRANSTON and his colleagues (CRANSTON et al. 1975a, b, 1976), in which they examined in rabbits the effect of salicylate on pyrogen fever and PGE content of cisternal CSF. When a steady state fever was obtained by an intravenous infusion of EP the PGE level in the cisternal CSF was found to increase and to remain high throughout the duration of the fe-

ver. However, when the authors infused salicylate in small doses during the EP infusion neither the latency, the rate of rise, nor the final fever reached was different,
yet the levels of PGE in the CSF did not rise at all. The authors do not deny the
ability to EP to stimulate prostaglandin synthesis; in fact they state "that
throughout the fever there was a release of prostaglandin into the c.s.f." However,
even though PGE is known to produce hyperthermia in rabbits in similar concentrations to that found in the CSF, because of the action of a sub-antipyretic dose
of salicylate they called into doubt the idea that prostaglandin synthesis forms an
essential link in the actions of pyrogen in the brain. There are two ways of explaining the dissociation found by CRANSTON et al. without having to question the role
of prostaglandin as mediators of pyrogen fever:

1. The prostaglandin which appears in the cisternal CSF represents only the
"tip of the iceberg" (FELDBERG and MILTON 1978). Pyrogens probably stimulate
prostaglandin synthesis not only in the PO/AH region but also in other areas of
the brain. In the rabbit, however, only a small fraction of the prostaglandins synthesised in the PO/AH region will appear in the cisternal CSF owing to the absence
of a foramen of Magendie. In the experiments of CRANSTON et al. the level of prostaglandin in the cisternal CSF during fever was very near to the threshold of sensitivity of their assay method; a slight reduction in prostaglandin synthesis might
have been sufficient to give negative results when assaying the CSF, but insufficient
to bring about a perceptible effect on the fever since in a sub-antipyretic dose synthesis of PGE in the PO/AH may not be fully inhibited.

2. The PGE detected in the cisternal CSF may have been derived to a great extent from synthesis activated by the pyrogen in injured or inflammatory tissue near
the site where the hollow needle used for the CSF collection pierced the atlanto-
occipital membrane. Such extraneous sources of PGE were suggested to be responsible for the great variation in prostaglandin activity of cisternal CSF observed in
cats after intravenous endotoxin injections (FELDBERG et al. 1973). It was pointed
out that as long as such extraneous sources are not rigidly excluded, a high level
of PGE in cisternal CSF is not always a sign of increased prostaglandin synthesis
in the PO/AH region.

The response of the new-born lamb to PGE and to pyrogen has also been used
to discount the prostaglandin theory. PITTMAN et al. (1975) found that prostaglandin injected into the cerebral ventricles of new-born lambs sensitized to *Salmonella
abortus equi* only produced hyperthermia in two out of ten lambs whereas intravenous injection of bacterial pyrogen produced fever in all of them. Injection of endotoxin directly into the cerebral ventricles of these same lambs produced fever in
every case. Similar results were obtained by PITTMAN et al. (1977a, b) when they
injected PGE_1 and PGE_2 directly into the PO/AH of the new-born lamb where
both prostaglandins failed to produce fever even though the same area of the hypothalamus is known to be highly reactive to bacterial pyrogen. It must be pointed
out, however, that fever resulting from direct injection into the ventricles or into
the hypothalamus is not the same as fever resulting from intravenous endotoxin,
as centrally applied endotoxin is almost certainly acting directly, producing a reaction similar to a local inflammatory reaction, in which case the fever is not mediated by EP. It could be that in the new-born lamb the PO/AH is very insensitive
to prostaglandins, hence there is no response to exogenously applied PGE but a

sufficiently large dose of endotoxin can promote a massive inflammatory response enabling enough PGE to be released and therefore to produce fever. It would be of interest to know whether the fever resulting from the endotoxin in the lamb insensitive to PGE is abolished by antipyretic agents. The absence of response of new-born lambs to PGE only applies to the first few days of life; thereafter they become sensitive to both PGEs and endotoxins.

It is important to remember the recent work of KASTING et al. (1978 a, b) and COOPER et al. (1979) on the possibility that a circulating endogenous antipyretic substance is present in the new-born lamb. The presence of such a substance would obviously complicate the observations made with pyrogens and prostaglandins. Another point to be made is that the sheep is far less sensitive to prostaglandins than, for example, the cat. BLIGH and MILTON (1973) infused PGE_1 into the sheep to obtain sustained hyperthermias, since a single injection did not affect body temperature, though it produced transient inhibitory effects on respiration, vasoconstriction and shivering (BLIGH and MILTON, unpublished work). Because of the very high ability of the sheep to maintain body temperature within narrow limits, the co-ordinated changes in heat loss and heat gain mechanisms produced by PGE had to be sustained long enough for sufficient extra heat to be gained to elevate the animal's temperature.

In 1975 VEALE and COOPER found that in rabbits in which the entire PO/AH region had been destroyed bilaterally, PGE_1 and EP no longer induced fever when injected into this region, so that in this respect there was no discrepancy with the theory that prostaglandins mediate pyrogen fever. However, when the injections were made into the cerebral ventricles PGE_1 was without effect whereas EP still produced fever. This was also the case when injections of EP were made intravenously, and although temperature rose more gradually it reached the same end point as in control rabbits. These results can only be explained on the assumption that, at least in the rabbit, in addition to the PO/AH region there is another secondary site or sites on which pyrogen can act to produce fever. The difference in effectiveness between prostaglandin and EPs upon intraventricular injection would mean that with this method of application the secondary site is not reached by the prostaglandin but is reached by the pyrogen. The reason may be that it lies some distance from the ventricular site of injection and that the prostaglandin is removed from the ventricular system or from the tissue site before reaching the site of action of the pyrogen. If pyrogens act on the PO/AH region through prostaglandin, the same mechanism of action would be expected at the secondary site. Unfortunately, however, the authors of this paper did not determine whether the fever which occurred after the destruction of the PO/AH was sensitive to antipyretic drugs. The suggestion that pyrogen fever is independent of prostaglandin would only be valid if this were shown. It is interesting to note with reference to this case that ROSENDORF and MOONEY (1971) described a secondary EP-sensitive site in the midbrain. Subsequently, CRANSTON and RAWLINS (1972) performed bilateral micro-infusion of salicylate into different regions of the rabbit brain during fever. They found that defervescence was obtained from two sites and from two sites only, when the infusions were made into the PO/AH region and into the midbrain in or near the aqueductal grey matter.

MYERS (1977) applied labelled ^3H 5-HT and ^{14}C PGE_2 into the PO/AH of rabbits. Bacterial pyrogen delivered by a push-pull perfusion system to this region caused simultaneous release of both isotopes. However, when sodium salicylate was perfused together with the pyrogen in a dose insufficient to prevent fever, the enhancement of PGE_2 release by the pyrogen was reduced in spite of the ensuing hyperthermia. 5-HT release was not affected. MYERS considered that this was sufficient evidence to dissociate the action of bacterial pyrogen and prostaglandin release; however, these results really tell us nothing, as the mechanisms involved in the release of previously applied pre-formed PGE_2 and of newly synthesised PGE have not yet been shown to be similar.

The results of STITT and HARDY (1975) and JELL and SWEATMAN (1977) do not indicate that there is any relationship between the effects of prostaglandins and electrical discharge patterns from thermosensitive units which are affected by warm and cold stimuli, or any relationship between PGE_2 effects and pyrogen effects on similar neurones; however the results of SCHOENER and WANG (1976) and GORDON and HEATH (1980) support the theory that prostaglandins are involved in fever. However, it should be realised that if pyrogens act by activating the synthesis of prostaglandin to produce fever and not directly on neurones one would not expect any similarity in action. Secondly, as was pointed out by MILTON in 1978, the neurones in the hypothalamus responsible for processing information are not necessarily thermosensitive – in fact it would be a disadvantage if they were so. Since the prostaglandin receptor may be on thermally insensitive units which are responsible for activating the efferent pathways, one would not necessarily expect prostaglandins to alter the electrical activity of thermal sensitive neurones though electrical changes might be picked up on the efferent side.

The differences in responses of the echidna and young chicks to bacterial pyrogen and to prostaglandins also present certain problems. BAIRD et al. (1974) and ARTUNKAL et al. (1975) showed that particularly at low ambient temperatures the prostaglandins produce falls in deep body temperature, not rises. However, in both species prostaglandins produce vasodilatation of the peripheral vessels of the legs as well as sedation, catatonia or sleep by acting on areas of the brain other than the PO/AH. Consequently, at low ambient temperature heat loss due to these effects could easily mask the hyperthermic effect of the prostaglandins on the PO/AH, whereas at high ambient temperature, passive heat loss during sleep or sedation would be minimised and therefore the effects of the prostaglandins on the hypothalamus would predominate. During endotoxin fever catatonia and sleep are not observed and therefore no heat loss would occur from such phenomena. ARTUNKAL et al. (1975, 1977) observed that the fever produced by injecting bacterial pyrogen into the chicken hypothalamus was unaffected by pre-treatment with indomethacin, though the duration of the fever was reduced; at the same time they noticed that the response to prostaglandin was increased. With reference to the effect of the antipyretic on the fever produced by bacterial pyrogen, the authors acknowledged that they do not know the degree of prostaglandin synthesis inhibition obtained in their experiments. This is of importance, for it is known that some species are far more sensitive to antipyretic drugs than others; this may depend upon a variety of factors, not only a direct effect on the enzymes but also on the pharmacokinetics of the drug. For example 4-Ac which is a very good antipyretic drug in cats, is a very poor antipyretic drug in rabbits. GANDER et al. (1972) showed that in the rabbit 4-Ac was metabolised so rapidly that in order to obtain antipyretic blood levels it was necessary to give the drug either repeatedly or by continuous infusion. In contrast, in the cat a single dose of 50 mg/kg i.p. will exert an antipyretic action for approximately 4 h (MILTON and WENDLANDT 1968).

CLARK and CUMBY (1976) suggest from their experiments, in which the time-course of antipyretic action of 4-Ac, salicylate and indomethacin in inhibiting arachidonic acid fever was different from that in inhibiting pyrogen fever, that if prostaglandins are involved in fever then antipyretics act not as prostaglandin synthesis inhibitors but at a step before prostaglandin synthesis. Consideration should, however, be given to the problem of equating synthesis of prostaglandin from infused exogenous substrate and synthesis of prostaglandin from cellular constituents. In addition, the long delay in inhibition of arachidonic hyperthermia may be due to pre-formed prostaglandins remaining available for some time after the administration of the antipyretic. Remember that the antipyretic drug was not given until the arachidonic fever had fully developed. The initial hyperthermia seen after salicylate can be explained when one considers that there is considerable evidence that prostaglandin hyperthermia is potentiated by antipyretics (see p. 280).

In the past 3 years the use of protein synthesis inhibitors which have antipyretic action has been investigated to attempt to determine the roles of endotoxin, endogenous pyrogen and prostaglandins in fever. The results obtained so far have been reviewed by MILTON and SAWHNEY (this volume, Chap. 11). The results obtained are inconsistent, and the conclusion to be reached is that so far they have not provided any evidence to determine one way or the other whether there is a relationship between prostaglandin synthesis and pyrogen fever. Taken together, all the evidence produced by the various authors who have cast doubt on the prostaglandin theory is not convincing.

The evidence for the involvement of prostaglandins in fever is far greater, i.e. that in the PO/AH there are PGE receptors, the activation of which produces coordinated changes in heat gain and heat loss mechanisms, resulting in hyperthermia. Fever results from activation of these receptors by a PGE, probably PGE_2, the synthesis and release of which are activated by circulating pyrogen. The antipyretic drugs act by inhibiting the fatty acid cyclo-oxygenase enzyme responsible for converting arachidonic acid to the prostaglandin, and by this mechanism inhibit the synthesis and release of the prostaglandin and so inhibit fever.

Acknowledgement. I wish to thank DOROTHY TODD for keeping me up to date with the literature and for organizing the references.

References

Artunkal AA, Marley E (1974) Hyper- and hypothermic effects of prostaglandin E_1 (PGE_1) and their potentiation by indomethacin, in chicks. J Physiol (Lond) 242:141–142 P

Artunkal AA, Marley E, Stephenson JD (1975) Dissociation of bacterial pyrexia from prostaglandin E activity. Br J Pharmacol 54:250–251 P

Artunkal AA, Marley E, Stephenson JD (1977) Some effects of prostaglandins E_1 and E_2 injected into the hypothalamus of young chicks: dissociation between endotoxin fever and the effects of prostaglandins. Br J Pharmac 61:39–46

Atkins E, Bodel PT (1974) Fever. In: Grant L, McClusky RT (eds) The inflammatory process, 2nd edn, vol III. Academic Press, New York, pp 467–514

Baird JA, Hales JRS, Lang WJ (1974) Thermoregulatory responses to the injection of monoamines, acetylcholine, and prostaglandins into a lateral cerebral ventricle of the echidna. J Physiol (Lond) 236:539–548

Baumann I, Bligh J, Vallenas A (1975) Temperature regulation in the alpaca. (Lama pacos): thermoregulatory consequences and inconsequences of injections of adrenaline, 5-hydroxytryptamine, carbamyl choline and prostaglandin E_1 into a lateral cerebral ventricle. Comp Biochem Pyhsiol [C] 50:105–109

Bernheim HA, Gilbert TM, Stitt JT (1980) Prostaglandin E levels in third ventricular cerebrospinal fluid of rabbits during fever and changes in body temperature. J Physiol (Lond) 301:69–78

Blatteis CM (1980) Ontogenetic development of fever mechanisms. In: Lipton JM (ed) Fever. Raven, New York, pp 177–188

Bligh J, Milton AS (1973) The thermoregulatory effects of prostaglandin E_1 when infused into a lateral cerebral ventricle of the Welsh Mountain Sheep at different ambient temperatures. J Physiol (Lond) 229:30–31 P

Breckenridge BMcL, Lisk RD (1969) Cyclic adenylate and hypothalamic regulatory functions. Proc Soc Exp Biol (NY) 131:934–935

Bundy GL (1975) Synthesis of prostaglandin endoperoxide analogues. Tetrahedron Lett 24:1957–1960

Cammock S, Dascombe MJ, Milton AS (1976) Prostaglandins in thermoregulation. Adv Prostaglandin Thromboxane Res 1:375–380

Clark WG, Cumby HR (1975a) Effects of prostaglandin antagonist SC.19220 on body temperature and on hyperthermic responses to prostaglandin E_1 and leucocytic pyrogen in the cat. Prostaglandins 9:361–368

Clark WG, Cumby HR (1975b) The antipyretic effect of indomethacin. J Physiol (Lond) 248:625–638

Clark WG, Cumby HR (1976) Antagonism by antipyretics of the hyperthermic effect of a prostaglandin precursor, sodium arachidonate in the cat. J Physiol (Lond) 257:581–595

Clark WG, Lipton JM (1979) Hyperthermic effect of prostacyclin injected into the third cerebral ventricle of the cat. Brain Res Bull 4:15–16

Clark WG, Cumby HR, Davis HE (1974) The hyperthermic effect of intracerebroventricular cholera toxin in the unanaesthetized cat. J Physiol (Lond) 240:493–504

Cooper KE, Grundman MJ, Honour AJ (1968) Observations on sodium salicylate as an antipyretic. J Physiol (Lond) 196:56–57 P

Cooper KE, Veale WL, Kasting N, Pittman QJ (1979) Ontogeny of fever. Fed Proc 38:35–38

Cranston WI, Hellon RF, Mitchell D (1975a) Fever and brain prostaglandin release. J Physiol (Lond) 248:27–28 P

Cranston WI, Hellon RF, Mitchell D (1975b) A dissociation between fever and prostaglandin concentration in cerebrospinal fluid. J Physiol (Lond) 253:583–592

Cranston WI, Duff GW, Hellon RF, Mitchell D (1976) Effect of a prostaglandin antagonist on the pyrexias caused by PGE_2 and leucocyte pyrogen in rabbits. J Physiol (Lond) 256:120–121 P

Cranston WI, Duff GW, Hellon RF, Mitchell D, Townsend Y (1976b) Evidence that brain prostaglandin synthesis is not essential in fever. J Physiol (Lond) 259:239–249

Crawford IL, Kennedy JI, Lipton JM, Ojeda SR (1979) Effects of central administration of probenecid on fever produced by leukocytic pyrogen and PGE_2 in the rabbit. J Physiol (Lond) 287:519–533

Crawshaw LI, Stitt JT (1975) Behavioural and autonomic induction of prostaglandin E_1 fever in squirrel monkeys. J Physiol (Lond) 244:197–206

Cremades-Campos A, Milton AS (1978) The effect on deep body temperature of the intraventricular injection of two prostaglandin endoperoxide analogues. J Physiol (Lond) 282:38 P

Cremades-Campos A, Milton AS (1982) Thermoregulatory responses of the conscious rabbit to intraventricular injections of cyclic AMP and prostaglandin E_2. J Physiol (Lond) 325:39 P

Dascombe MJ (1981) Hypothermia in rabbits after intrahypothalamic injections of N^6-2'-O-dibutyryl adenosine 3',5',-monophosphate. Br J Pharmacol 73:314–315 P

Dascombe MJ, Milton AS (1975) The effects of cyclic adenosine 3',5'-monophosphate and other nucleotides on body temperature. J Physiol (Lond) 250:143–160

Dascombe MJ, Milton AS (1976) Cyclic adenosine 3',5'-monophosphate in cerebrospinal fluid during thermoregulation and fever. J Physiol (Lond) 263:441–463

Dascombe MJ, Milton AS (1980) Thermoregulatory effects of guanosine 3',5'-monophosphate in the cat. Br J Pharmacol 70:154–155 P

Dascombe MJ, Milton AS (1981) Dissimilar effects on body temperature in the cat produced by guanosine 3',5'-monophosphate, acetylcholine and bacterial endotoxin. Br J Pharmacol 74:405–413

Dascombe MJ, Parkes J (1981) Effects of N^6-2'-O-dibutyryl adenosine 3',5'-monophosphate on body temperature in the restrained rat. Br J Pharmacol 72:565–566 P

Dascombe MJ, Milton AS, Nyemitei-Addo I, Pertwee RG (1980) Thermoregulatory effects of N^6-2'-O-dibutyryl adenosine 3',5'-monophosphate in the restrained mouse. Br J Pharmacol 70:543–549

Dey PK, Feldberg W, Gupta KP, Milton AS, Wendlandt S (1974a) Further studies on the role of prostaglandin in fever. J Physiol (Lond) 241:629–646

Dey PK, Feldberg W, Wendlandt S (1974b) Lipid A and prostaglandin. J Physiol (Lond) 239:102–103 P

Dey PK, Feldberg W, Gupta PK, Wendlandt S (1975) Lipid A fever in cats. J Physiol (Lond) 253:103–119

Duff GW, Cranston WI, Luff RH (1972) Cyclic 3',5'-adenosine monophosphate in central control of body temperature. Fifth Int Congr Pharmacol Abstr 360, p 60

Ewen L, Milton AS, Smith S (1976) Effects of prostaglandin $F_{2\alpha}$ and prostaglandin D_2 on the body temperature of conscious cats. J Physiol (Lond) 258:121–122 P

Feldberg W, Gupta KP (1972) Sampling for biological assay of cerebrospinal fluid from the third ventricle in the unanaesthetized cat. J Physiol (Lond) 222:126–129 P

Feldberg W, Gupta KP (1973) Pyrogen fever and prostaglandin activity in cerebrospinal fluid. J Physiol (Lond) 228:41–53

Feldberg W, Milton AS (1978) Prostaglandins and body temperature. In: Vane JR, Ferreira SH (eds) Inflammation. (Handbook of experimental pharmacology, vol 50/1). Springer, Berlin Heidelberg New York, pp 617–656

Feldberg W, Myers RD (1964) Effect on temperature of amines injected into the cerebral ventricles. A new concept of temperature regulation. J. Physiol (Lond) 173:226–237

Feldberg W, Saxena PN (1970) Mechanism of action of pyrogen. J Physiol (Lond) 211:245–261

Feldberg W, Saxena PN (1971a) Fever produced by prostaglandin E_1. J Physiol (Lond) 217:547–556

Feldberg W, Saxena PN (1971b) Further studies on prostaglandin E_1 fever in cats. J Physiol (Lond) 219:739–745

Feldberg W, Saxena PN (1975) Prostaglandins, endotoxin, and lipid A on body temperature in rats. J Physiol (Lond) 249:601–615

Feldberg W, Myers RD, Veale WL (1970) Perfusions from cerebral ventricle to cisterna magna in the unanaesthetized cat. Effect of calcium on body temperature. J Physiol (Lond) 297:403–417

Feldberg W, Gupta KP, Milton AS, Wendlandt S (1972) Effect of bacterial pyrogen and antipyretics on prostaglandin activity in cerebrospinal fluid of unanaesthetized cats. Br J Pharmacol 46:550–551 P

Feldberg W, Gupta KP, Milton AS, Wendlandt S (1973) Effect of pyrogen and antipyretics on prostaglandin activity in cisternal CSF of unanaesthetized cats. J Physiol (Lond) 234:279–293

Flower RJ (1974) Drugs which inhibit prostaglandin biosynthesis. Pharmacol Rev 26:33–67

Ford DM (1974) A selective action of prostaglandin E_1 on hypothalamic neurones in the cat which respond to brain cooling. J Physiol (Lond) 242:142–143 P

Gander GW, Chaffee J, Goodale F (1967) Studies on the antipyretic action of salicylate. Proc Soc Exp Biol Med 126:205–209

Gander GW, Milton AS, Goodale F (1972) The antipyretic effects of n-acetyl p-aminophenol. Fifth Int Congr Pharmacol, Abstr 452, p 76

Gordon CJ, Heath JE (1980) Effects of prostaglandin E_2 on activity of thermosensitive and insensitive single units in the preoptic/anterior hypothalamus of unanaesthetized rabbits. Brain Res 183:113–121

Gorman RR, Fitzpatrick FA, Miller OV (1978) Adv Cyclic Nucleotide Res 9:597–609

Hales JRS, Bennett JW, Baird JA, Fawcett AA (1973) Thermoregulatory effects of prostaglandins E_1, E_2, $F_{1\alpha}$, and $F_{2\alpha}$ in the sheep. Pflügers Arch Ges Physiol 339:125–133

Harvey CA (1976) The role of prostaglandins and monoamines in fever and thermoregulation. PhD thesis, London University

Harvey CA, Milton AS (1975) Endogenous pyrogen fever, prostaglandin release and prostaglandin synthetase inhibitors. J Physiol (Lond) 250:18–20 P

Harvey CA, Milton AS, Straughan DW (1975) Prostaglandin E levels in cerebrospinal fluid of rabbits and the effects of bacterial pyrogen and antipyretic drugs. J Physiol (Lond) 248:26–27 P

Holmes SW, Horton EW (1968) The distribution of tritium labelled prostaglandin E_1 injected in amounts sufficient to produce central nervous effects in cats and chicks. Br J Pharmacol 34:32–37

Hori T, Harada Y (1974) The effects of ambient and hypothalamic temperatures on the hyperthermic responses to prostaglandins E_1 and E_2. Pflügers Arch Ges Physiol 350:123–134

Horton EW, Main IHM (1967) Identification of prostaglandins in central nervous tissues of the cat and chicken. Br J Pharmacol 30:582–602

Jell RM, Sweatman P (1977) Prostaglandin-sensitive neurones in cat hypothalamus: relation to thermoregulation and to biogenic amines. Can J Physiol Pharmacol 55:560–567

Kandasamy B, Girault JM, Jacob J (1975) Central effects of a purified bacterial pyrogen, prostaglandin E_1 and biogenic amines on the temperature in the awake rabbit. In: Lomax P, Schönbaum E, Jacob J (eds) Temperature regulation and drug action. Karger, Basel New York, pp 124–132

Karim SMM (ed) (1979) Practical applications of prostaglandins and synthesis inhibitors. University Park Press, Baltimore

Kasting NW, Veale WL, Cooper KE (1978a) Suppression of fever at term of pregnancy. Nature 271:245–246

Kasting NW, Veale WL, Cooper KE (1978b) Evidence for a centrally active endogenous antipyretic near parturition in the sheep. In: Lederis K, Veale WL (eds) Current studies of hypothalamic functions. Karger, Basel New York, pp 63–71

Kasting NW, Veale WL, Cooper KE (1979) Development of fever in the newborn lamb. Am J Physiol 236:R 184–R 187

Kebabian JW, Bloom FE, Steiner AL, Greengard PE (1975) Neurotransmitters increase cyclic nucleotides in postganglionic neurones, immunocytochemical demonstration. Science 190:157–159

Laburn H, Mitchell D, Rosendorff C (1972) Effects of prostaglandin antagonism on sodium arachidonate fever in rabbits. J Physiol (Lond) 267:559–570

Laburn H, Rosendorff C, Wilies G, Woolf C (1979) A role for noradrenaline and cyclic AMP in prostaglandin E_1 fever. J Physiol (Lond) 240:49–50 P

Lipton JM, Fossler DE (1974) Fever produced in the squirrel monkey by intravenous and intracerebral endotoxin. Am J Physiol 226:1020–1027

Lipton JM, Welch JP, Clark WG (1973) Changes in body temperature produced by injecting prostaglandin E_1, EGTA and bacterial endotoxins into the PO/AH region and the medulla oblongata of the rat. Experientia 29:806–808

Malmsten C, Hamberg M, Svensson J, Samuelsson B (1975) Physiological role of an endoperoxide in human platelets: hemostatic defect due to platelet cyclo-oxygenase deficiency. Proc Natl Acad Sci USA 72:1446–1450

Milton AS (1972) Prostaglandin E_1 and endotoxin fever, and the effects of aspirin, indomethacin and 4-acetamidophenol. Adv Biosci 9:495–500

Milton AS (1978) The hypothalamus and the pharmacology of thermoregulation. In: Cox B, Morris ID, Weston AH (eds) Pharmacology of the hypothalamus. Macmillan, London, pp 105–134

Milton AS, Sawhney VK (1981) The effects of a protein synthesis inhibitor on the thermoregulatory responses to bacterial pyrogen, endogenous pyrogen and to prostaglandin E_2. In: Szelényi Z, Székely M (eds) Contributions to thermal physiology. Akademiai Kiadó, Budapest, pp 165–167

Milton AS, Wendlandt S (1968) The effect of 4-acetamidophenol in reducing fever produced by the intracerebral injection of 5-hydroxytryptamine and pyrogen in the conscious cat. Br J Pharmacol 34:215–216 P

Milton AS, Wendlandt S (1970) A possible role for prostaglandin E_1 as a modulator for temperature regulation in the central nervous system of the cat. J Physiol (Lond) 207:76–77 P

Milton AS, Wendlandt S (1971 a) Effects on body temperature of prostaglandins of the A, E, and F series on injection into the third ventricle of unanaesthetized cats and rabbits. J Physiol (Lond) 218:325–336

Milton AS, Wendlandt S (1971 b) The effect of different environmental temperatures on the hyperpyrexia produced by the intraventricular injection of pyrogen, 5-hydroxytryptamine and prostaglandin E_1 in the conscious cat. J Physiol (Paris) 63:340–342

Milton AS, Wendlandt S (1971 c) The effects of 4-acetamidophenol (paracetamol) on the temperature response of the conscious rat to the intracerebral injection of prostaglandin E_1, adrenaline and pyrogen. J Physiol (Lond) 217:33 P

Milton AS, Smith S, Tomkins KB (1977) Levels of prostaglandin F and E in the cerebrospinal fluid of cats during pyrogen-induced fever. Br J Pharmacol 59:447–448

Milton AS, Cremades-Campos A, Sawhney VK, Bichard A (1980) Effects of prostacyclin, 6-oxo-$PGF_{1\alpha}$ and endoperoxide analogues on the body temperature of cats and rabbits. In: Cox B, Lomax P, Milton AS, Schönbaum E (eds) Thermoregulatory mechanisms and their therapeutic implications. Karger, Basel New York, pp 87–92

Milton AS, Pertwee RG, Todd DA (1982) The effect of prostaglandin E_2 and pyrogen on thermoregulation in the MFI mouse. J Physiol (Lond) 322:59 P

Moncada S, Gryglewski RJ, Bunting S, Vane JR (1976) An enzyme isolated from arteries transforms prostaglandin endoperoxide to an unstable substance that inhibits platelet aggregation. Nature Lond 263:663–665

Myers RD (1977) New aspects of the role of hypothalamic calcium ions, 5-HT and PGE during normal thermoregulation and pyrogen fever. In: Cooper KE, Lomax P, Schönbaum E (eds) Drugs, biogenic amines and body temperature. Karger, Basel New York, pp 51–53

Myers RD, Sharpe LG (1968) Intracerebral injections and perfusions in the conscious monkey. In: Vagtlong H (ed) Use of non-human primates in drug evaluation. Texas Press, Austin, pp 450–465

Myers RD, Veale WL (1971) The role of sodium and calcium in the hypothalamus in the control of body temperature of the unanaesthetized cat. J Physiol (Lond) 212:411–430

Nistico G, Marley E (1973) Central effects of prostaglandin E_1 in adult fowls. Neuropharmacology 12:1009–1016

Nistico G, Marley E (1976) Central effects of prostaglandin E_2, A_1 and $F_{2\alpha}$ in adult fowls. Neuropharmacology 15:737–741

Nistico G, Rotiroti D (1978) Antipyretics and fever induced in adult fowls by prostaglandin E_1, E_2 and O-somatic antigen. Neuropharmacology 17:197–203

Philipp-Dormston WK, Siegert R (1974 a) Identification of prostaglandin E by radio-immunoassay in cerebrospinal fluid furing endotoxin fever. Naturwissenschaften 61:134–135

Philipp-Dormston WK, Siegert R (1974 b) Prostaglandins of the E and F series in rabbit cerebrospinal fluid during fever induced by Newcastle disease virus. E. coli-Endotoxin of endogenous pyrogen. Med Microbiol Immunol 159:279–284

Piper P, Vane J (1971) The release of prostaglandin from lung and other tissues. Ann NY Acad Sci 180:363–385

Pittman QJ, Veale WL, Cooper KE (1975) Temperature responses of lambs after centrally injected prostaglandins and pyrogens. Am J Physiol 228:1034–1038

Pittman QJ, Veale WL, Cockeram AW, Cooper KE (1976) Changes in body temperature produced by prostaglandins and pyrogens in the chicken. Am J Physiol 230:1284–1287

Pittman QJ, Veale WL, Cooper KE (1977 a) Effect of prostaglandin; pyrogen and noradrenaline, injected into the hypothalamus, on thermoregulation in new-born lambs. Brain Res 128:473–483

Pittman QJ, Veale WL, Cooper KE (1977 b) Absence of fever following intrahypothalamic injections of prostaglandins in sheep. Neuropharmacology 16:743–749

Potts WJ, East PF (1972) Effects of prostaglandin E_2 on the body temperature of conscious rats and cats. Arch Int Pharmacodyn 197:31–36

Rawlins MD, Rosendorff C, Cranston WI (1971) The mechanism of action of antipyretics. In: Wolstenholm GEW, Birch J (eds) Pyrogens and fever. Churchill Livingstone, Edinburgh London, pp 175–187

Rosendorff C, Mooney JJ (1971) Central nervous system sites of action of a purified leucocyte pyrogen. Am J Physiol 220:597–603

Rudy TA, Viswanathan CT (1975) Effect of central cholinergic blockade on the hyperthermia evoked by prostaglandin E_1 injected into the rostral hypothalamus of the rat. Can J Physiol Pharmacol 53:321–324

Rudy TA, Williams JW, Yaksh TL (1977) Antagonism of indomethacin of neurogenic hyperthermia produced by unilateral puncture of the anterior hypothalamic/preoptic region. J Physiol (Lond) 272:721–736

Sanner JH (1974) Substances that inhibit the actions of prostaglandins. Arch Intern Med 133:133–146

Saxena PN, Beg MMA, Singhal KC, Ahmad M (1979) Prostaglandin-like activity in the cerebrospinal fluid of febrile patients. Indian J Med Res 70:495–498

Schoener EP, Wang SC (1974) Sodium acetylsalicylate effectiveness against fever induced by leukocytic pyrogen and prostaglandin E_1 in the cat. Experientia 30:383–384

Schoener EP, Wang SC (1976) Effects of locally administered prostaglandin E_1 on anterior hypothalamic neurones. Brain Res 117:157–162

Splawinski JA (1972) Mediation of hyperthermia of prostaglandin E_2: A new hypothesis. Naunyn-Schmiedebergs Arch Pharmacol 297:95–97

Splawinski JA, Gorka Z, Zacny E, Wojtaszek B (1978) Hyperthermic effects of arachidonic acid, prostaglandins E_2 and $F_{2\alpha}$ in rats. Pflügers Arch Ges Physiol 374:15–21

Splawinski JA, Wojtaszek B, Swies J (1979) Endotoxin fever in rats: is it triggered by a decrease in breakdown of prostaglandin E_2. Neuropharmacology 18:111–115

Stitt JT (1973) Prostaglandin E_1 fever induced in rabbits. J Physiol (Lond) 232:163–179

Stitt JT, Hardy JD (1975) Microelectrophoresis of PGE_1 onto single units in the rabbits hypothalamus. Am J Physiol 229:240–245

Stitt JT, Hardy JD, Stolwijk AJ (1974) PGE_1 fever: its effect on thermoregulation at different low ambient temperatures. Am J Physiol 227:622–629

Stone E (1763) An account of the success of the bark of the willow in the cure of agues. Philos Trans 53:195–200

Székely M, Komáromi I (1978) Endotoxin and prostaglandin fever of newborn guinea-pigs at different ambient temperatures. Acta Physiol Acad Sci Hung 51:293–298

Vane JR (1957) A sensitive method for the assay of 5-hydroxytryptamine. Br J Pharmacol 12:344–349

Vane JR (1971) Inhibition of prostaglandin synthesis as a mechanism of action for aspirinlike drugs. Nature New Biol 23:232–235

Van Miert AS, Frens J (1968) The reaction of different animal species to bacterial pyrogens. Zentralbl Vet Met 15:532–543

Varagic VM, Beleslin DB (1973) The effect of cyclic N-2-O-dibutyryl-adenosine-3′,5′-monophosphate, adenosine triphosphate and butyrate on the body temperature of conscious cats. Brain Res 57:252–254

Veale WL, Cooper KE (1975) Comparison of sites of action of prostaglandin and leucocyte pyrogen in brain. In: Lomax P, Schönbaum E, Jacob J (eds) Temperature regulation and drug action. Karger, Basel New York, pp 218–226

Veale WL, Wishaw I (1976) Body temperature responses at different ambient temperatures following injections of PGE_1 and NA into the brain. Pharmacol Biochem Behav 4:143–150

Waller MB, Myers RD (1973) Hyperthermia and operant responding for heat evoked in the monkey by intrahypothalamic prostaglandin. Proc Soc Neurosci p.118

Wendlandt S (1972) Some factors involved in the control of body temperature and the action of pyrogens and pharmacologically active substances in modifying body temperature. PhD thesis, Lodon University

Williams JW, Rudy TA, Yaksh TL, Viswanathan CT (1977) An extensive exploration of the rat brain for sites mediating PG-induced hyperthermia. Brain Res 120:251–262

Willis AL, Davison P, Ramwell PW, Brocklehurst WE, Smith B (1972) Release and actions of prostaglandins in inflammation and fever: inhibition by anti-inflammatory and anti-pyretics drugs. In: Ramwell PW, Pharris BB (eds) Prostaglandins in cellular biology. Plenum, New York, pp 227–259

Woolf CJ, Willis GH, Laburn H, Rosendorff C (1975) Pyrogen and prostaglandin fever in the rabbit. I. Effects of salicylate and the role of cyclic AMP. Neuropharmacology 14:397–403

Woolf CJ, Willis GH, Rosendorff C (1976) Does cyclic AMP have a role in the pathogenesis of fever in the rabbit. Naturwissenschaften 63:94

Woolf CJ, Willis GH, Rosendorff C (1977) Pyrogen, prostaglandin, and cyclic AMP fevers in the rabbit. In: Cooper KE, Lomax P, Schönbaum E (eds) Drugs, biogenic amines and body temperature. Karger, Basel New York, pp 136–139

Ziel R, Krupp P (1976) Influence of endogenous pyrogen on cerebral prostaglandin-synthetase system. Experientia 32:1451–1452

Zor V, Kaneko T, Schneider HPG et al. (1969) Stimulation of anterior pituitary adenyl cyclase activity and adenosine $3',5'$-cyclic phosphate by hypothalamic extract and prostaglandin E_1. Proc Nat Acad Sci USA 63:918–925

CHAPTER 11

Protein Synthesis and Fever

A. S. MILTON and V. K. SAWHNEY

A. Introduction

Protein synthesis inhibitors have been used extensively to determine the importance of the synthesis of new protein in biological processes such as learning and
memory (SQUIRE and BARONDES 1974; DAVIS et al. 1980). A universal problem in
using these inhibitors appears to be that they have numerous side effects on various
cellular functions which make it difficult to conclude with certainty whether or not
the observed effects are specifically due to an inhibition of protein synthesis. Over
the past few years experimental evidence has accumulated to suggest that the
pathogenesis of fever may depend on the synthesis of a specific protein mediator.
Our objective in this chapter is to review the pertinent literature which has led to
the idea that protein synthesis is a prerequisite for the manifestation of fever.

B. Experimental Evidence

The protein synthesis inhibitor cycloheximide (Fig. 1) has been shown to exert an
antipyretic effect in febrile cancer patients who have no apparent bacterial, fungal
or viral infection (YOUNG and DOWLING 1975). These authors suggested that in
some types of neoplastic disease, either the tumour cells or other normal cells of
the body may produce an endogenous pyrogen and, in relation to this, cycloheximide may exert its antipyretic activity by inhibiting the production of this
pyrogenic protein.

BELESLIN and SAMARDŽIĆ (1975) have documented evidence which they believe
indicates that protein synthesis in the brain is an important factor in the maintenance of normal body temperature. The found that the intraventricular injection

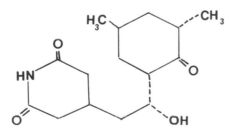

Fig. 1. Structure of cycloheximide

in cats of actinomycin D in a dose as low as 0.5 µg resulted in an irreversible hypothermia after a latency of several days. They postulated that a brain protein with a short biological half-life may be involved in the central mechanism of body temperature regulation. However, in view of the extreme toxicity of actinomycin D and the irreversible nature of the temperature change produced by this drug, one cannot be certain that the hypothermia reported was due to protein synthesis inhibition alone.

SIEGERT et al. (1975, 1976) first proposed the existence of a protein mediator in the pathway leading to the production of fever. They found that rabbits pretreated with intravenous cycloheximide (5 mg/kg) failed to develop a fever following the systemic administration of either exogenous or endogenous pyrogens even though the cerebrospinal fluid (CSF) levels of prostaglandin E and of cyclic AMP were elevated as in normal febrile animals. The dose of cycloheximide used in these experiments was shown to inhibit the incorporation of ^{14}C-labelled protein hydrolysate into brain protein by 30%–40% during a 3-h period following its administration. These original findings of SIEGERT and colleagues have since been confirmed in various laboratories. For example the systemic administration of cycloheximide to rabbits has been shown to prevent the febrile response to both exogenous pyrogens (STITT 1980; MILTON and SAWHNEY 1980a, b) and endogenous pyrogen (MILTON and TODD 1981; MILTON and SAWHNEY 1980b; HELLON et al. 1980).

Although SIEGERT et al. (1976) observed a slight fall in the body temperature of cycloheximide-treated rabbits, they did not consider the inhibition of fever by this drug to be due to a non-specific effect of the inhibitor. They found that cycloheximide did not prevent the hyperthermia due to exogenous overheating of the animals, and on the basis of this finding, SIEGERT et al. (1976) thought that cycloheximide did not affect normal thermoregulation in rabbits. In line with this, HELLON et al. (1980) also reported that cycloheximide does not affect central thermoregulatory mechanisms in the rabbit as it was found to have no effect on the central temperature responses to the intravenous administration of cold Hartman's solution.

Other experiments in which the specificity of the antipyretic effect of cycloheximide has been questioned have indicated that this inhibitor may have a general depressant effect on heat production. For example it was found to depress the metabolic response to cold stress in both rats (BARNEY et al. 1979) and rabbits (STITT 1980). STITT found that cycloheximide also impaired cold-induced thermogenesis following cooling of the PO/AH region of the brain. In addition, he reported that in a warm environment where pyrogen fever is produced primarily by a reduction in heat loss, cycloheximide failed to prevent the febrile response to intravenous *E. coli* endotoxin. STITT therefore concluded that the fever production pathway *per se* is unaffected by cycloheximide treatment. However, in conflict with this result, we have consistently found that the systemic pretreatment of rabbits with cycloheximide (5 mg/kg i.v.) at an ambient temperature of 30 °C does prevent the development of fever due to the subsequent administration of bacterial and endogenous pyrogens (MILTON and SAWHNEY 1980a, b) (Fig. 2).

There appear to be only three basic differences between the experiments reported by STITT (1980) and those of ours. They are: (1) that the bacterial pyrogens used

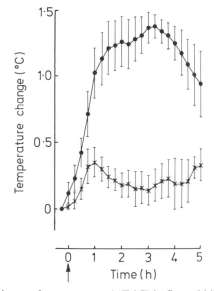

Fig. 2. Mean change in rectal temperature (ΔT °C) in five rabbits at an environmental temperature of $30° \pm 0.2$ °C. At the arrow shown, *Shigella dysenteriae* (1 µg/kg) was injected i.v. 90 min after pretreatment of the animals with either cycloheximide (5 mg/kg i.v.) or 0.9% NaCl (2 ml i.v.). Vertical lines define the S.E. of the mean. ●—● 0.9% NaCl + *S. dysenteriae*; ×—× cycloheximide + *S. dysenteriae*. (MILTON and SAWHNEY unpublished)

in the two studies were different; (2) the strain used by STITT was New Zealand White rabbits rather than the Dutch rabbits used by us; and (3) the time interval between the administration of cycloheximide and pyrogen was 3 h in the experiments of STITT whereas in our experiments it was only 90 min.

The bacterial pyrogen used in our studies was the "O" somatic antigen of *Shigella dysenteriae* and is different from the three bacterial pyrogens used by SIEGERT et al. (1976) which were *Escherichia coli* lipopolysaccharide, a synthetic double-stranded ribonucleic acid and Newcastle disease virus. However, it is thought that the induction of fever by various exogenous pyrogens proceeds via similar mechanisms in that endogenous pyrogen can be shown to be present in the blood and prostaglandin E (PGE) in cerebrospinal fluid of febrile animals, regardless of the exogenous pyrogen used to induce the fever (SIEGERT et al. 1976; HARVEY et al. 1975). Unless there is a real difference in the sensitivity of the two strains to cycloheximide, the most likely cause for the discrepancy between our finding and that reported by STITT is the difference in the time interval between the administration of cycloheximide and pyrogen. It is possible that by increasing this time interval, the inhibitory effect of cycloheximide had been reduced and a block of the febrile response was therefore no longer apparent.

It is generally accepted that exogenous pyrogens of bacterial or other origin do not act directly on the thermoregulatory structures within the CNS but, instead, they act indirectly to activate the production and release of endogenous pyrogens from various cells within the body (ATKINS 1960; BLIGH 1973; MILTON 1976). The in vitro formation and release of endogenous pyrogen (EP) from blood leucocytes has been shown to be susceptible to blockade by various inhibitors of RNA and protein synthesis, among which is cycloheximide (ATKINS and BODEL 1971).

The possibility that cycloheximide may interfere with pyrogen fever by preventing the production or release of endogenous pyrogen has been investigated using two different approaches. Either endogenous pyrogen has been prepared from rabbit peritoneal exudate cells (MILTON and SAWHNEY 1980 b) or endogenous pyrogen present in the serum or plasma from endotoxin-treated rabbits has been transferred to non-treated recipients (SIEGERT et al. 1976; MILTON and TODD 1981). In each of these experiments the febrile response to intravenously administered endogenous pyrogen was found to be abolished in the presence of cycloheximide. In addition, SIEGERT et al. (1976) and MILTON and TODD (1981) were able to show that endogenous pyrogen was still produced in cycloheximide-pretreated donor rabbits even though the febrile response was completely abolished. Thus, from all these experiments it appears that the antipyretic effect of cycloheximide is not due to an inhibition of the formation or release of endogenous pyrogen in vivo.

The possibility that cycloheximide may block the febrile response to systemically administered pyrogens by preventing the access of these pyrogens into the brain has also been investigated. CRANSTON et al. (1978) reported that intravenously administered cycloheximide attenuates the febrile response to the i.c.v. administration of endogenous pyrogen in the rabbit. In our laboratory we have found that intravenous cycloheximide significantly attenuated the febrile response to both i.c.v. endogenous pyrogen and to low doses of *Shigella dysenteriae* at an ambient temperature of 20 °C (MILTON and SAWHNEY 1980 b). However, the fevers due to a larger dose of bacterial pyrogen given by the same route at an ambient temperature of 20° or 30 °C were not affected by cycloheximide pretreatment (MILTON and SAWHNEY 1980 b). In contrast to this, cycloheximide did cause a partial inhibition of the fever due to the same high dose of centrally administered bacterial pyrogen at 5 °C. This inhibitory effect of cycloheximide may have been apparent at the low ambient temperature only because of its effect to interfere with cold-induced thermogenesis (STITT 1980). Since cycloheximide did attenuate the development of the febrile responses, when both endogenous pyrogen and a low dose of bacterial pyrogen were injected centrally, it seems unlikely that cycloheximide prevents the development of fevers due to systemically administered pyrogens by interfering with the transport of pyrogens into the brain. Interestingly, ANGEL and BURKETT (1971) have reported that cycloheximide has a disruptive effect on the blood-brain barrier function in the rat as was shown by an increased accumulation of cocaine in brain tissue of cycloheximide-treated rats.

In contrast to attenuation of the febrile response to i.c.v. leucocyte pyrogen, CRANSTON et al. (1978) reported that the hyperthermia produced by i.c.v. arachidonic acid in rabbits was not affected by cycloheximide pretreatment. The authors argued that this finding together with the results obtained by SIEGERT et al. (1976) demonstrated that metabolites of archidonic acid are unlikely to play an important role in the rise of body temperature during fever. However, in conflict with these results, a more recent report from the same laboratory has indicated that cycloheximide does block the hyperthermic effects of PGE_2 in rabbits and perhaps also attenuates the hyperthermic effects of arachidonic acid (HELLON et al. 1980). MILTON and SAWHNEY (1980 b), however, found that cycloheximide only caused a reduction of the hyperthermic responses to i.c.v. PGE_2 in rabbits kept at a low ambient temperature (5 °C); at higher ambient temperatures (20° and 30 °C), cycloheximide did not attenuate the responses to PGE_2. The hyperthermic response to arachidonic acid was only studied at an ambient temperature of 20 °C and, under these conditions, it was not affected by cycloheximide pretreatment. For the experiments reported by CRANSTON et al. (1978) and by HELLON et al. (1980), the environmental temperature was not stated.

A possible site of action of cycloheximide could be on the prostaglandin biosynthesis pathway. PONG et al. (1977) reported that cycloheximide inhibits the in vitro production of prostaglandins by methylcholanthrene-transformed mouse BALB/ 3T3 cells. This effect was due to a prevention of the deacylation of phospholipids, thus preventing the release of arachidonic acid.

Although our studies on the effects of cycloheximide on PGE_2 and arachidonic acid fevers suggest that cycloheximide prevents pyrogen fever by interfering with the release of arachidonic acid in the brain, the experiments of SIEGERT et al. (1976) do not support this mechanism.

Cycloheximide has also been shown to inhibit both the hyperactivity and hyperthermia that occur following the administration of L-tryptophan or 5-methoxy-N, N-dimethyltryptamine to rats treated with the monoamine oxidase inhibitor, tranylcypromine (GRAHAME-SMITH 1972). The inhibitory effects of cycloheximide on the hyperthermia and hyperactivity were dose dependent and were apparent following the administration of doses that produced an inhibition of brain protein synthesis greater than 60%–70%. As cycloheximide was found not to affect the rate of synthesis of brain 5-hydroxytryptamine (5-HT) in these experiments, it was concluded that this antibiotic inhibited the hyperactivity by virtue of its action on protein synthesis. In support of this conclusion emetine, a structurally similar protein synthesis inhibitor to cycloheximide (GROLLMAN 1966), was also found to inhibit the hyperactivity and hyperpyrexia in rats, whereas isoemetine, which is ineffective as an inhibitor of protein synthesis, had no such effect. GRAHAME-SMITH (1972) suggested that a brain protein with a short-biological half-life may be a specific mediator of the behaviourally excitant effects of brain 5-HT and 5-methoxy-N,N-dimethyltryptamine, or it may act as a regulating factor of the neuronal changes produced by these two compounds.

Cycloheximide is known to have many debilitating side effects which accompany its blocking action on protein synthesis. Among these are the production of severe metabolic acidosis, hypotension, gastrointestinal haemorrhage, vomiting, diarrhoea, and changes in plasma and cellular enzyme levels (YOUNG et al. 1963; YOUNG and DOWLING 1975; CH'IH et al. 1976; STITT 1980). In view of these toxic effects and the inability of cycloheximide-treated rats and rabbits to maintain a steady body temperature (BARNEY et al. 1979; STITT 1980), it is difficult to be certain that this protein synthesis inhibitor blocks pyrogen-induced fever by a specific action of the formation of a protein mediator of fever.

Recently, CRANSTON et al. (1981) reported on the effects of centrally administered cycloheximide on fever in rabbits. A 40-µg dose of cycloheximide injected into the cerebral ventricles was found to reduce the incorporation of radioactive leucine into hypothalamic protein by 94%. The same dose caused only a 25% reduction of the febrile response to i.c.v. endogenous pyrogen. The authors have in-

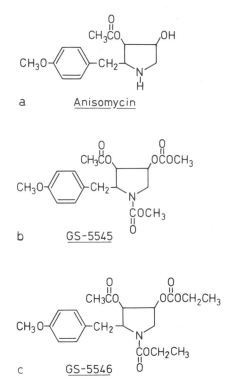

a   Anisomycin

b   GS-5545

c   GS-5546

Fig. 3 a–c. Structure of anisomycin (**a**) and of the inactive analogues Pfizer GS-5545 (**b**) and GS 5546 (**c**)

terpreted these results as indicating that the production of fever requires central protein synthesis. However, it could also be argued that these results, together with those reported by SIEGERT et al. (1976), indicate that there is no correlation between the degree of inhibition of protein synthesis in the brain and the attenuation of fever.

MYERS and RUWE (1980) studied the effects on fever in cats of a less toxic protein synthesis inhibitor, anisomycin (Fig. 3 a). Anisomycin is a highly effective inhibitor of eukaryotic protein synthesis (GROLLMAN and WALSH 1967) and is reported to be remarkably free of neuronal side effects (such as on action potentials and synaptic potentials) in *Aplysia* nervous tissue (SCHWARTZ et al. 1971). The mechanism of action of protein synthesis inhibition by anisomycin differs from that of cycloheximide. Anisomycin inhibits peptide bond formation, possibly by inhibiting the enzyme peptidyl transferase, whereas cycloheximide blocks translocation on the ribosomes but does not directly affect peptide bond formation (PESTKA 1971). The effects of anisomycin on protein synthesis are completely reversible and its duration of action is shortlived (PESTKA 1971; RUWE and MYERS 1979). RUWE and MYERS (1979) and MYERS and RUWE (1980) have reported that the systemic injection of anisomycin in conscious cats either completely inhibits or significantly delays the fevers produced by the subsequent intravenous and intrahypothalamic injections of typhoid vaccine. In addition, with the aim of determining whether the inhibition of protein synthesis within the hypothalamus attenuates pyrogen fever, RUWE and MYERS (1979) gave low doses of anisomycin bilaterally directly into the tissue of the PO/AH. The febrile response to the subsequent administration of endotoxin into the same loci was entirely abolished. It was not determined whether or not the inhibition of fever with the very low dose of anisomycin injected centrally was really due to a central action of this compound.

RUWE and MYERS (1979, 1980) have also investigated the effects of systemically and centrally administered anisomycin on the responses to intrahypothalamic PGE_2 and the monoamines in the cat. It was reported that systemically administered anisomycin does not modify the behavioural, autonomic, and hyperthermic responses to PGE_2, although a close examination of the trace shown by RUWE and MYERS (1980) appears to show an approximately 50% reduction of the hyperthermic response over the 2-h period following administration of the PGE_2. The hyperthermic response to 5-HT and the hypothermic responses to noradrenaline (NA) and dopamine (DA) were found to be unaffected by anisomycin pretreatment.

In our laboratory we have assessed the effects of systemically administered anisomycin on the febrile responses of cats to the i.c.v. administration of *Shigella dysenteriae* endotoxin and PGE_2 at a variety of ambient temperatures (MILTON and SAWHNEY 1981). The dose of anisomycin (15 mg/kg s.c.) used in our studies and the time interval (0.5 h) chosen for the administration of the protein synthesis inhibitor and the pyrogenic agent always greatly diminished the febrile responses to intravenous pyrogen. Similar doses of anisomycin when given subcutaneously to mice have been reported to cause approximately 80%–90% inhibition of brain protein synthesis during the first 2 h following its administration (FLOOD et al. 1974). At all environmental temperatures studied, anisomycin significantly attenuated the hyperthermic responses to PGE_2 as recorded by thermal response indices (TRI) (MILTON and WENDLANDT 1971) measured over a period of 2 h. In addition we found that the time course of action of anisomycin was a very important factor as the responses to i.c.v. bacterial pyrogen were attenuated only when anisomycin was injected 90 min after the pyrogen, i.e. just before the onset of the pyrogen hyperthermia. In experiments where the same dose of anisomycin had been injected before the pyrogen, the febrile response was not significantly altered.

To elucidate further the mechanism by which anisomycin inhibits fever produced by intravenous endotoxin, we have measured by radioimmunoassay, the CSF PGE_2 levels of cats treated with anisomycin (15 mg/kg s.c.) and bacterial pyrogen (*Shigella dysenteriae*, 2 μg/kg i.v.) (MILTON and SAWHNEY, unpublished work). Our results indicated that PGE_2 levels were still elevated after pyrogen injections even though the febrile responses were significantly attenuated. This finding that PGE_2 levels still increase in animals injected with anisomycin and pyrogen is consistent with the observations made by SIEGERT et al. (1976) in their studies with cycloheximide and pyrogen in the rabbit. It is also consistent with our own previous observation that anisomycin significantly reduces the hyperthermic effect of PGE_2 (MILTON and SAWHNEY 1981). Together, these results suggest that anisomycin may be acting at a site after PGE_2 in the pathway to fever.

RUWE and MYERS (1980) also reported that the thermoregulatory capacity of cats exposed to cold (10 °C) and warm (34 °C) environmental temperatures for a period of 1 h was unaffected by the subcutaneous administration of anisomycin.

The authors concluded that it is unlikely that anisomycin interferes with pyrogen fever by altering the monoamine receptor protein involved in the heat production pathway in the anterior hypothalamus. Instead they envisaged that an unknown protein factor within the preoptic anterior hypothalamus constitutes a link in the fever production pathway and acts either to affect the cellular mechanism involved in the synthesis or release of a hyperthermic substance, or to directly affect the receptors of neurones responsible for heat production. Unless a hyperthermic substance other than PGE_2 is involved, our results favour the latter mechanism of action.

Cranston et al. (1980 b) have shown that the intraventricular administration of anisomycin does not interfere with the thermoregulatory capacity of rabbits placed in a cold environment (9 °C), although the same dose does attenuate the febrile responses to endogenous pyrogen given either into the cerebral ventricles or intravenously. The dose of anisomycin used in these experiments was shown to cause an approximately 95% reduction in the incorporation of $[^{14}C]$ leucine into hypothalamic protein. In a short account of these experiments Cranston et al. (1980 a) had already demonstrated that the attenuation of fever by anisomycin was due to a central action, as the same dose of anisomycin when given intravenously did not affect the febrile response to intravenous endogenous pyrogen. Cranston et al. (1980 b) concluded that pyrogen fever may involve a step dependent on the synthesis of a hypothalamic protein with a rapid turnover.

By studying the febrile response of protein-deficient rabbits to *Pasturella multocida*, a Gram-negative bacteria pathogenic to rabbits, Hoffman-Goetz and Kluger (1979) have found that the first phase of the fever was completely abolished and instead the animals developed a hypothermia which lasted for 6–8 h. The second phase of the fever was also attenuated in the protein-deprived animals. Both protein-deprived and normal rabbits, however, responded to endogenous pyrogen with fevers of equal magnitude, and the authors suggested that the diminished febrile response to bacterial infection in the protein-deprived animals was due to an impairment in the synthesis or release, or both, of endogenous pyrogen. These results therefore seem to imply that just the first phase of a normal biphasic febrile response to bacterial pyrogen is dependent on the production of endogenous pyrogen.

The finding by Hoffman-Goetz and Kluger (1979) that protein-deficient rabbits exhibit undiminished fevers to the administration of endogenous pyrogen is in conflict with the numerous reports where protein synthesis inhibitors have been shown to attenuate endogenous pyrogen fever (Siegert et al. 1976; Cranston et al. 1978, 1980 b; Ruwe and Myers 1980; Milton and Sawhney 1980 b). Although the studies with anisomycin have indicated that the inhibition of fever with this compound correlates closely with its effect of inhibiting protein synthesis within the brain, the possibility still remains that some other pharmacological action of anisomycin, distinct from its effect on protein synthesis, may have been responsible for the observed inhibition of fever.

In the absence of a protein synthesis inhibitor relatively free of side effects on other bodily functions, it is difficult to determine with certainty whether or not the inhibition of fever seen with the available protein synthesis inhibitors is due specifically to an effect on a protein mediator of fever. To help in answering this question of specificity, we have recently been testing analogues of anisomycin which are relatively inactive as inhibitors of protein synthesis (Dr. Belcher, Pfizer, USA, personal communication). The two analogues GS-5545 and G 5-5546, the structures of which are shown in Fig. 3 b and c, were found to produce similar toxic effects to those produced by anisomycin in some of the cats. However, when administered in a similar dose to that of anisomycin, neither GS-5545 nor GS-5546 attenuated the febrile response or the rise in the PGE_2 levels in the CSF of cats subsequently injected with *Shigella dysenteriae* endotoxin intravenously (MILTON and SAWHNEY unublished work). These results with the analogues therefore appear to strengthen the idea that the inhibition of fever by anisomycin is due specifically to its effects to inhibit protein synthesis.

Both anisomycin and cycloheximide have been reported to have effects on central catecholamine-containing neurones. For example, FLEXNER et al. (1973) and SQUIRE et al. (1974) reported on the in vitro inhibition of brain tyrosine hydroxylase by cycloheximide, and similar findings have also been reported for anisomycin (SQUIRE et al. 1974; LUNDGREN and CARR 1978). Both protein synthesis inhibitors were found to increase the endogenous levels of tyrosine in the brain, probably as a result of a reduction of the incorporation of tyrosine into proteins. A decrease in NA synthesis could contribute to the hypothermia after cycloheximide in rabbits (FELDBERG and SAXENA 1971; CRANSTON et al. 1972) and indeed, the depletion of NA with α-methyltyrosine has been reported to attenuate the febrile response in rabbits (GIARMAN et al. 1968; TEDDY 1969).

C. Conclusions

In spite of the evidence that has accumulated to implicate a protein mediator and many other substances in the pathogenesis of fever, the exact sequence of events leading to the raised body temperature following the administration of a pyrogen is still uncertain. Since the original reports by SIEGERT et al. in 1975 and 1976, in which the existence of a protein mediator of fever was first postulated, numerous papers have appeared in the literature which have provided evidence both for and against this hypothesis. However, it still remains uncertain whether the inhibition of fever seen with cycloheximide is due to a specific action of this inhibitor on a putative protein mediator of fever, or due to some other non-specific toxic effect of the compound. The experiments with anisomycin have perhaps provided more convincing evidence to favour a role for an unknown protein factor in the genesis of fever. The data so far available suggest that anisomycin may be acting at a site after PGE_2 in the neurochemical pathway to fever, perhaps at receptors within the preoptic anterior hypothalamus which are involved in the production of heat.

References

Angel C, Burkett ML (1971) Effects of hydrocortisone and cycloheximide on blood-brain barrier function in the rat. Dis Nerv Syst 32:53–58

Atkins E (1960) Pathogenesis of fever. Physiol Rev 40:580–646

Atkins E, Bodel PT (1971) The role of leucocytes in fever. In: Westenholme GEW, Birch
   J (eds) Pyrogens and fever. Churchill Livingstone, Edinburgh London
Barney CA, Katovich MJ, Fregly MJ (1979) Effect of cycloheximide on temperature regu-
   lation in rats. Brain Res Bull 4:355–358
Beleslin DB, Samardžić R (1975) Inhibitors of protein synthesis and the central regulation
   of body temperature. Neuropharmacology 14:151–153
Bligh J (1973) Temperature regulation in mammals and other vertebrates. Elsevier, Amsterdam New York
Ch'ih JJ, Olszyna DM, Devlin TM (1976) Alteration in plasma and cellular enzyme and protein levels after lethal and non-lethal doses of cycloheximide in the rat. Biochem Pharmacol 25:2407–2408
Cranston WI, Hellon RF, Luff RH, Rawlins MD (1972) Hypothalamic endogenous noradrenaline and thermoregulation in the cat and rabbit. J Physiol (Lond) 223:59–67
Cranston WI, Dawson NJ, Hellon RF, Townsend Y (1978) Contrasting actions of cycloheximide on fever caused by arachidonic acid and by pyrogen. J Physiol (Lond) 285:35 P
Cranston WI, Hellon RF, Luff RH, Townsend Y (1980 a) Intracranial protein synthesis and
   the genesis of fever. J Physiol (Lond) 300:44 P
Cranston WI, Hellon RF, Townsend Y (1980 b) Suppression of fever in rabbits by a protein
   synthesis inhibitor, anisomycin. J Physiol (Lond) 305:337–344
Cranston W, Gourine VN, Townsend Y (1981) The effects of intracerebroventricular cycloheximide on protein synthesis and fever in rabbits. Br J Pharmacol 73:6–8
Davis HP, Rosenzweig MR, Bennett EL, Squire LR (1980) Inhibition of cerebral protein
   synthesis: dissociation of non-specific effects and amnesic effects. Behav Neural Biol
   28:99–104
Feldberg W, Saxena PN (1971) Effects of adrenoceptor blocking agents on body tempera-
   ture. Br J Pharmacol 43:543–554
Flexner LB, Serota RG, Goodman RH (1973) Cycloheximide and acetoxycycloheximide:
   inhibition of tyrosine hydroxylase activity and amnesic effects. Proc Nat Acad Sci USA
   70:354–356
Flood JF, Rosenzweig MR, Bennett EL, Orme AE (1974) Comparison of the effects of anisomycin on memory across six strains of mice. Behav Biol 10:147–160
Giarman NJ, Tanaka C, Mooney J, Atkins E (1968) Serotonin, norepinephrine and fever.
   Adv Pharmacol 6 A:307–317
Grahame-Smith DG (1972) The prevention by inhibitors of brain protein synthesis of the
   hyperactivity and hyperpyrexia produced in rats by monoamine oxidase inhibitor and
   the administration of L-tryptophan or 5-methoxy-N,N-dimethyltryptamine. J Neurochem 19:2409–2422
Grollman AP (1966) Structural basis for inhibition of protein synthesis by emetine and
   cycloheximide based on an analogy between ipecac alkaloids and glutarimide antibiotics. Proc Nat Acad Sci USA 56:1867–1874
Grollman AP, Walsh M (1967) Inhibitors of protein biosynthesis. II. Mode of action of anisomycin. J Biol Chem 242(13):3226–3233
Harvey CA, Milton AS, Straughan DW (1975) Prostaglandin E levels in cerebrospinal fluid
   of rabbits and the effects of bacterial pyrogen and antipyretic drugs. J Physiol (Lond)
   248:26–27 P
Hellon RF, Cranston WI, Townsend Y, Mitchell D, Dawson NJ, Duff GW (1980) Some
   tests of the prostaglandin hypothesis of fever. In: Lipton JM (ed) Fever. Raven, New
   York, pp 159–164
Hoffman-Goetz L, Kluger MJ (1979) Protein deprivation: its effects on fever and plasma
   iron during bacterial infection in rabbits. J Physiol (Lond) 295:419–430
Lundgren P, Carr A (1978) Effects of anisomycin and CNS stimulants on brain catechol-
   amine synthesis. Pharmacol Biochem Behav 9:559–561
Milton AS (1976) Modern views on the pathogenesis of fever and the mode of action of anti-
   pyretic drugs. J Pharm Pharmacol 28:393–399
Milton AS, Sawhney VK (1980 a) Dissimilar effects of cycloheximide on the febrile responses to the intravenous and intracerebrorentricular administration of various pyrogens.
   Br J Pharmacol 70:97 P

Milton AS, Sawhney VK (1980 b) The effects of a protein synthesis inhibitor on the thermoregulatory responses to bacterial pyrogen, endogenous pyrogen and to prostaglandin E_2. In: Szelényi Z, Székely M (eds) Advances in physiological sciences. Contributions to thermal physiology. Akademiai Kiodo, Budapest, pp 165–167

Milton AS, Sawhney VK (1981) The effects of anisomycin on the febrile responses to intracerebroventricular bacterial pyrogen and prostaglandin E_2 in cats. Br J Pharmacol 74:786 P

Milton AS, Todd D (1981) The effects of cycloheximide on endogenous pyrogen fever. Br J Pharmacol 72:543 P

Milton AS, Wendlandt S (1971) Effects on body temperature of prostaglandins of the A, E and F series on injection into the third ventricle of unanaesthetized cats and rabbits. J Physiol (Lond) 218:325–336

Myers RD, Ruwe WD (1980) Fever: intermediary neurohumoral factors serving the hypothalamic mechanism underlying hypothermia. In: Lipton JM (ed) Fever. Raven, New York, pp 99–110

Pestka S (1971) Inhibitors of ribosome functions. Annu Rev Microbiol 25:487–562

Pong SS, Hong SL, Levine L (1977) Prostaglandin production by methylcholanthrene-transformed mouse BALB/3 T 3. J Biol Chem 252(4):1408–1413

Ruwe WD, Myers RD (1979) Fever produced by intrahypothalamic pyrogen: effect of protein synthesis inhibition by anisomycin. Brain Res Bull 4:741–745

Ruwe WD, Myers RD (1980) The role of protein synthesis in the hypothalamic mechanism mediating pyrogen fever. Brain Res Bull 5:735–743

Schwartz J, Castellucci V, Kandel E (1971) Functioning of identified neurones and synapses in abnormal ganglion of *Aplysia* in absence of protein synthesis. J Neurophysiol 34:939–953

Siegert R, Philipp-Dormston WK, Radsak K, Menzel H (1975) Inhibition of Newcastle Disease Virus-induced fever in rabbits by cycloheximide. Arch Virol 48:367–373

Siegert R, Philipp-Dormston WK, Radsak K, Menzel H (1976) Mechanism of fever induction in rabbits. Infect Immun 14:1130–1137

Squire LR, Barondes SH (1974) Anisomycin, like other inhibitors of cerebral protein synthesis, impairs "long-term" memory of a discrimination task. Brain Res 66:301–308

Squire LR, Kuczenski R, Barondes SH (1974) Tyrosine hydroxylase inhibition by cycloheximide and anisomycin is not responsible for their amnesic effect. Brain Res 82:241–248

Stitt JJ (1980) The effect of cycloheximide on temperature regulation and fever production in the rabbit. In: Cox B, Lomax P, Milton AS, Schönbaum E (eds) Thermoregulatory mechanisms and their therapeutic implications. Karger, Basel New York London, pp 120–125

Teddy PJ (1969) The effects of alterations in hypothalamic monoamine content on fever in the rabbit. J Physiol (Lond) 204:140–141 P

Young CW, Dowling MD Jr (1975) Antipyretic effect of cycloheximide, an inhibitor of protein synthesis, in patients with Hodgkin's disease or other malignant neoplasms. Cancer Res 35:1218–1224

Young CW, Robinson PF, Sactor B (1963) Inhibition of the synthesis of protein in intact animals by acetoxycycloheximide and a metabolic derangement concomitant with this blockade. Biochem Pharmacol 12:855–865

CHAPTER 12

The Chemistry of the Non-Steroidal Antipyretic Agents: Structure-Activity Relationships

D. H. KIM, C. G. VAN ARMAN, and D. ARMSTRONG

A. Introduction

For a long time human fever has been considered to be a result of an alteration in the body's thermostat in the hypothalamus, in response to a variety of pyrogenic factors such as bacteria, viruses and fungi. Inflammation, caused by whatever means, has also been thought to cause similar alterations of the thermostat, resulting in fever (FELDBERG and MILTON 1979). These febrile responses have been considered to be a defence mechanism of the body against such foreign invaders.

MILTON and WENDLANDT in 1970 observed that injection of minute doses of prostaglandin E_1 (PGE_1) into the third ventricle of cats caused fever. They speculated that PGE_1 may act as a modulator in temperature regulation, and that the fever-lowering action of antipyretics may be due to their ability to inhibit the release of PGE_1 in the body.

In the following year, VANE demonstrated that aspirin-like drugs inhibit the synthesis of PG's in guinea-pig lung, and suggested that the antipyretic effect of aspirin (acetylsalicylic acid) is caused by its prevention of synthesis rather than by prevention of release (VANE 1971). Subsequently, FELDBERG and GUPTA (1973) and PHILLIP-DORMSTON and SIEGERT (1974) showed that PGE levels in the cerebrospinal fluid of cats and rabbits rose very significantly during pyrogenic fever and FELDBERG et al. (1973) and HARVEY et al. (1975) showed that the elevated PGE levels in the cerebrospinal fluid decreased when antipyretics were given. Since then, many reports have appeared supporting the theory that PGE_1 functions as a mediator of fever in the body (FELDBERG and MILTON 1979).

Pyrogen accelerates the synthesis and subsequent release of prostaglandins, and antipyretics bring the fever down by inhibition of prostaglandin synthesis. Such an explanation was originally proposed by VANE (1971) for anti-inflammatory and analgesic effects of aspirin-like drugs. The site of such pyretic action of PGE_1 was considered to be the preoptic/anterior hypothalamic region of the brain (VEALE and COOPER 1974). Inflammation caused by prostaglandins is, however, a local reaction. Although the prostaglandin theory of fever mediation was accepted with enthusiasm when first proposed, subsequently there appeared several reports showing evidence against such an explanation (PITTMAN et al. 1975; VEALE and COOPER 1975; CRANSTON et al. 1975, 1976).

An alternative explanation for the antipyretic action involves a competitive inhibition of the agonistic action of pyrogen at pyretic receptor sites by the antipyretic agent. In 1968, WIT and WANG, later supported by CRANSTON et al. (1971 a), CRANSTON and RAWLINS (1972) and LIN and CHAI (1972), first suggested that aspirin may compete with pyrogens at some specific receptors in the preoptic/ anterior hypothalamic region in effecting the antipyretic action. Probably the strongest evidence in support of the receptor theory is the finding of CLARK and COLDWELL (1972) that sodium salicylate and acetaminophen given in cats intraventricularly, 30 min before an intravenous (i.v.) injection of leukocytic pyrogen, caused parallel shifts to the right of the dose–response curve for the pyrogen. A similar shift was also observed with intravenously administered indomethacin (CLARK and CUMBY 1975). CLARK (1979) pointed out that although parallel shifts are consistent with competition between the pyrogen and antipyretics for receptors, they do not necessarily rule out competition at a step subsequent to pyrogen–receptor binding. Furthermore, SCHOENER and WANG (1975) observed that there was an alteration in the neuronal activity caused by pyrogen injected into one side of the anterior hypothalamus when aspirin was injected into the opposite side; the finding indicated that the antipyresis produced by aspirin was not necessarily due to competition with leukocytic pyrogen for a common receptor site. Apparently much more remains to be learned about antipyretic mechanisms.

B. Receptor Models for Antipyretic and Anti-Inflammatory Actions

Although the receptor models to be described have been proposed mainly for explanation of anti-inflammatory activity, they may also help in the understanding of antipyretic action, and thus in the designing of new antipyretic drugs.

In 1958, ADAMS and COBB reported that the anti-inflammatory activity of salicylates might be related to their capacities to uncouple oxidative phosphorylation. Numerous efforts were then made, especially by WHITEHOUSE and his colleagues, to explain the anti-inflammatory activity in terms of their uncoupling abilities (WHITEHOUSE and HASLAM 1962; WHITEHOUSE 1964) until the prostaglandin theory of VANE emerged in 1971. CRANSTON et al. (1971 b) showed that the antipyretic activity of salicylates was not well correlated with their ability to uncouple oxidative phosphorylation.

Agents such as aspirin and indomethacin that are anti-inflammatory, analgesic, and antipyretic prevent the synthesis of prostaglandins by inhibiting prostaglandin synthetase (fatty acid cyclooxygenase). This enzyme converts arachidonic acid into unstable cyclic endoperoxides, PGG_2 and PGH_2. PGH_2 is a common intermediate for the biosynthesis of a host of prostaglandins including PGE_2 which is considered to be a major causative factor in inflammation (SCHAAF 1977; GIBSON 1977).

In 1964, SCHERRER et al. proposed a hypothetical receptor site model for anti-inflammatory action based on structure–activity relationships of a number of different chemical series of anti-inflammatory compounds. The proposed receptor site is composed of a cationic site which interacts with the anionic centre (carboxylic acid group) of anti-inflammatory agents through ionic bonding, a flat area for the aromatic nucleus and a trough below the flat region. The trough accommodates the aromatic ring situated on the primary aromatic nucleus away from the anionic centre in a twisted antiplanar fashion (Fig. 1).

Almost simultaneously, but independently, SHEN proposed a similar receptor for the anti-inflammatory action of indomethacin after studying the structure–ac-

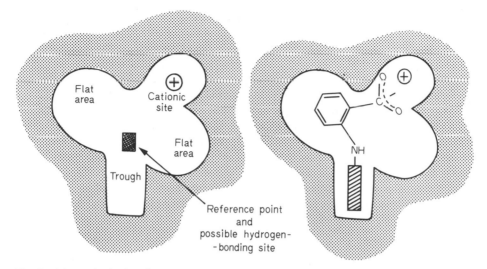

Fig. 1. A hypothetical anti-UV erythema receptor site model and its interaction with a fenamic acid, an anti-inflammatory agent. (SCHERRER et al. 1964)

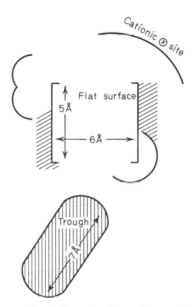

Fig. 2. "Receptor site" contour for indomethacin analogues. (SHEN 1965)

tivity relationship and the preferred configuration of indomethacin and related indoleacetic acids (SHEN 1965, 1967a). The main difference between the two receptor sites is the orientation of the through which accomodates the secondary aromatic ring. On the basis of the observation that the *cis*-indene analogue of indomethacin has higher anti-inflammatory activity compared with the *trans*-indene isostere (SHEN 1967b), SHEN proposed that the trough is oriented in opposite direction to the cationic centre (Fig. 2). The *cis*-indene analogue is about one-half as potent as indomethacin while the *trans* isomer is about one-tenth as active (see Sect. D.IV.5). However, OLSON et al. (1974) questioned the validity of SHEN's supporting evidence, saying that one-tenth of the activity of the extremely potent indomethacin still represents good activity, and thus the *trans* isostere still interacts with the receptor site quite well. The importance of the anti-planar conformation of the secondary aromatic ring in the *N*-arylanthranilic acids has also been questioned. WESTBY and BARFKNECHT (1973) observed that antiplanar *N*-(2,3-xylyl)-2-amino-3-toluic acid had the same order of anti-inflammatory activity as planar 5,6-dimethylacridan-4-carboxylic acid in the ultraviolet (UV) erythema assay. Another antiplanar analogue *N*-(2,3,6-trimethylphenyl)anthranilic acid was much more active than either of the two analogues. The authors concluded that factors other than the relative conformation of the aryl rings are more important in controlling anti-inflammatory activity. In an attempt to test the conformational requirement

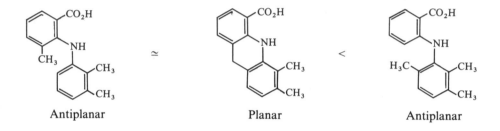

Antiplanar   Planar   Antiplanar

for SHEN's receptor model, OLSON et al. (1974) synthesized 10-chloro-2-methoxy-5-methyl-7H-pyrrolo[3,2,1-*de*]phenanthyrid-7-one-acetic acid as a conformationally rigid analogue of indomethacin. The compound was found to be inactive in the UV erythema assay. The inactivity is not inconsistent with the receptor site proposed by SHEN which requires the phenyl group of the aroyl portion to be antiplanar as well as *cis* with respect to the indole nucleus.

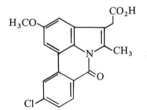

The proposed receptor sites were later presumed to be the active sites of prostaglandin synthetase (SHEN et al. 1974; SCHERRER 1974). SCHERRER suggested that the trough of the active site for an anti-inflammatory agent is the site where the oxygenation and cyclization of arachidonic acid is taking place in prostaglandin synthesis. Prostaglandin E_2 resembles closely the classical non-steroidal anti-inflammatory agents in the conformation as shown in Fig. 3 (SCHERRER 1974). HOYLAND and KIER (1972) using extended Hückel theory also predicted that in the energetically preferred conformer the two side chains are situated in intimately associated almost planar orientation.

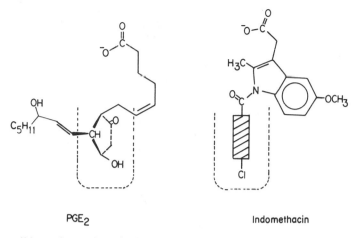

Fig. 3. A possible conformation of PGE$_2$ compared with indomethacin at the prostaglandin synthetase anti-inflammatory receptor (absolute configuration) (SCHERRER 1974)

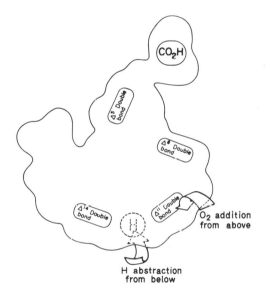

Fig. 4. Model of the fatty acid substrate binding site of prostaglandin synthetase. (GUND and SHEN 1977)

Further refinements of the proposed receptor site (Fig. 4) have been made by GUND and SHEN (1977). On the basis of conformational analysis of anti-inflammatory arylacetic acids, they put forward a detailed model for the active site of cyclooxygenase. As in the previous models, a carboxy binding centre is located adjacent to a broad hydrophobic binding region. Next to the hydrophobic region but away from the carboxylic centre, there is a hydrophobic groove which accommodates a part of the substrate. A π-electron acceptor site interacts with the Δ^8, Δ^{11}, and/or Δ^{14} double bonds from below. Hydrogen atom abstraction occurs stereo-

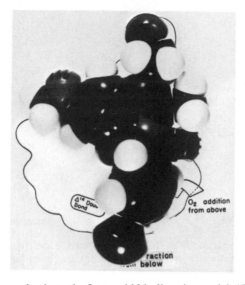

Fig. 5. Binding of indomethacin to the fatty acid binding site model. (GUND and SHEN 1977)

specifically from below. In the enzymatic oxidation of arachidonic acid, the addition of oxygen occurs from above. The binding of indomethacin to the receptor site is shown in Fig. 5.

C. Antipyretic Assay Methods

It is common practice in the pharmaceutical industry to screen large numbers of compounds first for effects against inflammation and pain, and of those found effective, usually only a few are further tested against fever. Methods of assay are fairly similar in many laboratories, and many will be found in the references in this chapter. Several animal species can be used, the most common being the rabbit and the rat. The rabbit is suitable for qualitative screening assays, as for example in testing intravenous solutions for contaminating pyrogens, because it is sensitive (COMMITTEE OF REVISION U.S.P. 1979); but its variability renders it less suitable for quantitative assays than the rat. For quantitative work the rat has less variability (but less sensitivity) than the rabbit (WINTER and NUSS 1963). A good assay method using yeast-induced fever in rats is that of LOUX et al. (1972). A still better method is by WINTER (1965) modified by VAN ARMAN and BOHIDAR (1978), described here:

Sprague–Dawley male rats, 170–190 g, body weight, in groups of six each, are injected subcutaneously with 2 ml of a 7.5% suspension of brewer's yeast in 0.5% methylcellulose solution. A rise in rectal temperature of about 2 °C or more occurs and persists for more than 24 h. It is measured by a rectal sensing probe having a rapid digital display. At 18 h after injection, the temperature is recorded. Test compounds are then given orally, suspended or dissolved in 0.5% methylcellulose. Temperature is recorded every 30 min for 2 h. The mean of the four readings after drug administration is calculated as the lowering of the fever in degrees Celsius. The ED_1 is that dose causing a 1 °C lowering. Note that this is also the dose causing

Table 1. Comparison of several drugs in antipyretic (yeast) and anti-inflammatory (carrageenan) assays in the same laboratory. (VAN ARMAN and BOHIDAR 1978)

Assay	Median effective oral doses (mg/kg)					
	Indo methacin	Sulindac	Di- flunisal	Phenyl- butazone	Aspirin	Thiaben- dazole
A Yeast-induced fever	1.3	2.9	24	24	45	83
B Carrageenan-induced oedema	2.7	5.5	9.8	27.7	89	200
B/A	2.1	1.9	0.4	1.2	2.0	2.4

roughly 50% alleviation of the fever, since the usual fever is 2 °C or somewhat more.

With this method, in 48 groups of six rats each, the dose–response line for indomethacin was $y = 1.63 \log x + 0.81$, in which y is lowering of fever in degrees Celsius and x is dose in mg/kg. The ED_1 was 1.31 mg/kg with 95% confidence limits of 1.23 and 1.39 mg/kg. The lambda value was 0.05, the g value 0.01, the coefficient of variation 11.9%, and $R_2 = 83.6\%$.

It is of interest to compare antipyretic effects in yeast-induced fever with anti-inflammatory effects tested by carrageenan-induced oedema in the same species (rat) in the same laboratory, for several drugs, as shown in Table 1 (VAN ARMAN and BOHIDAR 1978). Seeing the farily constant ratio of effects, one might be tempted to infer that the two different phenomena have similar mechanisms, but such inference would not hold if one considers a wider range of structures. For example, aminopyrine would have a median effective dose (ED_{50}) of 7.5 mg/kg in yeast-induced fever (SHEN and WINTER 1977) and 31 mg/kg in carrageenan-induced oedema (NIEMEGEERS et al. 1964), giving a ratio of 4.1; other examples such as steroids can be found yielding very high ratios.

D. Structure–Activity Relationships

I. Enolic Acids

Quinine is a major alkaloid of *Cinchona* bark. In the middle of the last century, it was the most popularly used antipyretic drug. It was and is especially important in controlling the fever of malaria. The *Cinchona* tree was limited to certain regions, mainly in the tropics, and, especially as the demand for the drug increased, the bark was expensive. Moreover, quinine has severe toxic side effects. Thus, in the late nineteenth century, a chemical search began for more efficient and readily available antipyretic agents. The search was naturally aimed at the synthesis of compounds with chemical structures similar to that of quinine.

KNORR found in 1884 a potent antipyretic compound which he named antipyrine. He thought mistakenly that it was a derivative of quinoline, and assigned dimethoxychinizin for the structure (KNORR 1883, 1884). However, he soon realized that the compound was not a quinoline derivative but a pyrazolone. Its analgesic activity was soon observed. Antipyrine was widely used, mainly as an analgesic, until, several decades later, its severe toxic effects were discovered. Over a thousand pyrazole derivatives were synthesized and tested for antipyretic activity, but occasionally also for analgesic effect. Aminopyrine (amidopyrine), which bears a dimethylamino group at the 4 position of antipyrine, was subsequently discovered to have potent antipyretic and analgesic activities. Although many related pyrazole derivatives have enjoyed sporadic popularity, only antipyrine and aminopyrine lasted in medical use until the 1970 s. These agents are no longer in therapeutic use because of their severe side effects, but they paved the way for the development of modern therapeutic agents in the control of inflammation, mild pain, and fever.

Continued search for improved analgesic–antipyretic drugs through molecular modification of antipyrine eventually led to the discovery of phenylbutazone, which was first synthesized in 1946 by STENZL (1950). It is one of the most widely

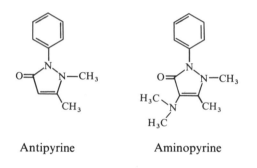

Antipyrine   Aminopyrine

used anti-inflammatory agents nowadays, and certainly one of the best in the pyrazole series. The antipyretic potency of phenylbutazone was less than that of antipyrine, but the effect was maintained unchanged over 2.5 h, whereas the effect of aminopyrine dropped off in 60–90 min (DOMENJOZ 1960). DOMENJOZ showed that oxyphenbutazone, a metabolite of phenylbutazone, had considerably greater

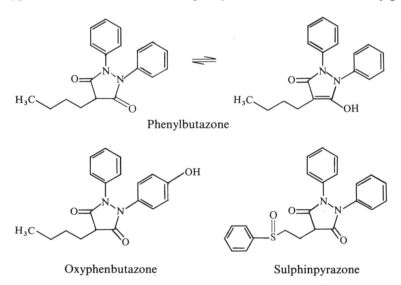

Phenylbutazone

Oxyphenbutazone   Sulphinpyrazone

antipyretic potency and duration of action than phenylbutazone, and equal to those of antipyrine in yeast-induced fever in rats. Sulphinpyrazone showed no antipyretic activity.

In phenylbutazone and related compounds, only minor variation in the structure could be made with retention of antipyretic and analgesic activity. In general, replacement of the butyl side chain or the phenyl rings with other functional groups resulted in a loss of both activities. The presence of enolizable hydrogen at the 4 position is essential for the biological activities, because the replacement of the proton with other groups such as alkyl or preparation of the enol ether caused loss of the activity. The carbocyclic analogue obtained by replacing both nitrogen atoms of phenylbutazone with carbon atoms was ineffective in inhibiting ultraviolet-induced erythema (BAVIN et al. 1955).

The pK_a values of phenylbutazone and related compounds with anti-inflammatory activity lie in the range 3.5–6.5. A much higher pK_a which one may assume for the carbocyclic analogue of phenylbutazone would explain its lack of activity. An excellent review on the structure–anti-inflammatory activity relationships for the pyrazolidinedione series has appeared (LOMBARDINO 1974).

CASADIO et al. (1972) obtained 4-prenyl-1,2-diphenyl-3,5-pyrazolidinedione (prenazone), an anti-inflammatory agent with a low ulcerogenic effect. It was obtained by converging the anti-inflammatory property of phenylbutazone with the anti-ulcer activity of some terpene compounds. The compound was almost equipotent with phenylbutazone in most of the standard animal assays for anti-inflammatory and analgesic activities. However, in the anti-UV-erythema test, prenazone was much less active than phenylbutazone. As an inhibitor of yeast-induced fever, prenazone was slightly less active than phenylbutazone in rats, but in mice it was equally active (BIANCHI et al. 1972).

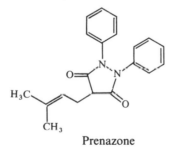

Prenazone

The pharmacological properties as well as the pK_a values of these compounds remained unchanged by the insertion of a carbonyl group between the two nitro-

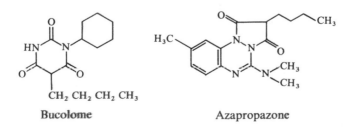

Bucolome   Azapropazone

gens in the pyrazolinediones, e.g. bucolome, which is a therapeutically effective anti-inflammatory agent (SENDA et al. 1967).

Azapropazone is a therapeutically useful non-steroidal anti-inflammatory analgesic agent which may be considered to be a pyrazolidinedione fused to a benzotriazine ring. The anti-inflammatory potency was approximately one-half that of phenylbutazone, and the antipyretic potency tested by the yeast-induced fever method was approximately one-quarter that of phenylbutazone (JONES 1976).

An anti-inflammatory agent studied in Japan, 1-phenyl-sulphonyl-5,5-diphenylhydantoin (PC-796), showed a more potent inhibitory effect on carrageenan-induced oedema in mice than did phenylbutazone. It was also more potent than phenylbutazone and aspirin against yeast-induced fever in the rat. The analgesic activity was mild. The pK_a was 5.0, close to that of phenylbutazone (NAKAMURA et al. 1970).

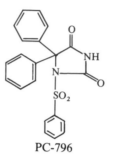

PC-796

In 1969, KADIN and WISEMAN discovered that 1,3-dioxoisoquinoline-4-carboxanilides are orally effective inhibitors of carrageenan-induced rat paw oedema. Some analogues, e.g. the p-chloroanilide of 2-methyl-1,3-dioxoisoquinoline-4-carboxylic acid (I), were as much as three times as potent as phenylbutazone in that assay. The anti-inflammatory potency was retained when the 1-oxo group in the ring of 1,3-dioxoisoquinoline-4-carboxanilide was replaced with a sulphoxide group to form 3,4-dihydro-2-alkyl-3-oxo-2 H-1,2-benzothiazine-4-carboxamide-1,1-dioxide. In this series, compounds such as the p-bromoanilide of 3,4-dihydro-2-methyl-3-oxo-2 H-1,2-benzothiazine-4-carboxylic acid (III) were as much as 1.5 times as potent as indomethacin (LOMBARDINO and WISEMAN 1971). These com-

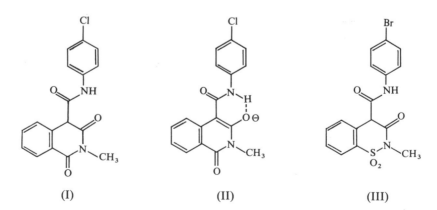

(I)   (II)   (III)

pounds are acids of moderate strength, having pK_a values in the range 4–6 measured in 2:1 dioxane–water. Stabilization of the enolate anion by internal hydrogen bonding with the neighbouring amide proton, as in II, was suggested to explain the enhanced activities.

In a further exploration for novel therapeutically effective anti-inflammatory agents, LOMBARDINO et al. (1971) investigated the 3-carboxamides of 2-alkyl-4-hydroxy-$2H$-1,2-benzothiazine-1,1-dioxide; one of these, 4-hydroxy-2-methyl-3-phenylcarbamoyl-$2H$-1,2-benzothiazine-1,1-dioxide (IV), was twice as potent as phenylbutazone when compared in the rat paw oedema anti-inflammatory test. The acidity of this compound and closely related analogues was in the range 6.4–8.6 on the pK_a scale, measured in 2:1 dioxane–water (LOMBARDINO et al. 1971). However, comparison by others (DiPASQUALE et al. 1973)

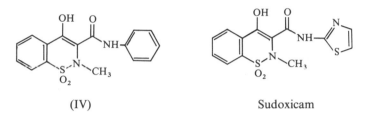

(IV)   Sudoxicam

of this compound with other anti-inflammatory agents indicated that IV had anti-inflammatory and antipyretic activities equivalent to those of phenylbutazone in the carrageenan-induced rat paw oedema, cotton-pellet-induced granuloma, prophylactic and therapeutic adjuvant-induced polyarthritis and yeast-induced fever in rats. Of the numerous analogues of the foregoing compound studied by LOMBARDINO et al., 4-hydroxy-2-methyl-3-(2-thiazoylcarbamoyl)-$2H$-1,2-benzothiazine-1,1-dioxide (sudoxicam) was almost three times more potent than indomethacin in the carrageenan-induced oedema assay, determined by dose–response comparison at four dose levels. The acid strength of sudoxicam (pK_a 5.3) was also increased by 2 pK_a units compared with the corresponding 3-phenylcarbamoyl compound (pK_a 7.3) (LOMBARDINO et al. 1972, 1973).

Dantrolene sodium is a therapeutically effective skeletal muscle relaxant (SNYDER et al. 1967; ELLIS et al. 1973) which is useful for the treatment of muscle spasticity. Recently, HARRISON (1975) demonstrated that this compound is highly effective in terminating and preventing the malignant hyperpyrexia syndrome induced in susceptible swine by exposure to halothane. The intravenous administration of the salt caused rapid loss of muscle rigor, immediate cessation of the increase in deep-muscle temperature followed by a rapid temperature decrease. Lately, dantrolene sodium has been introduced into clinical use in Canada for the treatment of malignant hyperthermic crises.

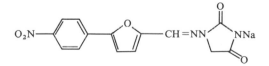

Dantrolene sodium

II. Salicylic Acid and Related Compounds

Although the use of naturally occurring salicylates may be traced back to ancient days, the antipyretic effect of salicylic acid was first recorded in 1763 by STONE who reported the successful treatment of malarial patients with a decoction of the bark of the white willow. It took sixty years until the active principle of the decoction was isolated and characterized as salicylic acid. In 1829, LEROUX isolated salicin in the pure state from willow bark, LÖWIG in 1835 obtained salicylic acid by the oxidation of salicylaldehyde, and PIRIA also obtained salicin in 1838 (review by GROSS and GREENBERG 1948). The demonstration of the antipyretic effect of salicylic acid was reported in 1875 by ZIMMERMANN, who showed that the fever produced by the injection of a putrid liquid into rabbits was reduced by oral administration of this drug.

Aspirin (acetylsalicylic acid) has been the most widely used antipyretic agent for the last eight decades, and still is the most popular drug for the control of not only fever but also arthritis and mild pain including headache. It was first prepared in 1853 by VON GERHARDT, but its therapeutic value had not been appreciated until 1899 when WITTHAUER, WOHLGEMUT and DRESER introduced it to medical practice. It was recommended as a substitute for salicylic acid, which had been in use widely for the treatment of fever and rheumatic disease but caused severe gastrointestinal irritation.

Numerous efforts have been made to improve the therapeutic value of salicylic acid and its acetyl derivative (aspirin) by structural modification. A variety of functional groups has been introduced to the phenyl ring of salicylic acid in the hope of enhancing its antirheumatic and antipyretic potency relative to its side effects. Most of such endeavours, however, have been direct toward improvement of anti-inflammatory and analgesic effects.

In 1958, CLARKE et al. reported a systematic investigation of various hydroxybenzoic acids for their therapeutic action of rheumatic fever. Of the three possible isomers of monohydroxybenzoic acid, only salicylic acid was effective.

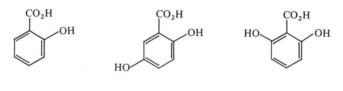

Salicylic acid   Gentisic acid   γ-Resorcylic acid

In the dihydroxybenzoic acid series, MEYER and RAGAN (1948) claimed that gentisic acid was as effective as salicylic acid and less toxic at about the same dose. This claim has been confirmed by others (ORY 1949; TESTONI and STRANO 1950; SCHAEFER et al. 1950). CLARKE et al. (1953), who treated 75 patients with acute rheumatic fever with gentisic acid and derivatives, also reported that sodium gentisate was more effective than sodium salicylate in the treatment of the acute, recurrent, and persistent forms of rheumatic fever. The disadvantage of sodium gentisate was its rapid elimination from the body so that it had to be administered at frequent intervals. REID et al. (1951) tried γ-resorcylic acid in seven rheumatic fever patients; it had about the same therapeutic effect as sodium salicylate at about one-tenth the dose. The effectiveness of γ-resorcylic acid in rheumatic fever patients was also shown by CLARKE et al. (1953), who reported that many manifestations of rheumatic fever were uniformly suppressed within 1–2 days of treatment. Pyro-catechuic acid was also useful in rheumatic fever, arresting the fever in 1–2 days at the dose of one-quarter to one-half the dose of salicylic acid. β-Resorcylic acid suppressed the fever of this disease less effectively than did gentisic acid, and pro-tocatechuic acid was ineffective (CLARKE et al. 1953).

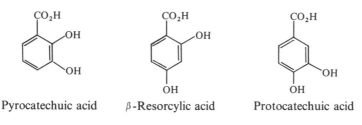

Pyrocatechuic acid   β-Resorcylic acid   Protocatechuic acid

The investigation then turned to two trihydroxybenzoic acids; 2,4,6-trihy-droxybenzoic acid (I) in a trial of 12 patients with rheumatic fever reduced the fever to normal in 6–10 days, and the antirheumatic potency was six to eight times greater than that of salicylic acid. 2,3,6-Trihydroxybenzoic acid (II) was superior to all other hydroxybenzoic acids studied in the treatment of rheumatic fever. The compound was free from side reactions, highly effective in small doses, and suppressed manifestations of severe rheumatic fever. Temperature fell to normal in 1–5 days even in severe forms of the disease (CLARKE et al. 1953).

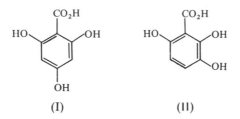

(I)   (II)

Simple substitution on the phenyl ring of salicylic and acetylsalicylic acid did not change the therapeutic profile of the parent compounds. As early as 1876, BUSS claimed that cresotinic acid had an antipyretic property and was effective in rheumatic conditions. The therapeutic value of m-cresotinic acid was reported to be similar to that of salicylic acid (STOCKMAN 1912). Amatin, the acetyl derivate of m-cresotinic acid, was also reported to be antipyretic (DOBNER 1930).

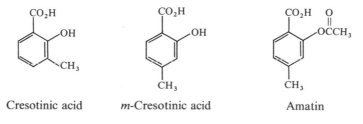

Cresotinic acid   m-Cresotinic acid   Amatin

Several hundred salicylic acid derivatives, most of which were derivatives of 4- and 5-arylsalicylic acids, were synthesized by a research group of the pharmaceutical company Merck, Sharp and Dohme in a project to develop improved salicylates (WALFORD et al. 1971; HANNAH et al. 1970, 1978). However, since their main interest was the analgesic and anti-inflammatory activities, unfortunately the structure–activity relationships with respect to antipyretic activity were not sought. Flufenisal, the first compound in clinical trial in the series, which was later withdrawn, had four to five times the potency of aspirin in the anti-inflammatory assays in rats; the analgesic potency was approximately double, but the fever-reducing potency only one-quarter that of aspirin (HANNAH et al. 1978).

The continued and persistent search was rewarded with the discovery of a better compound, diflunisal, by introduction of a second fluorine atom at the 2 position of the phenyl group. Diflunisal was approximately ten times as potent as aspirin in anti-inflammatory and analgesic activities and was relatively free of the side effect of gastric haemorrhage. However, the antipyretic potency did not improve to the same extent. Diflunisal was only slightly more active (1.4 times) than aspirin in the rat fever test (HANNAH et al. 1978; STONE et al. 1977). In the series of 4- and 5-heteroarylsalicylic acids, improvements over aspirin were observed in the anti-inflammatory and analgesic properties, but again the antipyretic activities of these compounds were disappointing. For example, 5-(N-pyrryl)salicylic acid (III) was more potent than aspirin, with less gastric toxicity in anti-inflammatory and analgesic tests, but it lacked the antipyretic potency of aspirin (JONES et al. 1978).

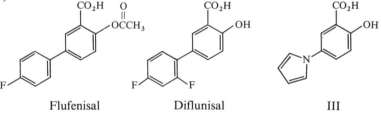

Flufenisal   Diflunisal   III

Fendosal (HP 129) possesses anti-inflammatory activity 1.4 times that of aspirin in carrageenan-induced rat paw oedema, and analgesic activity with longer duration of action. The antipyretic potency of fendosal was, however, only one-third of that of aspirin (LASSMAN et al. 1978).

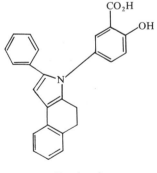

Fendosal

Woo (1963) reported that p-methoxycinnamic acid (IV) which he isolated from *Scrophularia* root showed good antipyretic and analgesic activities. The antipyretic activity was enhanced by combining the acid with known antipyretic agents. For example, *N*-(p-methoxycinnamoyl)-p-aminophenol (V) was twice as potent as aspirin in lowering temperature in rats with yeast-induced fever (LEE et al. 1968). Buu-Hội et al. (1970) found that VI is twice as active as acetylsalicylic acid.

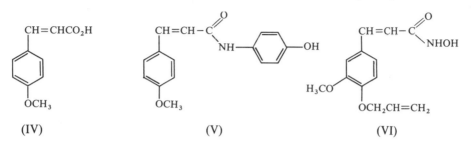

(IV)   (V)   (VI)

4-Hydroxyisophthalic acid (VII) and 2-hydroxyisophthalic acid (VIII) are by-products of the Kolbe–Schmitt process for the manufacture of salicylic acid. Both compounds exhibited antipyretic activity at least as potent as that of aspirin when tested in rabbits rendered febrile by *Proteus* pyrogen (COLLIER and CHESHER 1956).

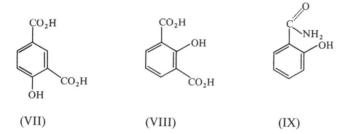

(VII)   (VIII)   (IX)

BAVIN et al. (1952) reported that antipyretic activity of salicylamide (IX) was rapid in onset but short in duration when tested in the yeast-induced fever in rats. In the study, some salicylamide derivatives, notably 2-ethoxysalicylamide, were found to have remarkable antipyretic activity, including a hypothermic effect in normal rats. Nevertheless, they concluded that salicylamide is a poorer anti-pyretic agent than aspirin. BULLER et al. (1957) studied the antipyretic effect of salicylamide on fever induced in the rat by Witte's peptone. Whereas aspirin reduced the fever approximately to normal at a dose of 200 mg/kg, salicylamide failed to reduce the fever at doses ranging from 50 to 300 mg/kg. A clinical study by VIGNEC and GASPARIK (1958) on the antipyretic effectiveness of salicylamide compared with aspirin in infants indicated that both drugs control fever equally well when used at the same dose level; salicylamide, however, has one advantage over aspirin. Because it is a chemically stable compound, the salicylam-ide can be used in a liquid suspension form which is especially important to infants. On the other hand, BOROVSKY (1960) in a careful study carried out with over two hundred infants and children, reported that salicylamide suspension produced only minor antipyretic responses, which were extremely transient. Aspirin generally produced a prompt and sustained antipyretic effect.

Recently, CRANSTON et al. (1971 b) studied several salicylic acid analogues for their antipyretic effects in the central nervous system. The compounds were injected directly into the lateral cerebral ventricle of febrile rabbits. The intraventricular route of administration was chosen in order to eliminate any differences between compounds in the rate of transport across the blood–brain barrier, and to reduce the possible influences of bodily activation, metabolism, and excretion. Only salicylic acid and acetylsalicylic acid (aspirin) produced an effect; the others did not, namely 2,4-dinitrophenol, sodium benzoate, salicylamide, 3-hydroxybenzoic acid, 4-hydroxybenzoic acid, and 5-hydroxybenzoic acid.

III. N-Arylanthranilic Acids

Since the first report on mefenamic acid by WINDER et al. in 1962, a large number of *N*-arylanthranilic acids and their derivatives have been screened for anti-inflammatory and analgesic activity and several have reached the market as therapeutic agents in the control of pain and inflammation. Mefenamic acid had one-half the potency of phenylbutazone in the UV erythema assay in guinea-pigs, but its antipyretic activity was equivalent to that of phenylbutazone. The relative antipyretic potencies in yeast-induced fever in the rat of several of the most potent anti-inflammatory *N*-arylanthranilic acids are shown below with their chemical structures. In this comparative study, the antipyretic activities were compared with that of phenylbutazone which scored 10 in comparison with 33–67 for indomethacin (WINDER et al. 1967). In a clinical trial with 71 children between 3 months and 15 years of age, the antipyretic potency of mefenamic acid was 2.5 times that of aspirin (SIMILÄ et al. 1977).

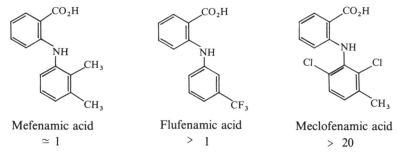

Mefenamic acid	Flufenamic acid	Meclofenamic acid
≃ 1	> 1	> 20

The pyridine derivative, clonixin, was also shown to have antipyretic activity slightly better than that of aspirin in the yeast-induced fever rat test. It had anti-inflammatory activity greater than that of aspirin, and approximately equal to those of phenylbutazone and flufenamic acid (WATNICK et al. 1971).

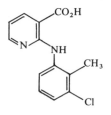

Clonixin

IV. Aryl- and Heteroarylalkanoic Acids and Related Compounds

1. Substituted Arylalkanoic Acids

In the early 1960s it was discovered that 4-t-butylphenylacetic acid (RD 10335) had potent anti-inflammatory, analgesic, and antipyretic activities (BOOTS PURE DRUG COMPANY 1967). The anti-inflammatory potency against UV erythema and analgesic potency against pressure-induced pain were four times those of aspirin; and against yeast-induced fever the antipyretic potency was two to four times that of aspirin. It was subsequently tried in rheumatic patients with remarkable results. However, a significant proportion of patients developed a skin rash, and the compound was withdrawn from the trial (BUCKLER and ADAMS 1968). Although it failed to reach the market, it opened up a new area for anti-inflammatory drug research which has proved very fertile.

The second compound selected by the Boots group for detailed pharmacology and human trial was ibufenac. The anti-inflammatory potency of ibufenac in the guinea-pig UV erythema assay was 2–4 times that of aspirin; the analgesic potency was 3.4 times, and the antipyretic activity 4 times that of aspirin (ADAMS et al. 1963, 1968). The introduction of a methyl group at the α-position to the carboxylic acid group in ibufenac produced ibuprofen, which showed a drastic improvement in the anti-inflammatory activity in animal models. The anti-inflammatory poten-

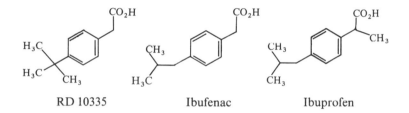

RD 10335   Ibufenac   Ibuprofen

cy of ibuprofen was 16–32 times that of aspirin. Ibuprofen was about 20 times more potent than aspirin in yeast-induced fever in the rat (ADAMS et al. 1967), a five-fold improvement over ibufenac.

Namoxyrate, the dimethylaminoethanol salt of 2-(4-biphenylyl)butyric acid, showed analgesic and antipyretic activities superior to those of aspirin in animal models. In the yeast-treated rat, namoxyrate reduced the fever by 2.3° in 1 h at 60 mg/kg given orally whereas aspirin reduced it by 1.75° in 1 h, at 240 mg/kg. The peak activity of namoxyrate was at 1 h, and that of aspirin between 1 and 3 h (EMELE and SHANAMAN 1967).

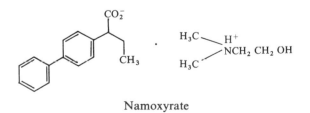

Namoxyrate

The displacement by halogen of a hydrogen atom next to the carboxylic acid group in the arylacetic acids improved the antipyretic activity much more than it did the anti-inflammatory and analgesic activities. Thus, fenclorac was 77 times more potent than aspirin, and more than twice as potent as indomethacin when tested against yeast-induced fever in rats, reducing the rectal temperature even at a dose of 0.11 mg/kg by 0.64°. It did not have a hypothermic effect on normal rats at anti-inflammatory doses as high as 18 mg/kg. The peak antipyretic activity of fenclorac occurred within 1 h after dosing, while peak effects of indomethacin and aspirin occurred after 1 h (Nuss et al. 1976). The anti-inflammatory activity of fenclorac in the carrageenan-induced paw oedema assay in rats, however, was only 13 times that of aspirin, and 0.3 times that of indomethacin. Its analgesic activity was only moderate (Nuss et al. 1976).

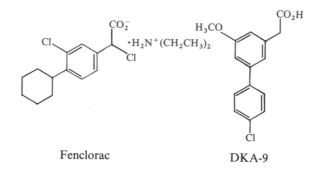

Fenclorac   DKA-9

Tamura et al. (1977) synthesized a series of 5-alkoxy-3-biphenylylacetic acids and related compounds as potential anti-inflammatory agents, among which DKA-9 was chosen for further evaluation. In the antipyretic test using rats with yeast-induced fever, it was more effective than aspirin but less so than ibuprofen. Its anti-inflammatory potency in the adjuvant-induced arthritis assay was approximately 25 times that of ibuprofen (Shibata 1977).

K 4277 is an analgesic–anti-inflammatory agent selected from a large number of 4-[(1-oxo-2-isoindolinyl)phenyl]alkanoic acids and derivatives (Nannini et al. 1973). It was 19 or 20 times more potent than phenylbutazone in inhibiting carrageenan-induced oedema, and in prevention of adjuvant-induced arthritis in the rat. Its analgesic potency in phenylquinone-induced writhing was 95 times that of phenylbutazone, but its antipyretic activity in reducing yeast-induced fever in rats was only 1.6 times that of phenylbutazone (Buttinoni et al. 1973).

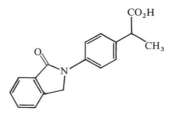

K 4277

The parent aromatic nucleus in the anti-inflammatory arylalkanoic acids may be replaced by an aromatic heterocyclic ring with retention of the biological activities. Fenclozic is an anti-inflammatory agent discovered by the adjuvant-induced arthritis assay by HEPWORTH et al. (1969). The potency of fenclozic in suppressing carrageenan-induced oedema in rats was comparable to that of phenylbutazone. In antipyretic evaluation in the rat, an oral dose of 100 mg/kg, administered immediately before the injection of *Pertussis* pyrogen, completely prevented the increase in body temperature. Lower doses of 50 and 25 mg/kg partially suppressed the temperature rise (NEWBOULD 1969; HEPWORTH et al. 1969).

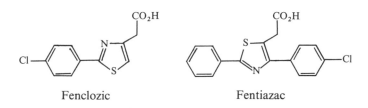

Fenclozic   Fentiazac

BROWN et al. (1974) found that fentiazac was one of the most active anti-inflammatory compounds in a large number of 2,4-diarylthiazole-5-acetic acids and related compounds. Its anti-inflammatory potency was five times more than that of phenylbutazone and comparable to indomethacin; it had analgesic activity slightly greater than that of aspirin (BROWN et al. 1968, 1974; MARMO et al. 1974; DAVIES et al. 1976). The antipyretic activity of fentiazac was greater than those of aspirin, phenylbutazone, and indomethacin, but less than those of mefenamic and flufenamic acids (MARMO et al. 1974).

BUCKLER et al. (1970) studied a series of aryltetrazolylalkanoic acids for anti-inflammatory activity. The most active compound in the series, 3-[5-(3,5-dichlorophenyl)]-2-tetrazolylpropionic acid (I) was 6.2 times as potent as phenylbutazone when tested by the carrageenan-induced abscess model in rats. These compounds were virtually devoid of hypothermic and analgesic activities.

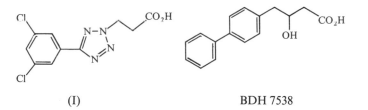

(I)   BDH 7538

BDH 7538 is a long-lasting anti-inflammatory agent, the potency of which is 0.6–0.7 times that of phenylbutazone in various animal models; however, when tested in rats treated with bacterial endotoxin, it was 2.5 times as potent as phenylbutazone (BARRON et al. 1968).

2. Alkyl- or Aryloxyarylalkanoic Acids and Related Compounds

In 1969, BUU-HÖI et al. discovered that 4-aryloxy-3-chlorophenylacetic acid (alclofenac) had pronounced analgesic, antipyretic, and anti-inflammatory properties.

In reducing fever of rabbits made hyperthermic by intravenous injection of anti-gonococcal vaccine, alclofenac was four to five times more potent than aspirin at a dose of 200 mg/kg. Alclofenac in adjuvant-induced polyarthritis of the rat was at least as effective as phenylbutazone. In a clinical trial with 14 patients with various diseases, it decreases the fever markedly (Buu-Hoï et al. 1969; Lambelin et al. 1970).

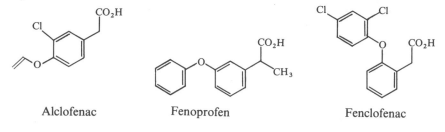

Alclofenac   Fenoprofen   Fenclofenac

Fenoprofen is an analgesic–antipyretic–anti-inflammatory agent structurally related to alclofenac (Nickander et al. 1971). Fenoprofen suppressed significantly the febrile state of patients with chronic disease and associated fever (Gruber 1974), and patients with influenza fever (Gruber and Collins 1972). A series of o-aryloxphenylacetic acids also exhibited the pharmacological properties of non-steroidal anti-inflammatory agents. Of a large number of compounds in this series, fenclofenac was selected for human trial. In the rat with established adjuvant arthritic disease, fenclofenac was more potent than phenylbutazone, but less active in acute anti-inflammatory tests. It reduced pyrogenic fever in rats, and was active in the mouse anti-writhing test (Atkinson et al. 1974). The parent compound, 2-phenoxyphenylacetic acid, was inactive in the adjuvant arthritic assay.

Leo 1028 which has a minimum effective dose of 13 mg/kg in carrageenan-induced rat paw oedema can be considered as a structural variant of alclofenac. However, it did not show any significant antipyretic effect at doses of 32 mg/kg in rats (Rohte 1971).

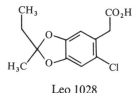

Leo 1028

Buu-Hoï et al. (1966) discovered that many of the alkoxyphenylacethydroxamic acids have anti-inflammatory and analgesic activities. A particularly interesting compound was 4-butoxyphenylacethydroxamic acid, which was effective against carrageenan-induced abscesses, and markedly more so than aspirin as an analgesic. When it was converted into the corresponding carboxamide (II), the anti-inflammatory activity was lost, but the analgesic activity remained unchanged. Further conversion to the corresponding carboxylic acid (III) caused loss of both activities. Both 4-butoxyphenylacethydroxamic acid (I) and 4-butoxphenylacetamide (II) showed antipyretic effects comparable to that of aspirin (Table 2, from Buu-Hoï et al. 1966). The same research group synthesized over two

Table 2. Pharmacological activities of 4-butoxyphenylacetic acid and its derivatives compared with those of aspirin. (From BUU-HÖI et al. 1966; LAMBELIN et al. 1968)

Number	Compounds	Relative potencies in:		
		Anti-inflammatory activity (carrageenan abscess)	Analgesic activity (writhing test)	Antipyretic activity (antigonococcal vaccine)
I	$CH_3CH_2CH_2CH_2O$—⟨ ⟩—CH_2C(=O)—NHOH	1.0	1.0	1.0
II	$CH_3CH_2CH_2CH_2O$—⟨ ⟩—CH_2C(=O)—NH_2	Inactive	1.0	1.0
III	$CH_3CH_2CH_2CH_2O$—⟨ ⟩—CH_2C(=O)—OH	0.3	In active	Not tested
	Aspirin	0.2	0.1	0.8

Table 3. Comparative antipyretic and anti-inflammatory potencies of 4-alkyloxyphenyl-hydroxamic acid and related compounds. (LAMBELIN et al. 1968)

Number	R	R_1	R_2	Relative [a] antipyretic potency ratio	Relative [b] anti-inflammatory potency ratio
I	NHOH	$H_3C(CH_2)_3O$	H	1	1
IV	NHOH	$H_3C(CH_2)_3S$	H	(Not tested)	0
V	NHOH	$H_3C(CH_2)_3O$	CH_3	0.8	1.6
VI	NHOH	$H_3C(CH_2)_3O$	OCH_3	(Not tested)	2.5
VII	NHOH	$H_3C(CH_2)_3O$	Cl	1	0.9
VIII	NHOH	$H_3C(CH_2)_3O$	Br	1	0.6
IX	NHOH	$H_3C(CH_2)_3O$	F	0.5	0.9
X	NHOH	$(H_3C)_3CO$	H	1	0.9
XI	NHOH	$H_3C(CH_2)_2O$	Cl	1.5	0.7
XII	NHOH	$H_2C=CHCH_2O$	H	2	1
XIII	NHOH	$H_2C=CHCH_2O$	Cl	1.7	1
XIV	OH	$H_3C(CH_2)_3O$	H	(Not tested)	0.3
Aspirin				0.8	0.25

[a] In rabbits with antigonococcal-vaccine-induced fever
[b] In carrageenan-induced abscess in rats

hundred compounds related to 4-butoxyphenylacethydroxamic acid, and studied their structure–activity relationships (LAMBELIN et al. 1968). In general, four types of pharmacological activity, i.e. anti-inflammatory, analgesic, antipyretic, and antispasmodic properties were present in variable degrees. Of those compounds prepared, only nine were tested for antipyretic activity in antigonococcal-vaccine-induced fever in rabbits. Table 3 lists the relative antipyretic and anti-inflammatory potencies of the compounds tested. The most potent antipyretic compound in the series was 4-allyloxyphenylacethydroxamic acid (XII), but the highest anti-inflammatory activity was observed with (VI) (Table 3) which was 2.5 times more potent than the parent compound in the carrageenan-induced abscess. The replacement of the oxygen with a sulphur atom eliminated the anti-inflammatory activity completely. The anti-inflammatory activity was also greatly diminished or eliminated by the removal of the hydroxylamine group to form the corresponding carboxamide or carboxylic acid.

3. Indanecarboxylic Acids and Related Compounds

JUBY et al. (1972 a) synthesized a series of indan-1-carboxylic acids and derivatives, and studied their structure–activity relationships for anti-inflammatory activities. The compounds in this series are different from other anti-inflammatory arylalkanoic acids, as the carboxylic acid group is held in an essentially rigid, out-of-plane conformation. The parent compound, indan-1-carboxylic acid, did not show any significant anti-inflammatory activity. A weak activity was, however, noticed when the 5 position of the parent compound was substituted with an open-chain aliphatic group, and the activity was improved greatly when the 5 aliphatic group was in cyclic form. TAI-284, 6-chloro-5-cyclohexylindan-1-carboxylic acid emerged as the most active compound in this series. When the absolute stereochemistry of the compound was established, the activity was found mostly in the isomer with the *S* configuration.

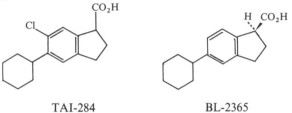

TAI-284   BL-2365

The same compound was also synthesized independently at about the same time by NOGUCHI et al. (1971). The potencies of TAI-284 in various anti-inflammatory and analgesic assays were approximately equal to those of indomethacin, but the antipyretic activity in rats with yeast-induced fever was much greater than that of indomethacin (KAWAI et al. 1971). BL-2365, which was chosen for human trial from the series of indan-1-carboxylic acids, showed an antipyretic effect in rats with yeast-induced fever 32 times as potent as that of aspirin, and one-half that of indomethacin. In various anti-inflammatory tests, BL-2365 was approximately one-half to one-quarter as active as indomethacin (PIRCIO et al. 1972).

The extension of the ethylene chain in bridging the aromatic nucleus and the acetic acid moiety seen in BL-2365 to a three carbon atom chain resulted in 1,2,3,4-tetrahydro-1-naphthoic acids (JUBY et al. 1972 b). Compared with BL-2365, the carboxylic acid group in the tetrahydronaphthoic acids is only partially restrained by the larger, more flexible cyclohexene ring. In this latter series, only the 6-cyclohexyl derivative showed any significant anti-inflammatory activity. No antipyretic test result was reported.

Among a large number of 1,3,4,9-tetrahydropyrano[3,4-b]indole-1-alkanoic acids synthesized by DEMERSON et al. (1975), prodolic acid was selected for further pharmacological study as an anti-inflammatory agent. Like other non-steroidal anti-inflammatory agents, prodolic acid showed antipyretic, analgesic and anti-inflammatory activities in several animal models. Prodolic acid was up to 17 times more potent than aspirin and approximately equipotent to phenylbutazone in chronic inflammations such as adjuvant arthritis. In reducing yeast-induced fever

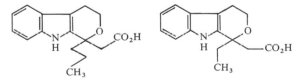

Prodolic acid   Etodolic acid

in rats, prodolic acid was 0.75 as potent as aspirin (MARTEL et al. 1974a). Continued investigation based on the structure–activity relationship of prodolic acid and its analogues has led DEMERSON et al. to synthesize etodolic acid. Etodolic acid was approximately 13 times more potent than prodolic acid in adjuvant arthritis. No antipyretic data was reported (MARTEL and KLICIUS 1976).

4. Aroylarylalkanoic Acids and Related Compounds

Further structural modification of phenothiazinealkanoic acids such as metiazinic acid (16,091 RP) led to the discovery of a new improved anti-inflammatory agent with a simpler chemical structure than the original compound. Ketoprofen (19,583 RP) thus obtained showed potency comparable to indomethacin in the carrageenan-induced oedema assay. The antipyretic activity of ketoprofen was even greater: it was three to four times as potent as indomethacin in reducing the yeast-induced fever in rats (JULOU et al. 1971).

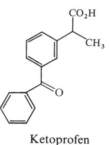

Ketoprofen

Suprofen was selected for detailed pharmacological study among a series of new compounds prepared with the general structure Het–CO–Ar–CH(CH$_3$)–CO$_2$H. It is a potent inhibitor of prostaglandin biosynthesis, and its analgesic potency determined by the writhing test in rats was 200 times that of aspirin, and 15 times and 6 times as potent as indomethacin and ketoprofen respectively (JANSSEN 1975; VAN DAELE et al. 1975). The antipyretic ED$_{50}$ (dose required to reduce the fever below 39° in 50% of the animals at the time of peak hyperthermia) of suprofen in rats with yeast-induced fever was 10 mg/kg, which is approximately 11 times less than that of aspirin, and about double that of indomethacin (NIEMEGEERS et al. 1975).

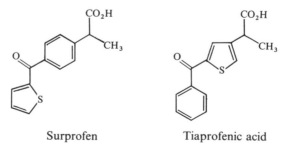

Surprofen   Tiaprofenic acid

The interchange of two aromatic rings in suprofen resulted in tiaprofenic acid which also showed potent anti-inflammatory and analgesic activities in animal and in human studies (CLÉMENCE et al. 1974). CARSON et al. (1971) prepared 5-p-chlorobenzoyl-1-methylpyrrole-2-acetic acid (I) and tolmetin in which the indole ring of indomethacin is replaced by a pyrrole ring. They felt that such compounds would also satisfy the requirement for the anti-inflammatory receptor site proposed by SHEN (see Sect. B). In carrageenan-induced oedema, both compounds

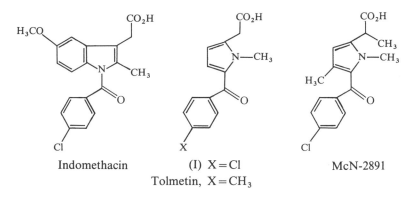

Indomethacin   (I) X = Cl   McN-2891
Tolmetin, X = CH₃

were approximately 0.4 times as potent as indomethacin, and significant analgesic and antipyretic activities were also observed with both. The anti-inflammatory activities were improved significantly by introduction of an additional methyl group next to the benzoyl moiety on the pyrrole ring. Thus, for example, McN-2891 had anti-inflammatory activity comparable to that of indomethacin. CARSON and WONG (1973) suggested that the improvement in the anti-inflammatory potency in the disubstituted aroylpyrroleacetic acid may be due to the steric influences of the substituents on the conformation of the aroyl group, causing the latter group to orient perpendicular to the pyrrole nucleus, thus being accommodated in the through of the anti-inflammatory receptor site more efficiently. Nevertheless, in detailed pharmacological evaluation of tolmetin and McN-2891, both compounds were less potent than indomethacin in various animal anti-inflammatory assays, and had greatly reduced ulcerogenic properties. In reducing yeast-induced fever in rats, both compounds were again much less potent then indomethacin; the relative potencies were tolmetin 1, McN-2891 3,4, and indomethacin 23 (WONG et al. 1973).

Another example of a non-steroidal anti-inflammatory–analgesic–antipyretic agent which bears the aroylphenylacetic acid structural skeleton is 5-benzoyl-1,2-

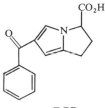

DPP

dihydro-3 *H*-pyrrolo[1,2-*a*]pyrrole-1-carboxylic acid (DPP). The compound showed potent analgesic, anti-inflammatory and antipyretic activity.

When given orally, in reducing the yeast-induced fever, DPP was 20 times as potent as aspirin. It inhibited carrageenan-induced paw oedema (37 times phenylbutazone) and cotton-pellet-induced granuloma with approximately double the potency of indomethacin (ROOKS et al. 1979).

UENO et al. (1976) and AULTZ et al. (1977 a) independently synthesized a series of 6,11-dihydrodibenz[*f,e*]oxapinacetic acids as potential anti-inflammatory and analgesic agents. These compounds may be considered as structural variants of ketoprofen, in which the benzoyl group is linked to the phenyl ring with a –O–CH$_2$– chain. In the structure–activity relationship study, it was revealed that the presence of the carbonyl moiety at the 11 position is essential for the activity.

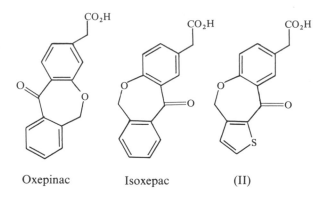

Oxepinac   Isoxepac   (II)

The position of the carboxylic acid side chain on the dibenz[*b,e*]oxepine ring plays a profound role in deciding the potency of anti-inflammatory activity. While oxepinac, which has the acetic acid moiety at the 3 position of 11-oxodibenz[*b,e*]oxepine, was twice as potent as indomethacin in the carrageenan-induced rat paw oedema test, its isomer with the acid moiety at the 1 position was inactive in a dose of 18 mg/kg or less (UENO et al 1976; TSUKADA et al. 1978; AULTZ et al. 1977 a). The anti-inflammatory potency of isoxepac in which the acid moiety is placed at the 2 position was in between the potencies of the two, and less than that of indomethacin. Compounds in this series had in general very low ulcerogenic activity. The anti-inflammatory potency was improved in (II) when one of the aromatic rings in the isoxepac was replaced with thiophene (AULTZ et al. 1977 b). The antipyretic effect of oxepinac when tested in rats with yeast-induced fever was approximately equal to that of indomethacin (TSUKADA et al. 1978).

5. Indoleacetic Acids and Analogues

Indomethacin is a therapeutically important anti-inflammatory–analgesic–antipyretic agent which was obtained as a result of screening more than 350 new indole derivatives (SHEN et al. 1963; WINTER et al. 1963).

Indomethacin was 20 times as potent as phenylbutazone in the carrageenan-induced rat paw oedema test (WINTER et al. 1963). The antipyretic potency of indomethacin when tested in febrile rats by different methods ranged from 10 to 18 times that of phenylbutazone, and measured in febrile rabbits was about

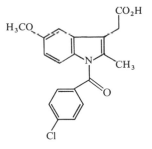

Indomethacin

20 times the potency of phenylbutazone (WINTER et al. 1963; CLARK and CUMBY 1975; VAN ARMAN and BOHIDAR 1978).

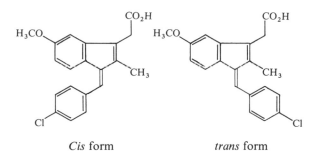

Cis form   *trans* form

The indene isostere of indomethacin can exist in two forms. The thermodynamically more stable *cis* isomer was about one half as potent as indomethacin in the carrageenan-induced oedema and cotton-pellet-induced granuloma assays, whereas the *trans* isomer was only one-tenth as active. The *cis* isomer was also active in the antipyretic and analgesic assays (SHEN 1967 b). Replacement of the chlorine at the 4 position of the *N*-benzoyl moiety of indomethacin with a pseudo-halogen, i.e. an azido group, resulted in zidomethacin. Its anti-inflammatory potency determined by the carrageenan oedema assay in the rat was slightly less than that of indomethacin, and its antipyretic potency against yeast-induced fever

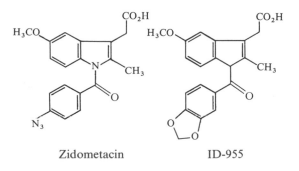

Zidometacin   ID-955

in the rat was approximately equal to that of indomethacin. However, the analgesic activity of zidomethacin was only one-fifth of that of indomethacin (TRICERRI et al. 1979).

A close analogue, ID-955, had a lower anti-inflammatory potency than that of indomethacin in animals, and one-tenth that of indomethacin in lowering the yeast-induced fever in rats (YAMAMOTO et al. 1969).

The movement of the nitrogen atom in the indole ring of indomethacin to different positions caused reduction in potency. Both 3-(4-chlorobenzoyl)-7-methoxy-2-methylindalizone-1-acetic acid (I) and 1-(4-chlorobenzoyl)-6-methoxy-2-methylindolizine-3-acetic acid (II), had approximately one-fifth the potency of indomethacin in the carrageenan-induced rat paw oedema test, and their analgesic activities were also less than that of indomethacin (CASAGRANDE et al. 1971).

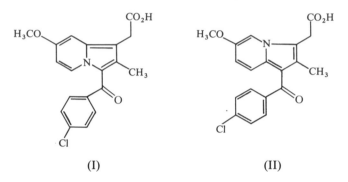

(I)   (II)

An indene analogue of indomethacin, sulindac, showed activity about one-half that of indomethacin in most anti-inflammatory assays. In the body the sulphoxide group in sulindac is reduced reversibly to form the corresponding sulphide which was shown to be the active metabolite. Thus the metabolite is generally twice as potent as the sulphoxide (sulindac) and as active as indomethacin (HUCKER et al. 1973). In yeast-induced fever, the antipyretic potency of sulindac was 0.6 times that of indomethacin. The active metabolite showed approximately 6 times the potency of sulindac (VAN ARMAN et al. 1976).

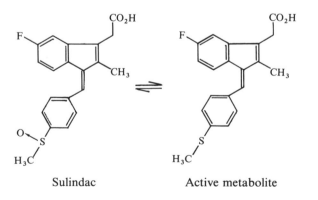

Sulindac   Active metabolite

JUBY and HUDYMA (1969) synthesized a series of 1-substituted-3-(5-tetrazolyl-methyl) indoles and homologues as tetrazole analogues of indomethacin. The most active compound in the tetrazole series was intrazole. The direct tetrazole analog of indomethacin, 1-(4-chlorobenzoyl)-5-methoxy-2-methyl-3-(5-tetrazoylmethyl)-indole, showed only weak activity in inhibiting carrageenan-induced foot oedema in rats. Further pharmacological study with intrazole showed that its activity against carragecnan-induced oedema was much less than that of indomethacin, but it was four times as potent as aspirin (FLEMING et al. 1969).

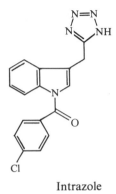

Intrazole

6. Polycycloaromatic Alkanoic Acids

In a search for improved antirheumatic drugs, HARRISON et al. (1970) observed that 2-napthylacctic acid had anti-inflammatory potency 0.6 times that of phenylbutazone. The potency was enhanced by the introduction of a small lipophilic group at the 6 position. The most active compound in the series, naproxen, was 55 times more potent then aspirin, or 11 times phenylbutazone, in the carrageenan-induced rat paw oedema assay. In reducing the fever caused by injection of yeast suspension into rats, naproxen was 22 times more potent than aspirin (HARRISON et al. 1970; ROSZKOWSKI et al. 1971; DORFMAN 1975). Among the series of 2-substituted benzothiazole acids prepared by WADA et al. (1973), 2-(p-dimethylaminophenyl-5-benzothiazoleacetic acid (I) was most active in carrageenan-induced rat paw oedema.

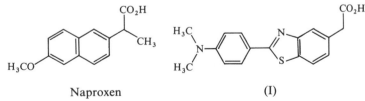

Naproxen   (I)

DURANT et al. (1965) discovered that α-(1-naphthyl)-2-furanpropionic acid (II) had anti-inflammatory activity when tested against UV erythema in the guinea-pig. It was one-quarter as potent as phenylbutazone when tested as a sodium salt. Numerous compounds were synthesized in the hope of improving the activity, but no better compound was found. From the structure–activity relationship, it was evident that the activity was associated with the 1-naphthylacetic acid moiety, and this activity was retained or enhanced by the introduction of a double bond or aromatic system linked to the α carbon atom by a methylene group. In antipyretic studies in rabbits using TAB- (typhoid–paratyphoid A and B)-vaccine as a pyretic agent, none of the compounds in the series showed a significant activity. A benzothiofen acetic acid, L 8109, showed anti-inflammatory, antipyretic, and analgesic activities in animal tests. Compared with phenylbutazone, the antiinflammatory potency de-

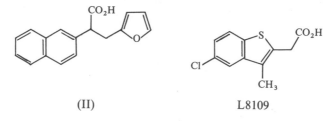

(II)   L8109

termined by carrageenan-induced oedema was about the same, and its antipyretic activity was about 2.5-fold (COLOT et al. 1974).

In a series of benzoxazolealkanoic acids studied by DUNWELL et al. (1975), benoxaprofen was chosen for preclinical pharmacological evaluation. The compound was five times more active than phenylbutazone in reducing the carrageenan-induced oedema, and three times more potent than aspirin as an antipyretic when tested by the yeast-induced fever in the rat (DUNWELL et al. 1975; CASHIN et al. 1977). Interestingly, benoxaprofen had only weak prostaglandin-synthesis-inhibiting property compared with other acidic anti-inflammatory agents (CASHIN et al. 1977).

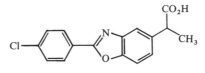

Benoxaprofen

R-803 is a derivative of benzofuran, which inhibited carrageenan-induced rat paw oedema with potency five times that of aspirin. The compound also had anti-pyretic and analgesic activities in animal testing (SWINGLE et al. 1975).

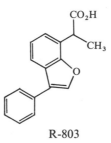

R-803

Among the carbazole-2-acetic acids, C-5720 had an antipyretic potency 16 times that of aspirin, 8 times that of phenylbutazone, and equal to indomethacin. In the carrageenan-induced oedema test in rats, C-5720 was equipotent to indomethacin, and about 30 times more potent than phenylbutazone or aspirin (RANDALL and BARUTH 1976).

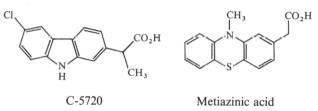

C-5720   Metiazinic acid

A large number of phenothiazinealkanoic acids and their derivatives were studied for anti-inflammatory activity (MESSER and FARGE 1967; MESSER et al. 1969). Metiazinic acid emerged as the most potent compound in the series, being three times more potent than phenylbutazone in the carrageenan-induced oedema test. The antipyretic potency of metiazinic acid in the yeast-induced rat fever test was five times that of phenylbutazone, and equipotent to that of indomethacin (JULOU and GUYONNET 1967; JULOU et al. 1969, 1971). Among a series of 4- and 5-argyl-naphthaleneacetic acids prepared as potential anti-inflammatory agents, the most active compound, 4-phenyl-1-naphthaleneacetic acid (III) was 62 times as potent as phenylbutazone in the guinea-pig UV erythema test. In the cotton-pellet-induced granuloma assay, (+)-α-methyl-5-phenyl-1-naphthaleneacetic acid (IV) was the most active of this series with potency 46 times that of phenylbutazone. Unfortunately, no antipyretic data are available (KALTENBRONN 1973).

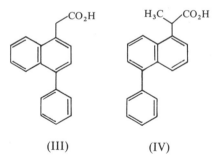

(III)   (IV)

A fluorenebutyric acid, furobufen, was developed as an anti-inflammatory agent. The potency of furobufen to inhibit carrageenan-induced rat paw oedema was comparable to that of phenylbutazone, and reduced completely the yeast-induced fever in rats at 100 mg/kg (MARTEL et al. 1974b).

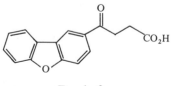

Furobufen

Naphthypramide was the most active anti-inflammatory compound in a series of α,α-disubstituted naphthylacetic amides (PALA et al. 1965), the potency of which was one-half that of phenylbutazone in the carrageenan-induced paw oedema assay (PALA et al. 1966; MARAZZI-UBERTI and TURBA 1966). In reducing yeast-induced fever in the rat, it was almost equipotent to phenylbutazone. It had a hypothermic effect when given to a normal rat (MARAZZI-UBERTI et al. 1966). It is worth noting that the corresponding acid was considerably less potent than naphthypramide in reducing oedema and fever in rats (PALA et al. 1966).

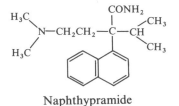

Naphthypramide

V. Non-Acidic Compounds

Most of the compounds so far discussed are acidic in chemical properties, having an ionizable acidic proton in their molecules. This proton may be in the form of a carboxylic acid, or an enolic (or potentially enolic) group such as β-diketone. Occasionally, isosteres of the carboxylic acid group, such as tetrazole, hydroxamic or sulphonic acid have been used as an alternative source of the proton. In general, the acidity of active non-steroidal anti-inflammatory–antipyretic agents falls in the range of pK_a 3.5–6.5 (UNTERHALT 1970). LOMBARDINO et al. (1975) determined pK_a values of 15 clinically effective acidic anti-inflammatory agents in a dioxane–water (2:1) mixture, and found that the pK_a values of almost all of these drugs fell within a fairly narrow range of 5.3–7.9.

In the search for new anti-inflammatory agents a large number of arylalkanoic acids were synthesized in the 1960s and early 1970s. However, all of these compounds had some degree of gastrointestinal irritant and ulcerogenic properties. These side effects seemed to be an inherent property of the acidic anti-inflammatory agents. Accordingly, a new trend began in the late 1960s in various pharmaceutical laboratories to look into non-acidic compounds as possibly being free from such side effects.

One of the earliest synthetic antipyretics, antipyrine, is a non-acidic compound discovered in 1884 by KNORR in a search for a new synthetic antipyretic drug that could be substituted for quinine (see Sect. D.I). Since its introduction into medical use, numerous pyrazolone derivatives have been synthesized and tested for antipyretic, analgesic, and anti-inflammatory activities in the hope of obtaining improved agents. Aminopyrine was a non-acidic pyrazolone derivative prepared from antipyrine. It was a therapeutically effective antipyretic and analgesic agent, slower in action but greater in potency than antipyrine, and was once used popularly for the control of rheumatic fever. Its gastric irritation was less than that caused by most acidic antipyretic–analgesic agents, but it induced agranulocytosis in a small percentage of cases.

Dipyrone is the methansulphonate derivative of aminopyrine, and thus more soluble in water than is aminopyrine. It is available for parenteral administration.

Dipyrone has similar pharmacological and toxicological properties to those of aminopyrine.

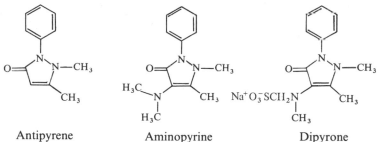

Antipyrene · Aminopyrine · Dipyrone

LINDNER (1973) reported an interesting structure–activity relationship between the antipyretic and analgesic activities of aminopyrine analogues. The replacement of the phenyl group in aminopyrine with a benzyl group to give Hoe 7694 im-

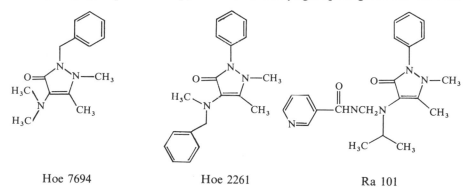

Hoe 7694 · Hoe 2261 · Ra 101

proved the analgesic activity, leaving the antipyretic potency unchanged; the exchange of one of the two methyl groups of the 4-dimethylamino group with a benzyl group giving Hoe 2261 eliminated the analgesic and anti-inflammatory activities almost completely, and the antipyretic potency was doubled. Ra 101 had antipyretic and anti-inflammatory activities superior to those of aminopyrine, but analgesic activity was practically unchanged (TUBARO and BANCI 1970).

A series of pyridazinone derivatives structurally related to aminopyrine was investigated by SATO et al. (1979).

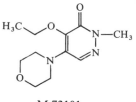

M 73101

In general, 4-alkoxy-2-methyl-5-morpholino-3(2 H)-pyridazinone had anti-inflammatory properties in animal models. The best compound in the series was M 73101. In an antipyretic test in rats in which fever was induced by an injection of a lipopolysaccharide (TTG) prepared from *Pseudomonas fluorescens*, it was less active than aminopyrine and almost equally active with tiaramide. The anti-inflammatory and analgesic activities of M 73101 were better than those of aminopyrine or phenylbutazone (SATO et al. 1979).

TANAKA et al. (1972) examined a series of 2-alkyl-4,5-diphenylpyrroles for anti-inflammatory activity. Bimetopyrole was selected for detailed pharmacological evaluation. It was 9.6 times more potent than phenylbutazone in the carrageenan-induced rat paw oedema assay, and suppressed aceticacid-induced writhing in mice. It reduced yeast-induced fever in rats completely in 2 h at a dose of 12 mg/kg; thus, the potency was 4.3 times that of phenylbutazone and 10.9 times that of aspirin (TANAKA and IIZUKA 1972; IIZUKA and TANAKA 1972).

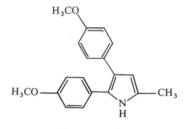

Bimetopyrole

Ditazol was the most active anti-inflammatory agent with very low toxicity among a series of 2-substituted-4,5-diphenyl-oxazoles synthesized by MARCHETTI et al. (1968). The antipyretic activity of ditazol was about the same as that of phenylbutazone in yeast-induced fever in rats. Its anti-inflammatory potency was

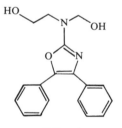

Ditazol

less than that of phenylbutazone in several assays; the drug also had some analgesic potency (CAPRINO et al. 1973).

Indoxole, discovered by SZMUSKOVICZ et al. (1966), is one of the relatively early non-acidic anti-inflammatory agents synthesized.

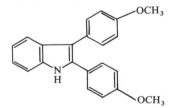

Indoxole

Table 4. Antipyretic, analgesic and anti-inflammatory potencies of pyrazole derivatives. (OSHIMA et al. 1969)

Structure	Antipyretic potency	Analgesic potency	Anti-inflammatory potency
Aminopyrine	1.0	1.0	1.0
	0.5	0.86	1.1
	0.5	0.48	1.3
Mepirizole	0.5	1.10	1.8

It was effective against carrageenan-induced oedema. Oral potency varied from 0.9 to 5.0 times that of phenylbutazone and 3 to 5 times that of aspirin, depending upon the vehicle used. Its antipyretic potency in rats with yeast-induced fever exceeded that of aspirin and phenylbutazone (GLENN et al. 1967).

Mepirizole (DA-398) was an analgesic and anti-inflammatory agent synthesized by NAITO et al. (1969). A study carried out with mepirizole and related compounds indicated that the antipyretic activities of these compounds in reducing fever induced by TTG pyrogen in rabbits were, in general, less than that of aminopyrine, but their anti-inflammatory and analgesic potencies were greater (Table 4; see OSHIMA et al. 1969).

Table 5. Analgesic, antipyretic and anti-inflammatory potencies of 1,3-disubstituted-5-amino-6-methyluracils. (SENDA et al. 1972)

R_1	R_2	A	Analgesic [a] potency	Antipyretic [b] potency		Anti-inflammatory [c] potency	
				100 mg/kg	200 mg/kg	100 mg/kg	200 mg/kg
Ph	Me	NMe_2	56		−0.1		65
Ph	Me	NEt_2	>300		−0.4		46
Ph	$CH_2=CHCH_2$	NMe_2	70	−0.7	−6.6		75
Me	Ph	NMe_2	46	−5.6	−7.7		44
Me	Ph	NEt_2	53	1.9	−5.0		45
Me	Ph	$NHCHMe_2$	73		−4.6		64
Me	Ph	$NHCH_2CH_2CH_3$	47		−5.5		48
Et	Ph	NMe_2	77		−5.6		37
Et	Ph	NEt_2	95		−5.5		57
$CH_2=CHCH_2$	Ph	NMe_2	45		−0.6	52	73
$P-MeOC_6H_4$	Me	NMe_2	>300		11.0		41
Me	$PhCH_2$	NMe_2	≅300		−8.9		38
Me	Me	NMe_2	29		−5.6		37
Aminopyrine			32	−4.1		69	86
Aspirin			49		−2.4		47

[a] Determined by the phenylbenzoquinone writhing method in mice (subcutaneous)
[b] Decreases in fever induced by a pyrogen obtained from *Pseudomonas fluorescens* in rats (oral)
[c] Reduction in rat hind-paw oedema induced by carrageenan (oral)

SENDA et al. (1972) synthesized a large number of 1,3-disubstituted-5-amino-6-methyluracil derivatives. They were structurally related to aminopyrine by having a six-membered uracil ring instead of the pyrazolone of aminopyrine. In general, the analgesic and anti-inflammatory activities of these uracil derivatives were less than those of aminopyrine. The relative analgesic, antipyretic, and anti-inflammatory activities of these compounds are shown in Table 5. The most active antipyretic compound in the series, 5-dimethylamino-1,6-dimethyl-3-phenyluracil was more potent than aminopyrine in reducing fever in rats, but its analgesic activity was less, and its anti-inflammatory activity was one-half that of aminopyrine (SENDA et al. 1972).

LANG et al. (1976) reported that various aryl-s-tetrazines, such as 3-(p-fluorophenyl)-s-tetrazine (I) had aspirin-like activity against carrageenan-induced oedema in rats, UV erythema in guinea-pigs, and adjuvant-induced arthritis in rats. These compounds also displayed analgesic activity in animal models. No antipyretic result was reported.

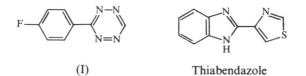

| (I) | Thiabendazole |

Thiabendazole is one of the most potent anthelmintic agents known, and is highly effective in the therapy of *S stercoralis* infections and of cutaneous larva migrans. During the clinical treatment of trichinosis, CAMPBELL (1971) first noticed its moderate anti-inflammatory and analgesic activities. When tested in rats, thiabendazole was approximately one-third to one-half as potent as aspirin in the antipyretic, carrageenan-induced oedema and adjuvant arthritis assays (VAN ARMAN and CAMPBELL 1975). Prompted by this observation, CLARK et al. (1978) synthesized a series of 2-(substituted phenyl)oxazolo[4,5-b]pyridines and 2-(substituted phenyl)oxazolo[5,4-b]pyridines. A few had activities comparable to those of phenylbutazone or indomethacin without producing gastrointestinal tract irritation. As antipyretics, the compounds were generally several times more potent than phenylbutazone. Pharmacological activities of five of the most active compounds in the series compared with aspirin and phenylbutazone are shown in Table 6, data being taken from CLARK et al. (1978).

ALMIRANTE et al. (1965) synthesized derivatives of imidazo[1,2-a]pyridine of the general structure II, and examined them for analgesic, anti-inflammatory, antipyretic, and muscle relaxant activities. A number of compounds in this series lowered the yeast-induced fever and, to some extent, the normal body temperature of rats. The unsubstituted parent compound

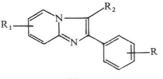

(II)

Table 6. Oxazolopyridine derivatives: median effective doses in antipyretic, anti-inflammatory and analgesic assays, mg/kg orally. (CLARK et al. 1978)

Assay	X=F, Y=H	X=CN, Y=H	X=Y=H	X=F	X=CN	Aspirin	Phenyl-butazone
Antipyretic	7	7.7	4.6	7.6	13	45	24
Anti-inflammatory	21	1.7	22	22	11	89	28
Analgesic	0.7	0.35	0.45	1.1	0.44	0.025	0.15

Table 7. Antipyretic effects in the rat of imidazo[1,2-a]pyridine derivatives at oral doses of 0.25 oral LD_{50}. (ALMIRANTE et al. 1965)

Number	R	R_1	R_2	Mean lowering of fever, °C over 6 h
IIA	H	H	H	1.08
IIB	o-SO_2CH_3	H	H	0.95
IIC	p-SCH_3	H	H	4.05
IID	p-SO_2CH_3	H	H	4.73
IIE	p-SO_2CH_3	5-CH_3	H	4.58
IIF	p-SO_2CH_3	H	$CH_2N(CH_3)_2$	1.78
	Aspirin			0.98
	Phenylbutazone			1.07

(II, where R = R_1 = R_2 = H) displayed only moderate activity, and monosubstitution in R with a methylthio, methylsulphoxy, or methylsulphonyl group appears to be necessary for high antipyretic potency. Further substitution in either R_1 or R_2 in an already active compound seemed to impart a negative influence, except in one case, in which R = SO_2CH_3, R_1 = CH_3, R_2 = H (IIE in Table 7). In this series there appears to be a greater structural specificity required for a high order of antipyretic activity than for anti-inflammatory or analgesic effects. Table 7 shows antipyretic effects, measured in yeast-induced fever in rats, of some imidazo[1,2-a] pyridine derivatives; the reader should be cautioned that the antipyretic effects were not measured at a uniform dose, but at a fixed fraction (0.25) of the lethal dose for each compound. Whereas alteration in the position of the methylsulphonyl group in the phenyl ring produced profound changes in antipyretic activity, as shown by a comparison of p-SO_2CH_3 (IID) with o-SO_2CH_3 (IIB, Table 7), such positional alteration of the methylsulphonyl group did not result in significant change in anti-inflammatory activity. 2-(p-Methylsulphonylphenyl)imidazo[1,2-α] pyridine (IID) and its dimethylaminomethyl Mannich base (IIF), emerged as the most interesting compounds in the various analgesic and anti-inflammatory assays (ALMIRANTE et al. 1965). ALMIRANTE et al. (1966) extended their work to include several related heterocyclic ring systems, i.e. imidazo[1,2-a]pyrimidine, 1 H-imidazo[1,2-d]tetrazole, imidazo[2,1-b]thiazole, 1 H-imidazo[1,2-b]-s-triazole, and imidazo[1,2-b]pyridazine. Since their earlier study had shown that the methylsulphonyl group substituted on the phenyl ring seemed to be necessary for a broad spectrum of activity, this group was kept unchanged in these new fused imidazole derivatives. 2-Phenylimidazo[1,2-a] pyrimidine with the methylsulphonyl group on the 2-phenyl ring at the *para* position showed highest antipyretic activity. None of the compounds prepared in this study, however, showed a spectrum of activity comparable to that of III,2-(p-methylsulphonylphenyl)imidazo[1,2-a]pyridine (ALMIRANTE et al. 1966).

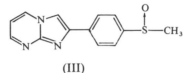

(III)

Benzydamine is a clinically useful anti-inflammatory agent obtained as a result of general pharmacological evaluation of a series of 1-substituted-3-dimethyl-aminoalkoxy-1 H-indazoles prepared by PLAZZO et al. (1966). The subsequent in-depth pharmacological study revealed that benzydamine possessed pharmacolog-

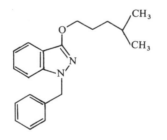

Benzydamine

ical properties in common with other non-steroidal anti-inflammatory agents. Its antipyretic potency in yeast-induced fever in rats was one-half that of aminopyrine; it lowered the yeast-induced fever in rats by 0.6–1.7° (mean decrease 1.2 °C) at dose of 100 mg/kg. No hypothermic effect on normal rats was observed at the same dose. It showed anti-inflammatory activity in various animal models, with a potency roughly that of phenylbutazone (SILVESTRINI et al. 1966).

Tiaramide which was studied by TAKASHIMA et al. (1972) exhibited anti-inflammatory, analgesic, and antipyretic activities when tested in experimental animals. In doses of 125 mg/kg, it reduced by 1 °C the fever induced in rats by yeast at 2 h.

Chinoin-127 was a more potent analgesic in the hot plate and writhing test than aspirin or phenylbutazone, and equally effective as an anti-inflammatory agent in various animal models. Its antipyretic activity tested by yeast-induced fever in the rat was approximately one-tenth that of indomethacin. The anti-inflammatory ac-

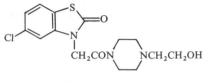

Tiaramide

tivity of this compound in the carrageenan-induced rat paw oedema tests, interestingly, was increased by simultaneous administration of indomethacin (KNOLL et al. 1979).

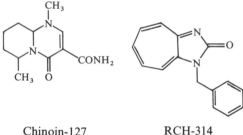

Chinoin-127   RCH-314

One of the rings of the bicyclic non-acidic antipyretic compounds may be enlarged to a seven-membered nucleus with retention of the pharmacological properties. MINAKAMI et al. (1964) found that 1-benzylcycloheptimidazol-2(1 H)-one (RCH-314) possessed potent analgesic and anti-inflammatory activities. Its antipyretic potency tested in rats with TTG-induced fever at 30 mg/kg was greater than that of aminopyrine. The analgesic potency of RCH-314 was two to three times that of aminopyrine.

KOBAYASHI and TAKAGI (1968) showed that 2-phenyl-6-dimethylamino-6 H-cycloheptoxazole (IV) synthesized by SOMA et al. (1967) had antipyretic, anti-inflammatory, and analgesic effects in animal tests. At an intraperitoneal (i.p.) dose of 2–5 mg/kg this compound showed a significant antipyretic effect on the fever induced by TTG in guinea-pigs. Its inhibitory potency on the oedema produced in the rat hind-paw by carrageenan was equivalent to that of phenylbutazone.

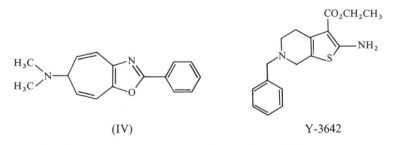

(IV)   Y-3642

Y-3642 (tinoridine) is a new structural type of anti-inflammatory–analgesic–antipyretic compound prepared by NAKANISHI et al. and extensively studied by the research group at the Yoshitomi Pharmaceutical Company in Japan (NAKANISHI et al. 1970 a, b, c, d, e). It was superior to aminopyrine in alleviating inflammatory pain, was comparable to aminopyrine in analgesic effects in the benzoquinone test, and markedly inhibited experimental oedema induced by various inflammatory agents. It reduced the fever from TTG in the rabbit with a potency higher than that of aminopyrine (NAKANISHI et al. 1970 c, e).

Some of the 1-benzylisoquinoline derivatives which have direct structural relationship with the spasmolytic, papaverine, showed weak but significant analgesic and antipyretic activities. The most active compound in the series was V, 5-(2-amino-3,4-dimethoxybenzyl)-1,3-dioxolo[4,5-g]isoquinoline (WEISBACH et al. 1968).

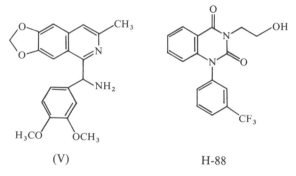

(V)   H-88

H-88 was selected over 400 new quinazoline-2,4-dione derivatives tested for anti-inflammatory, analgesic, and antipyretic effects. It inhibited increased vascular permeability and acute oedema of various origins. The potency was less than that of indomethacin, but greater than those of phenylbutazone and benzydamine. In antipyretic and analgesic assays, H-88 was two to four times more potent than aminopyrine and mefenamic acid (FUJIMURA 1973; FUJIMURA et al. 1974). This compound was unusual in that it exerted only negligible ulcerogenic activity, and surprisingly it prevented gastric ulcers induced by other non-steroidal anti-inflammatory agents such as indomethacin, phenylbutazone, and aspirin (FUJIMURA et al. 1974). Replacement of the hydroxy group by hydrogen to give 3-ethyl-1-[3-(trifluoromethyl)phenyl]-2,4-(1 *H*,3*H*)quinazolinedione removed the antipyretic and analgesic activities (FUJIMURA et al. 1974).

Proquazone was selected for detailed pharmacological evaluation as an anti-inflammatory and analgesic agent from nearly 50 compounds synthesized by COOMBS et al. (1973) in the series of 1-alkyl-4-aryl-2(1 *H*)-quinazolinones and

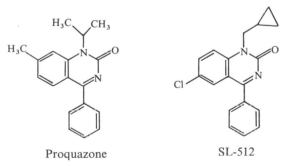

Proquazone   SL-512

quinazolinethiones. The acute anti-inflammatory effect of praquazone tested by carrageenan-induced oedema was equivalent to that of indomethacin. Praquazone and indomethacin reduced yeast-induced fever in rats in equal extent at a dose of 2.5 mg/kg. Praquazone had a more potent analgesic effect than that of indomethacin (TAKESUE et al. 1976).

KOMATSU et al. (1972) also investigated a series of quinazoline derivatives for potential anti-inflammatory agents, and selected SL-512 for further pharmacological investigation. In rats with yeast-induced fever it was comparable to phenylbutazone in its antipyretic potency; the anti-inflammatory effect on carrageenan-induced oedema in rats was also approximately equal to that of phenylbutazone (YAMAMOTO et al. 1973).

Anti-inflammatory and antipyretic activities were found in derivatives of 1,3-benzoxazin-4-one. The antipyretic potency of AP 67 (chlorthenoxazine) was 3.6 times that of aspirin (KADATZ 1957). TEOTINO et al. (1963) prepared a series of 2-alkylthioethyl-1,3-benzoxazin-4-ones, among which the 2-methylthioethyl and the corresponding sulphoxide showed antipyretic activities comparable to that of aspirin. The antipyretic activity was diminished greatly by further oxidation to the corresponding sulphone.

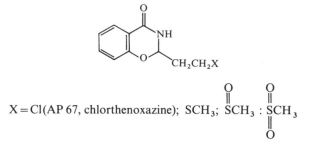

$$X = Cl(AP\ 67,\ chlorthenoxazine);\ SCH_3;\ \overset{O}{\underset{}{\overset{\|}{S}}}CH_3 : \overset{O}{\underset{O}{\overset{\|}{\underset{\|}{S}}}}CH_3$$

Antipyretic, analgesic, and anti-inflammatory activities can also be found in tricyclic compounds. Seclazone is an anti-inflammatory agent selected for clinical evaluation from a series of isoxazolo[3,2-b][1,3]benzoxazin-9-ones (REISNER et al. 1977a; BERGER et al. 1973). It completely abolished yeast-induced fever in rats at a dose of 300 mg/kg, which fact indicates about one-third to one-half of the antipyretic potency of aspirin (BERGER et al. 1973). While the introduction of a methyl group at the 2 position of seclazone (giving W-2395) raised the antipyretic activity to that of aspirin, the antipyretic activity of 3-methylseclazone was only one-quar-

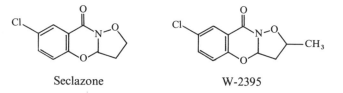

Seclazone   W-2395

ter of that of aspirin (BERGER et al. 1973; REISNER et al. 1977b; SOFIA et al. 1974). Seclazone and W-2395 inhibited adjuvant-induced polyarthritis and carrageenan-induced hind-paw oedema in rats, and analgesic activity in the Randall–Selitto test (BERGER et al. 1973; SOFIA et al. 1974). The metabolic study of seclazone in humans and animals revealed that it undergoes metabolic cleavage of the oxazine ring to form 5-chlorosalicylic acid which was excreted in free form and as conjugates with glucuronic acid and glycine (DOUGLAS et al. 1972). 5-Chlorosalicylic acid is the only hydrolytic product formed in the systemic circulation of rats after oral administration of the agent (EDELSON et al. 1972). These metabolic studies suggest that seclazone may be a pro-drug of 5-chlorosalicylic acid. In reducing yeast-induced fever in rats, W-2429 was approximately six times more potent than aspirin. At a dose of 12 mg/kg, it returned rectal temperature of febrile rats to the level of the control group. However, the compound also caused a significant and dose-dependent reduction in the rectal temperature of febrile rats following oral doses of 12–1,000 mg/kg. The effect of W-2429 in febrile rats may thus be a hypothermic effect rather than a true antipyretic action or a combination of both. W-2499 showed potent analgesic activity in a number of test procedures in mice and rats. On a mg/kg basis, the analgesic potency was considerably greater than that of aspirin, and superior or approximately equal to that of propoxyphene hydrochloride and codeine. In inhibiting carrageenan-induced oedema in the hind-paw of rats, its potency was approximately eight times that of aspirin, but it was totally ineffective against adjuvant-induced polyarthritis in rats (REISNER et al. 1977 b; SOFIA et al. 1977). The extension of the isoxazole portion of W-2429 to the six-membered oxazine to give 2,4-dihydro-(1,2)-oxazino[3,2-b]quinazolin-10(2H)one reduced all three pharmacological activities found with W-2429. The replacement of the isoxazole with a pyrrole ring to form pyrroloquinazolinone resulted in drastic reduction in the pharmacological activity (REISNER et al. 1977 b).

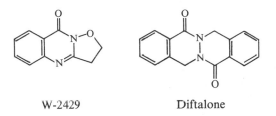

W-2429   Diftalone

Phthalazino[2,3-b]phthalazine-5,12-(7H,14H)-dione (diftalone) is a symmetrical tetracyclic compound with anti-inflammatory and antipyretic activities (BELLASIO and TESTA 1970; SCHIATTI et al. 1974). The anti-inflammatory potency of diftalone is greater than that of aspirin, approximately equal to that of phenylbutazone, but lower than that of indomethacin. Diftalone exhibited a limited but statistically significant antipyretic activity at doses of 20, 100, and 200 mg/kg but was less potent than aspirin or phenylbutazone (SCHIATTI et al. 1974).

There have been reported several anti-inflammatory antipyretic compounds which bear a ketonic group as a common structural feature. COOMBS et al. (1971) synthesized 2-morpholinomethylbenzophenone (VI) in their attempts to obtain compounds active on the central nervous system. The compound did not have any useful level of activity in the central nervous system, but had good anti-inflammatory activity. In the carrageenan-induced foot oedema test, it was approximately twice as active as phenylbutazone. Antipyretic activity against yeast-induced fever in rats was observed at 25 mg/kg orally. Attempts at improvement of the anti-inflammatory activity through molecular modification were not successful (COOMBS et al. 1971).

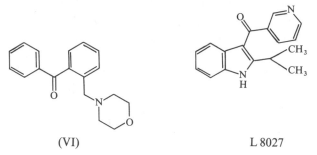

(VI)   L 8027

COLOT et al. (1973) reported that L 8027 had anti-inflammatory, antipyretic, and analgesic activities in animal models. Flazalone exhibited anti-inflammatory activity in a variety of animal tests. Administered orally to rats with yeast-induced fever, the drug had about half the antipyretic activity of sodium salicylate. In con-

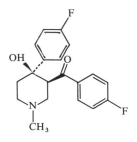

Flazalone

trast to a number of other non-steroidal anti-inflammatory agents, flazalone showed no analgesic activity in mice at doses up to 200 mg/kg i.p. in a modification of Grewal's method (DRAPER et al. 1972). The compound had a mild immunosuppressive property in that it inhibited graft rejection in goldfish (DRAPER et al. 1972; LEVY and McCLURE 1976).

Carisoprodol, an analogue of meprobamate, was originally synthesized as a tranquillizer and muscle relaxant (BERGER 1954). Carisoprodol differs from meprobamate in having an isopropyl group in place of the hydrogen atom on one of the carbamoyl nitrogens. Carisoprodol had a different profile of effects on the central nervous system (BERGER et al. 1959) and, in addition, an analgesic and anti-

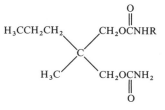

R = H: Meprobamate
R = CH(CH₃)₂: Carisoprodol

pyretic effect. In doses that did not produce ataxia, muscular relaxation or paralysis, it effectively relieved pain caused by injection of silver nitrate into the joints of rats. The antipyretic effect of carisoprodol on fever induced by injection of a TAB-vaccine was distinct at a dose of 200 mg/kg, but weaker than that of aspirin at 100 mg/kg. At 100 mg/kg carisoprodol was not antipyretic and did not have anti inflammatory activity (BERGER et al. 1960).

VI. Derivatives of Aniline and Aminophenol

Acetanilide was discovered before the turn of this century, and thus is among the oldest antipyretic drugs. The accidental discovery of its antipyretic effect occurred through an error made in filling a prescription; in 1886, CAHN and HEPP, the discoverers, named it antifebrin, and introduced it in medical practice. It soon proved to be excessively toxic, however, and was withdrawn from therapeutic use. It is hydrolyzed relatively easily to aniline which, like many other aromatic amines, produces methaemoglobin in the blood. Nevertheless, it served as the parent member of this group of drugs, and led to the discovery of the now widely used acetaminophen.

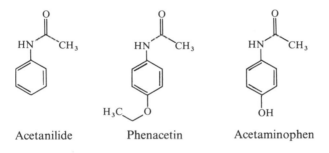

Acetanilide   Phenacetin   Acetaminophen

In a search for better drugs in this group, phenacetin (acetophenetidin) was discovered as one of the more satisfactory antipyretic and analgesic agents. It was introduced into therapy in 1887, and is still used, largely in analgesic therapy. N-acetyl-p-aminophenol (acetaminophen, paracetamol) is the major metabolite of phenacetin. It was first medically used by VON MERING in 1893, but for many years was not accepted widely. In the early 1950s, it was found that continued use of phenacetin could lead to severe renal papillary necrosis. Acetaminophen then replaced it as an analgesic and an antipyretic, and also replaced aspirin to some extent, especially for those patients who suffer from gastric irritation with aspirin, or have bleeding disorders (MIELKE et al. 1976). p-Aminophenol, one of the first derivatives prepared in the search for better antipyretics, had a strong antipyretic and analgesic activity, but was too toxic to be used as a therapeutic agent.

Although adequately controlled clinical trials are few in number, it is generally considered that acetaminophen and phenacetin are approximately as potent as aspirin as antipyretics and as analgesics (WARREN and WARREN 1946; COLGAN and MINTZ 1957; BEAVER 1965, 1966; KOCH-WESER 1976). These agents have only very weak anti-inflammatory activity, however, and thus are different from most other antipyretic agents.

MILTON and WENDLANDT (1965) showed that the fever produced by injection
of pyrogen into the lateral cerebral ventricles of conscious cats through a chronically implanted Collison cannula started to fall within 15 min after injection of
acetaminophen, reaching the control level in 1–2 h. Acetaminophen is as active as
aspirin in inhibiting the prostaglandin synthetase from brain tissue but it has only
very weak inhibitory activity against the synthetase from spleen. This marked difference in inhibitory activity of acetaminophen against the prostaglandin syn-
thetases of different tissues may partly explain the fact that acetaminophen is an
effective antipyretic, antagonizing the PG synthetase of brain, but is only weakly
anti-inflammatory (FLOWER and VANE 1972; FERREIRA and VANE 1974).

VII. Compounds of Natural Origin

Quinoline provided a rich source of medicinal agents during the early days of
chemical endeavours to obtain synthetic drugs. 2-Phenylcinchoninic acid (cinchophen) was introduced into medicine in 1906, and has been used mainly for the treatment of gout. It has also analgesic and antipyretic activities, but its tendency to
cause jaundice and other toxic symptoms has limited its utility.

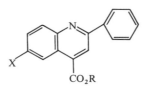

R=H, X=H: Cinchophen
R=CH$_2$CH$_3$, X=CH$_3$: Neocinchophen
R=CH$_2$CH=CH$_2$, X=H: Atoquinol

Neocinchophen was obtained in attempts to circumvent the toxicity of cinchophen. It was less toxic, but still had a potential for causing hepatic disease. The antipyretic effect of cinchophen was improved by forming an allyl ester to give atoquinol.

Cryogenine is an alkaloid isolated from *Heimia salicifolia;* its chemical structure has been established

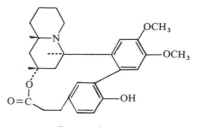

Cryogenine

by FERRIS et al. (1966). KAPLAN et al. (1967) demonstrated that cryogenine possesses significant anti-inflammatory activity at a dose of 100 mg/kg, given orally, against carrageenan-induced oedema in rats, in which test it had 0.86 times the anti-inflammatory potency of phenylbutazone. Cryogenine was also effective in reducing established adjuvant-induced arthritis. It had only slight antipyretic activity, however, in rats made febrile by peptone administration, although ROBICHAUD et al. (1964) had already demonstrated that it induces hypothermia in normothermic acclimatized animals. It had a low order of analgesic activity when tested by the rat tail-flick method (KAPLAN et al. 1967).

11-Desacetoxywartmannin is a mould metabolite which has been isolated from the culture filtrate of *Penicillium funiculosum*. The compound showed weak antifungal activity.

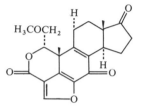

11-Desacetoxywartmannin

Unexpectedly, the compound showed potent anti-inflammatory activity. Its activity in inhibiting the carrageenan-induced paw oedema was equal to that of indomethacin and about six times that of phenylbutazone.

In established adjuvant arthritis, it showed a dose-dependent inhibition of primary and secondary arthritis. Like cryogenine, it lowered the rectal temperature in normothermic rats, but failed to reduce fever in rats (WIESINGER et al. 1974).

E. Conclusions

So far no systematic and comprehensive general study on the structure-activity relationships of antipyretic agents has appeared in the literature, and in only a few papers have the structure–activity relationships for compounds in any one series been described. Many antipyretic agents are reported to be more potent than aspirin, but it is still the most used.

The potencies are not absolutely parallel across all drugs studied for the three characteristic pharmacological properties – anti-inflammatory, analgesic, and antipyretic – which are found together in most of the non-steroidal anti-inflammatory agents; nevertheless, in general the antipyretic action does increase as the other two pharmacological properties increase. The anti-inflammatory potency appears somewhat better correlated with antipyretic potency than is the analgesic. The three properties may possibly be interrelated and work at least partly through a common mode of action, such as inhibition of prostaglandin synthesis. With respect to non-steroidal anti-inflammatory drugs, the sites of anti-inflammatory and analgesic actions are thought to be local, but the antipyretics may exert their actions in the central nervous system. That the dose–response lines found across the three kinds of assays are not always parallel may reflect the fact that the respective receptor sites may be different in nature and location.

It would be most useful to know enough about the mode of action of a drug to allow one to ascribe the antipyretic action to either a shift in the set-point temperature or a change in one or more of the thermoregulatory pathways. Naturally a shift in the set-point temperature will entail a change in heat loss or heat conservation mechanisms, but these latter may be affected without any change of the set-point temperature. Qualitative evidence for peripheral changes is often not difficult to obtain, as by observation of shivering, vasoconstriction, heat-seeking behaviour, cardio-acceleration, salivation, perspiration, etc. Clear deductions about the re-setting of the thermostat, however, are not so easy to obtain. If there were enough of such data obtained within each of several different classes of chemical structure, perhaps chemists would learn how to improve certain features of drugs.

References

Adams SS, Cobb R (1958) A possible basis for the antiinflammatory activity of salicylates and other non-hormonal anti-rheumatic drugs. Nature 181:773–774

Adams SS, Cliffe EE, Lessel B, Nicholson JS (1963) Some biological properties of "ibufenac", a new anti-rheumatic drug. Nature 200:271–272

Adams SS, Cliffe EE, Lessel B, Nicholson JS (1967) Some biological properties of 2-(4-isobutylphenyl)propionic acid. J Pharm Sci 56:1686

Adams SS, Hebborn P, Nicholson JS (1968) Some aspects of the pharmacology of ibufenac, a non-steroidal antiinflammatory agent. J Pharm Pharmacol 20:305–312

Almirante L, Polo L, Mugnaini A et al. (1965) Derivatives of imidazole. I. Synthesis and reactions of imidazo[1,2-a]pyridines with analgesic, antiinflammatory, antipyretic, and anticonvulsant activity. J Med Chem 8:305–311

Almirante L, Polo L, Mugnaini A et al. (1966) Derivatives of imidazole. II. Synthesis and reactions of imidazo[1,2-a]pyrimidines and other bi- and tricyclic imidazo derivatives with analgesic, antiinflammatory, antipyretic, and anticonvulsant activity. J Med Chem 9:29–33

Atkinson DC, Godfrey KE, Jordan BJ, Leach EC, Meek B, Nichols JD, Saville JF (1974) 2-(2,4-Dichlorophenoxy)phenylacetic acid (fenclofenac): one of a novel series of anti-inflammatory compounds with low ulcerogenic potential. J Pharm Pharmacol 26:357–358

Aultz DE, Helsley GC, Hoffman D, McFadden AR, Lassman HB, Wilker JC (1977a) Dibenz[b,e]oxepinalkanoic acids as nonsteroidal anti-inflammatory agents. 1. 6,11-Dihydro-11-oxodibenz[b,e]oxepin-2-acetic acids. J Med Chem 20:66–70

Aultz DE, McFadden AR, Lassman HB (1977b) Dibenz[b,e]oxepinalkanoic acids and nonsteroidal antiinflammatory agents. 2. Dihydro-10-oxofuro- and thieno[3,2-c][1]benzoxepin-8-acetic acids. J Med Chem 20:456–458

Barron DI, Copley AR, Vallance DK (1968) Anti-inflammatory and related properties of 4-(p-biphenylyl)-3-hydroxybutyric acid. Br J Pharmacol 33:396–407

Bavin EM, Drain DJ, Seymour DE, Waterhouse PD (1955) Anti-inflammatory compounds. Part I. The activity of a series of new compounds compared with phenylbutazone and cortisone. J Pharm Pharmacol 7:1022–1031

Bavin EM, Macrae FJ, Seymour DE, Waterhouse PD (1952) The analgesic and antipyretic properties of some derivatives of salicylamide. J Pharm Pharmacol 4:872–878

Beaver WT (1965) Mild analgesics: a review of their clinical pharmacology. Am J Med Sci 250:577–604

Beaver WT (1966) Mild analgesics: A review of their clinical pharmacology. Am J Med Sci 251:576–599

Bellasio E, Testa E (1970) Indagine Sulle Ftalazine III (1,2) – Sintesi di nuovi eterocicli diazotati a potenziale attività antiinfiammatoria ottenuti dal tetraidroftalazin-1-one. Farmaco [Sci] 25:305–313

Berger FM (1954) The pharmacological properties of 2-methyl-2-n-propyl-1,3 propanediol dicarbamate (miltown), a new interneuronal blocking agent. J Pharmacol Exp Ther 112:413–423

Berger FM, Kletzkin M, Ludwig BJ, Margolin S, Powell LS (1959) Unusual muscle relaxant and analgesic properties of N-isopropyl-2-methyl-2-propyl-1,3-propanediol dicarbamate (carisoprodol). J Pharmacol Exp Ther 127:66–73

Berger M, Kletzkin M, Ludwig BJ, Margolin S (1960) The history, chemistry and pharmacology of carisoprodol. Ann NY Acad Sci 86:90–107

Berger FM, Bates HM, Diamantis W, Kletzkin M, Plekss OJ, Sofia RD, Spencer HJ (1973) The pharmacological properties of seclazone (7-chloro-33a-dihydro-2H,9H-isoxazolo[3,2-b][1,3]benzoxazin-9-one). A new anti-inflammatory agent. Pharmacology 9:164–176

Bianchi C, Lumanchi B, Marazzi-Uberti E (1972) Pharmacological investigations of 4-prenyl-1,2-diphenyl-3,5-pyrazolidinedione (DA 2370). Part 1: Antiinflammatory, analgesic and antipyretic properties. Arzneim Forsch 22:183–191

Boots Pure Drug Company Ltd (1967) South African Patent 62/294

Borovsky MP (1960) Antipyretic activity of acetylsalicyclic acid and salicylamide suspension in pediatrics. A comparative clinical evaluation in two hundred six cases. Am J Dis Child 100:47/23–54/30

Brown K, Cavalla JF, Green D, Wilson AB (1968) Diaryloxazole and diarylthiazolealkanoic acids: Two novel series of non-steroidal anti-inflammatory agents. Nature 219:164

Brown K, Cater DP, Cavalla JF, Green D, Newberry RA, Wilson AB (1974) Nonsteroidal antiinflammatory agents. I. 2,4-Diphenylthiazole-5-acetic acid and related compounds. J Med Chem 17:1177–1181

Buckler JW, Adams SS (1968) The phenylalkanoic acids. Laboratory and clinical studies. Med Proc 14:574–578

Buckler RT, Hayao S, Lorenzetti OJ, Sancilio LF, Hartzler HE, Strycker WG (1970) Synthesis and antiinflammatory activity of some aryltetrazolylalkanoic acids. J Med Chem 13:725–729

Buller RH, Miya TS, Carr CJ (1957) The comparative antipyretic activity of acetylsalicylic acid and salicylamide in fever-induced rats. J Pharm Pharmacol 9:128–133

Buss CF (1876) On the antipyretic action of cresotinic acid. Klin Wochenschr 13:445

Buttinoni A, Cuttica A, Franceschini J, Mandelli V, Orsini G, Passerini N, Turba C, Tommasini R (1973) Pharmacological study on a new analgesic-antiinflammatory drug: α-[4-(1-oxo-2-iso-indolinyl)-phenyl]-propionic acid or K 4277. Arzneim Forsch 23:1100–1107

Buu-Höi NP, Lambelin G, Gillet C, Lepoivre C, Thiriaux J, Mees G (1966) Arylacethydroxamic acids: a new class of potent non-steroid anti-inflammatory and analgesic substances. Nature 211:752

Buu-Höi NP, Lambelin G, Gillet C, Roba J, Staquet M (1969) 4-Allyloxy-3-chlorophenylacetic acid, a new type of analgesic, antipyretic and antiphlogistic drug. Naturwissenschaften 56:330–331

Buu-Höi NP, Gillet CL, Lambelin GE, Roba JL, Thiriaux JE (1970) Synthesis and pharmacological properties of substituted cinnamohydroxamic acids. J Med Chem 13:211–213

Cahn A, Hepp P (1886) Das Anpifebrin, ein neues Fiebermittel. Centralbl Klin Med 7:561–564

Campbell WC (1971) Anti-inflammatory and analgesic properties of thiabendazole. JAMA 216:2143

Caprino L, Barrelli F, Falchetti R (1973) Pharmacological research on 4,5-diphenyl-2-bis(2-hydroxyethyl)aminoxazol(Ditazol), a new synthetic oxazole derivative as an antiinflammatory agent. Arzneim Forsch 23:1272–1277

Carson JR, Wong S (1973) 5-Benzoyl-1-methylpyrrole-2-acetic acids as antiinflammatory agents. 2. J Med Chem 16:172–174

Carson JR, McKinstry DN, Wong S (1971) 5-Benzoyl-1-methylpyrrole-2-acetic acids as antiinflammatory agents. J Med Chem 14:646–647

Casadio S, Pala G, Marazzi-Uberti E, Lumachi B, Crescenzi E, Donetti A, Mantegani A, Bianchi C (1972) Terpene compounds as drugs. X. 4-Prenyl-1,2-diphenyl-3,5-pyrazolidinedione (DA 2,370): a new antiinflammatory drug, with low ulcerogenic effects, derived from a series of terpenyl pyrazolidinediones. Arzneim Forsch 22:171–174

Casagrande C, Invernizzi A, Ferrini R, Miragoli G (1971) Indolizine analogues of indomethacin. Farmaco [Sci] 26:1059–1073

Cashin CH, Dawson W, Kitchen EA (1977) The pharmacology of benoxaprofen (2-[4-chlorophenyl]-α-methyl-5-benzoxazole acetic acid), LRCL 3794, a new compound with antiinflammatory activity apparently unrelated to inhibition of prostaglandin synthesis. J Pharm Pharmacol 29:330–336

Clark WG (1979) Mechanisms of antipyretic action. Gen Pharmacol 10:71–77

Clark WG, Coldwell BA (1972) Competitive antagonism of leukocytic pyrogen by sodium salicylate and acetaminophen. Proc Soc Exp Biol Med 141:669–672

Clark WG, Cumby HR (1975) The antipyretic effect of indomethacin. J Physiol (Lond) 248:625–638

Clark RL, Pessolano AA, Witzel B, Lanza T, Shen TY, Van Arman CG, Risley EA (1978) 2-(Substituted phenyl)oxazolo[4,5-b]pyridines and 2-(substituted phenyl)oxazolo[5,4-b]pyridines as non-acidic antiinflammatory agents. J Med Chem 21:1158–1165

Clarke NE, Mosher RE, Clarke CN (1953) Phenolic compounds in the treatment of rheumatic fever. I. A study of gentisic acid derivatives. Circulation 7:247–257

Clarke NE, Clarke CN, Mosher RE (1958) Phenolic compounds in chemotherapy of rheumatic fever. Am J Med Sci 235:7–22

Clémence F, LeMartret O, Fournex R, Plassard G, Dagnaux M (1974) Thiophene derivatives with antiinflammatory and analgesic activities. Eur J Med Chem 9:390–396

Colgan MT, Mintz AA (1957) The comparative antipyretic effect of N-acetyl-p-aminophenol and acetylsalicylic acid. J Pediatr 50:552–555

Collier HOJ, Chesher GB (1956) Antipyretic and analgesic properties of two hydroxyisophthalic acids. Br J Pharmacol 11:20–26

Colot M, Van Damme M, Dirks M, Beersaerts J, Deridder G, Charlier R (1973) Recherches dans la série des indoles. II. Propriétés anti-inflammatories et anti-arthritiques de 1'(isopropyl-2-indolyl)-3-pyridyl-3 cétone. Therapie 28:775–798

Colot M, Van Damme M, Dirks M, Beersaerts J, Charlier R (1974) Antiinflammatory and antiarthritic properties of 5-chloro-3-methylbenz[b]thiofen-2-acetic acid. Arch Int Pharmacodyn Ther 208:328–342

Committee of Revision (1979) Pyrogen test. In: The United States Pharmacopeia, Twentieth Revision, Mack, Easton, Pa, pp 902–903

Coombs R, Houlihan WJ, Nadelson J, Takesue EI (1971) Synthesis and antiinflammatory activity of tert-aminomethylbenzophenones. J Med Chem 14:1072–1074

Coombs RV, Danna RP, Denzer M et al. (1973) Synthesis and anti-inflammatory activity of 1-alkyl-4-aryl-2(1 H)-quinazolinones and quinazolinethiones. J Med Chem 16:1237–1245

Cranston WI, Rawlins MD (1972) Effects of intracerebral micro-injection of sodium salicylate on temperature regulation in the rabbit. J Physiol (Lond) 222:257–266

Cranston WI, Luff RH, Rawlins MD, Wright VA (1971 a) The influence of the duration of experimental fever on salicylate antipyresis in the rabbit. Br J Pharmacol 41:344–351

Cranston WI, Luff RH, Rawlins MD (1971 b) Antipyretic properties of some metabolic and structural analogues of sodium salicylate. J Physiol (Lond) 216:81 P–82 P

Cranston WI, Hellon RF, Mitchell D (1975) A dissociation between fever and PG concentration in the cerebrospinal fluid. J Physiol (Lond) 253:583–592

Cranston WI, Duff GW, Hellon RF, Mitchell D (1976) Effect of a PG antagonist on the pyrexia caused by PGE_2 and leucocyte pyrogen in rabbits. J Physiol (Lond) 256:120–121 P

Davies JE, Kellett DN, Pennington JC (1976) The anti-inflammatory and analgesic effects of Norvedan, a novel non-steroidal agent. Arch Int Pharmacodyn Ther 221:274–282

Demerson CA, Humber LG, Dobson TA, Martel RR (1975) Chemistry and antiinflammatory activities of prodolic acid and related 1,3,4,9-tetrahydropyrano[3,4-b]indole-1-alkanoic acids. 1. J Med Chem 18:189–191

DiPasquale G, Rassaert CL, Richter RS, Tripp LV (1973) The antiinflammatory effects of 4-hydroxy-2-methyl-3-phenylcarbamoyl-2H-1,2-benzothiazine-1,1-dioxide (W 7477). Arch Int Pharmacodyn Ther 203:92–100

Dobner J (1930) Amatin, ein neues, die Diaphorese nicht anregendes Antipyretikum. MMW 77:1103–1104

Domenjoz R (1960) The pharmacology of phenylbutazone analogues. Ann NY Acad Sci 86:263–291

Dorfman RI (1975) Chemistry and pharmacology of naproxen. Arzneim Forsch 25:278–281

Douglas JF, Edelson J, Ludwig BJ (1972) Metabolic fate of 7-chloro-3,3a-dihydro-2H,9H-isoxazolo[3,2-b][1,3]benzoxazin-9-one W-2354. Fed Proc 31:578

Draper MD, Petracek FJ, Klohs MW, McClure DA, Levy L, Ré ON (1972) p-Fluorophenyl-4-(p-fluorphenyl)-4-hydroxy-1-methyl-3-piperidyl ketone (Flazalone): A novel non-steroidal antiinflammatory agent. Arzneim Forsch 22:1803

Dreser H (1899) Pharmakologisches über Aspirin (Acetylsalicylsäure). Pfluegers Arch Ges Physiol 76:306–318

Dunwell DW, Evans D, Hicks TA, Cashin CH, Kitchen A (1975) 2-Aryl-5-benzoxazolealkanoic acid derivatives with notable antiinflammatory activity. J Med Chem 18:53–58

Durant GJ, Smith GM, Spickett RGW (1965) Nonsteroidal antiinflammatory agents. Some arylacetic acids. J Med Chem 8:598–603

Edelson J, Douglas JF, Ludwig BJ (1972) The absorption and distribution of 7-chloro-3,3a-dihydro-2H,9H-isoxazolo[3,2-b][1,3]benzoxazin-9-one, W-2354. Fed Proc 31:578

Ellis KO, Castellion AW, Honkomp LJ, Wessels FJ, Carpenter JF, Halliday RP (1973) Dantrolene, a direct acting skeletal muscle relaxant. J Pharm Sci 62:948–951

Emele JF, Shanaman JE (1967) Analgesic activity of namoxyrate (2-[4-biphenylyl]butyric acid 2-dimethylaminoethanol salt). Arch Int Pharmacodyn Ther 170:99–107

Feldberg W, Gupta KP (1973) Pyrogen fever and prostaglandin activity in cerebrospinal fluid. J Physiol (Lond) 228:41–53

Feldberg W, Milton AS (1979) Prostaglandins and body temperature. In: Vane JR, Ferreira SH (eds) Antiinflammatory drugs. (Handbook of experimental pharmacology, vol 50/I.) Springer, Berlin Heidelberg New York, pp 617–656

Feldberg W, Gupta KP, Milton AS, Wendlandt S (1973) Effects of pyrogen and antipyretics on prostaglandin activity in cisternal CSF of unaneasthetized cats. J Physiol (Lond) 234:279–303

Ferreira SH, Vane JR (1974) New aspects of the mode of action of nonsteroidal anti-inflammatory drugs. Ann Rev Pharmacol 14:57–73

Ferris JP, Boyce CB, Briner RC, Douglas B, Kirkpatrick JL, Weisbach JA (1966) Lythraceae alkaloids. Structure and stereochemistry of the major alkaloids of Decodon and Heimia. Tetrahedron Lett 3641–3649

Fleming JS, Bierwagen ME, Pircio AW, Pindell MH (1969) A new antiinflammatory agent, 1-(4-chlorobenzoyl)-3-(5-tetrazolylmethyl)indole (BL-R 743). Arch Int Pharmacodyn Ther 178:423–436

Flower RJ, Vane JR (1972) Inhibition of prostaglandin synthetase in brain explains the antipyretic activity of paracetamol (4-acetamidophenol). Nature New Biol 240:410–411

Fujimura H (1973) Pharmacological studies on some new quinazoline derivatives. (1). Antiinflammatory and some other properties. Jpn J Pharmacol [Suppl] 23:190

Fujimura H, Tsurumi K, Nozaki M, Hiramatsu Y, Tamura Y, Shimazawa T (1974) Pharmacological studies on H27 and H88, the new quinazoline-2,4-dione derivatives. I. Antiinflammatory, analgesic, and antipyretic activities. Nippon Yakurigaku Zasshi 70:673–695

Gibson KH (1977) Prostaglandins, thromboxanes, PGX: biosynthetic products from arachidonic acid. Chem Soc Rev 6:489–510

Glenn EM, Bowman BJ, Kooyers W, Koslowske T, Myers ML (1967) The pharmacology of 2,3-*bis*-(p-methoxyphenyl)indole (indoxole). J Pharmacol Exp Ther 155:157–166

Gross M, Greenberg LA (1948) The salicylates. A critical bibliographic review. Hillhouse, New Haven, pp 1–7

Gruber CM Jr (1974) Antipyresis with fenprofen. J Clin Pharmacol 14:215–218

Gruber CM Jr, Collins T (1972) Antipyretic effect of fenprofen. J Med Clin Exp 3:242–248

Gund P, Shen TY (1977) A model for the prostaglandin synthetase cyclooxygenation site and its inhibition by antiinflammatory arylacetic acids. J Med Chem 20:1146–1152

Hannah J, Ruyle WV, Kelly K, Matzuk A, Holtz WJ, Witzel BE, Winter CA, Silber RH, Shen TY (1970) Flufenisal – A new salicylate analog. Abstracts Joint Conference of the Chemical Institute of Canada and the American Chemical Society. Toronto, Canada, May 1970. No MEDI 18

Hannah J, Ruyle WV, Jones H, Matzuk AR, Kelly KW, Witzel BE, Holtz WJ, Houser RA, Shen TY, Sarett LH, Lotti VJ, Risley EA, Van Arman CG, Winter CA (1978) Novel analgesic-antiinflammatory salicylates. J Med Chem 21:1093–1099

Harrison GG (1975) Control of the malignant hyperpyretic syndrome in MHS swine by dantrolene sodium. Br J Anaesth 47:62–65

Harrison IT, Lewis B, Nelson P, Rooks W, Roszkowski A, Tomolonis A, Fried JH (1970) Nonsteroidal antiinflammatory agents. I. 6-Substituted 2-naphthylacetic acids. J Med Chem 13:203–205

Harvey CA, Milton AS, Straughan DW (1975) Prostaglandin E_1 levels in cerebral spinal fluid of rabbits and the effects of bacterial pyrogen and antipyretic drugs. J Physiol (Lond) 248:26–27P

Hepworth W, Newbould BB, Platt DS, Stacy GJ (1969) 2-(4-Chlorophenyl) thiazol-4-ylacetic acid ("Myalex"): A new compound with anti-inflammatory, analgesic and antipyretic activity. Nature Lond 221:582–583

Hoyland JR, Kier LB (1972) Preferred conformation of prostaglandin E_1. J Med Chem 15:84–86

Hucker HB, Stauffer SC, White SD et al. (1973) Physiologic disposition and metabolic fate of a new antiinflammatory agent, *cis*-5-fluoro-2-methyl-1-[p-methylsulfinyl)benzylindenyl]indene-3-acetic acid in the rat, dog, rhesus monkey, and man. Drug Metab Dispos 1:721–736

Iizuka Y, Tanaka K (1972) Antiinflammatory effect of bimetopyrol. II. Suppressive effect on adjuvant arthritis in rats. J Pharm Soc Jpn 92:11–18

Janssen PAJ (1975) Suprofen (R 25061), a new potent inhibitor of prostaglandin biosynthesis. Arzneim Forsch 25:1495

Jones CJ (1976) The pharmacology and pharmacokinetics of azapropazone – a review. Curr Med Res Opinion 4:3–15

Jones H, Fordice MW, Greenwald RB et al. (1978) Synthetic and analgesic-antiinflammatory activity of some 4- and 5-substituted heteroarylsalicylic acids. J Med Chem 21:1100–1104

Juby PF, Hudyma TW (1969) Preparation and antiinflammatory properties of some 1-substituted 3-(5-tetrazoylmethyl)indoles and homologs. J Med Chem 12:396–400

Juby PF, Goodwin WR, Hudyma TW, Partyka RA (1972a) Antiinflammatory activity of some indan-1-carboxylic acids and related compounds. J Med Chem 15:1297–1306

Juby PF, Goodwin WR, Hudyma TW, Partyka RA (1972b) Antiinflammatory activity and structure-activity relationship of some 1,2,3,4-tetrahydro-1-naphthoic acids and related compounds. J Med Chem 15:1306–1319

Julou L, Guyonnet J-C (1967) Propriétés anti-inflammatories de l'acide (méthyl-10-phénothiazinyl-2) acétique (16091 R.P.). CR Acad Sci [D] Paris 265:1007–1010

Julou L, Guyonnet J-C, Ducrot R, Bardone MC, Detaille GY, Laffargue B (1969) General pharmacological properties of metiazinic acid (16091 R.P.). Arzneim Forsch 19:1198–1206

Julou L, Guyonnet J-C, Ducrot R, Garret C, Bardone MC, Maignan G, Pasquet J (1971) Study of the pharmacological properties of a new anti-inflammatory drug: 2-(3-benzoylphenyl)-propionic acid (19583 R.P.). J Pharmacol (Paris) 2:259–286

Kadatz R (1957) Pharmakologische Eigenschaften des 2-(β-Chloroethyl)-2,3-dihydro-4-oxo-(benzo-1,3-oxazin), eines neuen Antiphlogisticum. Arzneim Forsch 7:651–653

Kadin SB, Wiseman BH (1969) Dioxoisoquinoline-4-carboxanilides – a new class of non-steroidal anti-inflammatory agents. Nature Lond 222:275–276

Kaltenbronn JS (1973) 4- and 5-Aryl-1-naphthaleneacetic acids as antiinflammatory agents. J Med Chem 16:490–493

Kaplan HR, Wolke RE, Malone MH (1967) Anti-inflammatory evaluation of cryogenine. J Pharm Sci 56:1385–1392

Kawai K, Kuzuna S, Morimoto S, Ishii H, Matsumoto N (1971) Antiinflammatory, analgesic, and antipyretic activities of 6-chloro-5-cyclohexylinden-1-carboxylic acid (TAI-284). Jpn J Pharmacol 21:621–639

Knoll J, Gyires K, Mészáros Z (1979) 1,6-Dimethyl-4-oxo-1,6,7,8,9a-hexahydro-4H-pyrido[1,2-a]pyrimidine-3-carboxamide (Chinoin-127), a potent non-narcotic analgesic and antiinflammatory agent. Arzneim Forsch 29:766–773

Knorr L (1883) Entwirkung von Acetessigester auf Phenylhydrazine. Ber 16:2597–2599

Knorr L (1884) Ueber die Constitution des Chinizin Derivatives. Ber 17:2032–2049

Kobayashi S, Takagi H (1968) Pharmacological studies of a new antiinflammatory compound, 2-phenyl-6-dimethylamino-6H-cyclohept oxazole. Arzneim Forsch 18:1352–1354

Koch-Weser J (1976 Acetaminophen. N Eng J Med 295:1297–1300

Komatsu T, Awata H, Sakai Y, Inukai T, Yamamoto M, Inaba S, Yamamoto H (1972) Novel quinazoline derivatives. I. Synthesis and preliminary pharmacological evaluation of an anti-inflammatory agent, SL-573. Arzneim Forsch 22:1958–1962

Lambelin G, Büu-Hoi NP, Brouihet H, Gautier M, Gillet C, Roba J, Thiriaux J (1968) Relationships between structure and four types of pharmacologic activity in arylacethydroxamic acids. Arzneim Forsch 18:1404–1408

Lambelin G, Roba J, Gillet C, Büu-Hoi NP (1970) Pharmacology of a new analgesic, antipyretic and anti-inflammatory agent, 4-allyloxy-3-chlorophenylacetic acid. Arzneim Forsch 20:610–618

Lang SA Jr, Johnson BD, Cohen E, Sloboda AE, Greenblatt E (1976) Aryl-s-tetrazines with antiinflammatory activity. J Med Chem 19:1404–1409

Lassman HB, Wilker JC, Anderson VB, Agnew MN, Allen RC, Novick WJ Jr (1978) Fendosal (HP 129): A potent antiinflammatory and analgesic compound. Agents Actions 8:209–217

Lee EB, Shin KH, Woo WS (1968) Synthesis and pharmacology of p-methoxycinnamic acid derivates. J Med Chem 11:1262–1263

Levy L, McClure D (1976) The pharmacology of flazalone: A new class of anti-inflammatory agent. J Pharmacol Exp Ther 198:473–480

Lin MT, Chai CY (1972) The antipyretic effect of sodium acetylsalicylate on pyrogen-induced fever in rabbits. J Pharmacol Exp Ther 180:603–609

Lindner E (1973) The antipyretic action of pyrazolones, derivatives of phenacetin and other new substances. In: Schönbaum E, Lomax P (eds) The pharmacology of thermoregulation. Symposium, San Francisco, 1972. Karger, Basel, pp 325–344

Lombardino JG (1974) Enolic acids with antiinflammatory activity. In: Scherrer AA, Whitehouse MW (eds) Antiinflammatory agents, chemistry, and pharmacology, vol 1. Academic Press, New York, pp 129–157

Lombardino JG, Wiseman EH (1971) Antiinflammatory 3,4-dihydro-2-alkyl-3-oxo-2H-1,2-benzothiazine-4-carboxamide 1,1-dioxides. J Med Chem 14:973–977

Lombardino JG, Wiseman EH (1972) Sudoxicam and related N-heterocyclic carboxamides of 4-hydroxy-2H-1,2-benzothiazine-1,1-dioxide. Potent nonsteroidal antiinflammatory agents. J Med Chem 15:848–849

Lombardino JG, Wiseman EH, McLamore WM (1971) Synthesis and antiinflammatory activity of some 3-carboxamides of 2-alkyl-4-hydroxy-2H-1,2-benzothiazine-1,1-dioxide. J Med Chem 14:1171–1175

Lombardino JG, Wiseman EH, Chiani J (1973) Potent antiinflammatory N-heterocyclic 3-carboxamides of 4-hydroxy-2-methyl-2H-1,2-benzothiazine-1,1-dioxide. J Med Chem 16:493–496

Lombardino JC, Otterness IG, Wiseman EH (1975) Acidic antiinflammatory agents – correlations of some physical, pharmacological and clinical data. Arzneim Forsch 25:1629–1635

Loux JJ, DePalma PD, Yankell SL (1972) Antipyretic testing of aspirin in rats. Toxicol Appl Pharmacol 22:672–675

Marazzi-Uberti E, Turba C (1966) α-isopropyl-α-(2-dimethylaminoethyl)-1-naphthylacetamide (naphthypramide, DA 992): A new antiinflammatory agent. I. Antiinflammatory activity and acute toxicity. Arch Int Pharmacodyn Ther 162:378–396

Marazzi-Uberti E, Turba C, Erba G (1966) α-isopropyl-α-(2-dimethylaminoethyl)-1-naphthylacetamide (naphthypramide, DA 992): A new antiinflammatory agent. II. Antipyretic, analgesic and C.N.S. depressant activity. Arch Int Pharmacodyn Ther 162:398–412

Marchetti E, Mattalia G, Rosnati V (1968) A new class of analgetic-antiinflammatory agents. 2-Substituted 4,5-diphenyloxazoles. J Med Chem 11:1092–1093

Marmo E, Rossi F, DiNola R, Cazzola F (1974) Experimentation of an anti-reactional, antalgic, and antipyretic drug (2-phenyl-4-chlorophenylthiazol-5-yl acetic acid). Gazz Med Ital 133:337–344

Martel RR, Klicius J (1976) Antiinflammatory and analgesic properties of etodolic acid in rats. Can J Physiol Pharmacol 54:245–248

Martel RR, Klicius J, Herr F (1974a) Investigation of 1,3,4,9-tetrahydro-1-propyl-pyrano[3,4-b]indole-1-acetic acid (prodolic acid), a new nonsteroidal anti-inflammatory agent, in rats. Agents Actions 4:370–376

Martel RR, Rochefort JG, Klicius J, Dobson TA (1974b) Antiinflammatory properties of furobufen. Can J Physiol Pharmacol 52:669–673

Messer M, Farge D (1967) Synthése des acides (méthyl-10-phénothiazinyl) acétiques. C R Acad Sci [C] 265:758–761

Messer PM, Farge D, Guyonnet J-C, Jeanmart C, Julou L (1969) Acidic derivatives of phenothiazin. Arzneim Forsch 19:1193–1198

Meyer K, Ragan C (1948) The antirheumatic effect of sodium gentisate. Science 108:281

Mielke CH Jr, Heiden D, Britten AF, Ramos J, Flavell P (1976) Hemostatis, antipyretics, and mild analgesics. Acetominophen vs. aspirin. JAMA 235:613–616

Milton AS, Wendlandt S (1965) The effect of 4-acetamidophenol in reducing fever produced by the intracerebral injection of 5-hydroxytryptamine and pyrogen in the conscious cat. Br J Pharmacol 34:215 P–216 P

Milton AS, Wendlandt S (1970) A possible role for prostaglandin E$_1$ as a modulator for temperature regulation in the central nervous system of the cat. J Physiol (Lond) 207:76–77 P

Minakami H, Takagi H, Kobayashi S (1964) Pharmacological studies of a new analgesic and antiinflammatory agent, 1-benzylcycloheptimidazol-2(1H)-one, (RCH-314). Life Sci 3:305–314

Naito T, Yoshikawa T, Kitahara S, Aoki N (1969) Studies on pyrimidinylpyrazoles. I. Syntheses of 1- and 2-pyrimidinyl-3-methylpyrazolin-5-one derivatives. Chem Pharm Bull (Tokyo) 17:1467–1478

Nakamura H, Kadokawa T, Nakatsuji K, Nakamura K (1970) Pharmacological studies of a new antiinflammatory drug, 1-phenylsulfonyl-5,5-diphenylhydantoin (PG-796) in experimental animals. I. Antiinflammatory, analgesic and antipyretic activity. Arzneim Forsch 20:1032–1046

Nakanishi M, Imamura H, Maruyama Y, Hoshino H (1970a) Studies on antiinflammatory agents. I. Some biological activities of thienopyridine derivatives. Yakugaku Zasshi 90:272–276

Nakanishi M, Imamura H, Maruyama Y (1970b) Studies on antiinflammatory agents. II. Analgesic and anti-edematous activities of 2-amino-3-ethoxycarbonyl-6-benzyl-4,5,6,7-tetrahydrothieno[2,3-c]pyridine. Yakugaku Zasshi 90:277–283

Nakanishi M, Imamura H, Maruyama Y (1970c) Studies on antiinflammatory agents. III. Effect of 2-amino-3-ethoxycarbonyl-6-benzyl-4,5,6,7-tetrahydro[2,3-c]pyridine (Y-3642) on pyretic reaction, vascular permeability and granuloma formation in experimental animals. Yakugaku Zasshi 90:284–290

Nakanishi M, Imamura H, Maruyama Y (1970 d) Pharmacological investigations of 2-amino-3-ethoxycarbonyl-6-benzyl-4,5,6,7-tetrahydrothieno[2,3-c]pyridine. Part I. Arzneim Forsch 20:998–1003

Nakanishi M, Imamura H, Ikegami K, Goto K (1970 e) Pharmacological investigations of 2-amino-3-ethoxycarbonyl-6-benzyl-4,5,6,7-tetrahydrathieno[2,3-c]pyridine. Part II. Arzneim Forsch 20:1004–1009

Nannini G, Giraldi PN, Malgora G et al. (1973) New analgesic-antiinflammatory drugs. Arzneim Forsch 23:1090–1100

Newbould BB (1969) The pharmacology of fenclozic acid (2-(4-chlorophenyl)-thiazol-4-glacetic acid; I.C.I. 54,450; "Myalex"); a new compound with anti-inflammatory, analgesic, and antipyretic activity. Br J Pharmacol 35:487–497

Nickander RC, Kraay RJ, Marshall WS (1971) Antiinflammatory and analgesic effects of fenoprofen. Fed Proc 30:563

Niemegeers CJE, Verbruggen FJ, Janssen PAJ (1964) Effect of various drugs on carrageenin-induced oedema in the rat hind paw. J Pharm Pharmacol 16:810–816

Niemegeers CJE, Lenaerts FM, Janssen PAJ (1975) The antipyretic effect of suprofen in rats with yeast-induced fever. Arzneim Forsch 25:1519–1524

Noguchi S, Kishimoto S, Minamida I, Obayashi M, Kawakita K (1971) 6-Chloro-5-cyclohexylinden-1-carboxylic acid (TAI-284), a new antiinflammatory agent. Chem Pharm Bull (Tokyo) 19:646–648

Nuss GW, Smyth RD, Breder CH, Hitchings MJ, Mir GN, Reavey-Cantwell NH (1976) The antiphlogistic, antinociceptive and antipyretic properties of fenclorac. Agents Actions 6:735–747

Olson DR, Wheeler WJ, Wells JN (1974) Rigid analogs of indomethacin. J Med Chem 17:167–171

Ory M (1949) Premiers essais thérapeutiques de l'acide gentisique dans les affections rheumatismales. Brux Med 29:1401

Oshima Y, Akimoto T, Tsukada W, Yamasaki T, Yamaguchi K, Kojima H (1969) Studies on pyrimidinylpyrazoles. IV. Pharmacological activities of 1-(4-methoxy-6-methyl-2-pyrimidinyl)-3-methyl-5-methoxypyrazole and its related compounds. Chem Pharm Bull (Tokyo) 17:1492–1497

Pala G, Casadio S, Bruzzese T, Crescenzi E, Marazzi-Uberti E (1965) Structure-activity relationships in antiinflammatory and analgesic compounds chemically related to α-isopropyl-2-(2-dimethylaminoethyl)-1-naphthylacetamide. J Med Chem 8:698–700

Pala G, Bruzzese T, Marrazi-Uberti E, Coppi G (1966) Synthesis and pharmacological evaluation of α-substituted 1-naphthylacetic acids. J Med Chem 9:603–605

Phillip-Dormston WK, Siegert R (1974) Prostaglandins of the E and F series in rabbit cerebrospinal fluid during fever induced by Newcastle disease virus, E. Coli-endotoxin or endogenous pyrogens. Med Microbiol Immunol (Berl) 159:279–284

Pircio AW, Bierwagen ME, Strife WE, Nicolosi WD (1972) Pharmacology of a new nonsteroidal antiinflammatory agent 5-cyclohexylindan-1-carboxylic acid. Arch Int Pharmacodyn Ther 199:151–163

Pittman QJ, Veable WL, Cooper KE (1975) Temperature responses of lambs after centrally injected PGs and pyrogens. Am J Physiol 228:1034–1038

Plazzo G, Carsi G, Baiocchi L, Silvestrini B (1966) Synthesis and pharmacological properties of 1-substituted 3-dimethylaminoalkoxy-1 H-indazoles. J Med Chem 9:38–41

Randall LO, Baruth H (1976) Analgesic and antiinflammatory activity of 6-chloro-α-methyl-carbazole-2-acetic acid (C-5720). Arch Int Pharmacodyn Ther 220:94–114

Reid J, Watson RD, Cochran JB, Sproull DH (1951) Sodium γ-resorcylate in rheumatic fever. Br Med J 2:321–325

Reisner DB, Ludwig BJ, Stiefel FJ, Gister S, Meyer M, Powell LS, Sofia RD (1977a) Synthesis and antiinflammatory activity of 3,3a-dihydro-2H,9H-isoxazolo[3,2-b][1,3]-benzoxazin-9-ones and related compounds. Arzneim Forsch 27:760–766

Reisner DB, Ludwig BJ, Simon E, Dejneka T (1977b) Pharmacological properties of 2,3-dihydro-9H-isoxazolo[3,2-b]quinazolin-9-one (W-2429). Arzneim Forsch 27:766–770

Robichaud RC, Malone MH, Schwarting AE (1964) Pharmacodynamics of cryogenine, an alkaloid isolated from Heimia salicifolia link and otto. Part I. Arch Int Pharmacodyn Ther 150:220–232

Rohte O (1971) Tierpharmakologische Versuche mit Leo 1028, einer neuen Substanz mit antiphlogistischen, analgetischen und antipyretischen Eigenschaften. Acta Pharmacol Toxicol [Suppl 4] 29:47

Rooks WH II, Tomolonis AJ, Maloney PJ, Wallach MB, Schuler ME (1979) The analgesic and antiinflammatory profile of ($\pm$)-5-benzoyl-1,2-dihydro-3H-pyrrolo[1,2-a]pyrrole-1-carboxylic acid (DPP). Fed Proc 38:1115

Roszkowski AP, Rooks WH II, Tomolonis AJ, Miller LM (1971) Antiinflammatory and analgesic properties of d-2-(6'-methoxy-2'-naphthyl)-propionic acid (Naproxen). J Pharmacol Exp Ther 179:114–123

Sato M, Tanizawa H, Fukuda T, Yuizono T (1979) Pharmacological investigations of 4-alkoxy-2-methyl-5-morpholino-3(2H)-pyridazinone derivatives. Jpn J Pharmacol 29:303–306

Schaaf TK (1977) Modulation of the arachidonic acid cascade. In: Clarke FH (ed) Annual reports in medicinal chemistry, vol 12. Academic Press, New York, pp 182–190

Schaefer LE, Rashkoff IA, Megibow RS (1950) Sodium gentisate in the treatment of acute rheumatic fever. Circulation 2:265–270

Scherrer RA (1974) Introduction to the chemistry of antiinflammatory and antiarthritic agents. In: Scherrer RA, Whitehouse MW (eds) Antiinflammatory agents, chemistry and pharmacology, vol 1. Academic Press, New York, pp 29–43

Scherrer RA, Winder CV, Short FW (1964) The antiinflammatory N-arylanthranilic acids. National Medicinal Chemistry Symposium (ACS Medicinal Chem Div) Abstract Proceedings, pp 11a–11i

Schiatti P, Selva D, Arrigoni-Martelli E, Lerner LJ, Diena A, Sardi A, Maffii G (1974) Antiinflammatory activity and other pharmacological properties of phthalazino-[2,3-b]-phthalazine-5,12(7H,14H)-dione (Diftalone). Arzneim Forsch 24:2003–2009

Schoener EP, Wang SC (1975) Observations on the central mechanism of acetylsalicylate antipyresis. Life Sci 17:1063–1068

Senda S, Izumi H, Fujimura H (1967) Über Uracil-Derivate und verwandte Verbindungen. Arzneim Forsch 17:1519–1523

Senda S, Hirota K, Banno K (1972) Pyrimidine derivatives and related compounds. 15. Synthesis and analgetic and antiinflammatory activities of 1,3-substituted 5-amino-6-methyluracil derivatives. J Med Chem 15:471–476

Shen TY (1965) Synthesis and biological activity of some indomethacin analogs. Excerpta Med Int Congr Ser 82:13–20

Shen TY (1967a) Anti-inflammatory agents. In: Rabinowitz JL, Myerson RM (eds) Topics in medicinal chemistry, vol 1. Interscience Publisher, New York, pp 29–78

Shen TY (1967b) Antiinflammatory arylacetic acid derivatives. Chim Ther 2:459–461

Shen TY, Windholz TB, Rosegay A et al. (1963) Non-steroid antiinflammatory agents. J Am Chem Soc 85:488–489

Shen TY, Ham EA, Cirillo VJ, Zanetti M (1974) Structure-activity relationship of certain prostaglandin synthetase inhibitors. In: Robinson HJ, Vane JR (eds) Prostaglandin synthetase inhibitors. Raven, New York, pp 19–31

Shen TY, Winter CA (1977) Clinical and biological studies on indomethacin, sulindac and their analogs. Adv Drug Res 12:89–246

Shibata Y (1977) Antiinflammatory, analgesic and other related actions of 4'-chloro-5-methoxy-3-biphenylacetic acid (DKA-9). Arzneim Forsch 27:2299–2308

Silvestrini B, Gorau A, Pozzatti C, Cioli V (1966) Pharmacological research on benzydamine – a new analgesic-antiinflammatory drug. Arzneim Forsch 16:59–63

Similä S, Kouvalainen K, Keinänen S (1977) Oral antipyretic therapy. Evaluation of mefenamic acid (short communication). Arzneim Forsch 27:687–688

Snyder HR, Davis CS, Bickerton RK, Halliday RP (1967) 1-[(5-arylfurfurylidene)amino]hydantoins. A new class of muscle relaxants. J Med Chem 10:807–810

Sofia RD, Diamantis W, Gordon R et al. (1974) Pharmacology of a new nonsteroidal antiinflammatory agent, 7-chloro-3,3a-dihydro-2-methyl-2H,9H-isoxazolo[3,2-b][1,3]benzoxazin-9-one (W-2395). Eur J Pharmacol 26:51–62

Sofia RD, Diamantis W, Ludig BJ (1977) Pharmacological properties of 2,3-dihydro-9*H*-isoxazolo[3,2-2β]quinazolin-9-one (W-2429). Arzneim Forsch 27:770–782

Soma N, Nakazawa J, Watanabe T, Sato Y, Sunagawa G (1967) Studies on seven-membered ring compounds. XXIII. Reaction of tropylium ions having fused heterocyclic system with various amines. Chem Pharm Bull (Tokyo) 15:627–633

Stenzl H, Staub A, Simon C, Baumann W (1950) 3-amino-5-pyrazolones. Helv Chem Acta 33:1183–1194

Stockman R (1912) The therapeutic action of cresotinic acid. J Pharmacol Exp Ther 4:97–108

Stone CA, Van Arman CG, Lotti VJ et al. (1977) Pharmacology and toxicology of diflunisal. Br J Clin Pharmacol 4:19S–29S

Stone E (1763) An account of the success of the bark of the willow – the cure of agues. Philos Trans R Soc Lond 53:195–200

Swingle KF, Scherrer RA, Grant TJ (1975) Antiinflammatory activity of α-methyl-3-phenyl-7-benzofuranacetic acid (R-803). Arch Int Pharmacodyn Ther 214:240–249

Szmuskovicz J, Glenn EM, Heinzelman RV, Hester JB Jr, Youngdale GA (1966) Synthesis and antiinflammatory activity of 2,3-*bis* (*p*-methoxyphenyl)indole and related compounds. J Med Chem 9:527–536

Takashima T, Kadoh Y, Kumada S (1972) Pharmacological investigations of benzothiazoline derivatives. Arzneim Forsch 22:711–715

Takesue EI, Perrine JW, Trapold JH (1976) The antiinflammatory profile of praquazone. Arch Int Pharmacodyn Ther 221:122–131

Tamura Y, Yoshimoto Y, Kunimoto K et al. (1977) Nonsteroidal antiinflammatory agents. 1. 5-Alkoxy-3-biphenylylacetic acids and related compounds as new potential antiinflammatory agents. J Med Chem 20:709–714

Tanaka K, Iizuka Y (1972) Antiinflammatory effect of bimetopyrol. I. Suppressive effect on acute inflammation. J Pharm Soc Jpn 92:1–10

Tanaka K, Iizuka Y, Yoshida N, Tomita K, Masuda H (1972) Diaryl pyrroles: a new series of antiinflammatory agents. Experientia 28:937–938

Teotino UM, Friz P, Gandini A, Bella DD (1963) Thioderivatives of 2,3-dihydro-4*H*-1,3-benzoxazin-4-one. Synthesis and pharmacological properties. J Med Chem 6:248–250

Testoni F, Strano A (1950) Clinical research on the treatment of acute articular rheumatism with sodium gentisate. Minerva Med 41 (II):450–456

Tricerri S, Panto E, Bianchetti A, Bossoni G, Venturini R (1979) Synthesis and preliminary pharmacological data on zidometacin, a new antiinflammatory compound. Eur J Med Chem 14:181–183

Tsukada W, Tsubokawa M, Masukawa T, Kojima H, Kasahara A (1978) Pharmacological study of 6,11-dihydro-11-oxodibenz[b,e]oxepin-3-acetic acid (oxepinac): a new antiinflammatory drug. Arzneim Forsch 28:428–438

Tubaro E, Banci F (1970) Pharmacology of a nicotinamidomethylaminopyrazolone (Ra 101). Arzneim Forsch 20:1019–1023

Ueno K, Kubo S, Tagawa H et al. (1976) 6,11-Dihydro-11-oxodibenz[b,e]oxepinacetic acids with potent antiinflammatory activity. J Med Chem 19:941–946

Unterhalt B (1970) Untersuchungen an neueren Antiphlogistica. Arch Pharm (Weinheim) 303:445–456

Van Arman CG, Bohidar NR (1978) Antiarthritics. In: Rubin AA (ed) New drugs – discovery and development. (Drugs and pharmaceutical sciences, vol 5). Dekker, New York, pp 1–27

Van Arman CG, Campbell WC (1975) Anti-inflammatory activity of thiabendazole and its relation to parasitic disease. Tex Rep Biol Med 33:303–311

Van Arman CG, Risley EA, Nuss GW, Hucker HB, Duggan DE (1976) Pharmacology of sulindac. In: Huskisson EC, Franchimont P (eds) Clinoril in the treatment of rheumatic disorders. Raven, New York, pp 9–36

Van Daele PGH, Boey JM, Sipido VK, DeBruyn MFL, Janssen PAJ (1975) Synthesis of α-methyl-4-(2-thienylcarbonyl)benzeneacetic acid, suprofen, and derivatives. Arzneim Forsch 25:1495–1501

Vane JR (1971) Inhibition of prostaglandin synthesis as a mechanism of action of aspirin-like drugs. Nature New Biol 231:232–235

Veale WL, Cooper KE (1974) Evidence for the involvement of prostaglandins in fever. In: Lederis K, Cooper KE (eds) Recent studies of hypothalamic function. Int Symp, Calgary, 1973. Karger, Basel, pp 359–370

Veale WL, Cooper KE (1975) Comparison of sites of action of PG E$_1$ leucocyte pyrogen in brain. In: Schönbaum E, Lomax P, Jacob J (eds) Temperature regulation and drug action. Karger, Basel, pp 218–226

Vignec AJ, Gasparik M (1958) Antipyretic effectiveness of salicylamide and acetylsalicylic acid in infants. A comparative study. JAMA 167:1821–1826

von Gerhardt C (1853) Untersuchungen über die wasserfreien organischen Säuren. Liebigs Ann 87:149–178

von Mering J (1893) Ueber die Function des Magens. Ther Monatsch (Berl) 7:201–204

Wada J, Suzuki T, Iwasaki M, Miyamatsu H, Ueno S, Shimizu M (1973) A new nonsteroidal antiinflammatory agent. 2-Substituted 5- or 6-benzothiazoleacetic acids and their derivatives. J Med Chem 16:930–934

Walford GL, Jones H, Shen TY (1971) Aza analogs of 5-(p-fluorophenyl) salicylic acid. J Med Chem 14:339–344

Warren MR, Warren HW (1946) The evaluation of antipyretics against pyrogen-induced fever. J Am Pharm Assoc 35:257–259

Watnick AS, Taber RI, Tabachnick IIA (1971) Anti-inflammatory and analgesic properties of clonixin [2-(2-methyl-3-chloroanilino)nicotinic acid]. Arch Int Pharmacodyn Ther 190:78–90

Weisbach JW, Kirkpatrick JL, Madso E, Douglas B (1968) Synthesis and pharmacology of some α-keto-, α-hydroxy-, and α-amino-1-benzylisoquinolines. J Med Chem 11:760–764

Westby TR, Barfknecht CF (1973) Acridan-4-carboxylic acids and N-aryl-2-amino-3-toluic acids as planar and antiplanar analogs of antiinflammatory N-arylanthranilic acids. J Med Chem 16:40–43

Whitehouse MW (1964) Biochemical properties of anti-inflammatory drugs. III. Uncoupling of oxidative phosphorylation in a connective tissue (cartilage) and liver mitochondria by salicylate analogues: relationship of structure to activity. Biochem Pharmacol 13:319–336

Whitehouse MW, Haslam JM (1962) Ability of some antirheumatic drugs to uncouple oxidative phosphorylation. Nature 196:1323–1324

Wiesinger D, Gubler HU, Haefliger W, Hauser D (1974) Antiinflammatory activity of the new mould metabolite 11-desacetoxy-wartmannin and of some of its derivatives. Experientia 30:135–136

Winder CV, Wax J, Scotti L, Scherrer RA, Jones EM, Short FW (1962) Anti-inflammatory, antipyretic and antinociceptive properties of N-(2,3-xylyl)anthranilic acid (mefenamic acid). J Pharmacol Exp Ther 138:405–413

Winder CV, Kaump DH, Glazko AJ, Holmes EL (1967) Pharmacology of the fenamates. Experimental observations on flufenamic, mefenamic, and meclofenamic acids. Ann Phys Med [Suppl] 7–49

Winter CA (1965) Anti-inflammatory testing method: Comparative evaluation of indomethacin and other agents. Int Congr Ser 82:190–202

Winter CA, Nuss GW (1963) Pyretogenic effects of bacterial lipopolysaccharide and the assay of antipyretic drugs in rats. Toxicol Appl Pharmacol 5:247–256

Winter CA, Risley EA, Nuss GW (1963) Anti-inflammatory and antipyretic activities of indomethacin, 1-(p-chlorobenzoyl)-5-methoxy-2-methylindole-3-acetic acid. J Pharmacol Exp Ther 141:369–376

Wit A, Wang SC (1968) Temperature-sensitive neurons in preoptic/anterior hypothalamic region: actions of pyrogen and acetylsalicylate. Am J Physiol 215:1160–1169

Witthauer K (1899) Aspirin, ein neues Salicylpräparat. Ther Mh 13:330

Wohlgemut J (1899) Über Aspirin (Acetylsalicylsäure). Ther Mh 13:276–278

Wong S, Gardocki JF, Pruss TP (1973) Pharmacologic evaluation of tolectin (tolmetin, McN-2559) and McN-2891, two antiinflammatory agents. J Pharmacol Exp Ther 185:127–138

Woo WS (1963) Pharmacologically active component in Scrophularia root, *p*-methoxycinnamic acid. I. Identification of *p*-methoxycinnamic acid and its antipyretic action. Yakhak Hoechi 7:55–57

Yamamoto H, Saito C, Okamoto T, Awata H, Inukai T, Hirohashi A, Yukawa Y (1969) Synthesis and pharmacology of a new potential anti-inflammatory drug, 1-(3′,4′-methylenedioxybenzoyl)-2-methyl-5-methoxy-3-indolylacetic acid (ID 955). Arzneim Forsch 19:981–984

Yamamoto H, Saito C, Inaba S, Awata H, Yamamoto M, Sakai Y, Komatsu T (1973) Novel quinazoline derivatives. II. A new antiinflammatory agent, SL-512. Arzneim Forsch 23:1266–1271

Zimmermann D (1875) Ein Beitrag zur Kenntnis der antifebrilen Wirksamkeit der Salicylsäure. Arch Exp Pathol Pharmakol 4:248–250

CHAPTER 13

Therapeutic Agents Affecting Body Temperature

R. G. PERTWEE

A. Introduction

This chapter surveys the effects on mammalian thermoregulation of general anaesthetics, barbiturates, narcotic analgesics, and phenothiazines, all of which can produce increases as well as decreases in deep-body temperature. In addition to an account of the various factors which influence the degree or direction of temperature change produced by single drug administration, this review contains discussions of how repeated drug administration can give rise to tolerance and of the thermoregulatory changes which may be precipitated by withdrawal of drug treatment. There are also discussions of possible sites and mechanisms of action, of drug effects on heat gain and heat loss mechanisms and of drug interactions giving rise to hyperthermic responses. Drug effects on human thermoregulation have been discussed separately. However, as will be seen, the human data are in general agreement with results obtained in animal experiments.

An important effect of general anaesthetics not discussed in this chapter is malignant hyperthermia. This has been reviewed in Chap. 17.

B. Effects of General Anaesthetics, Barbiturates, Narcotic Analgesics and Phenothiazines on Thermoregulation in Mammalian Species Other than Humans

I. Effects on Body Temperature

1. General Anaesthetics and Barbiturates

At ambient temperatures of 26 °C or less general anaesthetics and barbiturates can lower deep-body temperature in a wide range of species. Falls in deep-body temperature have been observed with pentobarbitone in cats (BANERJEE et al. 1968 b; EKSTRÖM 1951; FELDBERG and LOTTI 1967; FELDBERG and MYERS 1964; STRÖM 1950), dogs (CHATONNET and TANCHE 1959; EKSTRÖM 1951; HEMINGWAY 1941; KROG 1959), rabbits (FELDBERG and LOTTI 1967), rats (GEMMILL and BROWNING 1962; HERRMANN 1941; LOMAX 1966; ISOM et al. 1978), guinea-pigs and hamsters (BREESE et al. 1975), gerbils (BREESE et al. 1975; JÄRBE and HOLMGREN 1977), and mice (BREESE et al. 1975; DANDIYA and SELLERS 1961; HO 1976; MODAK et al. 1976; YAMAMOTO et al. 1978). Hypothermia has also been reported in one or more of these species following administration of amylobarbitone (BREESE et al. 1975; DAUDOVA 1961; HEMINGWAY 1941), thiopentone and secobarbitone (BREESE et al. 1975), phenobarbitone (BREESE et al. 1975; FLACKE et al. 1953; ROSENTHAL 1941), barbitone (Tahara 1962; Thauer 1943), ethanol (Abdallah and Roby 1975; Carvalho and Izquierdo 1977; Erickson et al. 1978; Flacke et al. 1953; Freund 1973; Järbe and Ohlin 1977; Kakihana 1977; Nikki et al. 1971; Pohorecky et al. 1974, 1976; Pohorecky and Jaffe 1975; Ritzmann and Tabakoff 1976a; Seed and Sechelski 1977; Strömbom et al. 1977; Werner 1941), paraldehyde (Herrmann 1941; Rosenthal 1941; Thauer 1943), chloralose (Breese et al. 1975; Feldberg and Lotti 1967; Feldberg and Myers 1964; Thauer 1943), urethane (Grant and Robbins 1949; Hauk and Ankermann 1963), diethyl ether (Hemingway 1948; Lindqvist et al. 1974; Paton and Speden 1965; Pertwee 1970), methoxyflurane (Mäkeläinen 1974; Nikki 1968; Nikki and Tammisto 1968; Paton and Speden 1965; Vapaatalo et al. 1975), halothane (Chambers et al. 1978; Eger et al. 1965; Feldberg and Lang 1970; Mäkeläinen et al. 1973a; Nikki 1968; Nikki and Tammisto 1968; Summers 1969; Vapaatalo et al. 1975), fluroxene and enflurane (Vapaatalo et al. 1975), cyclopropane (Eger et al. 1965), and nitrous oxide (Pertwee 1970).

The degree and rate of onset of hypothermia induced by general anaesthetics and barbiturates have been shown to be inversely related to ambient temperature (Krog 1959; Lomax 1966; Nikki 1968; Paton and Speden 1965; Pertwee 1970). It has also been shown that at thermally neutral ambient temperatures or above, body temperatures of drug-treated animals usually remain unaffected (Chambers et al. 1978; Freund 1973; Heroux et al. 1956; Mäkeläinen 1974; Mäkeläinen et al. 1973a; Nikki and Tammisto 1968; Pertwee 1970; Vapaatalo et al. 1975) or even rise above control levels (Freund 1973; Thauer 1943). The degree of hypothermia produced by general anaesthetics and barbiturates is influenced not only by ambient temperature but also by dose. Dose-related falls in body temperature have been observed for example in cats with pentobarbitone (Ekström 1951) and chloralose (Feldberg and Myers 1964), in rabbits with amylobarbitone (Daudova 1961), in rats with halothane, methoxyflurane (Nikki and Tammisto 1968), and ethanol (Carvalho and Izquierdo 1977), in gerbils with pentobarbitone (Järbe and Johansson 1977) and ethanol (Järbe and Ohlin 1977), and in mice with ethanol (Freund 1973). Dose-related hypothermia has also been observed in mice at an ambient temperature of 20 °C after exposure to diethyl ether, nitrous oxide, nitrogen, argon, dichlorodifluoromethane or chlorodifluoromethane (Pertwee 1970). With all six agents the threshold dose for hypothermia was found to be between one-third and one-fifth of the dose abolishing the righting reflex in 50% of a group of mice. (The loss of the righting reflex of mice is a commonly used, convenient end-point for onset of light anaesthesia). At the lower end of the effective dose range rectal temperatures fell to a new steady level within 60 min and the fall did not exceed 4 °C. At higher doses body temperature was usually still falling after 1 h and hypothermia was greater. With nitrous oxide, dichlorodifluoromethane, and chlorodifluoromethane, falls in temperature greater than 4 °C occurred only at doses equal to or greater than those abolishing the righting reflex.

The existence of a graded relationship between dose and degree of hypothermia suggests that general anaesthetics and barbiturates do not have an "all-or-none" effect on thermoregulation and that at some doses they can alter thermoregulation without completely abolishing it. This suggestion is supported by evidence reviewed by VON EULER (1961) and by BLIGH (1966, 1973) that in the presence of general anaesthetics thermoregulatory responses can still be activated, but only when body temperature has fallen or risen to a critical level. BLIGH proposed the existence of two distinct levels of body temperature control; a fine or narrow-band control which keeps body temperature within the normal range and a coarse or wideband control which becomes activated only if body temperature deviates markedly from the normal range. He also suggested that narrow-band control is more sensitive to general anaesthetics than the wide-band control system and that anaesthetics can inactivate narrow-band control while leaving wide-band control unaltered.

As well as affecting normal thermoregulation pentobarbitone and chloralose have also been shown to influence the effect of prostaglandins and endotoxins on body temperature. FELDBERG and SAXENA (1971) found that during the onset of pentobarbitone anaesthesia in cats injection of prostaglandin E_1 into the cerebrospinal fluid had no effect on body temperature when given at doses known to produce marked hyperthermia in unanaesthetized animals. More recently, DASHWOOD and FELDBERG (1977) showed that anaesthetic doses of pentobarbitone and chloralose could each reduce or prevent hyperthermic responses of cats to prostaglandin E_2 given intracerebroventricularly or to endotoxin (*Salmonella abortus-equi*) given intravenously. Pentobarbitone and chloralose were also reported to lessen the rise in concentration of prostaglandin E_2 in cerebrospinal fluid produced by the endotoxin.

2. Narcotic Analgesics
a) Effects

Narcotic analgesics have been shown to alter deep-body temperature in several species. Most experiments have been carried out with morphine which has been shown to produce temperature changes in monkeys, dogs, cats, rabbits, guineapigs, rats, and mice. In at least some of these species changes in body temperature have also been observed after treatment with heroin (MARTIN et al. 1977; THORNHILL et al. 1976), methadone (AHTEE et al. 1974; OKA 1977; KÄÄRIÄINEN and AHTEE 1976; SAARNIVAARA and MÄNISTÖ 1976; WARD et al. 1980), pethidine (AHTEE et al. 1974; BOTTING et al. 1978; GESSNER et al. 1974; JOUNELA et al. 1977; LEANDER et al. 1978; OKA 1977; SAARNIVARA and MÄNISTÖ 1976), cyclazocine (DOGGETT et al. 1975), and ketocyclazocine and ethylketocyclazocine (WARD et al. 1977, 1980).

In rats kept at ambient temperatures between 16° and 25 °C morphine can produce either hyperthermia or hypothermia. Systemic injections of morphine at doses ranging from 1.0 mg/kg to about 10 or 20 mg/kg usually cause hyperthermia (CHODERA 1963; COX et al. 1976a; FERRI et al. 1978; GUNNE 1960; HERRMANN 1941, 1942; KAAKKOLA and AHTEE 1977; LOTTI et al. 1965a, b; McGILLIARD et al. 1976; OKA et al. 1972; ROSENFELD and BURKS 1977; RUDY and YAKSH 1977; SAMANIN and VALZELLI 1972; SAMANIN et al. 1972; SHARKAWI 1972; SLOAN et al. 1962; SPRATTO and DORIO 1978; THORNHILL et al. 1978; WINTER and FLATAKER 1953). Higher doses usually produce a fall in body temperature (CHODERA 1963; COX et al. 1976a; FERRI et al. 1978; FULLER and BAKER 1974; GUNNE 1960; HAUBRICH and BLAKE 1971; HERRMANN 1942; KAAKKOLA and AHTEE 1977; LOMAX and KIRKPATRICK

1967; LOTTI et al. 1965a, 1966a, b; OKA and NOZAKI 1970; OKA et al. 1972; OKA 1977; PAOLINO and BERNARD 1968; ROSENFELD and BURKS 1977; SAMANIN and VALZELLI 1972; SAMANIN et al. 1972; SLOAN et al. 1962; SPRATTO and DORIO 1978; WARWICK et al. 1973; WARWICK and SCHNELL 1976). This hypothermia is sometimes followed by a transient rise in body temperature to above pre-injection levels (CHODERA 1963; COX et al. 1976a; GUNNE 1960; KAAKKOLA and AHTEE 1977; OKA et al. 1972; WARWICK and SCHNELL 1976).

As well as being affected by dose, the direction of the temperature change produced in rats by morphine can also be influenced by ambient temperature, by whether rats are restrained or free and by the strain of animal used. HERRMANN (1941) found that doses of morphine that induced hyperthermia at an ambient temperature of 25 °C lowered body temperature at 3 °C. PAOLINO and BERNARD (1968) showed that a dose of 50 mg/kg given intraperitoneally (IP) produced hypothermia at 5° and 24 °C but hyperthermia at 32 °C. MARTIN et al. (1977) and TRZCINKA et al. (1977) found that intraperitoneal injections of morphine given at doses in the range 15–50 mg/kg produced hypothermia in physically restrained rats and hyperthermia in unrestrained animals. OKA and NEGISHI (1977) reported that doses of 20 and 40 mg/kg subcutaneously (SC) produced either hyperthermia or hypothermia, depending on the strain of rat used. COX et al. (1979, 1980) also showed that the effect of morphine on body temperature could be influenced by the strain of animal used. Wistar rats were found to exhibit hyperthermia in response to a dose of 40 mg/kg whereas Sprague-Dawley rats showed only a transient rise in core temperature followed by a significant fall. At lower doses (5 and 20 mg/kg) both strains exhibited a hyperthermic response, the degree of hyperthermia produced showing a direct relationship to dose in the Wistar rats but an inverse relationship in the Sprague-Dawley animals. COX et al. (1979, 1980) have also observed a strain difference in the temperature response of rats to dextromoramide. However, the temperature effects of this drug were opposite to those of morphine. In Sprague-Dawley rats dextromoramide produced hypothermia at low doses (3.75 and 7.5 mg/kg) but hyperthermia at a higher dose (15 mg/kg). In Wistar rats the drug produced hyperthermia at the two lower doses and hypothermia at the highest dose.

In addition to affecting the direction of the temperature change produced in rats by morphine, dose level can also affect the degree or time course of the hyperthermia or hypothermia produced (CHODERA 1963; COX et al. 1980; GUNNE 1960; HERRMANN 1941, 1942; LOTTI et al. 1965a, b; MARTIN et al. 1977; OKA and NEGISHI 1977; ROSENFELD and BURKS 1977; SAMANIN et al. 1972). HERRMANN (1941) reported that morphine-induced hyperthermia was greater after a dose of 10 mg/kg than after 30 mg/kg. GUNNE (1960) found that the interval between injection of morphine and time of maximum hyperthermia increased with dose. The degree and duration of temperature changes produced by hypothermic doses of the drug were also found to increase with dose. Ambient temperature and age can also affect the degree of hypothermia induced in rats by morphine. OKA (1977) reported that morphine-induced hypothermia was greater at an ambient temperature of 12 °C than at 21 °C. He obtained similar results with methadone. Pethidine given subcutaneously at doses of 25 and 50 mg/kg produced hypothermia at 12 °C but had no effect at 21 °C. SPRATTO and DORIO (1978) found that young rats were more susceptible to the hypothermic effect of morphine than older animals.

As in rats so too in monkeys (EDDY and REID 1934; HOLTZMAN and VILLAR-REAL 1969, 1971; SMITH 1938), dogs (EDDY and REID 1934; GILBERT and MARTIN 1976; GREEN et al. 1943; HELFRICH 1934; HEMINGWAY 1938; WINTER and FLATAKER 1953), and guinea-pigs (GLAUBACH and PICK 1930; HELFRICH 1934; SCHULZ et al. 1974) morphine has been shown to produce both increases and decreases in deep-body temperature. In mice too both types of response have been observed (BAGDON and MANN 1965; BLOOM and DEWEY 1978; BOTTING et al. 1978; DOGGETT et al. 1975; FERNANDES et al. 1977; GLICK 1975; HELFRICH 1934; KÄÄRIÄINEN and AHTEE 1976; SAARNIVAARA and MÄNISTÖ 1976; WARD et al. 1977). GLICK (1975) reported that at an ambient temperature of 25 °C morphine injected intraperitoneally at doses of 1.25 or 2.5 mg/kg raised mouse body temperature whereas doses of 5.0 mg/kg or more produced a dose-related hypothermia. Morphine hypothermia in mice is sometimes followed by a transient hyperthermia (DOGGETT et al. 1975). In rabbits, although a hyperthermic response to morphine has been reported (HEL-FRICH 1934), the more usual response is hypothermia (EDDY 1932; DHAWAN 1960; GIRNDT and LIPSCHITZ 1931; KO 1937; MAYNERT and KLINGMAN 1962). The hypothermic response has been observed at ambient temperatures of up to 30 °C (DHAWAN 1960). Unlike rabbits, cats have usually been found to exhibit only hyperthermia in response to morphine (CLARK and CUMBY 1978; FRENCH et al. 1978 a, b; HELFRICH 1934; McCRUM and INGRAM 1951; MILTON 1975; STEWART and ROGOFF 1922). This is so even with systemically administered doses as high as 60 mg/kg (HELFRICH 1934), and at ambient temperatures as low as 5°–8 °C (STEW-ART and ROGOFF 1922). The degree of hyperthermia is related to dose (FRENCH et al. 1978 b; HELFRICH 1934; STEWART and ROGOFF 1922). FRENCH et al. (1978 a) did observe hypothermia in one cat given morphine intravenously at a dose of 1.0 mg/kg; six other cats given doses of 1.0–4.0 mg/kg showed only a hyperthermic response.

In rats the direction of the temperature change produced by morphine is influenced by physical restraint. Whether this is also true for other species is not yet known. However, it should be noted that the rabbit, a species which usually exhibits a hypothermic response to morphine, is normally kept restrained during measurement of body temperature whereas the cat, a species which usually shows a hyperthermic response to the drug, is normally kept unrestrained.

b) Role of Opiate Receptors

There is good evidence that changes in body temperature produced by narcotic analgesics are caused by interaction with opiate receptors. First, areas of the brain and spinal cord in which morphine can act to produce changes in deep-body temperature (see Sect. B.II.2) appear to contain high concentrations of opiate receptors (KUHAR et al. 1973). Second, COX et al. (1979) have found that the body temperature response of rats to narcotic analgesics depends on the configuration of the drug used. Dextromoramide was shown to alter body temperature whereas laevomoramide, its optical isomer, had no effect when administered in the same doses. Third, methionine enkephalin (L-tyrosylglycylglycyl-L-phenylalanyl-L-methionine), a putative endogenous opioid ligand for opiate receptors, has been shown to have effects on body temperature similar to those produced by morphine, (see Sect. B.VII). Finally, the effects of morphine on body temperature can be prevented by low doses of naloxone given either peripherally or by injection into the spinal subarachnoid space, cerebral ventricles or preoptic/anterior hypothalamic nuclei. Naloxone has been shown to antagonize morphine-induced hyperthermia in cats (CLARK 1977; CLARK and CUMBY 1978; FRENCH et al. 1978 b; MILTON 1975) and rats (FERRI et al. 1978; MARTIN et al. 1977; McGILLIARD et al. 1976; OKA and NEGISHI 1977; RUDY and YAKSH 1977; THORNHILL et al. 1978, 1980), and morphine-induced hypothermia in rats (BAIZMAN and WOLF 1975; FERRI et al. 1978; MARTIN et al. 1977; OKA 1977; WARWICK and SCHNELL 1976), and mice (WARD et al. 1980). There is also evidence that in rats naloxone can antagonize the temperature effects of dextromoramide (COX et al. 1979), heroin (MARTIN et al. 1977), pethidine and methadone (OKA 1977), and nalorphine can antagonize the effects of morphine (LOMAX and KIRKPATRICK 1967; LOTTI et al. 1965 b; SHARKAWI 1972).

In a few experiments naloxone has been found to enhance the effects of morphine on body temperature. In mice low doses of naloxone have been reported to potentiate the hypothermic effects of morphine and methadone (WARD et al. 1980). In rats naloxone has occasionally been found to enhance morphine-induced hyperthermia or to convert morphine-induced hypothermia into a hyperthermic response. COX et al. (1976 a) reported that hyperthermia produced in rats by morphine was enhanced and prolonged by the simultaneous administration of naloxone. THORNHILL et al. (1978) found that naloxone given subcutaneously at a dose of 1.0 mg/kg antagonized the hyperthermic effect of a low dose of morphine (5 mg/ kg SC) but tended to enhance the hyperthermic effect of a high dose (80 mg/kg). WARWICK and SCHNELL (1976) found that a dose of morphine which lowered the body temperature of naloxone-free rats, elicited a hyperthermic response in animals pre-treated with naloxone. Similar results have been obtained with nalorphine. LOTTI et al. (1965 b) reported that after treatment with nalorphine, the hypothermia normally produced by intrahypothalamic injections of morphine was replaced by a hyperthermic response.

Enhancement of hyperthermic responses to morphine induced by naloxone or nalorphine could be the result of a movement to the right of the dose–response curve for morphine. In rats low doses of morphine can produce hyperthermia whereas higher doses usually produce dose-related falls in body temperature. It is possible therefore that a naloxone-induced shift to the right of the morphine dose-response curve could cause a hypothermic response to be replaced by a hyperthermic one. There is evidence that in the hyperthermic dose range low doses of morphine can produce greater increases in body temperature than high doses. A rightward shift in the dose-response curve might therefore also cause a small increase in body temperature to be replaced by a larger increase. A similar hypothesis could be put forward to explain the observation (see Sect. B.V.2.a) that repeated administration of hyperthermic doses of morphine in rats sometimes enhances the hyperthermic effect of morphine: tolerance, like the administration of naloxone or nalorphine induces a rightward shift in the morphine dose-response curve.

c) Role of Prostaglandins

COLLIER et al. (1974) reported that morphine can stimulate prostaglandin production in rabbit brain homogenates enriched with sodium arachidonate. More recently, Scoto et al. (1979) found that brain homogenates prepared from rats which had received intracerebroventricular injections of a hyperthermic dose of methionine enkephalin contained greater concentrations of prostaglandin-like activity than control homogenates. Brains from rats which had been injected with methionine enkephalin daily for 8 days showed no such increases, suggesting that tolerance could develop. The effect was also prevented by pre-treatment with a systemic injection of naloxone. Prostaglandins can themselves produce hyperthermia when injected into brain or cerebrospinal fluid and these results are therefore consistent with the hypothesis that morphine produces hyperthermia by stimulating the production of prostaglandins. However, results of experiments with paracetamol and indomethacin, both inhibitors of prostaglandin synthetase, suggest that prostaglandins are not required for morphine-induced hyperthermia. Milton (1975) found that paracetamol and indomethacin could neither prevent nor reverse hypothermia induced in cats by morphine given either intravenously or directly into the cerebrospinal fluid. Clark and Cumby (1978) showed that a dose of indomethacin known to antagonize hyperthermic responses to sodium arachidonate had no significant effect on hyperthermia produced in cats by intraventricular injection of morphine. Rudy and Yaksh (1977) reported that in rats the hyperthermic effect of morphine administered intrathecally was not prevented by indomethacin.

3. Phenothiazines

Systemic administration of phenothiazines can cause both increases and decreases in body temperature. The direction of the change produced depends on ambient temperature. At temperatures below 30 °C phenothiazines have usually been shown to produce hypothermia. At higher ambient temperatures they may produce a rise, a fall or no change in body temperature. Most temperature experiments have been conducted with chlorpromazine. This drug has been shown to alter deep-body temperature in several species. In rats chlorpromazine-induced hypothermia has been observed after intraperitoneal administration (Boissier et al. 1967; Borbély et al. 1973; Chai and Lin 1977; Dandiya et al. 1960; Garattini et al. 1962; Jamieson and Van den Brenk 1961; Kollias and Bullard 1964; Kirkpatrick and Lomax 1971; Le Blanc 1958a, b; Le Blanc and Rosenberg 1957, 1958; Lin et al. 1978, 1979; Maier et al. 1955; Polk and Lipton 1975; Rudy and Wolf 1967; Saunders et al. 1974; Schaumkell 1955; Singh and Das 1976; Skobba and Miya 1969; Trzcinka et al. 1978; Tsoukaris-Kupfer and Schmidt 1972; Ulrich et al. 1967a; Weiss and Laties 1963; Wolfe et al. 1977; Yehuda and Wurtman 1972) after subcutaneous administration (Ankermann 1958; Binet and Decaud 1954, 1960; Courvoisier et al. 1953; Feller 1955; Giaja and Markovic-Giaja 1954; Hoffman 1958, 1959; Hoffman and Zarrow 1958; Shemano and Nickerson 1958) or after intravenous administration (Chai and Lin 1977; Kawashima et al. 1975).

Chlorpromazine-induced hypothermia has also been observed in monkeys (Chai et al. 1976), dogs (Brendel and L'Allemand 1955; Chatonnet and Tanche 1955, 1959; Courvoisier et al. 1953; L'Allemand et al. 1955), rabbits (Bächtold and Pletscher 1957; Cheymol and Levassort 1955; Fenters and Jeter 1961; Frommel et al. 1963; Jacob and Peindaries 1973; Lechat and Levassort 1969;

LIN 1979; NEUHOLD et al. 1957; REVOL 1959; WISLICKI 1960), guinea-pigs (CHEVIL-
LARD et al. 1958; FROMMEL et al. 1963; HALPERN and LIAKOPOULOS 1954; ULRICH
et al. 1967 a, b), hamsters and ground squirrels (HOFFMAN and ZARROW 1958), and
mice (BAGDON and MANN 1962; BOISSIER et al. 1967; COURVOISIER et al. 1953;
FENTERS and JETER 1961; FLACKE et al. 1953; FROMMEL et al. 1963; GOLDBERG et
al. 1973; LESSIN and PARKES 1957 a, b; LIU 1974; PARK et al. 1972; SPENCER and
WAITE 1968; TAVENDALE 1979; USINGER 1957; WITHERSPOON et al. 1957). Effective
hypothermic doses are about the same in all these species and range upwards from
about 1.0 or 2.0 mg/kg.

The degree of hypothermia produced by equivalent doses has been shown to
vary with species. COURVOISIER et al. (1953) reported that at 25 °C subcutaneous
injection of chlorpromazine at a dose level of 50 mg/kg produced maximum falls
in body temperature of 6.8 °C in mice and 2.1 °C in dogs. BOISSIER et al. (1967)
found that at 23 °C chlorpromazine (8, 16 or 32 mg/kg IP) produced a greater degree of hypothermia in mice than in rats. HALPERN and LIAKOPOULOS (1954) reported that at 10 °C, chlorpromazine (20 mg/kg) lowered the body temperature of
rats by 12 °C and of guinea-pigs by 3 °C. HOFFMAN and ZARROW (1958) showed
that at 23 °C chlorpromazine (10 mg/kg SC) produced maximum falls in body temperature of about 4 °C in rats and hamsters and 8 °C in ground squirrels. The
ground squirrels were studied at a time of year when they would normally have
been hibernating and preliminary results suggested that this species is less susceptible to the hypothermic effect of chlorpromazine when the drug is given during
the breeding season.

In rats the degree and duration of chlorpromazine-induced hypothermia is
thought to depend on a number of factors including ambient temperature (COUR-
VOISIER et al. 1953; GIAJA and MARKOVIC-GIAJA 1954; HALPERN and LIAKOPOULOS
1954; KOLLIAS and BULLARD 1964; LE BLANC and ROSENBERG 1957; SHEMANO and
NICKERSON 1958; YEHUDA and WURTMAN 1972), dose (BOISSIER et al. 1967; CHAI
and LIN 1977; HALPERN and LIAKOPOULOS 1954; HOFFMAN and ZARROW 1958; KA-
WASHIMA et al. 1975; KOLLIAS and BULLARD 1964; RUDY and WOLF 1967), route
of administration (CHAI and LIN 1977), age and body weight (ANKERMANN 1958;
HOFFMAN and ZARROW 1958; SAUNDERS et al. 1974), sex (HOFFMAN and ZARROW
1958) time of day (WOLFE et al. 1977), and the presence or absence of intact adrenal
glands (HOFFMAN 1959). LE BLANC and ROSENBERG (1957) found that the intensity
and duration of chlorpromazine-induced hypothermia was markedly less in rats
which had been kept at an ambient temperature of 6 °C for 7 or 28 days than in
control animals.

KOLLIAS and BULLARD (1964) studied the effect on rat body temperature of
chlorpromazine injected intraperitoneally at dose levels of 6.25 and 25 mg/kg. At
an ambient temperature of 23 °C both doses were hypothermic, the lower dose producing a fall in colonic temperature of about 4 °C and the higher dose a fall of
about 8 °C. At an ambient temperature of 28 °C the maximum fall in body temperature produced by the higher dose was only 1.5 °C. CHAI and LIN (1977) showed
that relatively low doses of chlorpromazine (10 μg) were needed to produce hypothermia when injections were made directly into rat cerebrospinal fluid. Higher
doses were needed for injections into the internal carotid artery, femoral vein or
peritoneal cavity. The drug was approximately seven times more potent by the in-

tra-arterial than by the intravenous route and about three times more potent intra-venously than intraperitoneally. HOFFMAN and ZARROW (1958) reported that fe-male rats were less susceptible than male rats to the hypothermic effect of a high dose of chlorpromazine. They also found that young male rats were less susceptible to the drug than older males. Differences in body weight may have influenced these results since the males were heavier than the females and the old animals heavier than the young. SAUNDERS et al. (1974) confirmed that the hypothermic response to chlorpromazine is greater in older rats than in young ones. After drug injection the brain concentration of chlorpromazine was the same in both age groups and it was suggested that tissue sensitivity to chlorpromazine may perhaps increase with age.

WOLFE et al. (1977) measured body temperature and brain and plasma concentrations of chlorpromazine in rats injected with chlorpromazine at various times of day. The rats were kept under a regular light–dark cycle. The degree of hypothermia produced by chlorpromazine varied with time of day and was greatest when the drug had been injected near the middle of the light phase. Brain and plasma concentrations of chlorpromazine did not show circadian variations. It is possible therefore that the temporal variations observed in the hypothermic response to chlorpromazine reflected time-dependent changes in tissue sensitivity to the drug. Alternatively, the ability of rats to resist a fall in body temperature, no matter how produced, may vary with time of day and perhaps also with age.

As in rats so too in other species the degree and duration of chlorpromazine-induced hypothermia can be influenced by ambient temperature (FENTERS and JETER 1961; HOFFMAN and ZARROW 1958; LIN 1979), dose (BOISSIER et al. 1967; CHEYMOL and LEVASSORT 1955; COURVOISIER et al. 1953; HALPERN and LIAKO-POULOS 1954; HOFFMAN and ZARROW 1958; L'ALLEMAND et al. 1955; WISLICKI 1960), route of administration (REVOL 1959), and sex (GOLDBERG et al. 1973; HOFF-MAN and ZARROW 1958). In mice for example, COURVOISIER et al. (1953) showed that chlorpromazine produced dose-related hypothermia when given subcutaneously at doses ranging from 2.0 to 50 mg/kg. GOLDBERG et al. (1973) reported that male mice which had been subjected to a 5-week isolation period showed a greater hypothermic response to chlorpromazine (1.5 and 3.0 mg/kg IP) than males which had been kept in a group until just before drug administration. The degree of chlorpromazine-induced hypothermia in female mice was not influenced by prior isolation.

Doses of chlorpromazine which provoke a fall in the body temperature of rats kept at ambient temperatures below 30 °C have been shown to elicit a hyperthermic response in animals kept at 36 °C or above (BINET and DECAUD 1960; SHEMANO and NICKERSON 1958; YEHUDA and WURTMAN 1972). The drug can also reduce survival time in heat (BINET and DECAUD 1954, 1960; KOLLIAS and BULLARD 1964). At ambient temperatures between 30° and 36 °C the body temperature of chlorpromazine-treated rats may either increase, decrease or remain unchanged. RUDY and WOLF (1967) simultaneously measured the effects in rats of chlorpromazine on the conditioned avoidance response and on body temperature. At an ambient temperature of 31 °C doses of chlorpromazine which disrupted the conditioned response produced increases in both peritoneal and hypothalamic temperatures. KOLLIAS and BULLARD (1964) carried out experiments with rats at an ambient temperature of 34 °C. Chlorpromazine-treated and control animals both experienced fatal hyperthermia. The drug-treated rats showed a greater degree of hyperthermia and also a shorter survival time. In contrast, SHEMANO and NICKERSON (1958) found that chlorpromazine produced hyperthermia in rats at 39 °C, hyperthermia at 30° and 33 °C and no significant change at 36 °C.

Although chlorpromazine produces hypothermia in mice at ambient temperatures below 30 °C, it has been shown to produce no change at 30 °C (USINGER 1957) or 32 °C (LESSIN and PARKES 1957a), and hyperthermia at 33 °C (GOLDBERG et al. 1973). At a higher ambient temperature the body temperature response of mice to chlorpromazine has been reported to vary with age. BAGDON and MANN (1962) measured body temperature changes in mice kept at an ambient temperature of 38 °C. Chlorpromazine produced hyperthermia in 10- and 15-day-old mice but hypothermia in 35- and 38-day-old animals. FENTERS and JETER (1961) also reported that chlorpromazine could lower mouse body temperature at a high ambient temperature (37 °C). In rabbits, chlorpromazine has been shown to produce hypothermia at ambient temperatures of 2° and 22 °C and hyperthermia at 32 °C (LIN 1979). However, the drug has also been reported to protect rabbits from fatal hyperthermia induced by exposure to an ambient temperature of 38 °C and to have no effect on body temperature of guinea-pigs kept at an ambient temperature of 43 °C (DECOURT et al. 1953).

It is possible that at ambient temperatures above 30 °C, the relationship between the temperature response to chlorpromazine and ambient temperature is influenced by stress. Rats attempting to avoid electric shocks (RUDY and WOLF 1967) showed hyperthermic responses at far lower doses than the lightly restrained rats of SHEMANO and NICKERSON (1958). Rats taped to boards were shown to experience fatal hyperthermia at a relatively low ambient temperature even in the absence of chlorpromazine (KOLLIAS and BULLARD 1964). In its presence they experienced even greater rises in body temperature and died earlier than untreated animals. Male mice which had been subjected to a prolonged isolation period showed a greater hyperthermic response to chlorpromazine at an ambient temperature of 33 °C than control animals, isolated only just before drug administration (GOLDBERG et al. 1973).

A few body temperature experiments have been carried out with phenothiazines other than chlorpromazine. At ambient temperatures below 30 °C rats have been shown to exhibit hypothermia in response to promethazine (BINET and DECAUD 1960; FELLER 1955; HALPERN and LIAKOPOULOS 1954; JAMIESON and VAN DEN BRENK 1961), perphenazine (MORPURGO 1962), pipamazine and triflupromazine (JAMIESON and VAN DEN BRENK 1961), trifluoperazine (JAMIESON and VAN DEN BRENK 1961; MORPURGO 1962), methoxypromazine, methotrimeprazine, acepromazine, and thiazinamium (BINET and DECAUD 1960), and trimeprazine (BINET and DECAUD 1960; JAMIESON and VAN DEN BRENK 1961). Diethazine was inactive except at high doses (BINET and DECAUD 1960; FELLER 1955). Promethazine has also been shown to produce hypothermia in mice (COURVOISIER et al. 1953) and acepromazine, perphenazine, methoxypromazine, methotrimeprazine, and prochlorperazine all induced marked hypothermia in rabbits (LECHAT and LEVASSORT 1969; REVOL 1959; VOTAVA 1973). MORPURGO (1962) reported that in rats chlorpromazine and perphenazine were more potent as hypothermic agents than trifluoperazine. Thioridazine had little or no activity. BINET and DECAUD (1960) showed that in rats kept at 4 °C, chlorpromazine and acepromazine were both highly effective as hypothermic agents. Methopromazine, methotrimeprazine, trimeprazine, promethazine, and thiazinamium were less effective. At an ambient temperature of 39 °C, the same phenothiazines produced an increase in rat body temperature. LECHAT and LEVASSORT (1969) found that in rabbits, thioridazine, thioproperazine, and prochlorperazine were markedly less effective in producing hypothermia than either chlorpromazine or methotrimeprazine. HOFMAN and RIEGLE (1977) showed that in sheep intramuscular injections of propiopromazine (1 mg/kg) produced hypothermia at an ambient temperature of 5 °C, hyperthermia at 35 °C and no effect at 25 °C. BAGDON and MANN (1965) reported that a high dose of the chlorpromazine metabolite, chlorpromazine sulphoxide, induced hyperthermia in 10-day-old mice at an ambient temperature of 38 °C.

II. Sites of Action

1. General Anaesthetics and Barbiturates

Little is yet known about the location of the sites at which general anaesthetics and barbiturates act to alter thermoregulation. Most experiments have been carried out with pentobarbitone. Whereas administration of this drug by systemic injection normally lowers body temperature of animals kept at ambient temperatures of 26 °C or less, injections into the cerebrospinal fluid or directly into the thermoregulatory centres of the preoptic/anterior hypothalamus have been reported to produce either hypothermia, hyperthermia or no change.

FELDBERG and MYERS (1964) using relatively high dose levels and injection volumes showed that both pentobarbitone and chloralose lowered the body temperature of cats when injected into the left lateral cerebral ventricle. Injection of chloralose into the third ventricle or directly into the hypothalamus of cats recovering from pentobarbitone anaesthesia suppressed shivering, lowered the respiratory rate and produced a renewed fall in body temperature (FELDBERG and MYERS 1965). Pentobarbitone has also been reported to lower cat body temperature after injection into the anterior hypothalamus (JACOBSON 1966). In rats kept at 10° or 34 °C, injection of pentobarbitone into the lateral hypothalamus was shown to produce a rise in body temperature (HUMPHREYS et al. 1976). However, at an ambient temperature of 23 °C the same treatment lowered body temperature. Changes in body temperature were also reported in rats kept at 10° or 23 °C after injection of pentobarbitone into the medulla oblongata (hypothermia) or the preoptic/anterior hypothalamic nuclei (hyperthermia). In contrast LOMAX (1966) reported that micro-injection of pentobarbitone into the hypothalamus or medulla oblongata had no effect on rat body temperature. Morphine injection into the same hypothalamic sites produced a marked hypothermia and it was concluded that the hypothermic effect of pentobarbitone is not the result of a direct action on the thermoregulatory centres in the hypothalamus. In monkeys pentobarbitone lowered body temperature slightly when injected into endotoxin-insensitive areas of the hypothalamus (LIPTON and FOSSLER 1974) and in sheep produced hyperthermia when injected into the third ventricle but not when injected into the cerebral aqueduct

(SEOANE and BAILE 1975). There was no change in body temperature when pento-barbitone was injected into the posterior hypothalamus of cats (JACOBSON 1966) or rats (HUMPHREYS et al. 1976) nor when it was injected into the mesencephalic reticular formation of rats (HUMPHREYS et al. 1976).

2. Morphine

BANERJEE et al. (1968 a) showed that low doses of morphine (25–100 µg) could in-crease rabbit body temperature when given intracerebroventricularly. Slightly higher doses had no effect on body temperature when given intraperitoneally. DETTMAR and COWAN (1980) have confirmed that intraventricular injections of morphine can produce hyperthermia in rabbits. In cats both intrahypothalamic (MILTON 1975) and intraventricular injections of morphine (BANERJEE et al. 1968 b; CLARK 1977; CLARK and CUMBY 1978; DETTMAR and COWAN 1980) have been shown to increase body temperature. The increases in temperature were sometimes preceded by a small fall. Intracerebroventricular injections of morphine have also been shown to produce hyperthermia in guinea-pigs and hypothermia in mice (DETTMAR and COWAN 1980). In rats morphine can alter body temperature either when injected into the cerebrospinal fluid (FERRI et al. 1978) or when injected di-rectly into the hypothalamus. LOTTI et al. (1965 a, b; 1966 a) found that at an am-bient temperature of 25 °C, injection of morphine sulphate (10–50 µg) into the preoptic/anterior hypothalamic nuclei of physically restrained rats produced a fall in body temperature. At a lower dose (4 µg) the drug has been shown to produce hyperthermia (COX et al. 1976 a). FERRI et al. (1978) found that intracerebroven-tricular injection of a dose of 2 µg morphine hydrochloride raised rat body temper-ature whereas a dose of 8 µg produced hypothermia. VAN REE et al. (1976) reported that injection of morphine into the anterior hypothalamus of rats produced hypo-thermia whereas injection into a more ventral area produced a rise in body temper-ature. LOTTI et al. (1965 a) found that doses of morphine producing a fall in rat body temperature when injected into the preoptic/anterior hypothalamic nuclei produced a rise in body temperature when injected into the region of the mammil-lary nuclei. No changes in body temperature have been observed after morphine injection into other sites adjacent to the preoptic/anterior hypothalamus (LOTTI et al. 1965 a) nor after injection into the medulla oblongata (TRZCINKA et al. 1977) or the arcuate nucleus (VAN REE et al. 1976).

As after systemic administration so too after intrahypothalamic injection the direction of the temperature change produced by morphine in rats seems to depend not only on dose but also on ambient temperature and on whether the rats used are restrained or free. PAOLINO and BERNARD (1968) reported that intrahypothala-mic injections of morphine produced hyperthermia at an ambient temperature of 32 °C, hypothermia at 5 °C and no change at 24 °C. TRZCINKA et al. (1977) found that micro-injection of morphine sulphate (50 µg) into the preoptic/anterior hypo-thalamic nuclei produced hypothermia in restrained rats and hyperthermia in un-restrained animals. MARTIN and MORRISON (1978) observed hyperthermia in unre-strained rats after intrahypothalamic injection of morphine but no change in the body temperature of restrained animals. THORNHILL et al. (1980) have also found that ambient temperature and physical restraint can influence the temperature response to central injection of morphine in rats.

The similarities between the temperature responses to systemic injection of morphine and the responses to intrahypothalamic injection provide strong evidence for the hypothesis that the effects on body temperature of peripherally administered morphine are mediated by sites located within the anterior hypothalamus. Further support for this hypothesis is given by results from experiments in which selective antagonists of morphine were used. It has been found that in rats nalorphine given directly into the preoptic/anterior hypothalamic nuclei can antagonize morphine-induced hypothermia (LOMAX and KIRKPATRICK 1967; LOTTI et al. 1965 b). It has also been reported that nalorphine can reverse morphine-induced hypothermia when injected into a posterior hypothalamic site (LOTTI et al. 1965 b). However, this was only observed in one of seven rats and in the remaining six animals no antagonism was detected when nalorphine was injected into sites adjacent to the preoptic/anterior hypothalamus even when these were situated in the region of the posterior hypothalamic nuclei. Nalorphine possesses weak agonist activity and is therefore not a pure antagonist. However, naloxone which lacks any detectable agonist activity has also been shown to antagonize the effects of morphine on body temperature. In cats naloxone given intraventricularly was found to prevent or reverse morphine-induced hyperthermia (CLARK 1977; CLARK and CUMBY 1978). In rats, systemic administration of naloxone has been shown to attenuate hyperthermia produced by injection of morphine directly into the preoptic/anterior hypothalamic nuclei (THORNHILL et al. 1980). Naloxone has also been reported to antagonize morphine-induced hyperthermia in rats when both drugs were injected into the hypothalamus (BAIZMAN and WOLF 1975).

RUDY and YAKSH (1977) have found that doses of morphine ranging from 2 to 45 µg can produce hyperthermia in rats when injected into the lumbar spinal subarachnoid space. The effect appeared to be dependent on dose but independent of ambient temperature. It could be completely reversed by the intraperitoneal injection of naloxone. However, intrathecal injections of naloxone even at a dose of 50 µg could only partially reverse hyperthermia produced by intraperitoneal injection of morphine. It was concluded that the hyperthermic effect of systemically administered morphine is mediated partly by an action on the spinal cord and partly by actions on brain regions such as the anterior hypothalamus not directly accessible to intrathecally injected naloxone. RUDY and YAKSH also suggested that intrathecally administered morphine probably produced hyperthermia by acting at a site within the substantia gelatinosa to modulate the passage of sensory information, thus altering the thermal information received by supraspinal regulatory centres.

FOSTER et al. (1967) conducted experiments using N-methylmorphine, a quaternary derivative of morphine expected to penetrate the blood–brain barrier at only a very low rate. The drug was shown to lower rat body temperature after microinjection into the preoptic/anterior hypothalamic nuclei but not after intravenous administration. Two other important differences in the properties of morphine and its N-methyl derivative were noted. First, although nalorphine antagonized morphine it failed to block the hypothermic response to N-methylmorphine. Second, tolerance is known to develop rapidly to the hypothermic effect of morphine (see

Sect. B.V.2.a) and yet there was no sign of tolerance to the N-methyl derivative in rats pre-treated either with morphine or N-methylmorphine nor of tolerance to morphine in rats pre-treated with N-methylmorphine. It is therefore not clear to what extent the results obtained with N-methylmorphine support the hypothesis that morphine alters thermoregulation mainly by acting at sites located within the central nervous system.

3. Chlorpromazine

REIGLE and WOLF (1971) reported that at an ambient temperature of 10 °C injection of 12.5–37.5 µg of chlorpromazine into the anterior hypothalamus of hamsters produced an immediate dose-dependent hypothermia. Chlorpromazine sulphoxide, a metabolite of chlorpromazine also lowered body temperature when injected into the anterior hypothalamus. However, the metabolite was far less potent than the parent compound and it was therefore concluded that the hypothermic response to chlorpromazine is mediated by a relatively specific drug–receptor interaction. CHAI et al. (1976) showed that chlorpromazine produced hypothermia in monkeys, both after intraventricular injection and after direct injection into the preoptic/anterior hypothalamus or medulla oblongata. Injections were also made into the posterior hypothalamus, mid-brain and pons. Of these injections only a small proportion produced a fall in body temperature, the remainder having no detectable effect. The drug was found to be at least seven times more potent when injected intraventricularly than when given intravenously. It was concluded that the hypothermic effect of peripherally injected chlorpromazine is mediated principally through central mechanisms located in the preoptic/anterior hypothalamus and medulla oblongata.

In rats there are reports both of hypothermic and hyperthermic responses to chlorpromazine when the drug is injected into the cerebrospinal fluid and also of hyperthermic responses after direct injection into brain tissue. CHAI and LIN (1977) found that injection of 10–40 µg of chlorpromazine into the third or fourth ventricle produced dose-related falls in body temperature. Much higher doses were required to produce hypothermia by systemic injection than by intraventricular injection, a finding consistent with their hypothesis that chlorpromazine-induced hypothermia is largely mediated by central mechanisms. In contrast, data from other experiments suggest that at least in rats chlorpromazine-induced hypothermia may be mediated mainly by peripheral mechanisms. In these experiments it was found that even at normal room temperatures rats exhibited a hyperthermic response to intraventricular or intrahypothalamic injections of chlorpromazine (KIRKPATRICK and LOMAX 1971; REWERSKI and GUMULKA 1969; REWERSKI and JORI 1968b; TRZCINKA et al. 1978; TSOUCARIS-KUPFER and SCHMITT 1972). REWERSKI and JORI (1968b) reported that injections of 0.5–60 µg chlorpromazine into the anterior hypothalamus of lightly anaesthetized rats produced a prolonged dose-related hyperthermia. A hyperthermic effect was also observed when the drug was injected into the third ventricle but not when it was injected into the posterior hypothalamus, thalamus or frontal lobes. Chlorpromazine sulphoxide also produced hyperthermia when injected into the anterior hypothalamus but was much less potent than chlorpromazine. In unanaesthetized rats too, injection of chlorpromazine into the preoptic/anterior hypothalamic nuclei has been shown to elicit hyperthermia (KIRKPATRICK and LOMAX 1971; TRZCINKA et al. 1978). It has also been shown that injections into various sites in the middle and posterior hypothalamus have no effect on body temperature (KIRKPATRICK and LOMAX 1971).

As well as showing that intrahypothalamic injections of chlorpromazine can produce hyperthermia in rats, KIRKPATRICK and LOMAX (1971) have found that N-methylchlorpromazine, a quaternary derivative of chlorpromazine expected to penetrate the blood–brain barrier only very slowly, has similar effects to chlorpromazine on rat body temperature not only when injected directly into the preoptic/anterior hypothalamic nuclei but also when given intraperitoneally. This finding was taken as additional evidence for the hypothesis that hypothermia produced by systemic injection of chlorpromazine is mediated largely at sites outside the central nervous system.

TRZCINKA et al. (1978) have found that injection of chlorpromazine into the medulla oblongata of rats can elicit hypothermia but only after destruction of the preoptic/anterior hypothalamic nuclei. In view of this observation it is interesting to note that CHAI and LIN (1977) reported that hypothermia produced in rats by intraperitoneal injection of chlorpromazine was potentiated by lesions of the anterior hypothalamus. Hypothermia was also enhanced by spinal lesions but not by lesions of the ventromedial nucleus of the hypothalamus. The lesions of the anterior hypothalamus and spinal cord also altered thermoregulatory responses to heat and cold.

The existence in the central nervous system of some sites showing a hypothermic response to chlorpromazine and of others showing a hyperthermic response could explain why intraventricular injections of the drug produced a fall in rat body temperature in one study but a rise in others. There are other possible explanations however, and further experiments are clearly needed if the question of whether systemically administered chlorpromazine exerts its effects on thermoregulation predominantly by central or peripheral mechanisms is to be resolved.

III. Effects on Heat Gain and Heat Loss Mechanisms

1. General Anaesthetics and Barbiturates

There is evidence that the hypothermia produced by general anaesthetics and barbiturates is caused both by decreases in heat production as measured by changes in oxygen consumption, respiratory rate or muscle tone and by increases in heat loss as measured by the presence of polypnoea (GRANT and ROBBINS 1949) or by increased skin blood flow in extremities such as the ear or foot. Cats given hypothermic doses of pentobarbitone or chloralose either intrahypothalamically or peripherally have been found to show reductions in respiratory rate, oxygen consumption and muscle tone (FELDBERG and LOTTI 1967; FELDBERG and MYERS 1964; JACOBSON 1966). Dogs experiencing hypothermia in response to pentobarbitone or amylobarbitone failed to shiver (HEMINGWAY 1941) and showed a decrease in oxygen consumption (CHATONNET and TANCHE 1959). In rabbits doses of amylobarbitone which lowered rectal temperature were also found to reduce oxygen consumption (DAUDOVA 1961). The effects of amylobarbitone on body temperature and

oxygen consumption were both dose related (40–100 mg/kg SC). Moreover, the reductions in oxygen consumption usually preceded the onset of hypothermia, suggesting that reduced heat production contributed towards the hypothermic effect
of the drug. In rats hypothermic doses of pentobarbitone (LOMAX 1966) and
urethane (HAUK and ANKERMANN 1963) have also been reported to lower oxygen
consumption. Pentobarbitone was also found to increase cutaneous blood flow in
the tail. JACOBSON (1966) reported that hypothermia induced in cats by intrahypothalamic injection of pentobarbitone was accompanied by vasodilatation as well
as by a reduction in oxygen consumption. Further evidence of drug-induced increases in skin blood flow in ear or paw has been obtained from experiments with
cats, dogs, and rabbits treated with pentobarbitone, chloralose, urethane, halothane or ether (FELDBERG and LOTTI 1967; GRANT and ROBBINS 1949; HEMINGWAY
1941, 1948; STRÖM 1950; SUMMERS 1969).

WEISS and LATIES (1963) and HUMPHREYS et al. (1976) have studied the effect
of pentobarbitone on behavioural thermoregulation. WEISS and LATIES found that,
in rats kept at an ambient temperature of 2 °C, hypothermic doses of pentobarbitone given intraperitoneally lowered the rate of bar-pressing for heat reinforcement. HUMPHREYS et al. (1976) made injections directly into the preoptic/anterior
hypothalamic nuclei of rats at a dose known to increase body temperature and
found that the drug reduced time spent on bar-pressing to escape heat. Injections
made into the medulla oblongata or lateral hypothalamus although altering body
temperature had no consistent effect on bar-pressing behaviour. The results obtained in both behavioural studies would suggest that rats do not attempt to compensate behaviourally for changes in body temperature produced by pentobarbitone.

Like the onset of hypothermia produced by general anaesthetics and barbiturates, recovery has been shown to be preceded or accompanied by changes in both
heat production and heat loss. Cats recovering from the hypothermic effects of
pentobarbitone, chloralose or halothane have been reported to exhibit hind-limb
muscle tremor, shivering, increased muscle tone and respiratory rate and constriction of ear vessels (DOMER and FELDBERG 1960; FELDBERG and MYERS 1964; SUM-
MERS 1969). In some of these experiments (FELDBERG and MYERS 1964) restoration
of normal body temperature was followed by a transient hyperthermia. Such an
effect was also observed by EKSTRÖM (1951). In rats (NIKKI and TAMMISTO 1968)
and mice (NIKKI 1968) shivering has been reported during recovery from both halothane and methoxyflurane hypothermia. Piloerection was also observed during
recovery from halothane in rats (NIKKI and TAMMISTO 1968). Rats recovering from
the hypothermic effects of halothane (MÄKELÄINEN et al. 1973 a) or
methoxyflurane (MÄKELÄINEN 1974) were found to have increased plasma concentrations of free fatty acids and glycerol. These increases were taken to indicate activation of non-shivering thermogenesis.

MÄKELÄINEN et al. (1973 a) found that the increases in plasma concentration of
free fatty acids and glycerol observed during recovery from halothane anaesthesia
were reduced in rats pre-treated with propranolol. On the other hand, pre-treatment with phenoxybenzamine had no effect. Propranolol was also reported to
abolish increases in plasma free fatty acids and glycerol normally observed during
recovery from fluroxene anaesthesia (VAPAATALO et al. 1975), to prolong shivering

during recovery from halothane anaesthesia (MÄKELÄINEN et al. 1973 a) and to delay reversal of hypothermia during recovery from methoxyflurane anaesthesia (MÄKELÄINEN 1974). It was concluded that non-shivering thermogenesis contributes towards restoration of body temperature during recovery from anaesthesia. It should be noted that plasma concentrations of free fatty acids were elevated not only after but also during administration of halothane or methoxyflurane. The increases that occurred during anaesthesia were attributed partly to increased release of catecholamines and partly to a direct action on adipose tissue; halothane and putative primary metabolites of halothane and methoxyflurane were all shown to stimulate lipolysis in vitro (MÄKELÄINEN 1974; MÄKELÄINEN et al. 1973 b; MÄKELÄINEN and ROSENBERG 1974).

2. Morphine

Morphine-induced increases in body temperature have been shown to be accompanied, in dogs, by shivering (HEMINGWAY 1938), in cats, by shivering (BANERJEE et al. 1968 b; CLARK and CUMBY 1978; MILTON 1975), increased motor activity (McCRUM and INGRAM 1951; MILTON 1975), and restlessness (CLARK and CUMBY 1978; STEWART and ROGOFF 1922) and, in rats, by tremor activity (RUDY and YAKSH 1977). Other signs of increased heat gain observed in morphine-treated rats include raised carbon dioxide production. (HERRMANN 1942), altered behavioural thermoregulation (Cox et al. 1976 a, b) and increased motor activity (SLOAN et al. 1962). GUNNE (1960) concluded that in rats morphine-induced increases in motor activity are not a cause of hyperthermia. He found that onset of peak hyperthermia generally preceded signs of excitement by 1–2 h and also that maximal temperatures sometimes occurred in rats which seemed totally immobile and even cataleptic. It was suggested that drug-induced increases in muscular tone might be an important source of extra heat production in morphine-treated rats.

Although it is likely that alterations in heat gain contribute towards morphine-induced hyperthermia in cats, dogs, and rats, it is less certain whether changes in heat loss are involved. In anaesthetized cats rises in body temperature produced by intraventricular injection of morphine were accompanied by constriction of ear vessels and hence presumably by a reduction in heat loss (BANERJEE et al. 1968 b). However, in conscious cats hyperthermic doses of the drug administered systemically have been reported to produce salivation (MILTON 1975) and panting (McCRUM and INGRAM 1951) as well as warm, sweating pads and signs of peripheral vasodilatation (STEWART and ROGOFF 1922). In unanaesthetized dogs a hyperthermic dose of morphine was also shown to produce peripheral vasodilatation and panting with no sign of reduced heat loss (HEMINGWAY 1938). In rats there is some evidence that decreases in heat loss may contribute towards morphine-induced hyperthermia. HERRMANN (1942) after measuring morphine-induced increases in heat production concluded that these increases were insufficient to account for the hyperthermic effect of the drug and that heat conservation must therefore also contribute. Cox et al. (1976 a) found that in rats morphine-induced increases in deep-body temperature were accompanied by falls in tail skin temperature, a change presumably reflecting a decrease in heat loss. Effects of hyperthermic doses of morphine on tail temperature have also been detected by RUDY and

YAKSH (1977) but not by WINTER and FLATAKER (1953). RUDY and YAKSH (1977) found that at 22 °C intrathecal injection of morphine was associated with a fall in rat tail temperature and also with the appearance of tremor activity. At 32 °C morphine affected only tail temperature whereas at 4 °C only tremor was observed. Presumably at 4 °C the rats were already fully vasoconstricted before drug injection whereas at 22° and 32 °C they were not. RUDY and YAKSH (1977) also found that morphine-treated rats kept at an ambient temperature of 22 °C could still respond to radiant heat applied to areas of the body other than the tail with an increase in tail skin temperature, suggesting that falls in tail temperature associated with the hyperthermia produced by morphine were not the result of a direct effect of the drug on vasomotor tone.

Like morphine-induced hyperthermia, morphine-induced hypothermia may be caused by changes in heat production. Hypothermic doses of morphine given to rats either systemically or directly into the preoptic/anterior hypothalamic nuclei have been shown to lower oxygen consumption (LOTTI et al. 1966b), decrease shivering measured electromyographically (BAIZMAN and WOLF 1975) and depress respiration (LOTTI et al. 1965a; SLOAN et al. 1962). Hypothermic doses of morphine can also reduce motor activity (SLOAN et al. 1962) and produce catalepsy in rats (COX et al. 1976a; LOTTI et al. 1965a, 1966b). However, these effects are thought not to play an important role in morphine-induced decreases in oxygen consumption or temperature (LOTTI et al. 1966b). There is evidence that there may be a cause and effect relationship between the effects of morphine on oxygen consumption and body temperature. LOTTI et al. (1966b) found that after morphine injection, the oxygen consumption of rats began to fall before deep-body temperature. It was also found that at the time of peak hypothermia, oxygen consumption was already returning towards pre-drug levels.

There is no evidence that changes in heat loss contribute towards the hypothermic effect of morphine. LOTTI et al. (1966b) studied the effect of hypothermic doses of morphine on rat tail blood flow and found that unlike chlorpromazine, morphine did not produce any increase in blood flow.

3. Phenothiazines

At ambient temperatures of 32 °C or less chlorpromazine has been shown to increase skin temperature in monkeys (CHAI et al. 1976), rabbits (LIN 1979), guinea-pigs (CHEVILLARD et al. 1958), and rats (CHAI and LIN 1977; KOLLIAS and BULLARD 1964; LE BLANC 1958a). The drug has also been shown to increase blood flow in rat tails (KOLLIAS and BULLARD 1964; LOTTI et al. 1966b). Skin temperature increases have been detected after injections into cerebrospinal fluid or brain (CHAI et al. 1976; CHAI and LIN 1977) as well as after systemic administration, however they have been observed only in the extremities of the body such as paw, tail or ear. In other parts of the body such as thigh (CHAI et al. 1976) or trunk (DANDIYA et al. 1960; LE BLANC 1958a; REIGLE and WOLF 1971; WEISS and LATIES 1963) skin temperature is not increased by chlorpromazine but instead passively follows drug-induced falls in deep-body temperature. The rises in skin temperature produced by chlorpromazine have been shown to occur immediately after injection and to precede the onset of hypothermia, supporting the hypothesis that increased heat loss from the extremities contributes towards chlorpromazine-induced hypothermia (CHAI et al. 1976; CHAI and LIN 1977; CHEVILLARD et al. 1958; LE BLANC 1958 a; LIN 1979). Increased evaporative heat loss from the respiratory tract may also contribute (CHAI et al. 1976; CHAI and LIN 1977; LIN 1979). After onset of hypothermia peripheral skin temperatures have been shown to return to their pre-injection values (CHAI et al. 1976; CHAI and LIN 1977; LE BLANC 1958 a; LIN 1979) where they remain even during recovery from hypothermia (CHAI et al. 1976; LE BLANC 1958 a). This would tend to minimize heat loss and hence hasten the recovery of deep-body temperature.

There is some evidence that chlorpromazine can affect heat production as well as heat loss. The drug has been shown to lower oxygen consumption in dogs (L'ALLEMAND et al. 1955), rabbits (LIN 1979), guinea-pigs (ULRICH et al. 1967 a, b), rats (COURVOISIER et al. 1953; DANDIYA et al. 1960; FELLER 1955; FILK et al. 1954; HADNAGY et al. 1958; HOFFMAN 1958; JAMIESON and VAN DEN BRENK 1961, KOLLIAS and BULLARD 1964; LETTAU et al. 1964; ULRICH et al. 1967 a), and mice (TAVENDALE 1979; USINGER 1957). In rats reductions in oxygen consumption have also been observed after administration of promethazine, trimeprazine, trifluoperazine and triflupromazine (JAMIESON and VAN DEN BRENK 1961). KOLLIAS and BULLARD (1964) reported that at a dose of 25 mg/kg, given intraperitoneally, chlorpromazine not only lowered oxygen consumption of rats but also abolished shivering. However, a lower hypothermic dose had no effect on shivering. In sheep, shivering was found to be abolished by a hypothermic dose of propiopromazine (HOFMAN and RIEGLE 1977). The same drug also increased ear temperature and respiratory evaporative heat loss.

In some experiments it was found that low hypothermic doses of chlorpromazine either had no effect on oxygen consumption (FELLER 1955) or even increased it (ANKERMANN 1958; CHATONNET and TANCHE 1959; CHEVILLARD et al. 1958; USINGER 1957). It is possible that at such doses drug-induced decreases in heat production were short lasting and therefore difficult to detect. Increases in oxygen consumption could reflect attempts to restore deep-body temperature to its pre-drug levels. Consistent with this suggestion are the results obtained by ULRICH et al. (1967 a) from experiments with guinea-pigs and rats. They observed that low hypothermic doses of chlorpromazine produced brief falls in oxygen consumption followed by longer lasting increases in which oxygen consumption rose above pre-drug levels.

The hypothesis that decreased heat production is a cause of hypothermia in chlorpromazine-treated animals was questioned by GIAJA and MARKOVIC-GIAJA (1954) who reported that in rats given chlorpromazine, falls in oxygen consumption could only be detected after onset of hypothermia. The report by FELLER (1955) that reductions in oxygen consumption of rats treated with chlorpromazine occurred only after deep-body temperature had fallen below 32 °C also fails to support the hypothesis. More recently there have been reports that in chlorpromazine-treated guinea-pigs (ULRICH et al. 1967 a), rats (KOLLIAS and BULLARD 1964; ULRICH et al. 1967 a), rabbits (LIN 1979), and mice (TAVENDALE 1979) reductions in oxygen consumption do precede hypothermia. It is likely therefore that under some conditions reductions in heat production do contribute towards chlorpromazine-induced hypothermia.

Like its effects on body temperature, the changes produced by chlorpromazine in heat production and heat loss appear to be related to ambient temperature (Dandiya et al. 1960; Kollias and Bullard 1964; L'Allemand et al. 1955; Lettau et al. 1964; Lin 1979; Usinger 1957). The drug has been reported to lower rat oxygen consumption at 23 °C but not at 28 °C (Kollias and Bullard 1964) and to have greater effects on rabbit oxygen consumption at 2 °C than at 22 °C (Lin 1979). Usinger (1957) found that chlorpromazine lowered mouse oxygen consumption at 20 °C but increased it at 30 °C. Kollias and Bullard (1964) studied the effects of chlorpromazine on thermoregulation in rats at several ambient temperatures. At 23 °C, the drug produced hypothermia accompanied by a lowering of heat production and increases in tail blood flow. At a higher ambient temperature, drug-treated rats exhibited smaller increases in tail blood flow than control animals, they also failed to salivate or to lick their fur. Licking behaviour and salivation which were observed in control animals serve to increase evaporative cooling from the body surface. It was concluded that chlorpromazine abolishes all mechanisms of temperature regulation for both heat and cold.

In rabbits as in rats there is evidence that chlorpromazine can affect heat loss mechanisms in the warm as well as in the cold (Lin 1979). At 32 °C, the drug produced hyperthermia accompanied by decreases both in ear temperature and in respiratory evaporative heat loss. At 22 °C, however, the drug produced hypothermia which was accompanied by a transient rise in ear temperature.

There have been several reports concerning the effects of chlorpromazine on behavioural thermoregulation. Le Blanc (1958 a) showed that chlorpromazine-treated rats kept at 21 °C adopted a cylindrically shaped posture with the extremities spread away from the body and became hypothermic. Control animals assumed a ball-shaped posture thereby reducing the proportion of body surface exposed to the environment. Lessin and Parkes (1957 b) observed that mice given hypothermic doses of chlorpromazine lay outstretched and made no attempt to crowd together, Schwartzbaum (1955) reported that chlorpromazine had no detectable effect on thermal preference in rats allowed to shuttle between warm and cool environments and Weiss and Laties (1963) found that chlorpromazine lowered the rate at which rats pressed a bar for heat reinforcement. The drug has also been found to reduce bar-pressing in experiments in which rats were trained to press a bar to escape heat (Polk and Lipton 1975). However, in the latter experiments rats were placed in the operant chamber only after onset of hypothermia and it is therefore not clear whether the behavioural changes observed reflected an effect of the drug on thermoregulation or an attempt to reverse chlorpromazine-induced hypothermia during recovery from the drug effect. It is also possible that the effects of chlorpromazine on bar-pressing for positive or negative heat reinforcement were not associated with a specific effect on thermoregulation but were instead caused by some less specific drug-induced change in bar-pressing behaviour. Taken together the behavioural data suggest that rats do not attempt to compensate behaviourally for falls in body temperature produced by chlorpromazine.

As well as affecting body temperature, chlorpromazine can also reduce motor activity. Several studies have been made to determine whether the two effects are causally related. Lessin and Parkes (1957 a) reported that there was a highly significant correlation between locomotor activity and body temperature in chlorpromazine-treated mice. Chlorpromazine had no effect on locomotor activity at 32 °C, an ambient temperature at which the drug did not lower body temperature. It was concluded that the effect of the drug on locomotor activity at ambient temperatures below 32 °C was probably a result and not a cause of hypothermia. In contrast, SPENCER and WAITE (1968) found that in hyperthyroid mice, chlorpromazine induced hyperthermia and that this was accompanied by a marked reduction of locomotor activity. They concluded that depression of activity by the drug does not depend on the presence of hypothermia. BORBÉLY et al. (1973) found that in rats with brain lesions chlorpromazine produced large falls in body temperature but had little effect on motor activity. CHAI and LIN (1977) reported that injections of chlorpromazine into rat cerebral ventricles produced a marked hypothermia but little apparent psychomotor depression. The results from both of these studies suggest that reduced motor activity is not a prerequisite for chlorpromazine-induced hypothermia.

IV. Neuropharmacology

1. General Anaesthetics and Barbiturates

a) Drug Interactions

Several of the drugs known to affect biosynthesis or fate of putative neurotransmitters have been found to influence the hypothermic effect of general anaesthetics and barbiturates. Falls in body temperature induced in rats by ether (LINDQVIST et al. 1974) and in mice by ethanol (STRÖMBOM et al. 1977) were reported to be prevented by pre-treatment with NSD 1015, an inhibitor of L-aromatic amino acid decarboxylase. Ethanol hypothermia was reduced by amphetamine (ABDALLAH and ROBY 1975) and ether hypothermia was prevented by pre-treatment with desipramine (REWERSKI and JORI 1968 a). Pre-treatment of rats for 5 days with p-chlorophenylalanine, an inhibitor of tryptophan hydroxylase was found to reduce the hypothermic effect of ethanol (FRANKEL et al. 1978). However, POHORECKY et al. (1976) found that a single pre-treatment with p-chloroamphetamine, also an inhibitor of tryptophan hydroxylase, enhanced the hypothermic effect of ethanol in rats. They also found that Lilly 110140 (fluoxetine), a drug thought to inhibit selectively the neuronal uptake of 5-hydroxytryptamine (5-HT), reduced ethanol hypothermia and concluded that the hypothermic effect of ethanol might be due to reduced stimulation by 5-HT of its receptors and that ethanol might act by somehow altering 5-HT metabolism. Tranylcypromine, pheniprazine, pargyline, nialamide, and amphetamine have all been shown to prevent the production of hypothermia by halothane in cats without altering the degree of anaesthesia produced (FELDBERG and LANG 1970; SUMMERS 1969). Tranylcypromine has also been shown to prevent hypothermia produced in cats by pentobarbitone or chloralose (FELDBERG and LOTTI 1967).

Tranylcypromine, phenipramine, and amphetamine were no more potent in preventing hypothermia when given directly into the lateral cerebral ventricles than when given peripherally and it was concluded (FELDBERG and LANG 1970) that after intraventricular administration these drugs had first to be absorbed into the bloodstream to produce their effect. Possibly they act at peripheral sympathetic nerve endings to increase the concentration of noradrenaline at postsynaptic adrenoceptors located on vascular smooth muscle and on sympathetically innervated organs of heat production and thereby counteract the effects of pentobarbitone, chloralose, and halothane on the production and loss of heat. Central sites of action could also be involved.

b) Effects on Temperature-Dependent Electrical Activities of Brain Neurones

A small proportion of cells in the central nervous system shows large increases or decreases in activity in response to a change in local temperature (for review see Chap. 9 of Bligh 1973). Some of these cells are thought to be primary temperature sensors whereas others may be thermoregulatory interneurones, themselves relatively insensitive to local temperature changes and driven by primary thermosensors. Murakami et al. (1967) found that in dogs (*encephale isolé*) both thiopentone and a mixture of chloralose and urethane could reduce the sensitivity to temperature of thermosensitive neurones in the preoptic area. No such effect was seen with ether which did however reduce the spontaneous firing rates of these cells. Eisenman and Jackson (1967) reported that in preoptic and septal areas of anaesthetized or decerebrate cats, methohexitone could reduce the effect of local temperature changes on the activity of cells thought to function as thermoregulatory interneurones. However, putative primary temperature sensors were relatively insensitive to the barbiturate. Jell and Gloor (1972) found that in preoptic and anterior hypothalamic areas of partially decerebrate cats only 2 of 30 thermosensitive cells studied decreased their sensitivity to local temperature change in the presence of anaesthetics (ether, chloralose, thiopentone or methohexitone). Of the remaining cells studied, 10 showed no change and 18 an increase in sensitivity. Finally, Nakayama and Hori (1973) reported that in the brain-stem reticular formation of urethane-anaesthetized rabbits, hexobarbitone reduced the response to local temperature change of cells thought to be thermoregulatory interneurones. Cells thought to be primary temperature sensors were not affected in this way by the drug.

2. Narcotic Analgesics

a) Drug Interactions and Brain Lesions

In 1968, Banerjee et al. (1968a) suggested that morphine might alter deep-body temperature in cats, rabbits, and rats by directly or indirectly activating serotoninergic mechanisms in the anterior hypothalamus. Subsequently, Haubrich and Blake (1971) reported that, albeit after systemic administration, p-chlorophenylalanine (pCPA) an inhibitor of the biosynthesis of 5-hydroxytryptamine (5-HT) abolished the hypothermic effect of morphine in rats when given at a dose producing 70% depletion of brain 5-HT. Similar results have been obtained from other rat experiments with pCPA (Oka and Nozaki 1970; Oka et al. 1972) and from studies with p-chloroamphetamine (Warwick et al. 1973) which like pCPA is an inhibitor of tryptophan hydroxylase. This enzyme catalyses the conversion of tryptophan to 5-hydroxytryptophan, the immediate precursor of 5-HT. Oka (1977) reported that pre-treatment with pCPA could prevent morphine hypothermia in rats both at ambient temperatures of 21° and 12 °C and could also shorten methadone hypothermia. It has also been reported that administration of 5-hydroxytryptophan (5-HTP), could restore the hypothermic effect of morphine in rats which had been pre-treated with pCPA (OKA et al. 1972).

Although results obtained with pCPA or p-chloroamphetamine support the hypothesis that morphine-induced hypothermia in rats depends in some way on neuronal release of 5-HT they do not support an involvement of 5-HT in morphine-induced hyperthermia. OKA and NEGISHI (1977) reported that in a strain of rats in which subcutaneously administered doses of morphine as high as 40 mg/kg produced only hyperthermia, pre-treatment with pCPA did not alter the temperature response to morphine. In a different strain of rats, a dose of morphine which was normally hypothermic produced a rise in body temperature in animals pre-treated with pCPA (OKA 1977). It was also found that morphine, pethidine, and methadone given at doses which by themselves had no effect on body temperature produced significant hyperthermia when given to rats which had also received pCPA. These effects of pCPA on the temperature responses of rats to narcotic analgesics could be abolished by 5-HTP (OKA 1977).

Electrolytic lesions of rat mid-brain raphé nuclei which reduce the fore-brain concentrations of 5-HT and of its primary metabolite 5-hydroxyindoleacetic acid have been reported to abolish the effect of morphine on body temperature (SAMANIN et al. 1972). Unlike pre-treatment with pCPA this method of reducing brain concentrations of 5-HT was found to abolish both the hypothermic and the hyperthermic responses to morphine. Lesioned rats were still able to respond to the hyperthermic action of dinitrophenol and to the hypothermic action of phentolamine. Neither of these drugs is thought to alter body temperature through serotoninergic mechanisms.

FULLER and BAKER (1974) found that rats pre-treated intraperitoneally with fluoxetine, a selective inhibitor of the neuronal uptake of 5-HT, exhibited an increased, prolonged hypothermia in response to morphine. In cats (FRENCH et al. 1978 a) fluoxetine has also been found to alter the effect of morphine on body temperature, in this case enhancing the hyperthermic response. These results provide further support for an involvement of 5-HT in the effects of morphine on body temperature. It has been suggested that morphine might alter the activity of serotoninergic pathways by facilitating release of 5-HT (HAUBRICH and BLAKE 1971). An alternative mechanism would be inhibition of neuronal uptake of 5-HT and indeed it has been shown that morphine can inhibit the in vitro uptake of 5-HT by synaptosomes prepared from rabbit brain (CIOFALO 1974) or from rat hypothalamus (WARWICK and SCHNELL 1976). However, there is little evidence to suggest that this action of morphine is responsible for its effects on body temperature (WARWICK et al. 1977). The in vitro concentrations of morphine needed to inhibit 5-HT uptake are high. Similar concentrations of the narcotic antagonist naloxone also inhibit synaptosomal uptake of 5-HT and yet naloxone does not alter body temperature in rats when given at a dose level at which morphine has been shown to produce marked hypothermia (WARWICK and SCHNELL 1976). Morphine-induced hypothermia in rats can be reversed by naloxone (see also Sect. B.I.2.b), but the effect of morphine on synaptosomal uptake of 5-HT is not reversed (WARWICK and SCHNELL 1976).

There have been several reports of experiments concerned with the effect of α-methyltyrosine (α-MT), an inhibitor of catecholamine biosynthesis, on morphine-induced changes in body temperature. HAUBRICH and BLAKE (1971) found that pre-treatment with α-MT significantly enhanced the hypothermic response to morphine in rats. The same pre-treatment also lowered brain concentrations of noradrenaline by 56%. It was concluded that enhancement of the hypothermic effect of morphine by α-MT was probably due to a depletion of catecholamines, resulting in reduced activity of central and peripheral noradrenergic pathways controlling the production and conservation of heat. In other experiments pre-treatment with α-MT was found to have no effect on morphine-induced hypothermia in rats (OKA et al. 1972). Morphine-induced hyperthermia was also found to be unaffected by this pre-treatment (OKA and NEGISHI 1977). OKA and NEGISHI (1977) also found that phenoxybenzamine and propranolol were without effect. These studies do not appear to support the involvement of dopaminergic or noradrenergic pathways in the body temperature changes produced by morphine in rats. However, negative findings with α-MT should be interpreted with particular caution since there are thought to be significant reserves of noradrenaline and dopamine stored in nerve endings and available for release (for review see GLOWINSKI 1975).

Other types of investigation have yielded results which support the involvement of dopaminergic pathways in the effects of morphine on body temperature. FRENCH et al. (1978a) reported that morphine-induced hyperthermia in cats was enhanced by pimozide, a selective dopamine antagonist. They proposed that in cat thermoregulation there may normally be a balance in the preoptic/anterior hypothalamic region between dopamine release, which would lower body temperature, and 5-HT release, which would raise it. Since morphine-induced hyperthermia was enhanced by fluoxetine as well as by pimozide they suggested that in the cat dopamine and 5-HT are both released from their nerve endings by morphine and that this produces a change in the balance between dopamine and 5-HT release in the hypothalamus and hence also a change in body temperature. In mice, haloperidol, a dopamine antagonist less selective than pimozide, was found to have no effect on morphine-induced hyperthermia although it did reduce morphine-induced hypothermia (GLICK 1975).

There are reports that the hyperthermic effect of morphine can be antagonized by the anticholinesterase physostigmine. However, antimuscarinic agents have also been shown to antagonize morphine-induced hyperthermia and the data are therefore difficult to interpret. GLICK (1975) found that hyperthermia produced by morphine in mice could be partially prevented by scopolamine and converted to a hypothermic effect by physostigmine. Scopolamine was found to have no effect on morphine-induced hypothermia. In rats too morphine-induced hyperthermia was shown to be antagonized by physostigmine (SHARKAWI 1972). Antagonism by the antimuscarinic agents scopolamine and atropine has also been reported (OKA and NEGISHI 1977). OKA et al. (1972) found that in rats scopolamine had no effect on morphine-induced hypothermia. More recently, however, KAAKKOLA and AHTEE (1977) reported that pre-treatment with scopolamine or atropine enhanced morphine-induced hypothermia in rats. The anticholinesterase neostigmine and the antimuscarinic agents methyl atropine and methscopolamine were shown to have no effect on morphine-induced changes in body temperature (KAAKKOLA and AH-

TEE 1977; SHARKAWI 1972). These drugs are all quaternary ammonium compounds and therefore expected to penetrate the blood–brain barrier only with difficulty. Possibly physostigmine, scopolamine, and atropine, all of which readily cross the blood–brain barrier, influence the effects of morphine by acting at sites located within the central nervous system. However, it should be noted that OKA and NEGISHI (1977) found that in rats morphine-induced hyperthermia was reduced not only by atropine and scopolamine but also by the quaternary analogues of these compounds.

b) Effects on Temperature-Dependent Electrical Activities of Brain Neurones

BALDINO et al. (1980) have studied the effects of iontophoretically applied morphine on hypothalamic thermosensitive neurones in rats anaesthetized with urethane. Rectal temperature was maintained at 37°–38 °C. Morphine was found to elevate the firing rate of 12 of 20 cells showing an increased firing rate in response to a rise in hypothalamic temperature. The drug reduced the firing rate of 6 of 7 cells showing a decreased firing rate in response to hypothalamic warming. Morphine was also found to alter the firing rates of 20 of 30 "temperature-insensitive" cells. It was concluded that morphine may lower body temperature by exerting actions both on warm-sensitive neurones, assumed to mediate heat dissipation responses, and on cold-sensitive neurones, assumed to mediate heat gain responses.

3. Phenothiazines

The phenothiazines possess several pharmacological properties which could account for their effects on thermoregulation. In particular they show antagonistic actions at dopaminergic receptors, serotoninergic receptors, α-adrenoceptors and muscarinic receptors. Any of these actions might give rise to changes in heat gain or heat loss since dopamine, 5-hydroxytryptamine, acetylcholine, and noradrenaline are all thought to act as neurotransmitters in central thermoregulatory pathways (for review see COX and LOMAX 1977). Heat loss could also be affected by antagonism of α-adrenoceptors located in vascular smooth muscle. Another pharmacological property of the phenothiazines is their local anaesthetic activity and it has been suggested that this could contribute to thermoregulatory changes observed after injection into brain or cerebrospinal fluid. Like chlorpromazine, the local anaesthetic procaine has been reported to cause hyperthermia when injected into the thermoregulatory centres in the rat (KIRKPATRICK and LOMAX 1971). The doses of procaine and chlorpromazine which produced comparable increases in deep-body temperature were found to be in the same ratio as those causing a comparable degree of nerve blockade in vitro.

There have been several studies of interactions between chlorpromazine and other drugs thought to influence the activity of thermoregulatory pathways in the central or peripheral nervous system. Chlorpromazine-induced hypothermia has been shown to be enhanced in rabbits by a hyperthermic dose of cocaine (WISLICKI 1960) and in rats by dibenamine and pyribenzamine (LE BLANC and ROSENBERG 1958) and by benserazide (LIN et al. 1978), an inhibitor of aromatic amino acid decarboxylase. It has also been reported that chlorpromazine-induced hypothermia can be enhanced by reducing brain concentrations of 5-HT in rabbits with 5,7-dihydroxytryptamine (LIN 1979) and in rats with lesions of dorsal and median raphé nuclei or with 5,6-dihydroxytryptamine or p-chlorophenylalanine (LIN et al. 1979). Rabbits pre-treated with 5,7-dihydroxytryptamine were found to lose heat more rapidly than control animals and such a change could well explain the effect of 5-HT depletion on the hypothermic response to chlorpromazine both in rabbits and rats. It should be noted that LIN et al. (1979) found chlorpromazine-induced hypothermia to be enhanced not only after 5-HT depletion but also after drug-induced increases in brain concentrations of this amine. They suggested that reduction and elevation of 5-HT concentrations could both result in suppression of the firing rate of 5-HT nerves and that it was this change in neuronal activity which led to facilitation of chlorpromazine-induced hypothermia.

Several drugs have been shown to reduce the effects of chlorpromazine on body temperature. BAGDON and MANN (1965) reported that pilocarpine antagonized the hyperthermic response of 10-day-old mice to chlorpromazine. Since chlorpromazine has antimuscarinic properties and since atropine, like chlorpromazine, can produce hyperthermia when injected into rat hypothalamus (KIRKPATRICK and LOMAX 1967) it is certainly possible that chlorpromazine-induced hyperthermia could result from an inhibitory effect on central cholinergic pathways. The hypothermic effect of chlorpromazine has also been found to be reduced by amphetamine in mice (LESSIN and PARKES 1957b) and rats (YEHUDA and WURTMAN 1972), by reserpine in rats (HOFFMAN 1958) and by 6-hydroxydopamine in rabbits (LIN 1979). It was found that, 2–6 weeks after injection of 6-hydroxydopamine into the third ventricle, rabbits showed decreases both in heat production and heat loss and yet were able to maintain normal body temperatures. When injected with chlorpromazine the animals pre-treated with 6-hydroxydopamine showed smaller changes in heat production and heat loss and smaller falls in deep-body temperature than control animals. Pre-treatment with 6-hydroxydopamine had no effect on the hyperthermic response of rabbits to chlorpromazine. In rats pre-treatment with reserpine (REWERSKI and JORI 1968b) or α-methyltyrosine (REWERSKI and GUMULKA 1969) has also been reported to have no effect on this response.

TSOUCARIS-KUPFER and SCHMITT (1972) reported that chlorpromazine reduced the hypothermic effect of clonidine in rats. Both drugs were given either intraperitoneally or intrahypothalamically. JACOB and PEINDARIES (1973) showed that injection of dopamine, noradrenaline or 5-HT into the lateral ventricles produced hyperthermia in rabbits. The effects of dopamine and 5-HT but not of noradrenaline were reduced by pre-treatment with hypothermic doses of chlorpromazine. Chlorpromazine has also been shown to prevent the hyperthermic responses of mice (BARNETT et al. 1972) and rats (MORPURGO and THEOBALD 1965; YEHUDA and WURTMAN 1972) to amphetamine. The antagonism was observed at normal room temperature but did not occur at 37 °C (YEHUDA and WURTMAN 1972). Chlorpromazine can hasten recovery from hypothermia caused by prior injection of reserpine in rats (COSTA et al. 1960) or mice (COOPER and SCHNIEDEN 1972; MORPURGO and THEOBALD 1965; WHITTLE 1967). WHITTLE (1967) found that this effect of chlorpromazine could be prevented by propranolol but not by phenoxybenzamine. COOPER and SCHNIEDEN (1972) observed that chlorpromazine was 8–15 times more effective in reversing reserpine-induced hypothermia when given directly into the cerebral ventricles than when given orally and also that the effect could be abolished by chlorisondamine. Taken together, these results suggest that the effect of chlorpromazine on reserpine-induced hypothermia could be initiated centrally. The effect may be mediated by the sympathetic nervous system and involve activation of β-adrenoceptors. Intact adrenal glands are also required for the full response to be elicited (COOPER and SCHNIEDEN 1972).

V. Effects of Repeated Administration

1. Barbiturates and Ethanol

Abrupt withdrawal after repeated administration of barbiturates or ethanol may be followed by the appearance of a withdrawal syndrome. TAGASHIRA et al. (1978) found that in rats withdrawal of phenobarbitone or barbitone was followed by a rise in body temperature. The drugs had been administered in the diet and hyperthermia was produced by withdrawal of the drugs after 7–10 days of treatment. The hyperthermia appeared within 24 h of withdrawal and lasted up to 48 h. BRICK and POHORECKY (1977) found that rats which had been maintained on an ethanol-containing diet for 6 weeks developed a preference for a warm environment (30 °C) when ethanol was withdrawn from the diet and the animals were placed in a T-maze with alley temperatures of 2°, 19°, and 30 °C. Ethanol withdrawal was not however followed by any detectable change in body temperature. The control rats preferred a temperature of 19 °C. Mice kept at normal room temperature and subjected to diets containing ethanol (RITZMANN and TABAKOFF 1976b) or phenobarbitone (TABAKOFF et al. 1978) were found to exhibit hypothermia lasting not more than 24 h (ethanol) or 44 h (phenobarbitone) when the drugs were withdrawn from the diet after 6–7 days. In the ethanol experiments placement of mice in the cold (4 °C) 5.5 h after withdrawal exacerbated the hypothermia whereas placement in the warm (34 °C) led to reversal of the hypothermia followed by onset of hyperthermia. Mice exposed to a temperature of 34 °C immediatelly after ethanol withdrawal exhibited only hyperthermia.

As well as affecting body temperature after withdrawal, the presence in the diet of ethanol (RITZMANN and TABAKOFF 1976b) or phenobarbitone (TABAKOFF et al. 1978) was found to result in the development of tolerance to the hypothermic effects of these drugs. Tolerance was observed in mice challenged with a single injection of ethanol (intracerebral or intraperitoneal) 24 h after its withdrawal from the diet or with phenobarbitone (intracerebral) 44 h after its withdrawal. Mice tolerant to ethanol also showed tolerance to the hypothermic effects of pentobarbitone and piribedil but not to the effect of clonidine (HOFFMAN and TABAKOFF 1977; TABAKOFF et al. 1977). Tolerance to the hypothermic effects of pentobarbitone (intracerebral or intraperitoneal) has also been detected in mice 3 days after subcutaneous implantation of a pentobarbitone pellet (HO 1976) and after 5 days of repeated administration of the drug by gavage (TABAKOFF et al. 1977). In rats tolerance to the hypothermic effect of ethanol has been observed after 5 days (FRANKEL et al. 1978) or 3 weeks (NIKKI et al. 1971) of repeated oral administration. FRANKEL et al. (1978) concluded that 5-hydroxytryptamine might be involved in the development of tolerance to the hypothermic effect of ethanol in rats since p-chlorophenylalanine appeared to slow down or even abolish onset of tolerance. However, their results are difficult to interpret since p-chlorophenylalanine by itself was found to alter body temperature.

Most hypotheses of drug dependence postulate that physical dependence is closely linked to pharmacodynamic tolerance (for review see KALANT et al. 1971). This type of tolerance develops in the presence of a drug and may result from adaptive biological changes which serve to compensate for the effects of the drug. Once pharmacodynamic tolerance has developed withdrawal of the drug is thought to precipitate an abstinence syndrome by upsetting the balance between the drug effects and the compensatory mechanisms. There is now evidence that, in mice, certain signs of tolerance to phenobarbitone or ethanol can be eliminated without affecting the development of physical dependence to these drugs. It was found that, after intracerebral administration of 6-hydroxydopamine, mice receiving diets containing ethanol (RITZMANN and TABAKOFF 1976 c) or phenobarbitone (TABAKOFF et al. 1978) no longer became tolerant to the effects of these drugs on body temperature or behaviour and yet still showed changes in body temperature and behaviour after drug withdrawal. The pre-treatment with 6-hydroxydopamine was shown to affect brain concentrations of noradrenaline but not those of dopamine or 5-hydroxytryptamine and it was therefore suggested (TABAKOFF et al. 1977) that noradrenergic systems are necessary for the expression of at least some forms of tolerance to barbiturates and ethanol.

2. Narcotic Analgesics

a) Tolerance

Development of tolerance to the hypothermic effect of morphine has been noted in monkeys and dogs (EDDY and REID 1934), rabbits (KO 1937), guinea-pigs (SCHULZ et al. 1974), rats (GUNNE 1960; HAUBRICH and BLAKE 1973; LOMAX and KIRKPATRICK 1967; LOTTI et al. 1966a; MAYNERT and KLINGMAN 1962; OKA et al. 1972; ROSENFELD and BURKS 1977; WARWICK et al. 1973, 1977), and mice (BLOOM and DEWEY 1978; FERNANDES et al. 1977). Tolerance was produced either by subcutaneous implantation of morphine base in pellet form (HAUBRICH and BLAKE 1973; SCHULZ et al. 1974; WARWICK et al. 1973, 1977) or by single or repeated morphine injection. Repeated injections were made using either a constant dose level (EDDY and REID 1934; FERNANDES et al. 1977; GUNNE 1960; KO 1937) or progressively greater doses (BLOOM and DEWEY 1978; EDDY and REID 1934; GUNNE 1960; MAYNERT and KLINGMAN 1962; OKA et al. 1972; ROSENFELD and BURKS 1977). Tolerant animals have been shown to exhibit either a reduced hypothermic response or even hyperthermia when given morphine at doses producing marked hypothermia in non-tolerant animals. Tolerance to morphine-induced hypothermia can develop rapidly. In rats it has been reported to occur within 5 h of a single morphine injection given subcutaneously, intravenously or directly into the preoptic/anterior hypothalamic nuclei (LOMAX and KIRKPATRICK 1967; LOTTI et al. 1966a; ROSENFELD and BURKS 1977).

Tolerance has been shown to develop not only to morphine-induced hypothermia but also to the hyperthermic effect of the drug. This type of tolerance has been observed in cats (FRENCH et al. 1978b) and rats (RUDY and YAKSH 1977) pre-treated with hyperthermic doses of morphine. Such pre-treatment does not always produce tolerance in rats. THORNHILL et al. (1978) found that repeated administration of hyperthermic doses of morphine in rats kept at 25°–27 °C did not produce tolerance but instead enhanced the hyperthermic effect of the drug. In other rat experiments (GUNNE 1960; WARWICK et al. 1973) morphine pre treatment was found to abolish only the hypothermic component of a biphasic temperature response to morphine. The hyperthermic component was unaltered or even enhanced. It has also been found that the hyperthermic response to morphine reaches its peak earlier in rats pre-treated with morphine than in control animals (GUNNE 1960; THORNHILL et al. 1978; WARWICK et al. 1973).

b) Withdrawal Effects

In animals rendered tolerant to the effects of morphine on body temperature, abrupt withdrawal of drug treatment is followed by a gradual loss of tolerance. SCHULZ et al. (1974) found that in guinea-pigs tolerance was lost 3–7 days after removal of subcutaneously implanted morphine pellets. In rats (GUNNE 1960; LOTTI et al. 1966a; ROSENFELD and BURKS 1977) and mice (FERNANDES et al. 1977) withdrawn from morphine after one or more injections, it took more than two weeks for tolerance to disappear.

Abrupt withdrawal of morphine treatment or administration of narcotic antagonists to animals pre-treated with morphine can give rise to withdrawal effects some of which may reflect disruption of thermoregulation (WEI et al. 1974). In rats withdrawal effects include teeth chattering, "wet dog" shakes, increased motor activity, piloerection, salivation, and escape behaviour (ARY and LOMAX 1976; ARY et al. 1976, 1977; COX et al. 1975, 1976b; LASKA and FENNESSY 1976, 1978; MARTIN et al. 1963; ROSENFELD and BURKS 1977; TSENG et al. 1975). These effects could all reflect alterations in activity of heat gain or heat loss mechanisms. So too could withdrawal-induced "wet dog" shakes in cats (FRENCH et al. 1978b) and shivering, tremor, piloerection and salivation induced by morphine withdrawal in monkeys (EDDY and REID 1934; HOLTZMAN and VILLARREAL 1969). Further support for a link between withdrawal effects and thermoregulation comes from the observation that ambient temperature can influence the occurrence of "wet dog" shakes, which is a possible heat gain mechanism, and escape behaviour, which is a possible heat loss mechanism. WEI et al. (1974) reported that the frequency of "wet dog" shakes induced by naloxone in rats pre-treated with morphine was greater in the cold than in the warm and also that naloxone-induced escape behaviour was enhanced in a hot environment.

More direct evidence for a withdrawal-induced change in thermoregulation is the observation that morphine withdrawal is often followed by a change in deep-body temperature. There are reports that dogs (MAYNERT and KLINGMAN 1962) and rabbits (KO 1937; MAYNERT and KLINGMAN 1962) pre-treated with morphine become hyperthermic after drug withdrawal or in response to a narcotic antagonist whereas monkeys (EDDY and REID 1934; HOLTZMAN and VILLARREAL 1969), cats (FRENCH et al. 1978b), mice (KAMEI and UEKI 1974), and rats (ARY and LOMAX 1976; ARY et al. 1976, 1977; BHARGAVA 1977; BHARGAVA and MATWYSHYN 1977; COX et al. 1975, 1976b; LAL et al. 1971; LASKA and FENNESSY 1976, 1978; LINSEMAN 1976; MAYNERT and KLINGMAN 1962; OKA and NOZAKI 1970; OKA et al. 1972;

Roffman et al. 1973; Rudy and Yaksh 1977; Tseng et al. 1975) exhibit hypothermia. Withdrawal hypothermia is sometimes preceded by a transient hyperthermia (Holtzman and Villarreal 1969, 1971; Kamei and Ueki 1974) which in monkeys has been shown to be enhanced by atropine (Holtzman and Villarreal 1971).

In monkeys pre-treated with morphine, hypothermia can be induced by abrupt withdrawal of drug treatment (Eddy and Reid 1934; Holtzman and Villarreal 1971), by physical restraint imposed 3–7 h after withdrawal (Holtzman and Villarreal 1969) or by injection of nalorphine (Holtzman and Villarreal 1969, 1971) and can be reversed by morphine (Holtzman and Villarreal 1969). Holtzman and Villarreal (1971) found that the falls in body temperature induced by physical restraint in monkeys pre-treated with morphine could also be reversed at least partially by codeine, pethidine, methadone, dextromoramide, levorphanol, and GP 1658. Atropine was also effective but amphetamine, methylatropine, and the optical isomers of levorphanol and GP 1658 were not. Atropine did not significantly alter hypothermia induced by nalorphine in monkeys pre-treated with morphine. Holtzman and Villarreal (1971) also found that monkeys pre-treated with morphine became markedly hypothermic when injected with the cholinesterase inhibitor physostigmine at a dose producing only a small fall in the body temperature of control animals. It was concluded that this effect was mediated by cholinergic mechanisms located outside the blood–brain barrier since the hypothermia was antagonized more effectively by methylatropine than atropine and could also be induced by neostigmine which, like methylatropine, is a quaternary ammonium compound.

In rats as in monkeys, hypothermia may be induced after morphine pre-treatment either by abrupt withdrawal (Bhargava 1977; Bhargava and Matwyshyn 1977; Lal et al. 1971; Roffman et al. 1973) or by injection of a narcotic antagonist. Nalorphine (Maynert and Klingman 1962), naloxone (Ary et al. 1977; Bhargava 1977; Bhargava and Matwyshyn 1977; Cox et al. 1975, 1976b; Laska and Fennessy 1976, 1978; Linseman 1976; Oka and Nozaki 1970; Oka et al. 1972; Rudy and Yaksh 1977; Tseng et al. 1975), and naltrexone (Ary and Lomax 1976; Ary et al. 1976) are all effective. Maynert and Klingman (1962) reported that nalorphine caused a decrease in the rectal temperatures of rats treated chronically with morphine. Oka et al. (1972) found that systemic administration of naloxone produced hypothermia in rats made tolerant to morphine by a series of morphine injections. Hypothermia was greater at an ambient temperature of 20 °C than at 30 °C. Intrathecal administration of naloxone to morphine-tolerant rats has also been found to lower body temperature (Rudy and Yaksh 1977). The hypothermia was accompanied by a marked rise in tail skin temperature. Naloxone had no effect on body temperature in non-tolerant rats (Oka et al. 1972; Rudy and Yaksh 1977). Laska and Fennessy (1976) reported that naloxone can lower rat body temperature when given only 24 h after the subcutaneous administration of a slowly-released preparation of morphine. It has also been found that naloxone (Cox et al. 1975) and naltrexone (Ary and Lomax 1976) can produce hypothermia in rats when injected systemically 72 h after subcutaneous implantation of morphine pellets. The naloxone-induced falls in body temperature could be reduced by injection of morphine into the preoptic/anterior hypothalamic nuclei, suggesting that withdrawal hypothermia is a response mediated by pathways situated in this part of the brain. At 45 days after pellet implantation naltrexone had no effect on body temperature. It is noteworthy however that a single injection of morphine could "resensitize" these animals to naltrexone (ARY and LOMAX 1976). This observation was taken to support the proposal of BRASE et al. (1976) that administration of an opiate to abstinent animals can restore the ability of narcotic antagonists to precipitate signs of withdrawal by uncovering "a latent, pre-existing state of physical dependence."

c) Neuronal Mechanisms in Rats

There have been several investigations into the part played by putative central neurotransmitters in the temperature responses to morphine or naloxone by rats pretreated with morphine. MEDON and BLAKE (1973) found that rats which had been made tolerant to the hypothermic effect of morphine showed unaltered hypothermic responses to intraventricular injections of 5-hydroxytryptamine, noradrenaline or pilocarpine. They concluded that tolerance to morphine-induced hypothermia was not caused by changes in postsynaptic sensitivity to putative transmitters in the thermoregulatory centres.

HAUBRICH and BLAKE (1973) reported that morphine could increase turnover of 5-hydroxytryptamine in rat brains during the 90 min period following drug injection (30 mg/kg SC). Morphine was also found to increase the steady-state brain concentration of 5-hydroxyindoleacetic acid (5-HIAA). Development of tolerance to the hypothermic effect of morphine was accompanied by a return to normal of the brain concentrations of 5-HIAA. However, turnover of 5-hydroxytryptamine in rat brains was greater in tolerant than in non-tolerant animals. LASKA and FENNESSY (1976, 1978) also found that rats pre-treated with morphine showed increases in brain 5-HIAA. However, when rats were pre-treated with naloxone instead of morphine, increases in brain 5-HIAA also occurred, suggesting that morphine-induced increases in this metabolite are not causally related to the development of morphine tolerance or dependence (LASKA and FENNESSY 1977). OKA et al. (1972) showed that in rats rendered tolerant to the hypothermic effect of morphine neither hyperthermia induced by morphine nor hypothermia induced by naloxone was altered by pre-treatment with α methyltyrosine. The temperature responses to morphine and naloxone were also unaffected by pre-treatment with p-chloroamphetamine or p-chlorophenylalanine at doses known to antagonize the hypothermic effect of morphine in non-tolerant animals (OKA and NOZAKI 1970; OKA et al. 1972; WARWICK et al. 1973). It was concluded that temperature responses of morphine-tolerant rats to morphine or naloxone are not mediated by adrenergic or serotoninergic mechanisms. It was also concluded that serotoninergic mechanisms are unlikely to be associated with the development of tolerance to the effects of morphine on rat thermoregulation (WARWICK et al. 1973).

In contrast to the experiments with α-methyltyrosine, other types of experiment have yielded results which suggest that, in rats pre-treated with morphine, hypothermia induced by withdrawal (LAL et al. 1971) or by naloxone (ARY et al. 1977; COX et al. 1975, 1976b) may be mediated by dopaminergic mechanisms and that these may be located in the hypothalamus. Pimozide, a selective dopamine antagonist has been shown to decrease naloxone-induced hypothermia in rats pre-treated with morphine (COX et al. 1975, 1976b). This effect was observed not only when pimozide was given intraperitoneally but also when it was injected directly into the preoptic/anterior hypothalamic nuclei. Pimozide was also found to antagonize naloxone-induced changes in behavioural thermoregulation and to increase naloxone-induced chewing, head shakes and writhing. In other experiments ARY et al. (1977) found that apomorphine decreased naloxone-induced "wet dog" shakes, teeth chatter, writhing, diarrhoea, and weight loss in rats pre-treated with morphine. It has also been found that the fall in body temperature produced in morphine-dependent rats by concurrent administration of hypothermic doses of apomorphine and naloxone was the same as the fall produced by naloxone alone (COX et al. 1975).

In morphine-tolerant rats exhibiting a hyperthermic response to a dose of morphine known to produce hypothermia in non-tolerant animals, it has been found that morphine-induced hyperthermia can be attenuated by treatment with either scopolamine or atropine (OKA and NOZAKI 1970; OKA et al. 1972). After administration of scopolamine, a prolonged hyperthermic response to morphine was replaced by a biphasic response consisting of a transient hypothermia followed by a brief hyperthermia. The hyperthermic response to morphine was also affected by methylscopolamine. Scopolamine had no effect on naloxone-induced hypothermia in morphine-tolerant rats or on morphine-induced hypothermia in non-tolerant animals. OKA et al. (1972) concluded that the hyperthermic response to morphine observed in rats tolerant to the hypothermic effect of morphine might well depend on activation of both central and peripheral cholinergic mechanisms.

3. Phenothiazines

Repeated administration of chlorpromazine has been reported to produce tolerance to chlorpromazine-induced hypothermia in rats (ANKERMANN 1958; SINGH and DAS 1976) and mice (LIU 1974). Similarly, repeated administration of perphenazine has been shown to produce tolerance to perphenazine-induced hypothermia in rabbits (VOTAVA 1973). With daily injections of chlorpromazine or perphenazine, tolerance was found to develop within 7 days. It has also been reported that rats can become tolerant to the effects of chlorpromazine on oxygen consumption (ANKERMANN 1958; COURVOISIER et al. 1953). COURVOISIER et al. (1953) found that rats subjected to daily injections of chlorpromazine (20 mg/kg SC) became tolerant within 36 days.

VI. Drug Interactions Producing Hyperthermia

1. Narcotic Analgesics

Administration of pethidine to rabbits pre-treated with a monoamine oxidase inhibitor can produce changes often ending in death. These changes include motor restlessness, hyperexcitability, shiver-like tremors and hyperthermia (ELTAYEB and OSMAN 1975; FAHIM et al. 1972; GONG and ROGERS 1971, 1973; JOUNELA et al. 1977; LOVELESS and MAXWELL 1965; MATTILA and JOUNELA 1973; NYMARK and NIELSEN 1963; OSMAN and ELTAYEB 1977; PENN and ROGERS 1971; SINCLAIR 1972 a; SINCLAIR and LO 1977). There may also be tachypnoea (ELTAYEB and OSMAN 1975; OSMAN and ELTAYEB 1977; SINCLAIR 1972 a), and profuse salivation (GONG and

ROGERS 1973; PENN and ROGERS 1971). Dextromethorphan (SINCLAIR 1973) and the pethidine analogue, ethoheptazine (SINCLAIR 1972b) can elicit a similar reaction. However levorphanol, codeine, pentazocine, levallorphan, nalorphine, anileridine, alphaprodine, piminodine, and dextropropoxyphene have been shown to be inactive (PENN and ROGERS 1971; SINCLAIR 1972b). In most but not all experiments morphine and methadone have also been shown to be inactive (PENN and ROGERS 1971; SINCLAIR 1972a, b). The finding that several highly effective narcotic analgesics failed to elicit fatal hyperthermia in animals pre-treated with a monoamine oxidase inhibitor suggests that this interaction does not involve opiate receptors. This conclusion is supported by reports (FAHIM et al. 1972; SINCLAIR 1972a) that the interaction between pethidine and monoamine oxidase inhibitors is not prevented by nalorphine or by chronic pre-treatment with morphine. Potentiation of pethidine by monoamine oxidase inhibitors through an effect on pethidine metabolism has also been discounted as a possible mechanism (SINCLAIR and Lo 1977).

There is evidence that the interaction between pethidine and monoamine oxidase inhibitors in rabbits may depend on increases in the concentration of 5-HT at the synapse. It has been shown that in rabbits pre-treated with a monoamine oxidase inhibitor the reaction to pethidine can be prevented by prior administration of p-chlorophenylalanine (ELTAYEB and OSMAN 1975; FAHIM et al. 1972; GONG and ROGERS 1971, 1973; MATTILA and JOUNELA 1973; OSMAN and ELTAYEB 1977) or 5-HT antagonists (ELTAYEB and OSMAN 1975; OSMAN and ELTAYEB 1977; SINCLAIR 1972a) and can be mimicked by inhibitors of neuronal uptake of 5-HT (SINCLAIR and Lo 1977) or by 5-hydroxytryptophan (ELTAYEB and OSMAN 1975; OSMAN and ELTAYEB 1977). Similar results have been obtained with dextromethorphan (SINCLAIR 1973). FAHIM et al. (1972) reported that pethidine evoked excitement and hyperthermia in rabbits pre-treated with lithium or yohimbine, drugs which were both expected to elevate brain concentrations of 5-HT. GONG and ROGERS (1973) showed that in pargyline-treated rabbits fatal hyperthermia induced by pethidine was not prevented when either reserpine or α-methyl-p-tyrosine was administered with the pargyline. Reserpine and α-methyl-p-tyrosine prevented pargyline-induced increases in brain catecholamine concentrations but did not prevent increases in 5-HT concentrations.

PENN and ROGERS (1971) proposed that pethidine can induce fatal hyperthermia in rabbits pre-treated with a monoamine oxidase inhibitor by blocking the neuronal uptake of 5-HT. This hypothesis was tested by SINCLAIR and Lo (1977). They found that, with one exception, drugs known to elicit fatal hyperthermia in rabbits tended to be more potent as inhibitors of 5-HT uptake in vitro than drugs which do not induce fatal hyperthermia. The exception to this rule was levorphanol which was found to be about equipotent with pethidine as an inhibitor of 5-HT uptake and yet not to interact with phenelzine. SINCLAIR and Lo (1977) noted that levorphanol had a marked depressant effect in rabbits and suggested that this could have blocked the development of fatal hyperthermia. MATTILA and JOUNELA (1973) have questioned the hypothesis that the interaction between pethidine and monoamine oxidase inhibitors depends on brain concentrations of 5-HT. They found that although p-chlorophenylalanine could prevent induction of hyperthermia and excitement by pethidine in phenelzine-treated rabbits, administration of

5-HTP along with p-chlorophenylalanine restored brain concentrations of 5-HT without also restoring the pethidine–phenelzine interaction.

Monoamine oxidase inhibitors have been shown to increase pethidine lethality in mice as well as rabbits (Ahtee et al. 1974; Botting et al. 1978; Brownlee and Williams 1963; Fuller and Snoddy 1975; Gessner 1973; Gessner and Soble 1973; Rogers 1971; Rogers and Thornton 1969). Jounela (1970) also detected an interaction between pethidine and a monoamine oxidase inhibitor but only in aggregated mice. In mice pre-treated with a monoamine oxidase inhibitor, death induced by pethidine has been found to be preceded by hyperthermia at an ambient temperature of 29 °C (Gessner 1973; Gessner and Soble 1973), by either hyperthermia or no change in body temperature at 25 °C (Ahtee et al. 1974; Jounela 1970; Leander et al. 1978) and by hypothermia at 22 °C or less (Botting et al. 1978; Gessner et al. 1974). Changes in body temperature could be prevented by methysergide (Botting et al. 1978) but not by pre-treatment with p-chlorophenylalanine (Gessner and Soble 1973). Rogers and Thornton (1969) reported that pre-treatment with iproniazid or tranylcypromine potentiated the acute lethality of morphine, pentazocine, and phenazocine as well as of pethidine. However in other studies pre-treatment with monoamine oxidase inhibitors was found to have no significant effect on the lethality of morphine, pentazocine, methadone, alphaprodine, anileridine or piminodine (Ahtee et al. 1974; Botting et al. 1978; Jounela 1970).

In mice as in rabbits there is evidence that enhancement of pethidine lethality by monoamine oxidase inhibitors depends on activation of serotoninergic pathways (Ahtee et al. 1974; Botting et al. 1978; Gessner and Soble 1973; Jounela 1970; Rogers 1971; Rogers and Thornton 1969). However, inhibition of serotoninergic neuronal uptake may not be involved. Fuller and Snoddy (1975) found that the lethality of fluoxetine in mice was unaffected by pre-treatment with a monoamine oxidase inhibitor even though this drug is about 40 times more potent than pethidine as an inhibitor of 5-HT uptake by synaptosomes (Sinclair and Lo 1977). Rogers and Thornton (1969) reported that the lethality of morphine in mice was enhanced by pre-treatment with monoamine oxidase inhibitors. Yet morphine is markedly less potent than either fluoxetine or pethidine as an inhibitor of 5-HT uptake in vitro (Sinclair and Lo 1977).

A feature of the interaction between pethidine and monoamine oxidase inhibitors which has yet to be explained is the finding that not all monoamine oxidase inhibitors can enhance pethidine lethality. In mice, pethidine lethality is increased by tranylcypromine (Botting et al. 1978; Fuller and Snoddy 1975; Gessner 1973; Gessner and Soble 1973; Rogers 1971; Rogers and Thornton 1969), phenelzine (Ahtee et al. 1974; Botting et al. 1978; Jounela 1970), and iproniazid (Botting et al. 1978; Rogers and Thornton 1969) but not by pargyline or clorgyline (Leander et al. 1978). In rabbits too, pethidine lethality is increased by tranylcypromine (Loveless and Maxwell 1965) and phenelzine (Jounela et al. 1977; Mattila and Jounela 1973; Sinclair 1972a; Sinclair and Lo 1977). Nialamide (Loveless and Maxwell 1965) and pargyline (Fahim et al. 1972; Gong and Rogers 1971, 1973; Penn and Rogers 1971) are also effective in rabbits but clorgyline is not (Jounela et al. 1977). Possible explanations for the absence of an interaction between pethidine and clorgyline are discussed by Jounela et al. (1977).

2. Chlorpromazine

The effect of chlorpromazine on body temperature can be markedly altered by pre-treatment with thyroxine. SKOBBA and MIYA (1969) found that rats which had been made hyperthyroid by repeated administration of thyroxine exhibited hyperthermia in response to chlorpromazine. The hyperthermia was accompanied by salivation and convulsions and ended in death. SPENCER and WAITE (1968) reported that hyperthyroid mice showed a reduced hypothermic response to chlorpromazine at an ambient temperature of 22 °C and a hyperthermic response at 26 °C. They obtained similar results with reserpine. PARK et al. (1972) showed that doses of chlorpromazine which were hypothermic in euthyroid mice did not lower body temperature in hyperthyroid animals. The hyperthyroid mice no longer responded to a low dose of chlorpromazine and experienced fatal hyperthermia after a high dose.

Like hyperthyroid animals, animals pre-treated with dinitrophenol can also become hyperthermic in response to chlorpromazine. SKOBBA and MIYA (1969) reported that chlorpromazine produced fatal hyperthermia in euthyroid rats pre-treated with dinitrophenol. TAVENDALE (1979) showed that mice pre-treated with dinitrophenol exhibited hyperthermia in response to doses of chlorpromazine which produced hypothermia in control animals. The rises in temperature were preceded by large increases in oxygen consumption, suggesting that the hyperthermia was caused at least in part by increased heat production. Chlorpromazine-induced increases in heat production have also been detected in rats pre-treated with dinitrophenol (FELLER 1955; POPOVIC 1954).

The effect of chlorpromazine on the body temperature of animals pre-treated with dinitrophenol or thyroxine seems to depend on ambient temperature. At ambient temperatures above 25 °C, the increases in body temperature produced by chlorpromazine are large (SKOBBA and MIYA 1969; SPENCER and WAITE 1968; TAVENDALE 1979). However, at lower ambient temperatures (PARK et al. 1972; SPENCER and WAITE 1968; TAVENDALE 1979) or after extracorporeal cooling (SKOBBA and MIYA 1969) hyperthermia is less marked and may even be replaced by hypothermia.

Like the effect of chlorpromazine on body temperature in mice pre-treated with reserpine (see Sect. B.IV.3) the effect of chlorpromazine in mice pre-treated with dinitrophenol has been shown (BLANCHARD and PERTWEE unpublished) to be abolished by a ganglion blocker (pentolinium) and also by a β-adrenoceptor antagonist (propranolol). Hyperthermia induced in mice by dinitrophenol was not prevented by propranolol. There is evidence therefore that, like the chlorpromazine–reserpine interaction, the chlorpromazine–dinitrophenol interaction may be mediated by the sympathetic nervous system which, by activating β-adrenoceptors could stimulate heat production and hence trigger the observed rises in body temperature.

VII. Effects of Methionine Enkephalin and β-Endorphin on Thermoregulation

The enkephalins are naturally occurring pentapeptides thought to be endogenous ligands for opiate receptors. They are found in several tissues including brain and spinal cord (for reviews see Beaumont and Hughes 1979; Hughes and Kosterlitz 1977). In cats, intracerebroventricular injections of methionine enkephalin have been found to elevate body temperature and also to produce shivering and vomiting (Clark 1977). In rats, too, intraventricular administration of methionine enkephalin has been found to alter body temperature (Ferri et al. 1978). A dose of 100 µg produced hyperthermia whereas 400 µg produced initial hypothermia followed by hyperthermia. On a molar basis morphine was more than 30 times more potent than methionine enkephalin in altering body temperature. This difference in potency may reflect the high susceptibility of the enkephalins to biological degradation. Metcalf et al. (1980) have reported that intracerebroventricular injections of an analogue of methionine enkephalin relatively resistant to biological degradation, [D-Ala]^2 methionine enkephalin, produces hyperthermia in unrestrained rabbits. Sedation, depressed respiratory rate and catalepsy were also observed. Bajorek and Lomax (1980) studied the effects of methionine enkephalin on body temperature in rats and gerbils. A dose of 100 µg given intraventricularly produced hypothermia in gerbils but had no effect on rat body temperature. A dose of 20 µg injected directly into the preoptic/anterior hypothalamus had no effect in either species. Cohn et al. (1980) were also unable to detect changes in rat body temperature after either intracerebroventricular or intracerebral injections of methionine enkephalin.

Both the hypothermic and the hyperthermic effects of methionine enkephalin have been shown to be antagonized by naloxone (Bajorek and Lomax 1980; Clark 1977; Ferri et al. 1978). Naloxone seems to be less effective as a methionine enkephalin antagonist than as an antagonist of morphine. A possible explanation for this difference is that there is a heterogeneous population of opiate receptors (Lord et al. 1977; Robson and Kosterlitz 1979) and that morphine interacts preferentially with one type of receptor (µ) and methionine enkephalin with another type (δ). Naloxone is thought to have a far lower affinity for the δ receptor than for the µ receptor.

Changes in body temperature can be produced not only by methionine enkephalin but also by β-endorphin, a large polypeptide which is found both in brain and pituitary gland and which contains the amino acid sequence of methionine enkephalin. Injection of β-endorphin into the cerebrospinal fluid of rats has been found to produce hyperthermia at doses below 10 µg (Holaday et al. 1977) and hypothermia at higher doses (Bloom et al. 1976; Brown and Vale 1980; Holaday et al. 1977; Tseng et al. 1977). The hypothermia may be followed by hyperthermia (Tseng et al. 1977) and can be reversed by naloxone (Bloom et al. 1976; Holaday et al. 1978 a). β-Endorphin is less resistant than methionine enkephalin to antagonism by naloxone. Possibly this is because unlike methionine enkephalin, β-endorphin has the same affinity for the putative µ and δ types of opiate receptor (Lord et al. 1977). Tseng et al. (1977) showed that rats subjected to repeated intracerebroventricular injections of β-endorphin rapidly became tolerant to the hypothermic effects both of β-endorphin and of morphine. It has also been shown that rats pre-treated with morphine can develop tolerance to the hypothermic effect of β-endorphin (Tseng et al. 1977) and to the effects on body temperature of methionine enkephalin (Ferri et al. 1978).

ROFFMAN et al. (1973) and DRAWBAUGH and LAL (1974) found that after rats had been subjected to a series of training sessions in which administration of morphine was paired with a conditional stimulus (CS), the animals became hypothermic when the combined morphine–CS treatment was withdrawn. This hypothermia could be reversed not only by morphine but also by the CS, given without morphine. In further studies in which a CS was paired with a hyperthermic dose of morphine, it was found that trained rats showed a hyperthermic response to the CS even in the absence of morphine (LAL et al. 1976; MIKSIC et al. 1975). The hyperthermic response to the CS could be prevented by naloxone. LAL et al. concluded that the effect of the CS on body temperature could have been caused by the release of an endogenous opioid ligand.

These results suggest first that endogenous opioid peptides may have a role in normal thermoregulation and second that they may also mediate thermoregulatory changes precipitated by withdrawal of morphine from dependent animals. Consistent with the first of these hypotheses is the observation that naloxone can produce small but statistically significant changes in rat body temperature. The doses of naloxone which have been shown to alter body temperature are greater than those needed to antagonize the effects of morphine on body temperature. However, they are not greater than those required to antagonize the effects of exogenously administered methionine enkephalin. GOLDSTEIN and LOWERY (1975) reported that in rats kept at ambient temperatures of 2° or 23 °C naloxone (10 mg/kg SC) opposed a temperature rise produced by saline injection. The size of the effect was small and they concluded that their results gave little support to the hypothesis that endogenous opioid ligands have an important role in normal thermoregulation. HOLADAY et al. (1978 b) found that at an ambient temperature of about 37 °C naloxone-treated rats (10 mg/kg IP) showed a slight increase in body temperature whereas saline-treated animals showed a fall. The naloxone-treated rats made a greater number of attempts to escape from the heat than control animals. ARY et al. (1976) found that naltrexone induced a dose-dependent hypothermia in rats but only at intraperitoneal doses 80–160 times greater than the dose (1.0 mg/kg) that precipitated hypothermia in morphine-dependent animals. They also found that rats given naltrexone at a dose of 160 mg/kg delayed escape from a heat lamp and thereby avoided hypothermia.

Although naloxone may affect thermoregulation in rats when given systemically at a dose of 10 mg/kg, lower doses have usually been found to alter body temperature only in morphine-dependent animals. However, there are exceptions. THORNHILL et al. (1978) reported that at ambient temperatures of 25°–27 °C, the rectal temperatures of rats given naloxone subcutaneously at doses of 1, 10, or 40 mg/kg were significantly lower than those of a group which had been injected with saline. The naloxone-treated rats were found to be calmer and less irritated by handling and insertion of the rectal probe than the control animals. FERRI et al. (1978) found that in rats kept at 21 °C naloxone produced hyperthermia when given subcutaneously at a dose of 3 mg/kg and hypothermia when given at a dose of 10 mg/kg. However, the effects were small and, like GOLDSTEIN and LOWERY (1975) they concluded that their results provide little support for the hypothesis that endogenous opioids normally function in the control of body temperature.

C. Effects of General Anaesthetics,
Barbiturates, Narcotic Analgesics and Phenothiazines
on Human Thermoregulation

I. General Anaesthetics and Barbiturates

Both general anaesthetics and barbiturates have been shown to alter body temperature in humans. Isbell et al. (1950) studied the effects of chronic administration of large doses of secobarbitone, amylobarbitone, and pentobarbitone on five former morphine addicts. Single doses of up to 2 g produced marked behavioural, psychological, and neurological changes but had little effect on rectal temperature. During the first three weeks of chronic administration of barbiturates at doses increasing progressively from 0.4 g to between 1.3 and 3.0 g per day, the average rectal temperatures were depressed by about 0.1 °C. Thereafter rectal temperatures were the same as they had been before the start of drug treatment, although daily fluctuations were greater. Abrupt drug withdrawal precipitated a marked abstinence syndrome. Four of the subjects developed psychoses during which rectal temperatures rose 0.5°–1.0 °C. In further experiments in which a larger number of subjects was included, hyperthermia after barbiturate withdrawal was again observed (Fraser et al. 1954). Withdrawal of alcohol after chronic administration has also been shown to alter body temperature in humans. In one study, six former morphine addicts were given daily oral doses of up to 489 ml ethyl alcohol (95%) for between 48 and 87 days (Isbell et al. 1955). During alcohol administration body temperature was little affected. However, after withdrawal severe abstinence syndromes developed and rectal temperatures rose, in one subject reaching a level of 41.4 °C. Gross et al. (1975) have also detected increases in body temperature after withdrawal of alcohol from human subjects who had been receiving large daily doses of the drug.

   Haight and Keatinge (1973) reported that in seven healthy male volunteers, ethanol (25–32 ml) taken by mouth after a period of hard exercise produced marked falls in blood glucose and rectal temperature, even at an ambient temperature of about 20 °C, and decreased the metabolic response to cold. The effects of ethanol on rectal temperature and on metabolic rate in the cold were probably caused by the hypoglycaemia since they could be prevented by pre-treatment with glucose. Ethanol had no effect on blood glucose, metabolic rate or body temperature when given to subjects who had not been exercising. Keatinge and Evans (1960) studied the effects of ethanol (75 ml, orally administered) on the thermoregulation of ten healthy subjects at rest and immersed up to the neck in cold water (15 °C). The drug was found to have no significant effect on rectal temperature. However, the rate of heat loss from the index finger of all subjects was marginally increased by ethanol and in seven of the subjects metabolic rate was decreased by the drug. Three of the subjects moved about after ethanol administration and did not show a fall in metabolic rate. It was also noted that in the ethanol experiments, subjects felt far less cold than in control experiments. More recent studies have confirmed that ethanol, administered in doses commonly taken "socially," i.e., absolute (100%) ethanol, 0.9–1.2 ml/kg or 70° proof (35%–40% v/v) whiskey, 1.87 ml/kg, has no significant effect on the deep-body temperature of resting subjects immersed in cold water (HOBSON and COLLIS 1977; MARTIN et al. 1977; MARTIN and COOPER 1978).

Much of the human data on general anaesthetics has been obtained clinically in the operating theatre and hence usually from patients who have received a combination of drugs. These can include drugs for pre-medication (e.g. atropine or scopolamine and narcotic analgesics or barbiturates), drugs for induction of anaesthesia (e.g. thiopentone) and drugs for skeletal muscle relaxation (e.g. succinylcholine, tubocurarine, and gallamine). All these drugs can affect thermoregulation when administered by themselves and their presence adds to the difficulties of determining how general anaesthetics affect human thermoregulation. Even so clinical observations made with anaesthetized patients have been largely consistent with those made experimentally with animals.

The degree of change in body temperature during anaesthesia has been reported to depend on depth of anaesthesia (SMITH 1962) and on ambient temperature (CLARK et al. 1954; MORRIS 1971; MORRIS and KUMAR 1972; MORRIS and WILKEY 1970). The direction of change in body temperature also seems to be related to ambient temperature. At ambient temperatures of 24 °C or less, body temperature often falls (ENGELMAN and LOCKHART 1972; GOLDBERG and ROE 1966; HARRISON et al. 1960; MORRIS 1971; NEWMAN 1971; SMITH 1962) whereas at higher ambient temperatures, body temperature can remain unchanged (MORRIS 1971) or even increase (CLARK et al. 1954; NAITO et al. 1974). There are exceptions, however. Ketamine has been reported to increase body temperature in 2- to 8-year-olds at 21°–24 °C (ENGELMAN and LOCKHART 1972) and in Ghana both halothane and ether were found to lower body temperature even though the ambient temperature was 28.7 °C (ELLIS and ZWANA 1977). The effects of anaesthetics on body temperature also depend on age, the very young being particularly susceptible (ENGELMAN and LOCKHART 1972; GOUDSOUZIAN et al. 1973; HARRISON et al. 1960; NAITO et al. 1974). It has also been found in some (GOLDBERG and ROE 1966; ROE et al. 1966) but not all studies (MORRIS and WILKEY 1970; MORRIS and KUMAR 1972) that patients more than 60 years old are more sensitive than younger adults to the effects of anaesthetics on body temperature.

The onset of anaesthesia in humans has been shown to be accompanied by dramatic rises in the skin temperature of extremities such as the thumb or great toe (ELLIS and ZWANA 1977; FOREGGER 1943) and recovery from anaesthesia by vasoconstriction (ROE et al. 1966) and also by onset of shivering and increased oxygen consumption (ROE et al. 1966; SOLIMAN and GILLIES 1972). ROE et al. (1966) reported that the size of post-operative increases in the oxygen consumption of patients who had experienced similar degrees of hypothermia during anaesthesia depended on the anaesthetic used. Increases in oxygen consumption above levels observed before anaesthesia ranged from 126% with halothane to 8% with methoxyflurane. In patients aged between 20 and 60 the post-operative increase in oxygen consumption was related to the degree of hypothermia experienced during anaesthesia. However, older patients showed relatively low post-operative increases in oxygen consumption in spite of having experienced the largest falls in deep-body temperature during anaesthesia. SOLIMAN and GILLIES (1972) in a study of 215 patients detected shivering during recovery from anaesthesia in only 39% of the patients. The incidence of shivering was greater after methoxyflurane (50%)

or halothane (42%) than after cyclopropane (20%) or nitrous oxide – pethidine – curare (10%). In 83 of the patients receiving halothane deep-body temperature was monitored. The tendency of these patients to shiver during recovery was found to depend on the degree of hypothermia experienced during anaesthesia.

II. Narcotic Analgesics

1. Single and Repeated Administration

A number of controlled investigations have been made into the effects of narcotic analgesics in humans. Most of these have been conducted with former heroin addicts. The results obtained from these investigations show that in humans as in other species narcotic analgesics can alter thermoregulation. After the administration of a single dose, narcotic analgesics have been shown to produce falls in deep body temperature of up to 0.6 °C (Isbell et al. 1948 a, b). With repeated administration tolerance develops (Isbell et al. 1948 b). Dependence may also develop and, after withdrawal of drug treatment, deep-body temperature has been shown to rise (Isbell et al. 1947, 1948 b; Martin et al. 1973). Isbell et al. (1948 b) reported that during the first few days of treatment with methadone (initially 20 mg/day) rectal temperature decreased by about 0.5 °C. With further drug administration it rose again to its initial level. After the first week of drug treatment rectal temperature remained 0.2°–0.4 °C above this initial level. Withdrawal of the methadone treatment precipitated an abstinence syndrome during which rectal temperature rose 0.5 °C. Withdrawal of morphine from morphine-dependent subjects was also found to provoke a rise in rectal temperature (0.6 °C). Martin et al. (1973) reported that during chronic methadone treatment (up to 100 mg/day) body temperature gradually increased to a new level. After withdrawal of the drug treatment there was a rise in body temperature. Two weeks later body temperature started to fall, eventually attaining subnormal levels. Gritz et al. (1976) found that high oral doses of the narcotic antagonist, naltrexone (up to 160 mg) produced slight falls in the sublingual temperatures of former heroin addicts. A similar observation has been made in rats (see Sect. B.VII). Nalorphine, too, has been shown to lower body temperature in humans (Wikler et al. 1953).

2. Drug Interactions

There are numerous reports concerning adverse, sometimes fatal, reactions to pethidine in patients treated with monoamine oxidase inhibitors (Denton et al. 1962; Palmer 1960; Papp and Benaim 1958; Pells Cocks and Passmore-Rowe 1962; Reid and Jones 1962; Shee 1960; Taylor 1962; Vigran 1964). Some of these patients exhibited large increases in body temperature after administration of pethidine (Denton et al. 1962; Palmer 1960; Reid and Jones 1962). Hyperthermia has also been observed in patients treated with monoamine oxidase inhibitors after administration of dextromethorphan (Rivers and Horner 1970; Shamsie and Barriga 1971).

III. Phenothiazines

Data derived mainly from case reports concerning adverse reactions of mentally ill patients to phenothiazines show that, in humans as in other mammalian species, this group of drugs can induce marked rises and falls in deep-body temperature. Falls in body temperature have been observed on numerous occasions in patients receiving chlorpromazine (GAUTIER et al. 1972; GLINOER et al. 1973; HAUGAN 1966; HOLLISTER 1966; IRVINE 1973; JONES and MEADE 1964; LOUGHNANE 1968; MELLERIO 1970; MITCHELL et al. 1959). Patients with myxoedema may be particularly susceptible (JONES and MEADE 1964; MITCHELL et al. 1959). Hypothermic doses of chlorpromazine in humans are of the same order as those that lower body temperature in other species. For example, in a number of healthy human subjects at an ambient temperature of about 19 °C, axillary, oral and rectal temperatures were lowered 1°–2 °C by intravenous doses of chlorpromazine ranging from 0.3 to 2.0 mg/kg (DOBKIN et al. 1954). It was also found that the skin of the drug-treated subjects was warm and dry but very pale and that the temperature of the extremities rose markedly after injection. Elevation in the temperature of extremities has also been observed in other species after administration of chlorpromazine and is thought to reflect increased heat loss (see Sect. B.III.3).

Rises in body temperature often to levels above 41 °C have been observed in patients receiving chlorpromazine (AYD 1956; CHILDERS 1961; GREENBLATT and GREENBLATT 1973; GREENLAND and SOUTHWICK 1978; HARDER et al. 1971) trifluoperazine (SHAPIRO 1967; WALKER 1959), mepazine (EXT 1958; FORD 1959), fluphenazine and promazine (ZELMAN and GUILLAN 1970), and methotrimeprazine and clopenthixol (HARDER et al. 1971). Hyperthermia has also been observed after combined administration of mepazine and prochlorperazine (MAHRER et al. 1958) or chlorpromazine and trifluoperazine (FORESTER 1978; ZELMAN and GUILLAN 1970). The rises in body temperature have sometimes ended in death (AYD 1956; CHILDERS 1961; EXT 1958; FORESTER 1978; ZELMAN and GUILLAN 1970). Phenothiazine-induced increases in body temperature have mostly been observed when ambient temperatures were high, usually above 32 °C (AYD 1956; EXT 1958; FORD 1959; FORESTER 1978; MAHRER et al.1958; SHAPIRO 1967; ZELMAN and GUILLAN 1970). Hyperthermia has also been observed in drug-treated patients during periods of increased motor activity consisting either of exercise (GREENBLATT and GREENBLATT 1973) or struggling in response to physical restraint (GREENLAND and SOUTHWICK 1978).

A frequently reported feature of phenothiazine-induced hyperthermia is absence of sweating (GREENBLATT and GREENBLATT 1973; MAHRER et al. 1958; SHAPIRO 1967; ZELMAN and GUILLAN 1970), a heat loss mechanism particularly important to humans at high ambient temperatures. Since the phenothiazines possess antimuscarinic activity it is possible that their hyperthermic activity in humans could be due in part to inhibition of sweating through a direct action on cholinergic receptors of the sweat glands. In view of this possibility it should be noted that several of the patients who experienced fatal hyperthermia after treatment with phenothiazines had also been given other drugs with antimuscarinic activity such as benztropine (FORESTER 1978; ZELMAN and GUILLAN 1970). It should also be noted that moderate doses of atropine can produce hyperthermia in humans and that this effect is thought to be due in part to a direct inhibitory effect on sweat glands (EXT 1958).

D. Concluding Summary

General anaesthetics, barbiturates and phenothiazines can produce either rises or falls in deep-body temperature, the direction of the change depending on ambient temperature. The effects of narcotic analgesics on body temperature seem to be more complex since the direction of change produced depends not only on ambient temperature but also on species and dose. In rats, the strain of animal used and degree of physical restraint are also important. How these factors influence the direction of change in body temperature produced by morphine remains to be elucidated.

Repeated administration of ethanol, barbiturates or phenothiazines can produce tolerance to the effect of these drugs on body temperature. Tolerance to morphine has also been demonstrated. However, in some experiments pre-treatment with morphine has been found to enhance the rise in body temperature produced by hyperthermic doses of morphine. In other experiments doses of morphine producing marked hypothermia in non-tolerant animals have been shown to provoke a hyperthermic response in animals pre-treated with morphine. A possible explanation for these observations is given in Sect. B.I.2.b. Repeated administration of morphine, ethanol, and barbiturates as well as producing tolerance can also give rise to dependence. Withdrawal effects include changes in body temperature. In morphine-dependent animals, other withdrawal signs may also reflect changes in thermoregulation.

Morphine is thought to lower body temperature by an effect on heat gain mechanisms. Effects on heat loss have not been detected. In rats, morphine seems to raise body temperature by affecting heat loss as well as heat gain mechanisms. In cats and dogs, however, only heat gain mechanisms seem to be involved. Indeed, these species usually exhibit signs of increased heat loss after treatment with hyperthermic doses of morphine. In contrast to morphine, general anaesthetics, barbiturates, and phenothiazines can lower body temperature by producing changes in both heat gain and heat loss. At ambient temperatures below thermal neutrality they have been shown to decrease heat production and to increase heat loss from the extremities. In addition, they may increase evaporative heat loss. There is also evidence that animals treated with pentobarbitone or chlorpromazine make no attempt to compensate behaviourally for falls in body temperature experienced. The hyperthermia produced by phenothiazines at ambient temperatures above thermal neutrality is caused by decreased heat loss. Increases in heat production may also contribute.

Results obtained from experiments with N-methylchlorpromazine and N-methylmorphine, both of which are thought to cross the blood–brain barrier only very slowly, are consistent with the hypotheses that chlorpromazine-induced hypothermia is produced by actions at peripheral sites and that morphine acts mainly at sites located within the central nervous system. However, these results should be interpreted with particular caution since the blood–brain barrier does not restrict movement of charged compounds into all parts of the central nervous system. Certain regions of the brain such as the area postrema and the ventral part of the median eminence of the hypothalamus are thought to be relatively accessible even to large polar molecules. Moreover, after N methylation pharmacological properties of a compound may be altered. For example, there are differences between the pharmacological properties of morphine and N-methylmorphine (see Sect. B.II.2). Also, N-methylation of atropine is known to confer strong ganglionic blocking activity. These reservations apply equally to interpretation of results obtained from experiments with neostigmine and methylscopolamine (see Sect. B.IV).

Experiments in which injections made into the cerebrospinal fluid or brain through stereotaxically implanted cannulae have provided convincing evidence that narcotic analgesics act primarily at sites located within the hypothalamus and spinal cord. Many of the changes in thermoregulation produced by morphine after systemic administration have also been produced when lower doses of the drug were given intracerebroventricularly, intrathecally or intrahypothalamically. Moreover, several of the factors known to alter body temperature responses to peripherally injected morphine (ambient temperature, dose, narcotic antagonists, tolerance, physical restraint) have also been shown to do so when the drug was injected into cerebral ventricles or brain tissue. Intracerebral or intracerebroventricular injections of pentobarbitone and chlorpromazine have also been shown to alter body temperature. However, although hypothermic responses were obtained in some experiments, in others body temperature either rose or was unchanged. The part played by central sites of action in body temperature changes produced by peripheral administration of these drugs is therefore unclear.

In the search for sites within the central nervous system at which peripherally administered drugs might act to alter thermoregulation it is important to bear in mind that, in addition to hypothalamic thermoregulatory centres, there are thought to be secondary extrahypothalamic control mechanisms. There is some evidence that the hypothalamic centres contain "narrow-band" temperature control mechanisms whereas the extrahypothalamic centres contain "wide-band" mechanisms (LIPTON 1973; see also Chap. 3). If this is so, low doses of general anaesthetics might well act primarily at sites located within the hypothalamus, thereby, abolishing narrow-band control but leaving wide-band control intact (see Sect. B.I.1). There is also evidence that one putative secondary control centre (in the medulla oblongata) usually responds minimally to direct administration of chlorpromazine because it is normally suppressed by control mechanisms located within the preoptic/anterior hypothalamic nuclei (TRZCINKA et al. 1978). It is therefore possible that some drugs when given by peripheral routes could reduce the influence of the preoptic/anterior hypothalamic nuclei on extrahypothalamic thermoregulatory mechanisms and alter thermoregulation by producing changes, not only within the hypothalamus but also within extrahypothalamic centres. It would then only be possible to mimic fully the effects on thermoregulation of systemic drug administration by making intracerebral injections at all the thermoregulatory centres involved.

Little is known about the mechanisms by which general anaesthetics, barbiturates, narcotic analgesics or phenothiazines alter thermoregulation. General anaesthetics and barbiturates could act by blocking synaptic transmission in thermoregulatory pathways. So too could the phenothiazines since they can antagonize the actions of several neurotransmitters thought to have a role in thermoregulation. The effects of narcotic analgesics on thermoregulation probably depend on the activation of opiate receptors. Serotoninergic, dopaminergic, and cholinergic pathways may all be involved in producing changes in body temperature caused either by single doses of morphine or by withdrawal of drug treatment. There is also evidence that morphine can produce hyperthermia by altering sensory input to supraspinal thermoregulatory centres. Finally, morphine and also certain general anaesthetics and barbiturates have been shown to alter the effects of temperature on the firing rates of warm- and cold-sensitive neurones in the brain.

References

Abdallah AH, Roby DM (1975) Antagonism of depressant activity of ethanol by DH-524; a comparative study with bemigride, doxapram, and d-amphetamine. Proc Soc Exp Biol Med 148:819–822

Ahtee L, Jounela AJ, Saarnivaara L, Simola I (1974) Interactions of some analgesics and antidepressants with phenelzine or reserpine in the mouse. Pharmacology 12:39–47

Ankermann H (1958) Die Beeinflussung des Stoffwechsels durch Chlorpromazin. Arzneim Forsch 8:81–83

Ary M, Lomax P (1976) Reinstatement of precipitated narcotic withdrawal hypothermia in the rat. Life Sci 18:1199–1202

Ary M, Chesarek W, Sorensen SM, Lomax P (1976) Naltrexone-induced hypothermia in the rat. Eur J Pharmacol 39:215–220

Ary M, Cox B, Lomax P (1977) Dopaminergic mechanisms in precipitated withdrawal in morphine dependent rats. J Pharmacol Exp Ther 200:271–276

Ayd FJ (1956) Fatal hyperpyrexia during chlorpromazine therapy. J Clin Exp Psychopathol 17:189–192

Bächtold H, Pletscher A (1957) Einfluß von Isonikotinsäurehydraziden auf den Verlauf der Körpertemperatur nach Reserpin, Monoaminen und Chlorpromazin. Experientia 13:163–165

Bagdon WJ, Mann DE (1962) Chlorpromazine hyperthermia in young albino mice. J Pharm Sci 51:753–755

Bagdon WJ, Mann DE (1965) Factors modifying chlorpromazine hyperthermia in young albino mice. J Pharm Sci 54:240–246

Baizman ER, Wolf HH (1975) Central mechanisms involved in morphine-induced hypothermia: differentiation by selective receptor blockade. Proc Fed Am Soc Exp Biol 34:787

Bajorek JG, Lomax P (1980) Comparative effects of met^5-enkephalin and morphine on body temperature of gerbils and rats. In: Cox B, Lomax P, Milton AS, Schönbaum E (eds) Thermoregulatory mechanisms and their therapeutic implications. Karger, Basel, pp 169–172

Baldino F, Beckman AL, Adler MW (1980) Effects of iontophoretically applied morphine on rat hypothalamic thermosensitive neurons. In: Cox B, Lomax P, Milton AS, Schönbaum E (eds) Thermoregulatory mechanisms and their therapeutic implications. Karger, Basel, pp 157–158

Banerjee U, Burks TF, Feldberg W, Goodrich CA (1968a) Temperature effects and catalepsy produced by morphine injected into the cerebral ventricles of rabbits. Br J Pharmacol Chemother 33:544–551

Banerjee U, Feldberg W, Lotti VJ (1968b) Effect on body temperature of morphine and ergotamine injecte1 into the cerebral ventricles of cats. Br J Pharmacol Chemother 32:523–538

Barnett A, Goldstein J, Taber RI (1972) Apomorphine-induced hypothermia in mice: a possible dopaminergic effect. Arch Int Pharmacodyn Ther 198:242–247

Beaumont A, Hughes J (1979) Biology of opioid peptides. Annu Rev Pharmacol Toxicol 19:245–267

Bhargava HN (1977) Rapid induction and quantitation of morphine dependence in the rat by pellet implantation. Psychopharmacology 52:55–62

Bhargava HN, Matwyshyn GA (1977) Brain serotonin turnover and morphine tolerance-dependence induced by multiple injections in the rat. Eur J Pharmacol 44:25–33

Binet P, Decaud J (1954) Irradiation infrarouge et chlorpromazine chez le rat blanc. CR Soc Biol (Paris) 148:1557–1559

Binet P, Decaud J (1960) Influence de la température ambiante sur la température réctale du rat traité par quelques dérivés de la phénothiazine. Therapie 15:253–257

Bligh J (1966) The thermosensitivity of the hypothalamus and thermoregulation in mammals. Biol Rev 41:317–367

Bligh J (1973) Temperature regulation in mammals and other vertebrates. Elsevier/North Holland, Amsterdam Oxford New York

Bloom AS, Dewey WL (1978) A comparison of some pharmacological actions of morphine and Δ^9-tetrahydrocannabinol in the mouse. Psychopharmacology 57:243–248

Bloom F, Segal D, Ling N, Guillemin R (1976) Endorphins: profound behavioral effects in rats suggest new etiological factors in mental illness. Science 194:630–632

Boissier JR, Simon P, Giudicelli JF (1967) Effets centraux de quelques substances adréno-et/ou sympatholytiques. 1. – Action sur la température rectale. Arch Int Pharmacodyn Ther 168:180–187

Borbély AA, Huston JP, Baumann IR (1973) Body temperature and behavior in chronic brain-lesioned rats after amphetamine, chlorpromazine, and γ-butyrolactone. In: Lomax P, Schönbaum E (eds) The pharmacology of thermoregulation. Karger, Basel, pp 447–462

Botting R, Bower S, Eason CT, Hutson PH, Wells L (1978) Modification by monoamine oxidase inhibitors of the analgesic, hypothermic and toxic actions of morphine and pethidine in mice. J Pharm Pharmacol 30:36–40

Brase DA, Iwamoto ET, Loh HH, Way EL (1976) Reinitiation of sensitivity to naloxone by a single narcotic injection in postaddicted mice. J Pharmacol Exp Ther 197:317–325

Breese GR, Cott JM, Cooper BR, Prange AJ, Lipton MA, Plotnikoff NP (1975) Effects of thyrotropin-releasing hormone (TRH) on the actions of pentobarbital and other centrally acting drugs. J Pharmacol Exp Ther 193:11–22

Brendel W, L'Allemand H (1955) Der Einfluß von Megaphen auf die Wärmeregulation. Arch Exp Pathol Pharmakol 225:87–90

Brick J, Pohorecky LA (1977) Ethanol withdrawal: altered ambient temperature selection in rats. Alcoholism 1:207–211

Brown M, Vale W (1980) Peptides and thermoregulation. In: Cox B, Lomax P, Milton AS, Schönbaum E (eds) Thermoregulatory mechanisms and their therapeutic implications. Karger, Basel, pp 186–194

Brownlee G, Williams GW (1963) Potentiation of amphetamine and pethidine by monoamine oxidase inhibitors. Lancet 1:669

Carvalho LP, Izquierdo I (1977) Changes in the frequency of electroencephalographic rhythms of the rat caused by single, intraperitoneal injections of ethanol. Arch Int Pharmacodyn Ther 229:157–162

Chai CY, Lin MT (1977) The enhancement of chlorpromazine-induced hypothermia by lesions in the anterior hypothalamus. Br J Pharmacol 61:77–82

Chai CY, Fann YD, Lin MT (1976) Hypothermic action of chlorpromazine in monkeys. Br J Pharmacol 57:43–49

Chambers DM, Jefferson GC, Ruddick CA (1978) Halothane-induced sleeping time in the mouse: its modification by benzodiazepines. Eur J Pharmacol 50:103–112

Chatonnet J, Tanche M (1955) Action de la chlorpromazine sur la régulation thermique du chien exposé au froid. CR Soc Biol (Paris) 149:716–719

Chatonnet J, Tanche M (1959) Chlorpromazine et régulation thermique. 1°-Zone de froid. Therapie 14:778–792

Chevillard L, Giono H, Laury MC (1958) Action comparée de quelques vasodilatateurs sur la température corporelle et le métabolisme respiratoire chez le cobaye. CR Soc Biol (Paris) 152:1074–1077

Cheymol J, Levassort C (1955) Hyperthermisants et chlorpromazine. CR Soc Biol (Paris) 149:475–480

Childers RT (1961) Hyperpyrexia, coma and death during chlorpromazine therapy. J Clin Exp Psychopathol 22:163–164

Chodera A (1963) The influence of marsilid on the temperature response in rats after morphine. Arch Int Pharmacodyn Ther 144:362–369

Ciofalo FR (1974) Methadone inhibition of ^{3}H-5-hydroxytryptamine uptake by synaptosomes. J Pharmacol Exp Ther 189:83–89

Clark WG (1977) Emetic and hyperthermic effects of centrally injected methionine-enkephalin in cats. Proc Soc Exp Biol Med 154:540–542

Clark WG, Cumby HR (1978) Hyperthermic responses to central and peripheral injections of morphine sulphate in the cat. Br J Pharmacol 63:65–71

Clark RE, Orkin LR, Rovenstine EA (1954) Body temperature studies in anaesthetized man: effect of environmental temperature, humidity and anesthesia system. JAMA 154:311–319

Cohn ML, Cohn M, Taube D (1980) Thyrotropin releasing hormone induced hyperthermia in the rat inhibited by lysine acetylsalicylate and indomethacin. In: Cox B, Lomax P, Milton AS, Schönbaum E (eds) Thermoregulatory mechanisms and their therapeutic implications. Karger, Basel, pp 198–201

Collier HOJ, McDonald-Gibson WJ, Saeed SA (1974) Morphine and apomorphine stimulate prostaglandin production by rabbit brain homogenate. Br J Pharmacol 52:116P

Cooper F, Schnieden H (1972) Study of the mechanisms of action of desipramine and chlorpromazine in reversing reserpine-induced hypothermia in mice. Br J Pharmacol 45:162–163P

Costa E, Garattini S, Valzelli L (1960) Interactions between reserpine, chlorpromazine and imipramine. Experientia 16:461–463

Courvoisier S, Fournel J, Ducrot R, Kolsky M, Koetschet P (1953) Propiétés pharmacodynamiques du chlorhydrate de chloro-3 (diméthylamino 3′propyl) 10-phénothiazine (4.560 R.P.). Arch Int Pharmacodyn Ther 92:305–361

Cox B, Lomax P (1977) Pharmacologic control of temperature regulation. Annu Rev Pharmacol Toxicol 17:341–353

Cox B, Ary M, Lomax P (1975) Dopaminergic mechanisms in withdrawal hypothermia in morphine dependent rats. Life Sci 17:41–42

Cox B, Ary M, Chesarek W, Lomax P (1976a) Morphine hyperthermia in the rat: an action on the central thermostats. Eur J Pharmacol 36:33–39

Cox B, Ary M, Lomax P (1976b) Dopaminergic involvement in withdrawal hypothermia and thermoregulatory behavior in morphine dependent rats. Pharmacol Biochem Behav 4:259–262

Cox B, Lee TF, Vale MJ (1979) Effects of morphine and related drugs on core temperature of two strains of rat. Eur J Pharmacol 54:27–36

Cox B, Lee TF, Vale MJ (1980) Comparative thermoregulatory effects of narcotic analgesics in two strains of rat. In: Cox B, Lomax P, Milton AS, Schönbaum E (eds) Thermoregulatory mechanisms and their therapeutic implications. Karger, Basel, pp 163–165

Dandiya PC, Sellers EA (1961) Mechanism of the hypnosis prolongation action of 5-hydroxytryptamine and some sympathomimetic amines. Arch Int Pharmacodyn Ther 130:32–41

Dandiya PC, Johnson G, Sellers EA (1960) Influence of variation in environmental temperature on the acute toxicity of reserpine and chlorpromazine in mice. Can J Biochem Physiol 38:591–596

Dashwood MR, Feldberg W (1977) Endotoxin fever, prostaglandin and anaesthesia. In: Cooper KE, Lomax P, Schönbaum E (eds) Drugs, biogenic amines and body temperature. Karger, Basel, pp 145–152

Daudova GM (1961) Changes in body temperature and oxygen consumption in rabbits following the administration of sodium amytal. Bull Exp Biol Med USSR 52:792–796

Decourt P, Brunaud M, Brunaud S (1953) Action d'un narcobiotique (chlorpromazine) sur la température centrale des animaux homéothermes soumis à des températures ambiantes supérieures, égales ou inférieures à leur température centrale normale. CR Soc Biol (Paris) 147:1605–1609

Denton PH, Borrelli VM, Edwards NV (1962) Dangers of monoamine oxidase inhibitors. Br Med J 2:1752–1753

Dettmar PW, Cowan A (1980) Comparative effects of centrally injected buprenorphine and morphine on body temperature. In: Cox B, Lomax P, Milton AS, Schönbaum E (eds) Thermoregulatory mechanisms and their therapeutic implications. Karger, Basel, pp 173–174

Dhawan BN (1960) Blockade of LSD-25 pyrexia by morphine. Arch Int Pharmacodyn Ther 127:307–313

Dobkin AB, Gilbert RGB, Lamoureux L (1954) Physiological effects of chlorpromazine. Anaesthesia 9:157–174

Doggett NS, Reno H, Spencer PSJ (1975) Narcotic agonists and antagonists as models for potential antidepressant drugs. Neuropharmacology 14:507–515

Domer FR, Feldberg W (1960) Tremor in cats: the effect of administration of drugs into the cerebral ventricles. Br J Pharmacol Chemother 15:578–587

Drawbaugh R, Lal H (1974) Reversal by narcotic antagonist of a narcotic action elicited by a conditional stimulus. Nature 247:65–67

Eddy NB (1932) Studies of morphine, codeine and their derivatives. I. General methods. J Pharmacol Exp Ther 45:339–359

Eddy NB, Reid JG (1934) Studies of morphine, codeine and their derivatives. VII. Dihydromorphine (paramorphan), dihydromorphinone (dilaudid) and dihydrocodeinone (dicodide). J Pharmacol Exp Ther 52:468–493

Eger EI, Saidman LJ, Brandstater B (1965) Temperature dependence of halothane and cyclopropane anesthesia in dogs: correlation with some theories of anesthetic action. Anesthesiology 26:764–770

Eisenman JS, Jackson DC (1967) Thermal response patterns of septal and preoptic neurons in cats. Exp Neurol 19:33–45

Ekström GA (1951) Note on the influence of small doses of nembutal upon the temperature regulation in cats. Acta Physiol Scand 22:345–347

Ellis FR, Zwana S (1977) A study of body temperatures of anaesthetized man in the tropics. Br J Anaesth 49:1123–1126

Eltayeb IB, Osman OH (1975) Furazolidone-pethidine interaction in rabbits. Br J Pharmacol 55:497–501

Engelman DR, Lockhart CH (1972) Comparisons between temperature effects of ketamine and halothane anesthesia in children. Anesth Analg 51:98–101

Erickson CK, Tyler TD, Harris RA (1978) Ethanol: modification of acute intoxication by divalent cations. Science 199:1219–1221

Euler C von (1961) Physiology and pharmacology of temperature regulation. Pharmacol Rev 13:361–398

Ext HJ (1958) Five cases of heat stroke observed in mentally ill patients treated with Pacatal during the hot weather spell. NY State J Med 58:1877–1881

Fahim I, Ismail M, Osman OH (1972) The role of 5-hydroxytryptamine and noradrenaline in the hyperthermic reaction induced by pethidine in rabbits pretreated with pargyline. Br J Pharmacol 46:416–422

Feldberg W, Lang WJ (1970) Effects of monoamine oxidase inhibitors and amphetamine on hypothermia produced by halothane. Br J Pharmacol 38:181–191

Feldberg W, Lotti VJ (1967) Body temperature responses in cats and rabbits to the monoamine oxidase inhibitor tranylcypromine. J Physiol (Lond) 190:203–220

Feldberg W, Myers RD (1964) Temperature changes produced by amines injected into the cerebral ventricles during anaesthesia. J Physiol (Lond) 175:464–478

Feldberg W, Myers RD (1965) Hypothermia produced by chloralose acting on the hypothalamus. J Physiol (Lond) 179:509–517

Feldberg W, Saxena PN (1971) Further studies on prostaglandin E_1 fever in cats. J Physiol (Lond) 219:739–745

Feller K (1955) Die Wirkung einiger Phenothiazinderivate, insbesondere Megaphen, auf den Gasstoffwechsel der weißen Ratte. Arch Exp Pathol Pharmakol 226:269–277

Fenters JD, Jeter WS (1961) Effect of variation in body temperature on antibody production in rabbits and mice. J Bacteriol 82:156–157

Fernandes M, Kluwe S, Coper H (1977) Quantitative assessment of tolerance to and dependence on morphine in mice. Arch Pharmacol 297:53–60

Ferri S, Arrigo-Reina R, Santagostino A, Scoto GM, Spadaro C (1978) Effects of met-enkephalin on body temperature of normal and morphine-tolerant rats. Psychopharmacology 58:277–281

Filk H, Ritter K, Stürmer E, Loeser A (1954) Studien zur Stoffwechselwirkung eines Phenothiazinabkömmlings ("Megaphen"). Klin Wochenschr 32:265–266

Flacke W, Mülke G, Schulz R (1953) Beitrag zur Wirkung von Pharmaka auf die Unterdrucktoleranz. Arch Exp Pathol Pharmakol 220:469–476

Ford WL (1959) Heat stroke with mepazine therapy. Am J Psychiatry 116:357

Foregger R (1943) Surface temperatures during anaesthesia. Anesthesiology 4:392–402

Forester D (1978) Fatal drug-induced heat stroke. JACEP 7:243–244

Foster RS, Jenden DJ, Lomax P (1967) A comparison of the pharmacologic effects of morphine and N-methyl morphine. J Pharmacol Exp Ther 157:185–195

Frankel D, Khanna JM, Kalant H, Le Blanc AE (1978) Effect of p-chlorophenylalanine on the acquisition of tolerance to the hypothermic effects of ethanol. Psychopharmacology 57:239–242

Fraser HF, Isbell H, Eisenman AJ, Wikler A, Pescor FT (1954) Chronic barbiturate intoxication. Further studies. Arch Intern Med 94:34–41

French ED, Vasquez SA, George R (1978a) Potentiation of morphine hyperthermia in cats by pimozide and fluoxetine hydrochloride. Eur J Pharmacol 48:351–356

French ED, Vasquez SA, George R (1978b) Thermoregulatory responses of the unrestrained cat to acute and chronic intravenous administration of low doses of morphine and to naloxone precipitated withdrawal. Life Sci 22:1947–1954

Freund G (1973) Hypothermia after acute ethanol and benzyl alcohol administration. Life Sci 13:345–349

Frommel E, Ledebur I, Beguin M (1963) De l'antagonisme de la nalorphine envers la chlorpromazine. Arch Int Pharmacodyn Ther 143:52–77

Fuller RW, Baker JC (1974) Further evidence for serotonin involvement in thermoregulation following morphine administration from studies with an inhibitor of serotonin uptake. Res Commun Chem Pathol Pharmacol 8:715–718

Fuller RW, Snoddy HD (1975) Inhibition of serotonin uptake and the toxic interaction between meperidine and monoamine oxidase inhibitors. Toxicol Appl Pharmacol 32:129–134

Garattini S, Giachetti A, Jori A, Pieri L, Valzelli L (1962) Effect of imipramine, amitriptyline and their monomethyl derivatives on reserpine activity. J Pharm Pharmacol 14:509–514

Gautier J, Bagros P, Lamisse F, Royer A (1972) Hypothermies accidentelles au cours des comas toxiques. Sem Hop Paris 48:481–502

Gemmill CL, Browning KM (1962) Effects of pentobarbital on temperature and heart rate of rats subjected to cold. Am J Physiol 203:758–761

Gessner PK (1973) Antagonism of the tranylcypromine-meperidine interaction by chlorpromazine in mice. Eur J Pharmacol 22:187–190

Gessner PK, Soble AG (1973) A study of the tranylcypromine-meperidine interaction: effects of p-chlorophenylalanine and L-5-hydroxytryptophan. J Pharmacol Exp Ther 186:276–287

Gessner PK, Clarke CC, Adler M (1974) The effect of low environmental temperature on the tranylcypromine-meperidine interaction in mice. J Pharmacol Exp Ther 189:90–96

Giaja J, Markovic-Giaja L (1954) La chlorpromazine et la thermorégulation. CR Soc Biol (Paris) 148:842–844

Gilbert PE, Martin WR (1976) Sigma effects of nalorphine in the chronic spinal dog. Drug Alcohol Depend 1:373–376

Girndt O, Lipschitz W (1931) Über die Wirkung des Morphins auf die Körpertemperatur. Arch Exp Pathol Pharmakol 159:249–258

Glaubach S, Pick EP (1930) Über die Beeinflussung der Temperaturregulierung durch Thyroxin. I. Mitteilung. Arch Exp Pathol Pharmakol 151:341–370

Glick SD (1975) Hyperthermic and hypothermic effects of morphine in mice: interactions with apomorphine and pilocarpine and changes in sensitivity after caudate nucleus lesions. Arch Int Pharmacodyn Ther 213:264–271

Glinoer D, Ectors M, Paulet P, Thys JP, Cornil A (1973) Etude clinique de 39 observations d'hypothermie accidentelle de l'adulte. Acta Clin Belg 28:40–55

Glowinski J (1975) Properties and functions of intraneuronal monoamine compartments in central aminergic neurons. In: Iversen LL, Iversen SD, Snyder SH (eds) Handbook of psychopharmacology, vol 3. Plenum, New York, pp 139–167

Goldberg MJ, Roe CF (1966) Temperature changes during anesthesia and operations. Arch Surg 93:365–369

Goldberg ME, Dubnick B, Hefner M, Salama AI (1973) Influence of chlorpromazine on brain serotonin turnover and body temperature in isolated aggressive mice. Neuropharmacology 12:249–260

Goldstein A, Lowery PJ (1975) Effect of the opiate antagonist naloxone on body temperature in rats. Life Sci 17:927–931

Gong SNC, Rogers KJ (1971) Role of brain monoamines in the fatal hyperthermia induced by pethidine or imipramine in rabbits pretreated with pargyline. Br J Pharmacol 42:646 P

Gong SNC, Rogers KJ (1973) Role of brain monoamines in the fatal hyperthermia induced by pethidine or imipramine in rabbits pretreated with a monoamine oxidase inhibitor. Br J Pharmacol 48:12–18

Goudsouzian NG, Morris RH, Ryan JF (1973) The effects of a warming blanket on the maintenance of body temperatures in anaesthetized infants and children. Anesthesiology 39:351–353

Grant R, Robbins ME (1949) Effect of ethyl carbamate on temperature regulation. Proc Fed Am Soc Exp Biol 8:59–60

Green HD, Nickerson ND, Lewis RN, Brofman BL (1943) Consecutive changes in cutaneous blood flow, temperature, metabolism and hematocrit readings during prolonged anesthesia with morphine and barbital. Am J Physiol 140:177–189

Greenblatt DJ, Greenblatt GR (1973) Chlorpromazine and hyperpyrexia. Clin Pediat 12:504–505

Greenland P, Southwick WH (1978) Hyperthermia associated with chlorpromazine and full-sheet restraint. Am J Psychiatry 135:1234–1235

Gritz ER, Shiffman SM, Jarvik ME, Schlesinger J, Charuvastra VC (1976) Naltrexone: physiological and psychological effects of single doses. Clin Pharmacol Ther 19:773–776

Gross MM, Lewis E, Best S, Young N, Feuer L (1975) Quantitative changes of signs and symptoms associated with acute alcohol withdrawal: incidence, severity and circadian effects in experimental studies of alcoholics. Adv Exp Med Biol 59:615–631

Gunne LM (1960) The temperature response in rats during acute and chronic morphine administration. A study of morphine tolerance. Arch Int Pharmacodyn Ther 129:416–428

Hadnagy C, Eperjessy A, Kiss Á, Csegedy J, Dézsi Z, Hantz A, Erdei P (1958) Die Wirkung des Largactils auf die Gewebsatmung und auf einige enzymatische Prozesse des intermediären Kohlenhydratstoffwechsels. Arch Int Pharmacodyn Ther 117:395–403

Haight JSJ, Keatinge WR (1973) Failure of thermoregulation in the cold during hypoglycaemia induced by exercise and ethanol. J Physiol (Lond) 229:87–97

Halpern BN, Liakopoulos P (1954) Action comparée de la prométhazine et de la chlorpromazine sur la témperature chez le rat et le cobaye. CR Soc Biol (Paris) 148:955–959

Harder A, Modestin J Steiner H (1971) Verlauf der Körpertemperatur bei Neuroleptika-Injektionskuren. Schweiz Med Wochenschr 101:828–831

Harrison GG, Bull AB, Schmidt HJ (1960) Temperature changes in children during general anaesthesia. Br J Anaesth 32:60–68

Haubrich DR, Blake DE (1971) Modification of the hypothermic action of morphine after depletion of brain serotonin and catecholamines. Life Sci 10:175–180

Haubrich DR, Blake DE (1973) Modification of serotonin metabolism in rat brain after acute or chronic administration of morphine. Biochem Pharmacol 22:2753–2759

Haugan S (1966) Aksidentell hypotermi under neurolepticumbehandling. Nord Med 75:377–380

Hauk F, Ankermann H (1963) Die Thermoregulation in der Urethan-Narkose. Acta Biol Med Ger 11:203–209

Helfrich LS (1934) The effect of morphine sulphate on temperature of various animals. Arch Int Pharmacodyn Ther 49:259–261

Hemingway A (1938) The effect of morphine on the skin and rectal temperatures of dogs as related to thermal polypnea. J Pharmacol Exp Ther 63:414–420

Hemingway A (1941) The effect of barbital anesthesia on temperature regulation. Am J Physiol 134:350–358

Hemingway A (1948) Rate of recovery of temperature-regulating responses after ether anesthesia. Am J Physiol 152:663–670

Heroux O, Hart JS, Depocas F (1956) Metabolism and muscle activity of anesthetised warm and cold acclimated rats on exposure to cold. J Appl Physiol 9:399–403

Herrmann JB (1941) Effects of certain drugs on temperature regulation, and changes in their toxicity, in rats exposed to cold. J Pharmacol Exp Ther 72:130–137

Herrmann JB (1942) The pyretic action on rats of small doses of morphine. J Pharmacol Exp Ther 76:309–315

Ho IK (1976) Systematic assessment of tolerance to pentobarbital by pellet implantation. J Pharmacol Exp Ther 197:479–487

Hobson GN, Collis ML (1977) The effects of alcohol upon cooling rates of humans immersed in 7.5 degrees C water. Can J Physiol Pharmacol 55:744–746

Hoffman RA (1958) Temperature response of the rat to action and interaction of chlorpromazine, reserpine and serotonin. Am J Physiol 195:755–758

Hoffman RA (1959) Influence of the adrenal gland on hypothermic response of the rat to chlorpromazine, reserpine and serotonin. Am J Physiol 196:876–880

Hoffman PL, Tabakoff B (1977) Alterations in dopamine receptor sensitivity by chronic ethanol treatment. Nature 268:551–553

Hoffman RA, Zarrow MX (1958) Hypothermia in the rat, hamster, ground squirrel and pigeon following chlorpromazine. Am J Physiol 193:547–552

Hofman WF, Riegle GD (1977) Effects of electroanesthesia and a phenothiazine tranquilizer on thermoregulation in the sheep. Am J Vet Res 38:403–406

Holaday JW, Law PY, Tseng LF, Loh HH, Li CH (1977) β-Endorphin: pituitary and adrenal glands modulate its action. Proc Natl Acad Sci USA 74:4628–4632

Holaday JW, Tseng LF, Loh HH, Li CH (1978 a) Thyrotropin releasing hormone antagonizes β endorphin hypothermia and catalepsy. Life Sci 22:1537–1544

Holaday JW, Wei E, Loh HH, Li CH (1978 b) Endorphins may function in heat adaptation. Proc Natl Acad Sci USA 75:2923–2927

Hollister LE (1966) Overdoses of psychotherapeutic drugs. Clin Pharmacol Ther 7:142–146

Holtzman SG, Villarreal JE (1969) Morphine dependence and body temperature in rhesus monkeys. J Pharmacol Exp Ther 166:125–133

Holtzman SG, Villarreal JE (1971) Pharmacologic analysis of the hypothermic responses of the morphine-dependent rhesus monkey. J Pharmacol Exp Ther 177:317–325

Hughes J, Kosterlitz HW (1977) Opioid peptides. Br Med Bull 33:157–161

Humphreys RB, Hawkins M, Lipton JM (1976) Effects of anesthetic injected into brainstem sites on body temperature and behavioral thermoregulation. Physiol Behav 17:667–674

Irvine RE (1973) Hypothermia. Mod Geriatr 3:464–470

Isbell H, Wikler A, Eddy NB, Wilson JL, Moran CF (1947) Tolerance and addiction liability of 6-dimethylamino-4-4-diphenyl-heptanone-3 (methadon). JAMA 135:888–894

Isbell H, Eisenman AJ, Wikler A, Frank K (1948 a). The effects of single doses of 6-dimethylamino-4-4-diphenyl-3-heptanone (amidone, methadon or "10820") on human subjects. J Pharmacol Exp Ther 92:83–89

Isbell H, Wikler A, Eisenman AJ, Daingerfield M, Frank K (1948 b) Liability of addiction to 6-dimethylamino-4-4-diphenyl-3-heptanone (methadon, "amidon" or "10820") in man. Archs Intern Med 82:362–392

Isbell H, Altschul S, Kornetsky CH, Eisenman AJ, Flanary HG, Fraser HF (1950) Chronic barbiturate intoxication. An experimental study. Arch Neurol Psychiatry 64:1–28

Isbell H, Fraser HF, Wikler A, Belleville RE, Eisenman AJ (1955) An experimental study of the etiology of "rumfits" and delirium tremens. QJ Stud Alcohol 16:1–33

Isom GE, McCarthy TA, Eells JT, Wimer ER (1978) Influence of intracerebroventricular injections of N6, O 2'-dibutyryl adenosine 3'5'-cyclic monophosphate on sodium pento barbital-induced narcosis in rats. Neuropharmacology 17:53–58

Jacob J, Peindaries R (1973) Central effects of monoamines on the temperature of the conscious rabbit. In: Lomax P, Schönbaum E (eds) The pharmacology of thermoregulation. Karger, Basel, pp 202–216

Jacobson FH (1966) Hypothalamic site of the metabolic reduction by pentobarbital. Proc Fed Am Soc Exp Biol 25:515

Järbe TUC, Holmgren B (1977) Discriminative properties of pentobarbital after repeated noncontingent exposure in gerbils. Psychopharmacology 53:39–44

Järbe TUC, Johansson JO (1977) Pentobarbital diazepam and bemegride: their effects on open-field behaviour in the Gerbil (Meriones unguiculatus). Arch Int Pharmacodyn Ther 225:88–97

Järbe TUC, Ohlin GC (1977) Interactions between alcohol and other drugs on open-field and temperature measurements in Gerbils. Arch Int Pharmacodyn Ther 227:106–117

Jamieson D, Van den Brenk HAS (1961) Relation of mast cell changes to hypothermia in the rat. Biochem Pharmacol 7:35–46

Jell RM, Gloor P (1972) Distribution of thermosensitive and nonthermosensitive preoptic and anterior hypothalamic neurons in unanesthetized cats, and effects of some anesthetics. Can J Physiol Pharmacol 50:890–901

Jones IH, Meade TW (1964) Hypothermia following chlorpromazine therapy in myxoedematous patients. Gerontol Clin 6:252 256

Jounela AJ (1970) Influence of phenelzine on the toxicity of some analgesics in mice. Ann Med Exp Biol Fenn 48:261–265

Jounela AJ, Mattila MJ, Knoll J (1977) Interaction of selective inhibitors of monoamine oxidase with pethidine in rabbits. Biochem Pharmacol 26:806–808

Kaakkola S, Ahtee L (1977) Effect of muscarinic cholinergic drugs on morphine-induced catalepsy, antinociception and changes in brain dopamine metabolism. Psychopharmacology 52:7–15

Kääriäinen I, Ahtee L (1976) Effect of narcotic analgesics on the striatal homovanillic acid content in mice; relation to antinociceptive effect. Med Biol 54:56–61

Kakihana R (1977) Endocrine and autonomic studies in mice selectively bred for different sensitivity to ethanol. Adv Exp Med Biol 85 A:83–95

Kalant H, Le Blanc AE, Gibbins RJ (1971) Tolerance to, and dependence on, some non-opiate psychotropic drugs. Pharmacol Rev 23:135–191

Kamei C, Ueki S (1974) Naloxone-induced abstinence syndromes in morphine-treated mice. Jpn J Pharmacol 24:655–657

Kawashima K, Wurzburger RJ, Spector S (1975) Correlation of chlorpromazine levels in rat brain and serum with its hypothermic effect. Psychopharmacol Commun 1:431–436

Keatinge WR, Evans M (1960) Effect of food, alcohol and hyoscine on body temperature and reflex responses of men immersed in cold water. Lancet 2:176–178

Kirkpatrick WE, Lomax P (1967) The effect of atropine on the body temperature of the rat following systemic and intracerebral injection. Life Sci 6:2273–2278

Kirkpatrick WE, Lomax P (1971) Temperature changes induced by chlorpromazine and N-methyl chlorpromazine in the rat. Neuropharmacology 10:61–66

Ko B (1937) The effect of morphine hydrochloride on temperature of rabbits under chronic intoxication. Jpn J Med Sci IV Pharmacol 10:202–203

Kollias J, Bullard RW (1964) The influence of chlorpromazine on physical and chemical mechanisms of temperature regulation in the rat. J Pharmacol Exp Ther 145:373–381

Krog J (1959) Notes on rectal temperature variations in dogs during nembutal anaesthesia. Acta Physiol Scand 45:308–310

Kuhar MJ, Pert CB, Snyder SH (1973) Regional distribution of opiate receptor binding in monkey and human brain. Nature 245:447–450

Lal H, Puri SK, Karkalas Y (1971) Blockade of opioid-withdrawal symptoms by haloperidol in rats and humans. Pharmacologist 13:263

Lal H, Miksic S, Smith N (1976) Naloxone antagonism of conditioned hyperthermia: an evidence for release of endogenous opioid. Life Sci 18:971–975

L'Allemand H, Brendel W, Usinger W (1955) Über den Mechanismus der Chlorpromazin-(Megaphen-)Wirkung auf die Temperaturregulation. Anaesthetist 4:36–41

Laska FJ, Fennessy MR (1976) Physical dependence in the rat induced by slow release morphine: dose-response, time course and brain biogenic amines. Clin Exp Pharmacol Physiol 3:587–598

Laska FJ, Fennessy MR (1977) Dissociation of increased 5-hydroxyindoleacetic acid levels and physical dependence: the effects of naloxone. Clin Exp Pharmacol Physiol 4:515–523

Laska FJ, Fennessy MR (1978) Induction of physical dependence on cyclazocine and pentazocine in the rat. Eur J Pharmacol 48:57–65

Leander JD, Batten J, Hargis GW (1978) Pethidine interaction with clorgyline, pargyline or 5-hydroxytryptophan: lack of enhanced pethidine lethality or hyperpyrexia in mice. J Pharm Pharmacol 30:396–398

Le Blanc J (1958a) Chlorpromazine hypothermia in rats. J Appl Physiol 13:237–238

Le Blanc JA (1958b) Role of adrenaline and noradrenaline on response of cold-acclimatized animals to chlorpromazine. Proc Soc Exp Biol Med 98:406–407

Le Blanc J, Rosenberg F (1957) Hypothermic effect of chlorpromazine, histamine and serotonin, and acclimatization to cold. Proc Soc Exp Biol Med 96:482–483

Le Blanc J, Rosenberg F (1958) Effect of dibenamine and pyribenzamine on hypothermia of chlorpromazine. Proc Soc Exp Biol Med 97:95–97

Lechat P, Levassort C (1969) Modification of rabbit body temperature induced by the simultaneous injection of gonococcus vaccine and various phenothiazine neuroleptics. Pharmacology 2:100–112

Lessin AW, Parkes MW (1957a) The relation between sedation and body temperature in the mouse. Br J Pharmacol Chemother 12:245–250

Lessin AW, Parkes MW (1957b) The hypothermic and sedative action of reserpine in the mouse. J Pharm Pharmacol 9:657–662

Lettau HF, Sellers EA, Schönbaum E (1964) Modification of drug-induced hypothermia. Can J Physiol Pharmacol 42:745–755

Lin MT (1979) Effects of brain monoamine depletion on chlorpromazine-induced hypothermia in rabbits. Can J Physiol Pharmacol 57:16–23

Lin MT, Chow CF, Chern YF (1978) The effect of a decarboxylase inhibitor, benserazide, on both thermoregulation and chlorpromazine-induced hypothermia in rats. J Pharm Pharmacol 30:759–761

Lin MT, Chern YF, Chow CF, Li YP (1979) Effects of brain serotonin alterations on hypothermia produced by chlorpromazine in rats. Pharmacology 18:128–135

Lindqvist M, Kehr W, Carlsson A (1974) Effect of pentobarbitone and diethyl ether on the synthesis of monoamines in rat brain. Arch Pharmacol 284:263–277

Linseman MA (1976) Effects of lesions of the caudate nucleus on morphine dependence in the rat. Pharmacol Biochem Behav 5:465–472

Lipton JM (1973) Thermosensitivity of medulla oblongata in control of body temperature. Am J Physiol 224:890–897

Lipton JM, Fossler DE (1974) Fever produced in the squirrel monkey by intravenous and intracerebral endotoxin. Am J Physiol 226:1022–1027

Liu RK (1974) Hypothermic effects of marihuana, marihuana derivatives and chlorpromazine in laboratory mice. Res Commun Chem Pathol Pharmacol 9:215–228

Lomax P (1966) The hypothermic effect of pentobarbital in the rat: sites and mechanisms of action. Brain Res 1:296–302

Lomax P, Kirkpatrick WE (1967) The effect of N-allylnormorphine on the development of acute tolerance to the analgesic and hypothermic effects of morphine in the rat. Med Pharmacol Exp 16:165–170

Lord JAH, Waterfield AA, Hughes J, Kosterlitz HW (1977) Endogenous opioid peptides: multiple agonists and receptors. Nature 267:495–499

Lotti VJ, Lomax P, George R (1965a) Temperature responses in the rat following intracerebral microinjection of morphine. J Pharmacol Exp Ther 150:135–139

Lotti VJ, Lomax P, George R (1965b) N-allylnormorphine antagonism of the hypothermic effect of morphine in the rat following intracerebral and systemic administration. J Pharmacol Exp Ther 150:420–425

Lotti VJ, Lomax P, George R (1966a) Acute tolerance to morphine following systemic and intracerebral injection in the rat. Int J Neuropharmacol 5:35–42

Lotti VJ, Lomax P, George R (1966b) Heat production and heat loss in the rat following intracerebral and systemic administration of morphine. Int J Neuropharmacol 5:75–83

Loughnane T (1968) Hypothermia in a young adult. Lancet 2:455–456

Loveless AH, Maxwell DR (1965) A comparison of the effects of imipramine, trimipramine and some other drugs in rabbits treated with a monoamine oxidase inhibitor. Br J Pharmacol Chemother 25:158–170

Mäkeläinen A (1974) Methoxyflurane and lipid and carbohydrate metabolism in rats. Acta Anaesthesiol Scand 18:144–152

Mäkeläinen A, Rosenberg P (1974) The effects of halothane and methoxyflurane metabolites on lipolysis in vitro. Acta Anaesthesiol Scand 18:153–160

Mäkeläinen A, Nikki P, Vapaatalo H (1973a) Halothane-induced lipolysis in rats. Acta Anaesthesiol Scand 17:170–178

Mäkeläinen A, Vapaatalo H, Nikki P (1973b) Halothane-induced lipolysis in vitro in the rat. Acta Anaesthesiol Scand 17:179–183

Mahrer PR, Bergman PS, Estren S (1958) Atropine-like poisoning due to tranquilizing agents. Am J Psychiatry 115:337–339

Maier A, Forster F, Schaff G (1955) Effet de la chlorpromazine sur la durée de survie du Rat blanc séjournant à basse température (+5 °C) ou à la neutralité thermique (+31 °C). CR Soc Biol (Paris) 149:568–570

Martin GE, Morrison JE (1978) Hyperthermia evoked by the intracerebral injection of morphine sulphate in the rat: the effect of restraint. Brain Res 145:127–140

Martin GE, Pryzbylik AT, Spector NH (1977) Restraint alters the effects of morphine and heroin on core temperature in the rat. Pharmacol Biochem Behav 7:463–469

Martin S, Cooper KE (1978) Alcohol and respiratory and body temperature changes during tepid water immersion. J Appl Physiol 44:683–689

Martin S, Diewold RJ, Cooper KE (1977) Alcohol, respiration, skin, and body temperature during cold water immersion. J Appl Physiol 43:211–215

Martin WR, Wikler A, Eades CG, Pescor FT (1963) Tolerance to and physical dependence on morphine in rats. Psychopharmacologia 4:247–260

Martin WR, Jasinski DR, Haertzen CA, Kay DC, Jones BE, Mansky PA, Carpenter RW (1973) Methadone – a reevaluation. Arch Gen Psychiatry 28:286–295

Mattila MJ, Jounela AJ (1973) Effect of p-chlorophenylalanine on the interaction between phenelzine and pethidine in conscious rabbits. Biochem Pharmacol 22:1674–1676

Maynert EW, Klingman GI (1962) Tolerance to morphine. I. Effects on catecholamines in the brain and adrenal glands. J Pharmacol Exp Ther 135:285–295

McCrum WR, Ingram WR (1951) The effect of morphine on cats with hypothalamic lesions. J Neuropathol Exp Neurol 10:190–203

McGilliard KL, Tulunay FC, Takemori AE (1976) Antagonism by naloxone of morphine – and pentazocine – induced respiratory depression and analgesia and of morphine-induced hyperthermia. In: Kosterlitz H (ed) Opiates and endogenous opioid peptides. Elsevier/North Holland, Amsterdam Oxford New York, pp 281–288

Medon PJ, Blake DE (1973) Temperature effects on intraventricular serotonin, norepinephrine and pilocarpine in the morphine-tolerant rat. Life Sci 13:1395–1402

Mellerio F (1970) Principales modifications électroencéphalographiques observées au cours des intoxications aiguës par neuroleptiques. Acta Psychiatry Belg 70:730–742

Metcalf G, Dettmar PW, Watson T (1980) The role of neuropeptides in thermoregulation. In: Cox B, Lomax P, Milton AS, Schönbaum E (eds) Thermoregulatory mechanisms and their therapeutic implications. Karger, Basel, pp 175–179

Miksic S, Smith N, Numan R, Lal H (1975) Acquisition and extinction of a conditioned hyperthermic response to a tone paired with morphine administration. Neuropsychobiology 1:277–283

Milton AS (1975) Morphine hyperthermia, prostaglandin synthetase inhibitors and naloxone. J Physiol (Lond) 251:27–28 P

Mitchell JRA, Surridge DHC, Willison RG (1959) Hypothermia after chlorpromazine in myxoedematous psychosis. Br Med J 2:932–933

Modak AT, Weintraub ST, McCoy TH, Stavinoha WB (1976) Use of 300-msec microwave irradiation for enzyme inactivation: a study of effects of sodium pentobarbital on acetylcholine concentration in mouse brain regions. J Pharmacol Exp Ther 197:245–252

Morpurgo C (1962) Influence of phenothiazine derivatives on the accumulation of brain amines induced by monoamine oxidase inhibitors. Biochem Pharmacol 11:967–972

Morpurgo C, Theobald W (1965) Influence of imipramine-like compounds and chlorpromazine on the reserpine-hypothermia in mice and the amphetamine-hyperthermia in rats. Med Pharmacol Exp 12:226–232

Morris RH (1971) Operating room temperature and the anesthetized, paralyzed patient. Arch Surg 102:95–97

Morris RH, Kumar A (1972) The effect of warming blankets on maintenance of body temperature of the anesthetized, paralysed adult patient. Anesthesiology 36:408–411

Morris RH, Wilkey BR (1970) The effects of ambient temperature on patient temperature during surgery not involving body cavities. Anesthesiology 32:102–107

Murakami N, Stolwijk JAJ, Hardy JD (1967) Responses of preoptic neurons to anesthetics and peripheral stimulation. Am J Physiol 213:1015–1024

Naito H, Yamazaki T, Nakamura K, Matsumoto M, Namba M (1974) Skin and rectal temperatures during ether and halothane anesthesia in infants and children. Anesthesiology 41:237–241

Nakayama T, Hori T (1973) Effects of anesthetic and pyrogen on thermally sensitive neurons in the brainstem. J Appl Physiol 34:351–355

Neuhold K, Taeschler M, Cerletti A (1957) Beitrag zur zentralen Wirkung von LSD. Versuche über die Lokalisation von LSD-Effekten. Helv Physiol Pharmacol Acta 15:1–7

Newman BJ (1971) Control of accidental hypothermia. Anaesthesia 26:177–187

Nikki P (1968) Influence of some cholinomimetic and cholinolytic drugs on halothane shivering in mice. Ann Med Exp Biol Fenn 46:521–530

Nikki P, Tammisto T (1968) Halothane-induced heat loss and shivering in rats. Acta Anaesthesiol Scand 12:125–134

Nikki P, Vapaatalo H, Karppanen H (1971) Effect of ethanol on body temperature, postanaesthetic shivering and tissue monoamines in halothane-anaesthetised rats. Ann Med Exp Biol Fenn 49:157–161

Nymark M, Nielsen IM (1963) Reactions due to the combination of monoamine oxidase inhibitors with thymoleptics, pethidine or methylamphetamine. Lancet 2:524–525

Oka T (1977) Role of 5-hydroxytryptamine in morphine-, pethidine- and methadone-induced hypothermia in rats at low ambient and room temperature. Br J Pharmacol 60:323–330

Oka T, Negishi K (1977) Effect of neurohumoral modulators on the morphine-induced hyperthermia in non-tolerant rats. Eur J Pharmacol 42:225–229

Oka T, Nozaki M (1970) The effects of parachlorophenylalanine on non-tolerant rats and of cholinergic blocking drugs on tolerant rats to morphine. Jpn J Pharmacol 20:455–457

Oka T, Nozaki M, Hosoya E (1972) Effects of p-chlorophenylalanine and cholinergic antagonists on body temperature changes induced by the administration of morphine to nontolerant and morphine-tolerant rats. J Pharmacol Exp Ther 180:136–143

Osman OH, Eltayeb IB (1977) Hyperpyrexic interaction between debrisoquine and pethidine in rabbits. J Pharm Pharmacol 29:143–146

Palmer H (1960) Potentiation of pethidine. Br Med J 2:944

Paolino RM, Bernard BK (1968) Environmental temperature effects on the thermoregulatory response to systemic and hypothalamic administration of morphine. Life Sci 7:857–863

Papp C, Benaim S (1958) Toxic effects of iproniazid in a patient with angina. Br Med J 2:1070–1072

Park S, Happy JM, Prange AJ (1972) Thyroid action on behavioral-physiological effects and disposition of phenothiazines. Eur J Pharmacol 19:357–365

Paton WDM, Speden RN (1965) An analysis of the kinetics of anaesthesia of mice. Br J Pharmacol Chemother 25.88–103

Pells Cocks D, Passmore-Rowe A (1962) Dangers of monoamine oxidase inhibitors. Br Med J 2:1545–1546

Penn RG, Rogers KJ (1971) Comparison of the effects of morphine, pethidine and pentazocine in rabbits pretreated with a monoamine oxidase inhibitor. Br J Pharmacol 42:485–492

Pertwee RG (1970) The effects of anaesthetic gases at high pressure on thermoregulation. PhD thesis, Oxford University

Pohorecky LA, Jaffe LS (1975) Noradrenergic involvement in the acute effects of ethanol. Res Commun Chem Pathol Pharmacol 12:433–447

Pohorecky LA, Jaffe LS, Berkeley HA (1974) Effects of ethanol on serotoninergic neurons in the rat brain. Res Commun Chem Pathol Pharmacol 8:1–11

Pohorecky LA, Brick J, Sun JY (1976) Serotoninergic involvement in the effect of ethanol on body temperature in rats. J Pharm Pharmacol 28:157–159

Polk DL, Lipton JM (1975) Effects of sodium salicylate, aminopyrine and chlorpromazine on behavioral temperature regulation. Pharmacol Biochem Behav 3:167–172

Popovic V (1954) La chlorpromazine et la poïkilothermie expérimentale. CR Soc Biol (Paris) 148:845–846

Reid NCRW, Jones D (1962) Pethidine and phenelzine. Br Med J 1:408

Reigle TG, Wolf HH (1971) The effects of centrally administered chlorpromazine on temperature regulation in the hamster. Life Sci 10:121–132

Revol L (1959) Effets comparés de divers psychotropes sur la température du lapin. Therapie 14:804–810

Rewerski WT, Gumulka W (1969) The effect of α-MT on hyperthermia induced by chlorpromazine. Int J Neuropharmacol 8:389–391

Rewerski W, Jori A (1968 a) Effect of desipramine injected intracerebrally in normal or reserpinized rats. J Pharm Pharmacol 20:293–296

Rewerski WJ, Jori A (1968 b) Microinjection of chlorpromazine in different parts of rat brain. Int J Neuropharmacol 7:359–364

Ritzmann RF, Tabakoff B (1976 a) Ethanol, serotonin metabolism, and body temperature. Ann NY Acad Sci 273:247–255

Ritzmann RF, Tabakoff B (1976 b) Body temperature in mice: a quantitative measure of alcohol tolerance and physical dependence. J Pharmacol Exp Ther 199:158–170

Ritzmann RF, Tabakoff B (1976 c) Dissociation of alcohol tolerance and dependence. Nature 263:418–420

Rivers N, Horner B (1970) Possible lethal reaction between nardil and dextromethorphan. Can Med Assoc J 103:85

Robson LE, Kosterlitz HW (1979) Specific protection of the binding sites of D-Ala^2-D-Leu^{5}enkephalin (δ-receptors) and dihydromorphine (μ-receptors). Proc R Soc Lond [Biol] 205:425–432

Roe CF, Goldberg MJ, Blair CS, Kenney JM (1966) The influence of body temperature on early postoperative oxygen consumption. Surgery 60:85–92

Roffman M, Reddy C, Lal H (1973) Control of morphine-withdrawal hypothermia by conditional stimuli. Psychopharmacologia 29:197–201

Rogers KJ (1971) Role of brain monoamines in the interaction between pethidine and tranylcypromine. Eur J Pharmacol 14:86–88

Rogers KJ, Thornton JA (1969) The interaction between monoamine oxidase inhibitors and narcotic analgesics in mice. Br J Pharmacol 36:470–480

Rosenfeld GC, Burks TF (1977) Single-dose tolerance to morphine hypothermia in the rat: differentiation of acute from long-term tolerance. J Pharmacol Exp Ther 202:654–659

Rosenthal FE (1941) Cooling drugs and cooling centres. J Pharmacol Exp Ther 71:305–314

Rudy TA, Wolf HH (1967) Relation of chlorpromazine-evoked hypothermia to disruption of conditioned avoidance-escape behavior. J Pharmacol Exp Ther 156:397–406

Rudy TA, Yaksh TL (1977) Hyperthermic effects of morphine: set point manipulation by a direct spinal action. Br J Pharmacol 61:91–96

Saarnivaara L, Männistö PT (1976) Effects of lithium and rubidium on antinociception and behaviour in mice. I. Studies on narcotic analgesics and antagonists. Arch Int Pharmacodyn Ther 222:282–292

Samanin R, Valzelli L (1972) Serotoninergic neurotransmission and morphine activity. Arch Int Pharmacodyn Ther [Suppl] 196:138–141

Samanin R, Kon S, Garattini S (1972) Abolition of the morphine effect on body temperature in midbrain raphe lesioned rats. J Pharm Pharmacol 24:374–377

Saunders DR, Paolino RM, Bousquet WF, Miya TS (1974) Age-related responsiveness of the rat to drugs affecting the central nervous system. Proc Soc Exp Biol Med 147:593–595

Schaumkell KW (1955) Über die Morphokinese und das Strukturbild der Rattenschilddrüse nach Gaben von N-(3'-Dimethylamino)-propyl-3-chlorphenothiazin (Megaphen Bayer) unter verschiedenen experimentellen Bedingungen. Arch Exp Pathol Pharmakol 225:381–401

Schulz R, Cartwright C, Goldstein A (1974) Reversibility of morphine tolerance and dependence in guinea-pig brain and myenteric plexus. Nature 251:329–331

Schwartzbaum JS (1955) Effects of reserpine and chlorpromazine on nest building and thermal preference in rats. Proc Soc Exp Biol Med 90:275–277

Scoto GM, Spadaro C, Spampinato S, Arrigo-Reina R, Ferri S (1979) Prostaglandins in the brain of rats given, acutely, and chronically, a hyperthermic dose of met-enkephalin. Psychopharmacology (Berlin) 60:217–219

Seed JR, Sechelski J (1977) Tryptophol levels in mice injected with pharmacological doses of tryptophol, and the effect of pyrazole and ethanol on these levels. Life Sci 21:1603–1610

Seoane JR, Baile CA (1975) Feeding and temperature changes in sheep following injections of barbiturates, Ca^{++}, or Mg^{++} into the lateral, third of fourth ventricle or cerebral aqueduct. J Dairy Sci 58:515–520

Shamsie SJ, Barriga C (1971) The hazards of use of monoamine oxidase inhibitors in disturbed adolescents. Can Med Assoc J 104:715

Shapiro MF (1967) Despair, trifluoperazine, exercise, and temperature of 108 °F. Am J Psychiatry 124:705–707

Sharkawi M (1972) Morphine hyperthermia in the rat: its attenuation by physostigmine. Br J Pharmacol 44:544–548

Shee JC (1960) Dangerous potentiation of pethidine by iproniazid and its treatment. Br Med J 2:507–509

Shemano I, Nickerson M (1958) Effect of ambient temperature on thermal responses to drugs. Can J Biochem Physiol 36:1243–1249

Sinclair JG (1972a) The effect of meperidine and morphine in rabbits pretreated with phenelzine. Toxicol Appl Pharmacol 22:231–240

Sinclair JG (1972b) Ethoheptazine – monoamine oxidase inhibitor interaction in rabbits. Can J Physiol Pharmacol 50:923–926

Sinclair JG (1973) Dextromethorphan – monoamine oxidase inhibitor interaction in rabbits. J Pharm Pharmacol 25:803–808

Sinclair JG, Lo GF (1977) The blockade of serotonin uptake into synaptosomes: relationship to an interaction with monoamine oxidase inhibitors. Can J Physiol Pharmacol 55:180–187

Singh PP, Das PK (1976) Role of catecholamines in the hypothermic activity of cannabis in albino rats. Psychopharmacology (Berlin) 50:199–204

Skobba T, Miya TS (1969) Hyperthermic responses and toxicity of chlorpromazine in L-thyroxine sodium-treated rats. Toxicol Appl Pharmacol 14:176–181

Sloan JW, Brooks JW, Eisenman AJ, Martin WR (1962) Comparison of the effects of single doses of morphine and thebain on body temperature, activity and brain and heart levels of catecholamines and serotonin. Psychopharmacologia 3:291–301

Smith PK (1938) The relation of acetanilid and other drugs to analgesia in monkeys. J Pharmacol Exp Ther 62:467–474

Smith NT (1962) Subcutaneous, muscle and body temperatures in anesthetized man. J Appl Physiol 17:306–310

Soliman MG, Gillies DMM (1972) Muscular hyperactivity after general anaesthesia. Can Anaesth Soc J 19:529–535

Spencer PSJ, Waite R (1968) The effects of chlorpromazine and reserpine in hyperthyroid mice. Br J Pharmacol Chemother 32:419–420 P

Spratto GR, Dorio RE (1978) Effect of age on acute morphine response in the rat. Res Commun Chem Pathol Pharmacol 19:23–36

Stewart GN, Rogoff JM (1922) Influence of morphine on normal cats and on cats deprived of the greater part of the adrenals, with special reference to body temperature, pulse, and respiratory rate and blood sugar content. J Pharmacol Exp Ther 19:97–130

Ström G (1950) Influence of local thermal stimulation of the hypothalamus of the cat on cutaneous blood flow and respiratory rate. Acta Physiol Scand [Suppl 70] 20:47–112

Strömbom U, Svensson TH, Carlsson A (1977) Antagonism of ethanol's central stimulation in mice by small doses of catecholamine-receptor agonists. Psychopharmacology (Berlin) 51:293–299

Summers RJ (1969) Effects of MAO inhibitors on the hypothermia produced in cats by halothane. Br J Pharmacol 37:400–413

Tabakoff B, Ritzmann RF, Hoffman PL (1977) Role of catecholamines in the development of tolerance to barbiturates and ethanol. Adv Exp Med Biol 85 B:155–168

Tabakoff B, Yanai J, Ritzmann RF (1978) Brain noradrenergic systems as a prerequisite for developing tolerance to barbiturates. Science 200:449–451

Tagashira E, Izumi T, Yanaura S (1978) Experimental barbiturate dependence. Psychopharmacology (Berlin) 57:137–144

Tahara M (1962) Studies on the summation of the body temperature lowering effects due to combined use of sodium barbiturate and morphine hydrochloride and its mechanism in rabbits. J Keio Med Soc 39:371–378

Tavendale R (1979) The effects of Δ^9-tetrahydrocannabinol on temperature regulation in mice. PhD thesis, University of Aberdeen

Taylor DC (1962) Alarming reaction to pethidine in patients on phenelzine. Lancet 2:401–402

Thauer R (1943) Der Einfluß der Narkose auf die normale Wärmeregulation und das Fieber, zugleich ein Beitrag zur Frage des zentralen Wärmeregulationsmechanismus (Wärmezentrum). Pfluegers Arch Ges Physiol 246:372–410

Thornhill JA, Hirst M, Gowdey CW (1976) Changes in diurnal temperature and feeding patterns of rats during repeated injections of heroin and withdrawal. Arch Int Pharmacodyn Ther 223:120–131

Thornhill JA, Hirst M, Gowdey CW (1978) Changes in the hyperthermic responses of rats to daily injections of morphine and the antagonism of the acute response by naloxone. Can J Physiol Pharmacol 56:483–489

Thornhill JA, Cooper KE, Veale WL (1980) Effects of restraint and ambient temperature on core temperature responses to morphine in the rat. In: Cox B, Lomax P, Milton AS, Schönbaum E (eds) Thermoregulatory mechanisms and their therapeutic implications. Karger, Basel, pp 159–162

Trzcinka GP, Lipton JM, Hawkins M, Clark WG (1977) Effects on temperature of morphine injected into the preoptic/anterior hypothalamus, medulla oblongata, and peripherally in unrestrained and restrained rats. Proc Soc Exp Biol Med 156:523–526

Trzcinka GP, Lipton JM, Hawkins M, Clark WG (1978) Differential effects on temperature of chlorpromazine injected into PO/AH and medulla oblongata of the rat. Arch Int Pharmacodyn Ther 232:111–116

Tseng LF, Loh HH, Wei ET (1975) Effects of clonidine on morphine withdrawal signs in the rat. Eur J Pharmacol 30:93–99

Tseng L, Loh HH, Li CH (1977) Human β-endorphin: development of tolerance and behavioral activity in rats. Biochem Biophys Res Commun 74:390–396

Tsoucaris-Kupfer D, Schmitt H (1972) Hypothermic effect of α-sympathomimetic agents and their antagonism by adrenergic and cholinergic blocking drugs. Neuropharmacology 11:625–635

Ulrich WD, Maess M, Wirth J (1967 a) Untersuchungen zur Frage der Chlorpromazinwirkung. I. Respiratorischer Stoffwechsel und Körpertemperatur bei Behaglichkeitstemperatur nach Gabe von Chlorpromazin. Arch Int Pharmacodyn Ther 167:80–89

Ulrich WD, Wirth J, Maess M (1967 b) Untersuchungen zur Frage der Chlorpromazinwirkung. II. Die Temperaturregulation unter Chlorpromazin. Arch Int Pharmacodyn Ther 167:90–99

Usinger W (1957) Respiratorischer Stoffwechsel und Körpertemperatur der weißen Maus in Narkose und unter Chlorpromazin. Pfluegers Arch Ges Physiol 265:365–381

Van Ree JM, Spaapen-Kok WB, De Wied D (1976) Differential localization of pituitary-adrenal activation and temperature changes following intrahypothalamic microinjection of morphine in rats. Neuroendocrinology 22:318–324

Vapaatalo H, Mäkeläinen A, Nikki P (1975) Effects of some inhalation anesthetics on thermoregulation and metabolic processes. In: Jacob J, Lomax P, Schönbaum E, (eds) Temperature regulation and drug action. Karger, Basel, pp 319–324

Vigran IM (1964) Dangerous potentiation of meperidine hydrochloride by pargyline hydrochloride. JAMA 187:953–954

Votava Z (1973) Tolerance and withdrawal effects after one week administration of perphenazine in rabbits. In: Ban TA, Boissier JR, Heimann H et al. (eds) Psychopharmacology, sexual disorders and drug abuse. Elsevier/North Holland, Amsterdam Oxford New York, pp 377–382

Walker MFC (1959) Stimulation of tetanus by trifluoperazine overdosage. Can Med Ass J 81:109–110

Ward SJ, Metcalf G, Rees JMH (1977) The comparative pharmacology of morphine, ketocyclazocine and 2′-hydroxy-5,9-dimethyl-2-allyl-6,7-benzomorphan in rodents. J Pharm Pharmacol [Suppl] 29:54 P

Ward SJ, Metcalf G, Rees JMH (1980) The effects of proposed μ- and κ-opiate agonists on body temperature in mice. In: Cox B, Lomax P, Milton AS, Schönbaum E (eds) Thermoregulatory mechanisms and their therapeutic implications. Karger, Basel, pp 166–168

Warwick RO, Schnell RC (1976) Studies relating morphine hypothermia with serotonin reuptake in the rat hypothalamus. Eur J Pharmacol 38:329–335

Warwick RO, Blake DE, Miya TS, Bousquet WF (1973) Serotonin involvement in thermoregulation following administration of morphine to nontolerant and morphine-tolerant rats. Res Commun Pathol Pharmacol 6:19–32

Warwick RO, Bousquet WF, Schnell RC (1977) Effect of acute and chronic morphine treatment on serotonin uptake into rat hypothalamic synaptosomes. Pharmacology 15:415–427

Wei E, Tseng LF, Loh H, Way EL (1974) Similarity of morphine abstinence signs to thermoregulatory behaviour. Nature 247:398–400

Weiss B, Laties VG (1963) Effects of amphetamine, chlorpromazine and pentobarbital on behavioral thermoregulation. J Pharmacol Exp Ther 140:1–7

Werner HW (1941) The effects of benzedrine, coramine, metrazol and picrotoxin on body temperature and gaseous metabolism in rabbits depressed by alcohol. J Pharmacol Exp Ther 72:45

Whittle BA (1967) Reversal of reserpine-induced hypothermia by pharmacological agents other than antidepressants. Nature 216:579–580

Wikler A, Fraser HF, Isbell H (1953) N-allylnormorphine: effects of single doses and precipitation of acute "abstinence syndromes" during addiction to morphine, methadone or heroin in man (post-addicts). J Pharmacol Exp Ther 109:8–20

Winter CA, Flataker L (1953) The relation between skin temperature and the effect of morphine upon the response to thermal stimuli in the albino rat and the dog. J Pharmacol Exp Ther 109:183–188

Wislicki L (1960) Intensification of chlorpromazine hypothermia by cocaine. Arch Int Pharmacodyn Ther 124:302–309

Witherspoon JD, Short HW, Hiestand WA (1957) Influence of ascorbic acid and chlorpromazine on body temperature and resistance of mice to drowning. Proc Soc Exp Biol Med 95:560–561

Wolfe GW, Bousquet WF, Schnell RC (1977) Circadian variations in response to amphetamine and chlorpromazine in the rat. Commun Psychopharmacol 1:29–37

Yamamoto I, Ho IK, Loh HH (1978) The antagonistic effects of 5-ethyl-5-(3-hydroxy-1-methylbutyl)-barbituric acid on pentobarbital narcosis in both naïve and tolerant mice. Life Sci 22:1103–1112

Yehuda S, Wurtman RJ (1972) The effects of D-amphetamine and related drugs on colonic temperatures of rats kept at various ambient temperatures. Life Sci 11:851–859

Zelman S, Guillan R (1970) Heat stroke in phenothiazine-treated patients: a report on three fatalities. Am J Psychiatry 126:1787–1790

CHAPTER 14

Capsaicin Type Pungent Agents Producing Pyrexia

J. SZOLCSÁNYI

A. Introduction

The object of this chapter is to review the effects of capsaicin-like pungent agents, with special attention to the unique, irreversible impairment in thermoregulation induced by these drugs. In the light of recent findings it is a promising possibility that these compounds are useful tools in studies of temperature regulation. In this context evidence for the concept that these compounds form a new class of specifically acting drugs, namely, the selective sensory neurone blocking agents, is presented and discussed in detail.

Over a hundred years chemical challenge of the thermoregulatory "black box" by means of pyrogens and antipyretics has supplied the corner-stone of conceptual models for the regulating circuit (LIEBERMEISTER 1875; MITCHELL et al. 1970; CABANAC and MASSONETT 1974). It seems to be tempting to challenge these models from the input side by means of pungent agents. The important question is what is the "signal-to-noise ratio?" What are the gains and what are the limits when capsaicin or its congeners are used? Experimental evidence to clarify their site of action as well as effects not strictly related to thermal reflexes are summarized from this point of view.

Before dealing with the topic in detail it is necessary to define the meaning of pungent agents or pungency. These words are commonly used to characterize peppers or pepper-like compounds producing a burning sensation. Their precise definition, however, is not an easy task. On the one hand, pungency is the most appropriate word to denote the biting sensory effect elicited by "pepper-flavoured" compounds (NEWMAN 1954a). On the other hand, this word is generally used in a broader sense, and compounds producing a simple unpleasant pricking pain ("irritants") could also be called pungent agents. On the tongue capsaicin and piperine, the pungent principles in paprika and black pepper, respectively, elicit in near-threshold concentrations a simple, pleasantly warm sensation and nothing else. A burning sensation develops only if higher concentrations are tasted. Most irritants even in threshold concentrations produce an unpleasant, sometimes ill-defined "pricking" feeling which in the case of some compounds – e.g. mustard oil, allyl alcohol, or eugenol – is also mixed with a "hot" feeling.

For the sake of clarity the term pungent agent is used in this review to denote compounds which elicit a simple warm sensation at threshold concentration and produce burning pain at higher concentrations only. The prototypes of this group are capsaicin and piperine.

B. Historical Background

Peppers have always been, and still are the most important condiments in the world. This aspect of pungent agents as well as the interesting history of peppers and related substances lie outside the scope of this review.

The first experimental results as to the effect of pungent agents on thermoregulation were reported from Hungarian laboratories (Högyes 1878). Högyes observed that capsicol, the pungent oily extract of paprika (*Capsicum annuum*) caused a fall in body temperature when introduced into the stomach of dogs. He tested the effect of capsicol on different preparations (e.g. on frog heart, nerve–muscle preparation) and concluded that the site of action of the extract was primarily the sensory nerves.

Some fifty years later Stary reported the oral administration of pungent extracts of red pepper, black pepper, or ginger to lower the body temperature of the rabbit (Stary 1925). The response was attributed to stimulation of warm-sensitive fibres in the alimentary tract. Heubner completed a classification of different types of irritants („Reizstoffe") in the same year (Heubner 1925). On the basis of findings obtained with two synthetic pungent congeners of capsaicin he put the peppers and related substances into the category of pure neural stimulants („reine Nervenreizgifte").

All these authors established that inflammation with signs of tissue damage cannot be evoked by treatment with pungent agents. The reactive hyperaemia, however, is one of the most characteristic effects which they produce. Thus, pungent agents are known as *rubefacients* or, owing to their therapeutic application, they are commonly referred to as *counter-irritants*.

Interestingly, this rubefacient property of these compounds was the source of a recent development in the thermoregulatory effect of pungent agents. N. Jancsó in the early 1940 s discovered the activation of reticulo-endothelial system by histamine (Jancsó 1947). For this purpose he started to use pungent agents. In the course of these experiments he made a remarkable discovery. After repeated application of pungent agents of acylamide type, e.g. by instillation into the eye of a guinea-pig, the pain and inflammation produced by pain-producing chemical agents were abolished for days. The mechanical sensitivity of the area remained intact, e.g. the corneal reflex to gentle touch was readily elicited. This phenomenon has been called *local capsaicin desensitization*.

In one chapter of his excellent monograph Jancsó (1955) published for the first time the early findings on pungent agents he had obtained in collaboration with his wife. A short abstract in Hungarian (Jancsó and Jancsó-Gábor 1949) and some parts of his wife's dissertation (Jancsó-Gábor 1947) provide evidence that the discovery of local capsaicin desensitization was made much earlier. In the book mentioned above he reported that a similar desensitizing effect could also be produced by parenteral capsaicin pre-treatment in the mouse (*general capsaicin desensitization*). In these pre-treated mice the hypothermic response to pungent agents was also abolished.

This observation was the corner-stone of the thermoregulatory part of capsaicin research, the detailed analysis of which was performed under his direction from 1963 until his death in 1966.

Results of this period were presented by him at three meetings (JANCSÓ 1965; JANCSÓ and JANCSÓ-GÁBOR 1965; JANCSÓ et al. 1966) and published in extenso in two papers (JANCSÓ-GÁBOR et al. 1970a, b).

Having been myself a co-worker of Professor N. JANCSÓ, it is my intention to describe the historical background in order to make clear his pioneering role in this field. I have felt it particularly necessary since he published only two full papers in international journals about the effects of capsaicin or other pungent agents (PÓRSZÁSZ and JANCSÓ 1959; JANCSÓ et al. 1961). His wife and myself as co-workers in these experiments later made an attempt to publish the findings obtained during his last years according to his views (JANCSÓ 1968; JANCSÓ et al. 1967, 1968; JAN-CSÓ-GÁBOR et al. 1970a, b).

A review about capsaicin in general was published by MOLNÁR (1965). This thorough survey covers a complete list of references on the pharmacological effects of capsaicin up to 1965. The monograph written by GLATZEL (1968) gives a full account of the effect of spices on human subjects. A recent minireview published by VIRUS and GEBHART (1979) gave an account of some thermoregulatory and other effects of capsaicin discussing the possible involvement of substance P and 5-hydroxytryptamine in its actions.

C. Chemical Structure

I. Natural Pungent Substances

1. Capsaicin

The chemical structure of capsaicin is: N-(3-methoxy-4-hydroxybenzyl)-8-methyl-6-*trans*-nonenoicamide, which corresponds to 8-methyl-6-*trans*-nonenoyl-vanillyl-amide (Fig. 1).

The substance is the pungent principle of the red pepper (*Capsicum annuum*). There are about fifty varieties of red peppers, and several names are in use to differentiate among them (paprika, chili, cayenne pepper, pimento etc.). Crude extracts containing capsaicin – official pharmaceutical products in a number of countries – are called capsicin (Tinctura capsici), or capsicol. The capsaicin content of pepper pods of different origin varies in the range 0.21%–1.43% (LUCKNER et al. 1969) and in dried products 0.02%–0.5% (NEWMAN 1953a; LUCKNER et al. 1969). Some closely related similarly pungent vanillylamides (capsaicinoids) were also found in "natural capsaicin" (STICHER et al. 1978). The threshold concentrations of capsaicin on the tongue in producing lukewarm and definite painful burning sensations are 2×10^{-7} and $> 10^{-6}$ g/ml, respectively (SZOLCSÁNYI and JANCSÓ-GÁBOR 1975b; SZOLCSÁNYI 1977a).

2. Piperine and Chavicine

The chemical structure of piperine is: N-5-(3,4-methylenedioxyphenyl)penta-2,4-*trans,trans*-dienoyl piperidine, in shorter form piperinoylpiperidide (Fig. 1). The substance is one of the two isomers which are responsible for the pungency of black pepper (*Piper nigrum*). The 2,4-*cis,cis* isomer of the above structure is present in

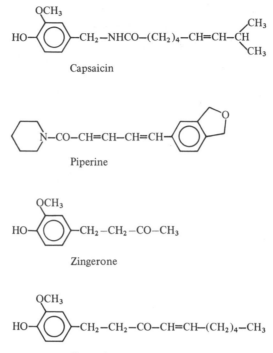

Fig. 1. Chemical structure of natural pungent agents

the molecule of the piperidide of chavicic acid, namely chavicine (Newman 1953 b). Ground black pepper contains 4.6%–9.8% piperine. Its threshold concentration on the human tongue is 3×10^{-6} g/ml (Szolcsányi and Jancsó-Gábor 1975 b).

3. Zingerone and Other Natural Pungent Agents

Zingerone and shogaol, two pungent principles of ginger (*Zingiber officinale*) were isolated from the pungent extract (gingerol) of the rhizoma. The chemical structure of zingerone is: 4(4-hydroxy-3-methoxyphenyl)-butan-2-one and that of shogaol (4-hydroxy,3-methoxyphenyl)-3-oxo-dec(5)en (Fig. 1). Zingerone in threshold concentration of 1×10^{-3} g/ml elicits a simple lukewarm sensation on the tongue without any sign of pricking pain, paraesthesia etc.

According to List and Hackenberger (1973) valleral and isovallerals, the sensory stimulant principles of the mushroom *Lactarius vellereus* possess a capsaicin-like pungency. More information is needed, however, in respect to their sensory effects to decide whether they are non-specific irritants or pungent agents.

II. Synthetic Congeners

An attempt to survey all of the synthetic compounds which, on account of their pungency have been synthesized in order to substitute natural condiments, is beyond the scope of this chapter. Reviews focused on this aspect of chemistry of "pepper-flavoured" substances have already been published (NEWMAN 1953 a, b, c, d, 1954 a, b; GOVINDARAJAN 1977).

Synthetic analogues listed in Table 1 have been tested in animal experiments from the point of view of the object of this review. For references of preparation of compounds in groups I, V–VIII, and X–XIII see NEWMAN (1954 a, b). A systematic approach to reveal the characteristics of the pharmacological receptor site for capsaicin (SZOLCSÁNYI and JANCSÓ-GÁBOR 1975 b, 1976) has been made with the kind help of HEGYES and FÖLDEÁK (1974), who synthesized the derivatives of homovanillic acid listed in groups II–IV. Compounds No. 40 and No. 41, the two phenylethylamide derivatives (group IX) were prepared by ISSEKUTZ et al. (1955) and SIMON (unpublished), respectively. Nonanoyl vanillylamide (No. 3) is commercially available as "synthetic capsaicin."

D. Heat Loss Responses Produced by Pungent Agents

In different mammalian species the immediate response to capsaicin and other capsaicin-like pungent agents is an activation of heat loss mechanism and consequently a fall in body temperature. Thus, in the following section the acute thermoregulatory effects produced by parenterally or enterally given pungent agents are summarized.

I. Effects on the Mouse

The first experiments of JANCSÓ dealing with the effect of capsaicin and other pungent substances on body temperature were performed on mice (JANCSÓ 1955). It turned out that capsaicin and piperine are highly potent agents in producing a fall in body temperature (Table 2). A dose of 50 µg capsaicin given intraperitoneally (IP) caused a temperature fall of 5°–7 °C in a reproducible manner, without any sign of desensitization. Subcutaneous (SC) injection, slow intravenous infusion, or intragastric administration were also effective. The temperature-lowering effect of capsaicin (50–60 µg SC) at ambient temperature of 21 °C or 4.5°–6 °C was about the same.

The hyperthermia produced by high ambient temperature of 37 °C was less pronounced on capsaicin-treated mice than that of the controls. Furthermore, mice survived the lethal hypothermic response produced by large doses of capsaicin or piperine provided they were put in heated box (30°–35 °C).

On the basis of these findings as well as those obtained on guinea-pigs it has been concluded that, under the effect of capsaicin, thermoregulatory mechanisms control body temperature at a subnormal level. Consequently this hypothermic response resembled fever "in the negative direction" (JANCSÓ 1955).

Considering the well-known "hot" property of capsaicin and piperine, it has been assumed that these substances activate the heat loss mechanisms by exciting warm-sensitive and other nerve endings. Therefore, a series of pungent or non-pungent congeners of capsaicin and piperine as well as some other sensory stimulants were tested on mice and guinea-pigs. Indeed, the temperature-lowering effect of the acylamide congeners ran parallel with their pungency (Table 2a). Moreover, struc-

Table 1. Chemical structure of synthetic congeners of pungent agents

	No.[a]	R	Relative pungency[b]
I. Vanillylamides			

OCH$_3$

HO—⟨○⟩—CH$_2$—NHCO—R

	No.[a]	R	Relative pungency[b]
	1	Ethyl	2
	2	Hexyl	396
	3	Octyl	644
	4	1-Octenyl	714
	5	Nonyl	1,000
	6	9-Decenyl	XP

II. Homovanilloylamides
a)

OCH$_3$

HO—⟨○⟩—CH$_2$—CONH—R

	No.	R	Relative pungency
	7	Isobutyl	8
	8	Octyl	1,000
	9	Decyl	1,000
	10	Dodecyl	52
	11	Tetradecyl	25
	12	Hexadecyl	3
	13	Octadecyl	0
	14	Cyclohexyl	123
	15	Cyclododecyl	49

b)

OCH$_3$

HO—⟨○⟩—CH$_2$—CO—R

	No.	R	Relative pungency
	16	Dibutylamine	2
	17	Piperidine	1
	18	Azacyclooctane	9
	19	Azabicyclo(3.2.2)-nonane	6
	20	Dicyclohexylamine	0

III. Homovanilloylesters

OCH$_3$

HO—⟨○⟩—CH$_2$—COO—R

	No.	R	Relative pungency
	21	Methyl	4
	22	Propyl	11
	23	Octyl	172
	24	Nonyl	75
	25	Dodecyl	16
	26	N-Diethyl-3-aminopropyl	1

IV. Homovanilloylthioester

OCH$_3$ S

HO—⟨○⟩—CH$_2$—C—O—R

	No.	R	Relative pungency
	27	Octyl	1

Table 1 (continued)

	No.[a]	R	Relative pungency[b]
V. Homovanillylamides			
OCH$_3$			
HO—〈 〉—CH$_2$—CH$_2$—NHCO—R	28	Hexyl	6
	29	1-Octenyl	7
	30	Nonyl	17
VI. Guaiacylamides			
OCH$_3$			
HO—〈 〉—NHCO—R	31	Isopropyl	+
	32	Nonyl	+ + +
	33	9-Decenyl	+ + +
VII. Homoveratrylamides			
OCH$_3$			
CH$_3$O—〈 〉—CH$_2$—NHCO—R	34	Hexyl	0
	35	1-Octenyl	0
	36	Nonyl	0
VIII. Benzylamides			
〈 〉—CH$_2$—NHCO—R	37	Ethyl	0
	38	Hexyl	0
	39	1-Octenyl	0
IX. Phenylethylamides			
R			
R—〈 〉—CH$_2$—CH$_2$—NHCO—(CH$_2$)$_7$—CH$_3$	40	H	0
	41	OH	36
X. 4-Oxyphenylamides			
R$_1$—O—〈 〉—NHCO—R$_2$	42	R$_1$ = H R$_2$ = Nonyl	+ +
	43	R$_1$ = Heptanoyl R$_2$ = Hexyl	+
	44	R$_1$ = Nonanoyl R$_2$ = Octyl	+ +
	45	R$_1$ = 2-Nonenoyl R$_2$ = 1-Nonenyl	+
XI. Alkylamides			
CH$_2$=CH—(CH$_2$)$_8$—CONH—R	46	2-OH-ethyl	1
	47	3-OH-propyl	2

Table 1 (continued)

	No.[a] R		Relative pungency[b]

XII. Piperinoylamides

O–◯–CH=CH—CH=CH—CO—R

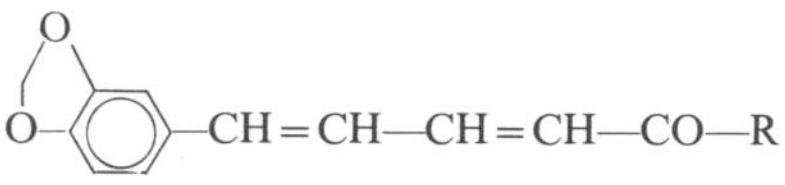	48	3-OH-propylamine	+ +
	49	Pyrrolidine	+ +
	50	Tetrahydroquinoline	0
	51	4-Aminoquinoline	0

XIII. Different structures

CH_2=CH—$(CH_2)_8$—CON⬠

| 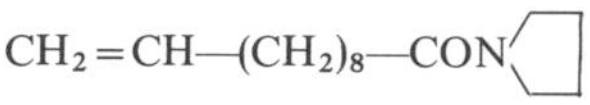 | 52 | 10-Undecenoylpyrrolidide | + + |

CH_2=CH—$(CH_2)_8$—CON⬡

| 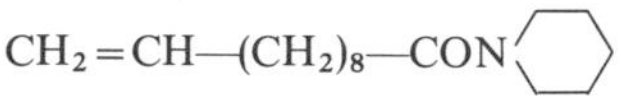 | 53 | 10-Undecenoylpiperidide | + |

OCH₃ structure: HO–◯–NHCO—$(CH_2)_8$—CH_3 with OCH_3 and CH_3O

| 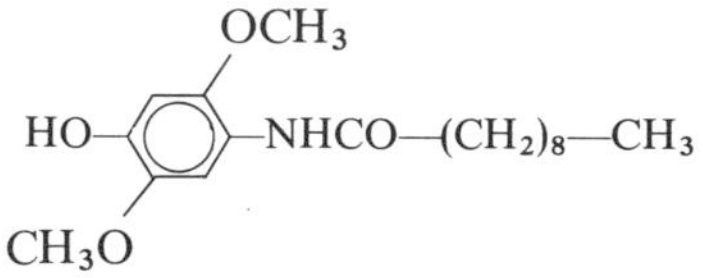 | 54 | Decanoyl-4-oxy-2,5-dimethoxyphenylamide | 0 |

CH_3O–◯–CH—CH—NHCO—$(CH_2)_8$—CH=CH_2 with OCH_3 OCH_3 CH_3

| 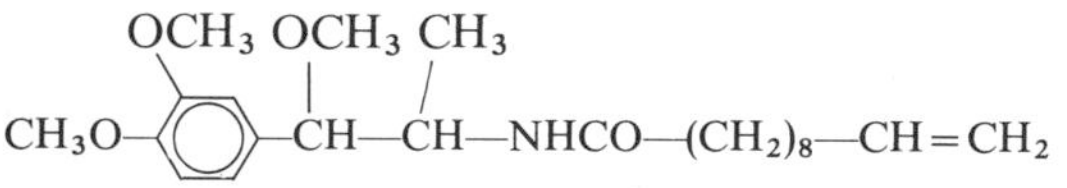 | 55 | 10-Undecenoyl-10-oxy-2-amino-isoeugenol-methylether | 0 |

CH_2=CH—$(CH_2)_8$—CO—N⬡N—CO—$(CH_2)_8$—CH=CH_2

| 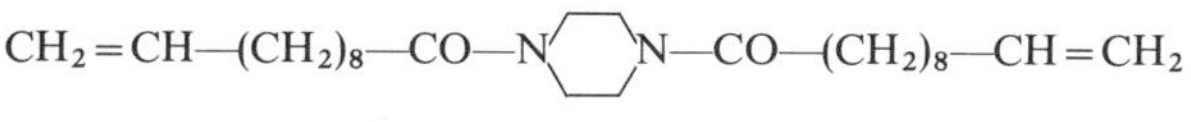 | 56 | 1,4-Di-10-Undecenoyl-piperazine | 0 |

[a] Reference numbers of the compounds in the text
[b] Numbers refer to the relative pain-producing effect on the eye of rat (Szolcsányi and Jancsó-Gábor 1975 b). XP = extremely pungent. Crosses denote estimated pungency on the human tongue according to Széki (1936):
+ + + = 6×10^{-5} g/ml produces burning sensation;
+ + = 6×10^{-5} g/ml ineffective but 3×10^{-3} g/ml produces burning sensation;
+ = barely detectable effect is produced by 3×10^{-3} g/ml

turally unrelated compounds possessing some pungent activity (e.g. zingerone, allyl alcohol, guajacol, isoeugenol, isochavibetol) produced also a deep fall in body temperature.

The effect of capsaicin on heat production and heat loss was analysed by Isse-kutz et al. (1950 a, b). By using a calorimeter and measuring the rectal temperature they calculated the metabolic rate and the overall activity of heat loss mechanism ("circulation index"). Capsaicin (1.4 mg/kg SC) produced a lasting vasodilatation

Table 2. The effect of pungent and non-pungent acylamides on the body temperature of the mouse and guinea-pig. (JANCSÓ 1955)

Compound	No.	Pungency[a]	Dose (mg/kg)[b]	T (°C)
a) Mouse				
Capsaicin		+ + + +	2.5 s.c.	5.0–7.0
			5 s.c.	10.0
Piperidine (piperinoyl piperidide)		+ + + +	25 p.o.	8.0
			15 s.c.	10.0
Decanoyl guaiacylamide	32	+ + +	700 p.o.	10.0
10-Undecenoyl guaiacylamide	33	+ + +	300 p.o.	4.0
			1,000 p.o.	14.6
10-Undecenoyl-3-propanolamide	47	+ + +	500 p.o.	9.0
10-Undecenoyl-2-ethanolamide	46	+ + +	500 p.o.	2.8
Piperinoyl-3-propanolamide	48	+ +	700 p.o.	11.5
Piperinoyl-pyrrolidide	49	+ +	600 p.o.	11.6
Nonanoyl-4(nonanoyloxy)phenylamide	44	+ +	1,000 p.o.	4.2
Heptanoyl-4(heptanoyloxy)phenylamide	43	+	600 p.o.	3.8
2-Nonenoyl-4(2-nonenoyloxy)phenylamide	45	+	800 p.o.	0.9
Piperinoyl-4-aminoquinoline	51	0	600 p.o.	0.9
Piperinoyl-tetrahydroquinoline	50	0	600 p.o.	1.0
10-Undecenoyl-1-oxy-2-amino-isoeugenol-methylether	55	0	650 p.o.	1.0
b) Guinea-pig				
Capsaicin		+ + + +	0.45 s.c.	4.4
Piperinoyl-3-propanolamide	48	+ +	30 p.o.	4.3
Decanoyl-4-oxyphenylamide	42	+ +	70 p.o.	4.2
10-Undecenoyl-pyrrolidide	52	+ +	80 p.o.	4.8
Isobutyryl-guaiacylamide	31	+	130 p.o.	1.3
10-Undecenoyl-piperidide	53	+	60 p.o.	0.4
Decanoyl-4-oxy-2,5-dimethoxyphenylamide	54	0	75 p.o.	Ø
1,4-Di-10-undecenoyl-piperazine	56	0	75 p.o.	0.6

[a] Crosses denote estimated pungency on the human tongue according to SZÉKI (1936):
  + + + = 6×10^{-5} g/ml produces burning sensation;
  + + = 6×10^{-5} g/ml ineffective but 3×10^{-3} g/ml produces burning sensation;
  + = barely detectable effect is produced by 3×10^{-3} g/ml
[b] s.c. = subcutaneous administration; p.o. = peroral administration into the stomach

and heat production fell by 50%–60% at an ambient temperature of 21 °C. In a warm environment of 33 °C vasodilatation was already present and a very slight, uncertain (10%), decrease in metabolic rate was found even if seven times higher dose was used. In a cool environment the effect of capsaicin was sometimes prevented by urethane (1 g/kg) but it remained unchanged if the animal was pre-treated with the antihistaminic agent pyribenzamine. The conclusion drawn from these experiments was that capsaicin does not decrease the metabolic rate in a primary way and its effect is based on excitation of "terminal heat receptors." The response is not mediated through liberation of histamine.

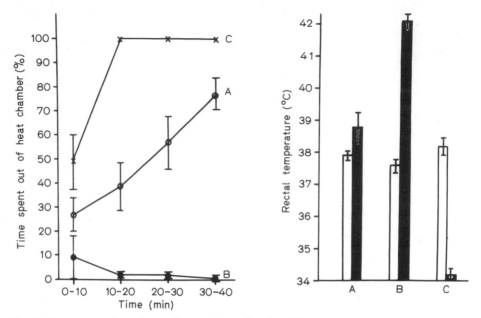

Fig. 2. Escape reaction of rats from a heat chamber (39°–41 °C) measured over 10 min periods, and their rectal temperatures before (white columns) and after (black columns) exposure. *A*, normal controls ($n=11$); *B*, rats desensitized by capsaicin ($50+100$ mg/kg SC) 20 days before the experiment ($n=11$); *C*; rats treated with capsaicin (1 mg/kg SC) 10 min before the experiment ($n=5$). (Szolcsányi and Jancsó-Gábor 1975)

II. Effects on the Rat

A temperature-lowering effect of capsaicin in the rat has been reported from different laboratories (Jancsó 1955; Jancsó-Gábor et al. 1970a, b; Szolcsányi and Jancsó-Gábor 1973, 1975a; Meeter 1973; Nakayama 1976, 1979, personal communication; Hori 1980). A subcutaneous dose of 100–200 µg/kg caused a fall of about 1 °C at an ambient temperature of 24 °C (Szolcsányi and Jancsó-Gábor 1973). The response accompanied by vasodilatation was dose dependent up to 10 mg/kg and after 50–80 mg/kg the hypothermic response lasting for several hours was followed by hyperthermia (Jancsó-Gábor et al. 1970a; Szolcsányi and Jancsó-Gábor 1973; Meeter 1974, personal communication; Nakayama 1979, personal communication). In newborn rats 5–10 µg capsaicin SC produced a sudden fall of 1°–2 °C in rectal temperature (Hori and Tsuzuki 1978a). In cool environments a rapid decrease in oxygen consumption was also observed (Szolcsányi 1967; Meeter 1974, personal communication). Even after a high dose of capsaicin (16 mg/kg), however, oxygen consumption did not fall below the basal metabolic rate (Szolcsányi and Jancsó-Gábor 1973), indicating that the increase in heat production produced by a cool ambient temperature was abolished in this way. Disruption of other heat conserving, mechanisms like piloerection and shivering were also striking.

The thermoregulatory behaviour of rats provided further evidence for the suggestion that the hypothermic response induced by capsaicin is the result of a coor-

Table 3. Pungency and impairment of thermoregulation of the rat caused by capsaicin and some chemically related compounds

Compound	No.	Pungency	Dose (mg/kg)[a]	Impairment of thermo-regulation	References
Capsaicin		Extreme	15–75 s.c.	Marked, irreversible	[1, 2, 3]
2-Nonenoyl vanillylamide	4	Extreme	15–75 s.c.	Marked, irreversible	[1, 3]
Heptanoyl vanillylamide	2	Strong	75 i.p.	Pronounced	[3]
Propionyl vanillylamide	1	Slight	250–500 i.p.	Slight	[2, 3]
Decanoyl guaiacylamide	32	Strong	125 i.p.	Pronounced	[1, 3]
Decanoyl-4-oxyphenylamide	42	Slight	125 i.p.	Moderate	[1, 2, 3]
Nonenoyl benzylamide	39	None	500 i.p.	None	[2, 3]
Homovanilloyl octylamide	8	Extreme	15–75 s.c.	Marked, irreversible	[4]
Homovanilloyl isobutylamide	7	Moderate	100–200 i.p.	Uncertain	[4]
Homovanilloyl nonylester	24	Strong	200 i.p.	None	[4]
Homovanilloyl octylester	23	Strong	200 i.p.	None	[4]
Homovanilloyl propylester	22	Moderate	200 i.p.	None	[4]
Piperine		Strong	75 i.p.	Pronounced, irreversible	[1, 2, 3]

[1] JANCSÓ (1965); [2] JANCSÓ-GÁBOR et al. (1970a); [3] SZOLCSÁNYI and JANCSÓ-GÁBOR (1973); [4] SZOLCSÁNYI and JANCSÓ-GÁBOR, unpublished observation
[a] s.c. = subcutaneous administration; i.p. = intraperitoneal administration

dinated heat loss response. The escape reaction from a warm environment was markedly increased during the fall in body temperature (Fig. 2). Capsaicin induced escape-like locomotion and prone body extension even at cold ambient temperatures (SZOLCSÁNYI and JANCSÓ-GÁBOR 1975a; SZOLCSÁNYI 1975). Subcutaneous injection of capsaicin gave rise to a decreased heat reinforcement response and an increased heat escape behaviour in an operant bar-pressing apparatus (HORI and HARADA 1977; HORI 1980).

Besides capsaicin other naturally occuring pungent agents, e.g. piperine (JANCSÓ 1955), zingerone; their pungent congeners listed in Table 3 as well as allyl alcohol greatly decrease body temperature. Their effects are prevented by capsaicin desensitization suggesting a common site of action with capsaicin (JANCSÓ-GÁBOR et al. 1970a; SZOLCSÁNYI and JANCSÓ-GÁBOR 1973).

III. Effects on the Guinea-pig

As in other species the hypothermic response to capsaicin (0.2-0.45 mg/kg SC) was accompanied by signs of a coordinated heat loss response. Vasodilatation, indicated by reddening of skin of the nose, ears, and paws, prone body extension, faster and deeper respiration, were observed until the body temperature reached its lowest level. Thereafter signs of vasoconstriction and shivering were observed, leading to a rapid recovery (JANCSÓ-GÁBOR 1947; JANCSÓ 1955; JANCSÓ-GÁBOR et al 1970a). Compounds related to capsaicin or piperine produced similar effects.

Again, their potency was dependent on their pungency and non-pungent congeners were ineffective (Table 2b).

The temperature-lowering effect of capsaicin cannot be attributed to release of histamine, since pyribenzamine pre-treatment did not alter the response to capsaicin (Issekutz et al. 1950b). According to these authors, transection of the spinal cord at the tenth or third thoracic level 4–5 days before the experiment, did not prevent the fall in body temperature produced by capsaicin, if the substance was injected into the lower part of the body. Therefore the fall in body temperature produced by capsaicin was thought to be due to spinal reflexes. This assumption, however, cannot be accepted, since the high dose used in these experiments (3 mg/kg) could gain access to the upper part of the body through the circulation and could elicit heat loss responses above the lesion.

IV. Effects on Other Animal Species

In dogs Högyes (1878) observed a fall in rectal temperature when capsicol – the pungent extract of paprika – was introduced into the stomach.

Oral administration of extracts from capsicum, pepper, and ginger were reported by Stary (1925) to lower the body temperature of the rabbit. The last extract was, however, slightly effective. A fall in body temperature was produced also after parenteral injections (Jancsó 1955). The sensitivity of this species to capsaicin was, however, relatively low. According to Nakayama (1979 personal communication) skin vasodilatation and increase in respiration accompanied the fall in body temperature. Local cooling of the hypothalamus antagonized these effects.

Capsaicin given to the cat (3–10 mg/kg SC or IP) produced vasodilatation, panting, and sweating of the paws while body temperature dropped (Szolcsányi 1975). Vasodilatation, panting and/or inhibition of shivering accompanied the fall in body temperature in goats as well. The response was dose dependent and reproducible if 0.1 or 0.2 mg/kg were used. Panting did not always occur in the cold but was reproducible in thermoneutral environments (Frens 1976, 1977, 1978).

In experiments designed to desensitize hibernators Mrosovsky (1974) observed that the golden-mantled ground squirrel (Citellus lateralis) responded to capsaicin (10 mg/180–270 g) with a temperature fall of about 3 °C. Thus, these hibernators were not as sensitive to capsaicin as the rat.

V. Effects on Human Subjects

The characteristics and mechanism of warm or hot sensation and vasodilatation elicited by these substances at the site of topical application are reviewed in Sect. H.

It is worth mentioning here that profuse sweating with flushing of the face is a common experience after intake of spicy "hot" foods. Under experimental conditions Heubner (1925) reproduced this phenomenon by applying undecylenoyl and nonenoyl vanillylamides (No. 4 and 6) on the tongue. Detailed analysis of this so-called gustatory sweating was performed by Lee (1954), who used chilli and pepper for this purpose. There was a close correspondence between regions affected by thermal and gustatory sweating, the latter being shown to be cholinergic in nature. Warming the body facilitated, while cooling the body inhibited or abolished the gustatory sweat secretion. Mustard elicited no sweating. These findings seem to support the role of warm-receptors in the reaction.

E. Long-Term Thermoregulatory Changes Induced by Pungent Agents

I. Desensitization to Pungent Agents by Capsaicin

The word desensitization has different meanings depending on the agent or stimulus to which the reduced or abolished sensitivity is intended. In context with "desensitized animals" *the term desensitization is confined in this review to denote a condition of reduced sensitivity or complete loss of sensitivity to the effect of pungent agents.* It is never used here in the sense of desensitization of a pharmacological receptor site like the "capsaicin receptor" proposed by KEELE (1962) in order to explain the mechanism of common chemical sense. This distinction must be understood since the findings of the last years have revealed that the chemical insensitivity is only one sign of the sensory neurone blocking action of capsaicin which is characterized by an impaired physiological function of the affected neurones, as will be discussed in Sect. H.

1. Desensitization of the Rat

A single subcutaneous injection of capsaicin (50–75 mg/kg) rendered the rats insensitive for months to the hypothermic effect of subsequent SC injection of 5–10 mg/kg capsaicin. A similar effect has been achieved by successive injections of increasing doses up to 50–70 mg/kg within 1–3 days (JANCSÓ-GÁBOR et al. 1970a; SZOLCSÁNYI and JANCSÓ-GÁBOR 1973). In newborn rats 1–4 days after birth repeated injections of increasing doses of 5–10 µg caused desensitization to the hypothermic effect of 1 mg capsaicin (HORI and TSUZUKI 1978a). Increments in the dose have the advantage of preventing or diminishing the incidence of lethal response, which may occur after the first doses. Furthermore, ether anaesthesia or diazepam pre-treatment (MEETER 1973) is also useful for this purpose. The reason of the lethal response has not been analysed in detail, but reflex respiratory failure, bradycardia, hypotension, and other reflexes evoked by capsaicin might be responsible for it. Since interoceptors responsible for the respiratory and circulatory effects of capsaicin can also be desensitized (SZOLCSÁNYI and JÁNOSSY 1971; SZOLCSÁNYI 1975) further subcutaneous injections in increasing doses are well tolerated.

The decrease in oxygen consumption in cool environments (SZOLCSÁNYI and JANCSÓ-GÁBOR 1973) and vasodilatation (MEETER, personal communication 1974; NAKAYAMA 1976 and personal communication 1979) elicited by subcutaneous capsaicin were also absent in rats pre-treated with high doses of capsaicin. The deep fall (4°–8 °C) in body temperature produced by piperine, zingerone, homovanilloyl dodecylamide (No. 10) or decanoyl vanillylamide (No. 5) were also abolished in this way (SZOLCSÁNYI and JANCSÓ-GÁBOR 1973). The general anaesthetic effect of SC zingerone was also absent in desensitized rats (JANCSÓ-GÁBOR 1978).

2. Desensitization of Other Animal Species

A schedule for desensitization of mice was described by Jancsó (1955). Daily subcutaneous capsaicin starting from 4 µg and increasing by 2–4 µg up to a final dose
of 70–100 µg (about 5 mg/kg) produced an insensitivity to the effect of 50 µg capsaicin given intraperitoneally. The hypothermic response to decenoyl vanillylamide
(No. 33), histamine, isoeugenol, or isochavibetol was also diminished or abolished.
The insensitivity lasted, however, only for 1–3 days. Schedules starting with higher
doses (Alarie and Keller 1973) and reaching a final dose of 50–70 mg/kg might
give rise an irreversible effect in this species as well.

In guinea-pigs injection of capsaicin produces a severe, sometimes lethal
bronchospasm (Jancsó 1955; Molnár et al. 1969 b). Irreversible desensitization
against capsaicin (1–2 mg/kg SC) can be achieved by a total dose of 30–40 mg capsaicin given subcutaneously in a schedule of increasing doses up to 7–10 mg within
7–24 h (Jancsó-Gábor et al. 1970 a). Long-term treatment with daily subcutaneous injections of 0.2 mg for 6 months was ineffective (Jancsó-Gábor 1947;
Jancsó-Gábor et al. 1970 a). This finding clearly shows that the prerequisite of the
irreversible desensitizing effect is the high blood concentration and not the slow accumulation of capsaicin in the body.

Unsuccessful attempts were made to desensitize ground squirrels (Mrosovsky
1974) and cats (Szolcsányi 1975) by parenteral capsaicin. Efficient protection
against the acute effects of capsaicin would be necessary to achieve success in these
species.

II. Impairment in Thermoregulation After Capsaicin Desensitization

1. Thermoregulation in Cool, Cold, and Thermoneutral Environments

Following the desensitizing pre-treatment, described in the foregoing section,
pyrexia ensued in all three species (mice, rats, and guinea-pigs) at room temperature. Rectal temperature rose above 40 °C in mice (Jancsó 1955) and guinea-pigs
(Jancsó-Gábor et al. 1970 a). In the latter case the pyrexia sometimes lasted for
6-10 days. In rats during the first two days after the pre-treatment rectal temperature in a cool environment and oxygen consumption at a thermoneutral temperature (30 °C) exceeded the control values by 1.6 °C and 10 ml/dm^{-2}/h^{-1}, respectively (Szolcsányi and Jancsó-Gábor 1973).

In contrast to this first period, the core temperature of rats in cool (Jancsó-Gábor et al. 1970 a, b; Meeter 1973; Szolcsányi and Jancsó-Gábor 1973, 1975 a;
Nakayama 1976; Arai 1976; Cabanac et al. 1976, 1977; Hori and Tsuzuki
1978 b) and metabolic rate in cool and thermoneutral environments (Szolcsányi
and Jancsó-Gábor 1973; Székely and Szolcsányi 1979) did not differ from that
of the controls, provided they were left undisturbed. At cool ambient temperatures
selection of a higher ambient temperature (Szolcsányi 1978) and heat reinforcement behaviour (Cabanac et al. 1976, 1977; Hori and Harada 1977; Hori and
Tsuzuki 1978 b) also remained unimpaired. Rectal temperature of the guinea-pigs
also returned to the control level (Jancsó-Gábor et al. 1970 a).

In desensitized rats and guinea-pigs painful stimuli or repeated handling
elicited an enhanced emotional hyperthermia up to 41°–42 °C accompanied by vi-

olent oscillations in skin temperature. In rats adrenalectomy combined with guanethidine or reserpine pre-treatment prevented this enhanced emotional hyperthermic response (JANCSÓ 1965; JANCSÓ-GÁBOR et al. 1970a; SZOLCSÁNYI and JANCSÓ-
GÁBOR 1973).

The circadian rhythm of body temperature is another interesting point. The
periodicity of the daily rhythm of blinded rats persisted after desensitization and
the daytime minimum level corresponded to the control value. The maximum temperature at night, however, was higher by 0.9 °C (NAKAYAMA et al. 1979). At night
the metabolism of rats is 25% higher than in the daytime independent of activity
(HEUSNER 1956). Consequently, a hypothesis was put forward that the 24 h rhythm
in set-point is responsible for this effect (ASCHOFF 1970). The lack of proportional
shift after desensitization seems to contradict this simple explanation.

Rats exposed to 10 gC for 2 h, to 1 °C for 1.5 h (JANCSÓ-GÁBOR et al. 1970a)
or to 2 °C for 1 h (MEETER 1973) showed piloerection and shivering, and rectal temperature did not differ significantly from that of the controls. Recently both
NAKAYAMA and ARAI have confirmed the conclusion that desensitized rats maintain their body temperature in the cold (NAKAYAMA 1979, personal communication; ARAI 1976).

2. Thermoregulation at High Ambient Temperatures

Capsaicin-desensitized rats and guinea-pigs were no longer able to protect themselves against overheating but responded with pronounced hyperthermia to high
ambient temperatures of 32°–40 °C even many months or over a year after the pre-
treatment (JANCSÓ 1965; JANCSÓ-GÁBOR et al. 1970a; SZOLCSÁNYI and JANCSÓ-GÁ-
BOR 1973, 1975a; SZOLCSÁNYI 1975, 1978; MEETER 1973; NAKAYAMA 1976; ARAI
1976; CABANAC et al. 1976, 1977; HORI and HARADA 1977; BENEDEK and OBÁL
1979, personal communication). Normal rats responded to heat exposure by
vasodilatation, salivation and with behavioural heat dissipating responses, which
include grooming, escape-like locomotion and prone body extension. These
reactions were absent in fully desensitized rats (JANCSÓ-GÁBOR et al. 1970a; SZOL-
CSÁNYI and JANCSÓ-GÁBOR 1973, 1975a; SZOLCSÁNYI 1975, 1978; MEETER 1973,
1974, personal communication; NAKAYAMA 1976; HORI and HARADA 1977; HORI
1980). The loss of function was dose dependent in the range of 20–70 mg/kg capsaicin given in a single subcutaneous injection (JANCSÓ 1965; JANCSÓ-GÁBOR et al.
1970a). Thus, the inability to regulate against heat ran parallel with the degree of
desensitization to the hypothermic effect of capsaicin.

Increased heat production in desensitized rats can be excluded as the cause of
their enhanced hyperthermic response, since their basal metabolic rate and the rise
in oxygen consumption at 35 °C did not differ from those of the controls (SZOL-
CSÁNYI and JANCSÓ-GÁBOR 1973).

In respect of the heat dissipating mechanisms the behavioural thermoregulatory responses and the role of salivary glands were analysed in detail. Rats were
put in a heated chamber (39°–41 °C) from where they were able to escape into a
cooler (25°–26 °C) compartment (SZOLCSÁNYI and JANCSÓ-GÁBOR 1975a). Figure 2 shows that control rats (A) spent progressively more time in the cooler compartment and consequently their rectal temperature rose only slightly. In contrast,
desensitized rats (B) after initial orientation remained in the inner compartment at

the higher temperature. They exhibited no sign of restlessness, prone body extension, or saliva spreading, although their rectal temperature rose to over 42 °C. It is also shown in Fig. 2 that, under the acute stimulatory effect of capsaicin, rapid, and complete escape reaction occurred (C). Pre-treatment with a single dose of 5 mg/kg capsaicin 7 days before the experiment inhibited this escape reaction whereas pre-treatment with its non-desensitizing pungent congener, homovanilloyl octylester (No. 23), did not cause any change in the response (Szolcsányi 1975, 1978).

Since the signals for thermoregulatory behaviour are thermal discomfort and thermal comfort (Cabanac 1972) these findings clearly show, that in desensitized rats there is a lack of sensitivity to discomfort when the body temperature is high. Studying the thermopreference of 52 desensitized rats fully confirmed this conclusion (Szolcsányi 1978). All control rats chose the lower ambient temperature if they had the opportunity to select between 30° and 35 °C or 35° and 40 °C. Similar thermopreference was not found if desensitized (50 + 100 mg/kg) rats were exposed to these ambient temperatures. On the other hand, after desensitization the selection between 5 °C differences in cool environments (in the range 10°–25 °C) corresponded to the control responses, i.e. both groups of animals avoided the cooler temperature of 10° or 15 °C.

Heat escape behaviour under operant bar-pressing conditions was severely impaired after desensitization, while behavioural response to cold remained unchanged (Hori 1980). The same holds good for rats pre-treated at an age of 8–10 days, and tested 80 days later (Hori and Tsuzuki 1978 b).

Conflicting results were obtained by Cabanac et al. (1976, 1977) in respect of the thermoregulatory operant behaviour of seven rats pre-treated with capsaicin. In these experiments, however, the degree of desensitization was not checked by capsaicin injection, instead the animals were put in a hot box, where some of them died. Consequently those rats were omitted from the experiments in which the desensitization was more complete (the largest dose of capsaicin was in the range 17–45 mg/kg). Furthermore, for some reason the bar-pressing response of the pre-treated rats was higher at 25° and 30 °C than that of the controls. Consequently, raising the ambient temperature from thermoneutral (30 °C) to 35 °C gave rise in control rats to a more than 9-fold increase in duration of bar-pressing, meanwhile pre-treated rats responded only by a 1.6-fold increase, the statistical significance of which was not indicated. Therefore, these results are far from suggesting convincingly an intact cooling reinforcement behaviour in desensitized rats.

Neither is their suggestion that the impaired heat tolerance in desensitized animals is due to a defect in the effector, saliva secreting, ability is acceptable. Salivation to pilocarpine was readily elicited in desensitized rats (Jancsó-Gábor et al. 1970 a) and grooming after handling did not differ from that of the controls. The enhanced hyperthermia of desensitized rats at warm ambient temperatures (32°–40 °C) was characteristic if rectal temperatures of desalivated rats were compared (Obál et al. 1979).

In desensitized rats the weight of salivary glands was not decreased but that of the controls was heavier if they were kept at warm temperatures. Consequently, the lack of salivation is merely one sign of the lack of counter-regulation against overheating.

III. Structure–Activity Relationship

The structure–activity relationship of 50 congeners of capsaicin and piperine was analysed in two series of tests in order to reveal some characteristics of the molecular interactions responsible for the irreversible desensitizing effect of capsaicin. From the thermoregulatory point of view the tolerance against heat was tested on the pre-treated animals. Table 3 shows a brief account of these results and their sources. The impairment of thermoregulation was most pronounced after pre-treatment with the most pungent acylamides having a long carbon chain. Esteric analogues, however, were ineffective in spite of the fact that their pungency was strong. In respect of the pain producing and desensitizing effect, most of the experiments were performed by local application of the compounds in order to avoid metabolic modification of the molecules in the organism. The hypothetical molecular interactions of capsaicin at the site of action (SZOLCSÁNYI and JANCSÓ-GÁBOR 1975b, 1976) will be discussed in Sect. H, since the results of the two series of experiments fit in well with each other.

F. Interaction with Fever, Drugs, and Neurotransmitters

On the basis of evidence described in Sects. D, E, G, and H of this chapter, capsaicin has been used as a pharmacological tool to reveal the role of warm-sensors in thermoregulatory changes induced by pyrogens and drugs. In conjunction with the above, further information has been gained about the effects of capsaicin as well.

I. Interaction with the Effects of Pyrogens and Antipyretics

Fever produced by purified *Escherichia coli* lipopolysaccharide or yeast suspension given subcutaneously was markedly enhanced in rats desensitized by capsaicin. The upper febrile level was dependent on the degree of desensitization. Sodium salicylate, phenylbutazone, acetanilide, and aminopyrine antipyretics abolished the febrile responses in desensitized animals (JANCSÓ 1965; SZOLCSÁNYI and JANCSÓ-GÁBOR 1973). Intrapreoptic micro-injection of the lipopolysaccharide was also effective (NAKAYAMA 1976).

In control and capsaicin-desensitized (30 + 60 mg/kg SC) rats the temporal sequence of the biphasic febrile response induced by intravenous *E. coli* (IV) pyrogen (10 µg/kg) were surprisingly the same, in spite of the fact that in the latter group the rise in core temperature was higher by 1.5 °C than that of the controls. Increase in oxygen consumption and brown fat thermogenesis as well as vasoconstriction took part in the rising phase. Both vasodilatation and a decrease in metabolic rate were responsible for the falling phase. As in the controls there was a characteristic negative correlation between the initial body temperature and febrile response. In capsaicin-desensitized rats, however, it was shifted to a higher level. It has been suggested that in both groups the neurohumoral sequence of events elicited by the pyrogen follows each other in the same order (SZÉKELY and SZOLCSÁNYI 1979). The enhancement of febrile response in desensitized animals has been explained by inactivation of hypothalamic warm-sensors which results in a lack of signal for counter-regulation against the rise in core temperature produced by pyrogens (JANCSÓ 1965; SZOLCSÁNYI and JANCSÓ-GÁBOR 1973; SZÉKELY and SZOLCSÁNYI 1979).

Another approach was made by FRENS (1976, 1977, 1978). In the goat, capsaicin (0.1 mg/kg) was injected at the time when temperature was expected to start rising. The effect of *E. coli* pyrogen overcame the hypothermic effect of capsaicin but not that produced by 5-hydroxytryptamine (5-HT) injected into the cerebral ventricle. In half of the experiments the hypothermic effect of capsaicin was completely absent. The rise in temperature over the pre-injection level was, however, slightly lower when the effects of capsaicin and pyrogen were combined $(0.7° \pm 0.3 °C)$ than in experiments with pyrogen alone $(1° \pm 0.3 °C)$.

It is worth mentioning that capsaicin injected subcutaneously at the plateau of the pyrexic response produced by preoptic injection of *E. coli* pyrogen (NAKAYAMA 1979, personal communication) or subcutaneous yeast suspension (unpublished observation) resulted in a similar fall in body temperature as in the control rats.

Findings with capsaicin favour the concept that the site of action of pyrogens and antipyretics is not the hypothalamic warm-sensors. Electrophysiological findings seem to contradict this assumption, since the responsiveness of high Q_{10} warm-sensitive units of the preoptic/anterior hypothalamic area (PO/AH) to hyothalamic heating was decreased by pyrogens (WIT and WANG 1968 b; CABANAC et al. 1968; EISENMAN 1969, 1974; SCHOENER and WANG 1975). EISENMAN (1969) pointed out, however, the neural drive to elevate core temperature should not originate from these neurones, since their firing rate was unaffected at normal core temperature following pyrogen administration. There are synapses on capsaicin-sensitive preoptic neurones (SZOLCSÁNYI et al. 1971) and the warm-sensitive neurones of the preoptic area receive excitatory inputs from other warm-sensors of the body (WIT and WANG 1968 a; HELLON 1970; GUIEU and HARDY 1970). The special characteristics of these neurones are that peripheral warming not only increases their firing rate but at the same time the responsiveness of these neurones to hypothalamic warming is diminished (BOULANT and BIGNALL 1973; BOULANT and HARDY 1974; BOULANT and GONZALEZ 1977). If it is considered that during development of fever warm-sensors throughout the body are activated, the decreased slope in thermosensitivity of the preoptic warm-sensors might be a sign of the enhanced input. In any case, the marked difference in the height of fever between control and desensitized animals provides evidence for the *important role of warm-sensors in counteracting the elevation of body temperature produced by pyrogens*.

II. Interactions with Neurotransmitters and Drugs

There is evidence in favour of the transmitter role of 5-HT in the heat loss pathway in the anterior hypothalamus of the rat (FELDBERG and LOTTI 1967; MYERS and YAKSH 1968; BLIGH 1972; MURAKAMI 1973). Depletion of 5-HT pools by p-chlorophenylalanine (pCPA) produces an impairment in thermoregulation (REID et al. 1968; GIARMAN et al. 1968; COOPER 1972) apparently similar to that found in animals desensitized by capsaicin.

Depletion of 5-HT by pre-treatment with pCPA inhibited, while pre-treatment with the 5-HT precursor, 5-hydroxytryptophan enhanced the hypothermic effect of capsaicin (1 mg/kg SC). In contrast to the behaviour of capsaicin-desensitized rats, the escape reaction of pCPA-treated animals from a heat chamber was more pronounced than that of the controls (SZOLCSÁNYI and JANCSÓ-GÁBOR 1975a). These findings provide evidence for the presence of serotonergic neurones in the physiological heat loss pathway of the rat, but not in the neural pathway of warm-sensation and escape reaction. It has been suggested that warm-sensors are not serotonergic neurones (SZOLCSÁNYI and JANCSÓ-GÁBOR 1975a). In agreement with this assumption the sequence of sites of action the "heat sensor pathway" has been proposed by FRENS (1977) as follows: capsaicin→pyrogen→5-HT→integration.

In similar experiments an interposed cholinergic synapse in the heat loss pathway from the warm-sensors has not been verified (MEETER 1973). Atropine (50 mg/kg IP) had no effect on subcutaneous capsaicin. In the case of intraventricular injections similar results were obtained. Atropine (50 µg) had no effect on capsaicin (2 µg) although it abolished the hypothermic response to carbachol (25 µg). Under cold exposure, but not at room temperature, intracerebroventricular atropine (50 µg) elicited a fall in body temperature, which was significantly greater in capsaicin-desensitized rats. It has been assumed that atropine blocked the input from peripheral cold-sensors. Peripheral warm-sensors exert a moderating influence which is lacking in capsaicin-desensitized rats.

Micro-injections of prostaglandin E_2 (PGE_2) into the preoptic area (10–20 ng) or into the lateral ventricle (SZOLCSÁNYI and JANCSÓ-GÁBOR 1975a) or preoptic injection of PGE_1 (20–200 ng), (NAKAYAMA 1979, personal communication) provoked a rise in rectal temperature of desensitized rats and in the controls. Thus, thermoregulatory response induced by these putative mediators of fever (MILTON and WENDLANDT 1971; MILTON 1976) seems not to be mediated by the warm-sensors.

The hyperthermia produced by dinitrophenol (25 mg/kg SC) was enhanced and the hypothermic effect of urethane (0.8 g/kg IP) promethazine (5–10 mg/kg SC), histamine (50–100 mg/kg IP), magnesium sulphate (100–400 mg/kg IP) remained unaltered after capsaicin desensitization. Slightly greater falls in rectal temperature were found in response to chlorpromazine (2–10 mg/kg SC) and pentobarbitone (5–20 mg/kg IV). On the other hand, the hypothermia produced by low doses of allyl alcohol (5–10 mg/g IV) was completely abolished (SZOLCSÁNYI and JANCSÓ-GÁBOR 1973; SZOLCSÁNYI 1975). An inhibition of the temperature-lowering effect of subcutaneous 5-IIT (6 mg/kg) was also reported (MAKARA et al. 1965). It is remarkable that up to now capsaicin desensitization has been found to inhibit the fall in core temperature produced by only those compounds with strong sensory stimulant (hot) properties.

G. Action of Capsaicin on Hypothalamic Warm-Sensors

The following lines of evidence suggest that the warm-sensors of the preoptic/anterior hypothalamic area (PO/AH) are stimulated and desensitized by capsaicin.

I. Effect of Intrahypothalamic Injection of Capsaicin

1) In rats, micro-injection of capsaicin (0.5–25 µg) into the PO/AH caused a prompt dose-dependent fall (0.2°–2.0 °C) in body temperature and abolished

shivering. With repeated injections of high doses (25 µg) the hypothermic effect of capsaicin gradually diminished and finally vanished (JANCSÓ-GÁBOR et al. 1970 b; SZOLCSÁNYI and JANCSÓ-GÁBOR 1973). These results have been confirmed by MEETER (1973), NAKAYAMA (1976, 1979, personal communication), and ARAI (1976) who demonstrated that intraventricular and intrahypothalamic capsaicin injection, respectively, elicited skin vasodilatation, as well. Increased heat escape response and decreased heat reinforcement response caused by preoptic injection of capsaicin suggest that the thermoregulatory behaviour is also affected in this way (HORI and HARADA 1977). Micro-injection of 5 µg of capsaicin produced a fall in rectal temperature even in the 1-day-old rat, placed in a thermoneutral environment. A smaller effect was obtained in response to a subsequent injection (HORI and SHINOHARA 1978, 1979; HORI and TSUZUKI 1978 a). In the rabbit intraventricular injection of capsaicin (2 mg) produced vasodilatation of the ear and a fall in hypothalamic and rectal temperatures (NAKAYAMA 1979, personal communication).

Investigating the effect of capsaicin on rats from another point of view, a transient slight fall in blood pressure has been reported following intraventricular injection of capsaicin (10 µg). A desensitizing effect was observed after which the blood pressure remained at the same level as before the injections (CORREA and GRAEFF 1974).

In conscious and slightly anaesthetized (1 g/kg urethane) rats dominantly cortical synchronization was observed (ARAI 1976); in awake immobilized rats cortical desynchronization was observed (BENEDEK et al. 1980) in response to preoptic injection of capsaicin. Both effects were absent after desensitization. Experiments are still in progress to clarify the mechanism of these electroencephalographic (EEG) changes.

2) After strong parenteral desensitization the intrahypothalamic (JANCSÓ-GÁBOR et al. 1970 b; NAKAYAMA 1976) or intraventricular (MEETER 1973) capsaicin produced no change in thermoregulation. Usually higher subcutaneous doses were required (up to repeated injections of 80–100 mg/kg) until complete abolition of the effects of intracerebral injections occurred. This indicates that, although capsaicin can reach both peripheral and central warm-sensors, low doses predominantly attack the peripheral ones (MEETER 1973).

3) Rats desensitized by hypothalamic injections with doses of 35–200 µg, exhibited a behaviour similar to rats pre-treated parenterally with capsaicin. The regulation of these rats against overheating of their bodies was impaired, as indicated by the enhanced hyperthermia in warm environments and the pronounced emotional hyperthermia to painful stimuli in cool environments (JANCSÓ-GÁBOR et al. 1970 b; SZOLCSÁNYI and JANCSÓ-GÁBOR 1973).

Two important differences in thermal responses were observed, however, between the parenterally and intrahypothalamically desensitized groups. In the latter case the fall in body temperature caused by subcutaneous injection of capsaicin was inhibited but not abolished (JANCSÓ-GÁBOR et al. 1970 b). Furthermore, intraventricular pre-treatment (100–250 µg) retarded but failed to block the heat escape reaction (SZOLCSÁNYI 1975, 1978). The incompleteness of the desensitizing effect might be due to a difficulty of access to all central warm-sensors by intracerebral injection. Another explanation would be that desensitization of the hypothalamic warm-sensors does not disrupt all heat loss mechanisms triggered by extrahypothalamic warm-sensors. The finding that after extensive bilateral PO/AH lesions the fall in rectal temperature produced by subcutaneous capsaicin was only inhibited but never abolished, favours the latter assumption (SZOLCSÁNYI and JANCSÓ-GÁBOR 1975a).

4) Impaired regulation against heat exposure (40 °C) was observed in cats pretreated intrahypothalamically with a total dose of 800–1,200 μg capsaicin. No panting, only a moderate increase in respiratory rate was observed during four hours exposure although their rectal temperature rose above 41.5 °C. Solvent-treated and untreated cats started to pant within 30–90 min and their rectal temperature stabilized between 40° and 41 °C (JANCSÓ 1965; SZOLCSÁNYI unpublished).

II. Action on Hypothalamic Thermosensitive Neural Responses

1) The fall in rectal temperature and cease in shivering elicited by local heating of the PO/AH (from 1° to 4 °C above the initial temperature) were markedly inhibited or abolished in rats strongly desensitized by subcutaneous capsaicin (JANCSÓ-GÁBOR et al. 1970b).

2) Recently the effect of capsaicin on hypothalamic units was also tested. In adult rats anaesthetized with urethane 17 warm-sensitive units out of 21 were excited by 1 mg/kg subcutaneous capsaicin (NAKAYAMA et al. 1978a).

In Fig. 3 the increase in firing rate to local heating of the PO/AH and the opposite response to cooling precede the activation produced by capsaicin at constant PO/AH temperature. The activity of all six cold-sensitive neurones – which increased firing rate in response to PO/AH cooling – were inhibited by capsaicin. No effect of capsaicin was observed on six thermally insensitive neurones. Similar results were obtained on newborn rats in response to 5 μg capsaicin given subcutaneously (HORI and SHINOHARA 1978, 1979).

The proportion of thermosensitive neurones in the PO/AH was decreased after systemic capsaicin desensitization. While in control rats out of 136 units 22.1% were warm-sensitive and 6.6% cold-sensitive, in desensitized rats out of 290 units the corresponding figures were 9.7% and 2.7%, respectively. Furthermore, in desensitized rats some warm-sensitive units lost their thermosensitivity with repeated thermal stimulations (HORI 1980) resembling to the responses of incompletely desensitized animals to chemically evoked painful stimuli (JANCSÓ 1968; SZOLCSÁNYI et al. 1975).

Activation of warm-sensitive units in the PO/AH by heating the skin (BOULANT and BIGNALL 1973; BOULANT 1974) or spinal cord (GUIEU and HARDY 1970; BOULANT and HARDY 1974) and inhibition of their activity by pyrogen (CABANAC et al. 1968; EISENMAN 1969; SCHOENER and WANG 1975) or progesterone (NAKAYAMA et al. 1975) is always accompanied by an inverse influence on the cold-sensitive units. Thus, irrespective of whether some cold sensitive neurones have a direct thermal sensitivity (NAKAYAMA et al. 1978b) or not, they seem to have a prevailing inhibitory synaptic input from warm-sensitive neurones of the PO/AH. The effects of capsaicin have provided evidence for this assumption. It is worth mentioning that noxious stimulation of the skin did not induce a consistant effect on thermosensitive units in the preoptic area (MURAKAMI et al. 1967).

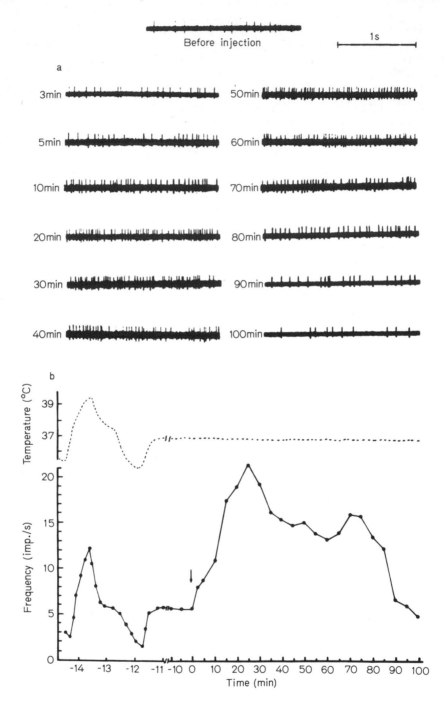

Fig. 3 a, b. Response of PO/AH warm-sensitive neurones to capsaicin. **a** reproduced from tape records. **b** discharge frequency response to change in PO/AH temperature and subcutaneous injection (*arrow*) of capsaicin (1 mg/kg body weight) at constant temperature. (Nakayama et al. 1978 b)

III. Ultrastructural and Biochemical Changes in the PO/AH Induced by Capsaicin

The long-lasting sensory neurone blocking effect of capsaicin is accompanied by ultrastructural changes in mitochondria of the small, B type of sensory neurones in the spinal, trigeminal, and vagal ganglia (Joó et al. 1969; SZOLCSÁNYI et al. 1975; SZOLCSÁNYI 1975).

In one type of PO/AH neurone in the area just beneath the anterior commissure a similar swelling of mitochondria was observed from 2 days to 5 months after SC capsaicin pre treatment. This cell type was characterized by its smaller size and thinner cytoplasm containing rough endoplasmic reticulum rather than free ribosomes. No alteration in fine structure of other nervous or glial elements was observed. Neither karyolysis nor other signs of cell disintegration were present. It has been suggested that the nerve cells with impaired mitochondria are the warm-sensors in the PO/AH (SZOLCSÁNYI et al. 1971; SZOLCSÁNYI and JANCSÓ-GÁBOR 1973).

Fluorescence microscopical study of the hypothalamus of capsaicin-desensitized rats revealed a disappearance of perivascular central adrenergic fibres in the mid-sagittal line, beneath the anterior commissure. Other central or peripheral adrenergic fibres remained untouched by the pre-treatment (CSILLIK et al. 1971). Cell bodies or axon terminals of capsaicin-responsive adrenergic fibres were not present in the PO/AH from where warm-sensitive units have been picked up by microelectrodes (MURAKAMI et al. 1967; WIT and WANG 1968a; GUIEU and HARDY 1970). Furthermore, physiological and pharmacological findings on rats do not support a selective role for noradrenaline in heat loss activation (BECKMAN 1970; BLIGH 1972; HELLON 1975; VAN ZOEREN and STRICKER 1976). Therefore, further experiments are needed to reveal the functional significance of this finding.

The effect of capsaicin on the adenylate cyclase activity of the particulate cell fraction of different brain regions was investigated by G. JANCSÓ and WOLLEMANN (1977) and HORVATH et al. (1979). There was a progressive enhancement in basal adenylate cyclase activity in the preoptic area of capsaicin-desensitized rats. No change in activity was observed one hour after the first injection (50 mg/kg SC), while at the eighth day after the pre-treatment (50 + 100 mg/kg) the activity was about ten-fold as compared with the controls. The adenylate cyclase activity of the cerebellum or parietal cortex remained unchanged. The enhanced activity of the preoptic area was markedly inhibited by in vitro addition of capsaicin ($10^{-7} - 10^{-5} M$) or 5-HT ($10^{-5} M$). On the other hand, in the presence of capsaicin there was an enhancement in adenylate cyclase activity in brain regions of the controls and in the cerebellum or cortex of desensitized rats. Capsaicin did not influence the phosphodiesterase activity of the brain regions investigated. In vitro specific ^{3}H-labelled capsaicin binding to the particulate cell fraction was highest in the preoptic area (SZEBENI et al. 1978). In the light of the impairment in thermoregulation produced by capsaicin, it has been assumed that adenylate cyclase is involved in maintaining normal thermoregulatory function.

The highly interesting region-selective biochemical changes and the above assumption merit further comment. The most powerful activation of the heat loss pathway is during the first hour after capsaicin injection. The fact that at that time no change in adenylate cyclase activity has been observed seems not to favour the neurotransmitter role of cyclic adenosine 5′-monophosphate (AMP) in the heat loss pathway. Neither a release of cyclic AMP into the cerebralospin fluid nor a hypothermic effect specific for this particular purine base has been verified (DASCOMBE and MILTON 1975, 1976; MILTON and DASCOMBE 1977). On the other hand, the long-term development in enhancement of adenylate cyclase activity might be related to the recovery from the first hyperthermic phase which occurs after desensitization. The lack of permanent pyrexia after desensitization of warm-sensors cannot be explained by any of the engineering models of thermoregulation. Involvement of synaptic plasticity (GRAGG 1972) synaptic reorganization and bio-chemical events in the analysis of the effect of capsaicin might help to clarify how the set-point is really adjusted in thermal homeostasis.

H. Action of Pungent Agents on Sensory Receptors

It has always been obvious that sensory nerve endings are activated by pungent agents. The crucial part of the question is how far their stimulatory and desensitiz-ing effects are specific. Consequently this section will review briefly all known sen-sory effects elicited by pungent agents, not only findings which support a site of action on warm-receptors.

I. Capsaicin Desensitization and Sensation

1) Protective reflexes elicited by a large number of chemically unrelated pain-pro-ducing substances were abolished for days after local application of capsaicin (lo-cal desensitization). Protective reflexes to mechanical, thermal, or electrical stimuli were readily elicited from the desensitized areas. Desensitization by parenteral cap-saicin injections resulted in a similar selective insensitivity of the skin and outer mu-cous membranes throughout the body. This effect lasted for months in guinea-pigs or rats (JANCSÓ 1955, 1960; JANCSÓ and JANCSÓ-GÁBOR 1959; JANCSÓ et al. 1961). These data form the basis for concluding that mechanically and chemically induced pain are mediated by different mechanisms.

These experiments were confirmed and analysed further on the eye of the rat (JANCSÓ 1968; MAKARA 1970; SZOLCSÁNYI et al. 1975; SZOLCSÁNYI and JANCSÓ-GÁ-BOR 1976; JANCSÓ-GÁBOR 1976), on the ear of the rat (JANCSÓ-GÁBOR 1976) and on the respiratory airways of mice (ALARIE and KELLER 1973).

In rats, pain reaction or corticosterone mobilization elicited by subcutaneous formaldeyhde (1%–3%), intraperitoneal acetic acid (0.35%), acetylcholine (16 mg/kg) or intra-arterial KCl, remained unchanged after capsaicin desensitiza-tion. Therefore, different mechanisms for deep and superficial chemonociception have been suggested (MAKARA et al. 1967b; MAKARA 1970). These invasive treat-ments and agents, however, are by no means appropriate tools to identify differ-ences between sensory receptors. Furthermore, after local or systemic desensitiza-tion, strong inhibition in pain reaction evoked by intra-arterial bradykinin, acetyl-choline, chloracetophenone (GÖRES and JUNG 1959; RICCIOPPO et al. 1974; JANCSÓ-GÁBOR 1976), or even KCl (BARAZ et al. 1968a, b) has been reported from different laboratories. The latency of foot-licking response to being placed on a hot plate

(53 °C) was slightly increased in desensitized rats for four days (SZOLCSÁNYI 1976) and in contrast to the controls, selection of a moderately warm floor temperature (35 °C) instead of a higher one (46 °C) was abolished. Irreversible impairment in pain reaction to noxious heating was obtained after neonatal (HOLZER et al. 1979) or intrathecal (YAKSH et al. 1979) capsaicin pretreatment.

2) In a self-experiment the facial skin was desensitized by treatment with alcoholic capsaicin solution. Pain sensation and hyperemia evoked by capsaicin or ammonia were eliminated in the desensitized skin area whereas "the sensitivity to touch, slight tickling and needle pricking" remained normal (JANCSÓ 1960).

The exposed base of cantharidine blisters (KEELE and ARMSTRONG 1964) were also desensitized by capsaicin to the pain-producing effects of capsaicin, bradykinin, and acetylcholine. Pain sensation produced by KCl remained unchanged. The effectiveness of KCl has been attributed to axonal stimulation of different fibres including those which conduct impulses from mechanical nociceptors (SZOLCSÁNYI 1977a).

The sensitivity of the human tongue was tested by psychophysical methods before and after capsaicin desensitization. Taste sensitivity (quinine, glucose, ascorbic acid, and NaCl), tactile threshold (5-10 mg), difference limen to cool or tactile stimuli as well as recognition threshold, and concentration of menthol were not altered by the pre-treatment. No paraesthesia or any peculiar sensation were felt and pin-prick or pinching the tongue elicited pain sensation as before.

The pungent sensation induced by capsaicin or zingerone and the pricking feeling in response to aqueous mustard oil were abolished. Mustard oil in higher concentration was felt as sweet, but capsaicin elicited no sensation. There was a pronounced disturbance in difference limen between warm temperatures indicating that different sets of receptors are responsible for sensation of cold or warmth on the human tongue. Furthermore, it turned out that the loss of chemical sensitivity is a sensation- and receptor-specific effect, since taste and cool sensation elicited by chemical means were not disturbed by capsaicin desensitization (SZOLCSÁNYI and JANCSÓ-GÁBOR 1973; SZOLCSÁNYI 1977a).

II. Electrophysiological Recordings from Exteroceptive Nerves

The first experiments in this line revealed that desensitization produced by parenteral capsaicin pre-treatment is peripheral in nature. Action potentials recorded from the saphenous and auricle nerves of control rats upon topical or subcutaneous application of capsaicin to the innervated area, were absent in desensitized animals. The effect of mustard oil was also strongly inhibited, whereas spikes evoked by tactile stimuli or pinching the skin were readily elicited in an unchanged pattern (PÓRSZÁSZ and JANCSÓ 1959; JANCSÓ et al. 1967).

Multi-fibre sensory discharges in the ciliary nerve of the excised cat eye were produced by light tactile stimuli to the cornea or by cooling its surface, as well as by different irritants including nonanoyl vanillylamide (No. 5). Threshold concentration of the pungent agent was 10^{-7}–10^{-6} M. None of the other substances stimulated the preparation after nonanoyl vanillylamide treatment although both cooling and tactile stimuli produced activation as before (GREEN and TREGEAR 1964).

In a preparation dissected from the recurrent laryngeal nerve of the cat containing only a few fibres, action potentials were elicited by stimulating the nerve endings of the larynx with nonanoyl vanillylamide, ω-chloracetophenone or ice-cold saline. In low concentration the chemicals produced no response on cold-sensitive fibres. Nonanoyl vanillylamide in a concentration of 10^{-4} M stimulated 8 out of 15 fibres which responded also to cold stimuli. Desensitizing effects to cold or chemical stimuli were not observed (Dirnhuber et al. 1965).

Capsaicin given in arterial injection (0.02–20 μg) to the innervated skin area excited the slowest-conducting C_2 fibres as detected by the collision technique (Douglas et al. 1960) on the saphenous nerve of the cat. A$\alpha\beta$, Aδ, as well as C_1 groups of fibres were activated by mechanical stimuli but no sign of excitation was observed after injection of capsaicin (Szolcsányi 1975, 1976, 1977a).

The C_2 group comprises the majority of fibres conducting impulses from the polymodal nociceptors, which respond to noxious heating, moderate-to-strong mechanical stimuli and to irritant chemicals (Bessou and Perl 1969; Burgess and Perl 1973; Torebjörk and Hallin 1974). A further characteristic feature of these sense organs is the increase in their excitability after mild stimulation, particularly after heat stimuli (Perl 1976; Lynn 1977). Therefore, the well known sensitizing effect of capsaicin to heating (Heubner 1925; Jancsó 1960) was analysed further.

In rats the frequency of action potentials evoked by SC injection of capsaicin was enhanced by rapid warming of the skin areas, while sudden cooling had a blocking effect. On human skin painted with a 1% solution of capsaicin in alcohol the threshold for thermal pain was shifted from 45°–46 °C to 30°–31 °C. On the basis of these findings as well as others reviewed in Sects. D, E of this paper it has been suggested that sensation produced by capsaicin is mediated by stimulating polymodal nociceptors and warm-receptors. The retained sensitivity to mechanical pain and noxious heat stimuli was explained (Szolcsányi 1975, 1976, 1977a) by the possibility that the mechanical nociceptors (Burgess and Perl 1973) and some heat nociceptors (Iggo and Ogawa 1971; Martin and Manning 1969) which belong to the Aδ group of fibres, remained intact.

Direct evidence has been obtained for the stimulatory and desensitizing effects of capsaicin on polymodal nociceptors in a systematic study on single fibres in the rabbit ear. Among slowly conducting fibres neither low-threshold C mechanoreceptors, high-threshold C mechanoreceptors, Aδ mechanical nociceptors, or cold-receptors were activated with concentrations of capsaicin which consistently stimulated polymodal nociceptors given by close arterial injection. Following higher desensitizing doses the response of polymodal nociceptors to chemical, mechanical, or noxious heat stimuli was diminished or abolished (Szolcsányi, unpublished observation).

In another single-fibre study nonanoyl vanillylamide, capsaicin, and different irritants were tested by topical application on the skin of the cat. The two potent pungent agents activated, then desensitized to irritants the "moderate-to-high-threshold C mechanoreceptors." High-threshold Aδ mechanoreceptors, low-threshold C mechanoreceptors and "very-high-threshold C mechanoreceptors" were unaffected (Foster and Ramage 1976). Since there is no indication in this procedure that the sensitivity of these mechanoreceptor units were tested to noxious heating, the capsaicin-sensitive units might be identical to polymodal nociceptors. The effect of capsaicin on single warm-sensitive fibres has not been tested.

III. Effects on Interoceptors

Since the pioneering work of PÓRSZÁSZ et al. (1955) and TOH et al. (1955) capsaicin has been used extensively for identification of reflexogenic areas, "silent" interoceptors in the cardiovascular, and respiratory systems.

1. Vagal Interoceptors

The reflex triad of vasodilatation, bradycardia, and apnoea has been evoked by stimulating the vagal receptors of the pulmonary circulation with capsaicin in different animal species (PÓRSZÁSZ et al. 1955, 1957; BEVAN 1962; COLERIDGE et al. 1964a; MOLNÁR and GYÖRGY 1967; MAKARA et al. 1967a; MITCHELL et al. 1967; TODA et al. 1972; RUSSEL and LAI-FOOK 1979). In cats and dogs similar chemoreflexes were also evoked from the sinus caroticus and aortic arch (TOH et al. 1955, PÓRSZÁSZ et al. 1957; MITCHELL et al. 1967; BRENDER and WEBB-PEPLOE 1969; RICCIOPPO et al. 1974) and from the coronary arteries (OSADCHII et al. 1967).

By testing a wide range of chemically very different pungent agents and nonpungent congeners (capsaicin, piperine, zingerone, and compounds No. 2, 3, 4, 7, 8, 10, 22, 23, 30, 36, 46, 47, 50) a close relationship was found between the pain-producing potency (tested on the eye) and interoceptor-stimulating potency (chemoreflex triad elicited from the pulmonary circulation). In rats desensitized with capsaicin or homovanilloyl dodecylamide (No. 10) the reflex triad to injection of capsaicin, piperine, zingerone, or undecenoyl-3-aminopropanol (No. 47) were strongly inhibited or completely abolished, while vagal reflexes elicited by phenyldiguanide from the systemic vascular bed or the carotid sinus reflex, or the effect of stimulation the central end of the cut vagal nerve remained practically unchanged (SZOLCSÁNYI and JÁNOSSY 1971; SZOLCSÁNYI 1975). The triad elicited by 5-HT was also inhibited even in animals which were incompletely desensitized to the effect of capsaicin (MAKARA et al. 1967a).

Studies on single vagal fibres revealed that capsaicin-stimulated nerve endings of the slowest-conducting fibres have the following common characteristics:

a) Unlike arterial baroreceptors or atrial receptors, which are concentrated in localized areas the capsaicin-sensitive endings are widely distributed in the wall of pulmonary artery, thoracic aorta and its branches, in the peripheral portion of the bronchial and pulmonary circulation, being in the latter case near the juxtapulmonary capillaries ("type J receptor"), in the coronary circulation ("epicardial receptors"), as well as in the wall of large veins (COLERIDGE et al. 1965, 1973; COLERIDGE and COLERIDGE 1972, 1977; ARMSTRONG and LUCK 1974).

b) They have either no spontaneous activity or only a sparse, irregular background, having no obvious relationship to the cardiac or respiratory cycle.

c) Conduction velocity of the majority of fibres is less than 2 m/s corresponding to the conduction velocity of unmyelinated C fibres.

d) Besides capsaicin they are sensitive to other chemical agents, e.g. to phenyldiguanide.

e) A high degree of mechanical distortion is required to excite them. Their threshold may be lowered in certain circumstances, e.g. as a result of pulmonary congestion (COLERIDGE and COLERIDGE 1972).

The functional role of these sensory nerve endings is not yet clarified. Since only this group of vagal sensory endings is stimulated by capsaicin, they should be responsible for the vagal reflexes described above to injection of capsaicin. Type J receptors probably mediate dyspnoeic sensation in response to pulmonary congestion (PAINTAL 1977). Pulmonary stretch receptors highly sensitive to veratrum alkaloids (COLERIDGE et al. 1965), ventricle pressure receptors (COLERIDGE et al. 1964 b), and the rapidly adapting "irritant" receptors (ARMSTRONG and LUCK 1974) were not excited by capsaicin. A slight enhancement of the pre-existing spontaneous discharge was noted in only one-third of the "irritant" receptors in response to a higher dose of capsaicin (ARMSTRONG and LUCK 1974). This might be due to pulmonary hypertension which was invariably elicited by this dose of capsaicin (MOLNÁR and GYÖRGY 1967).

2. Non-Vagal Pressor Chemoreflexes

In response to intra-arterial capsaicin non-vagal pressor chemoreflexes were elicited from splanchnic, iliacal, or coronary areas (TOH et al. 1955; OSADCHII et al. 1967; GÖRES and JUNG 1959; BARAZ et al. 1968 a; SANOILENKO 1970; BRENDER and WEBB-PEPLOE 1969; WEBB-PEPLOE et al. 1972). These responses have been considered as one sign of the chemonociceptive reflex (LIM et al. 1962), although another possibility has also been proposed (WEBB-PEPLOE et al. 1972).

IV. Local Efferent Function of Capsaicin-Sensitive Sensory Nerve Endings

1. Skin and Exteroceptive Mucous Membranes

JANCSÓ et al. (1967) provided the first experimental evidence that antidromic electrical stimulation of sensory nerves or orthodromic stimulation of sensory nerve endings by pain-producing substances elicits not only vasodilatation (antidromic vasodilatation) but other signs of inflammation as well (neurogenic inflammation). Capsaicin-sensitive nerve endings (JANCSÓ et al. 1967, 1968; JANCSÓ-GÁBOR and SZOLCSÁNYI 1969, 1970, 1972; SZOLCSÁNYI et al. 1976) of C fibres (SZOLCSÁNYI 1975, 1977 b; CHAHL and LADD (1976) mediated the response. Orthodromic stimulation of the capsaicin-sensitive sensory nerve endings (polymodal nociceptors) with different pain-producing substances elicits inflammation purely, dominantly, or partly through the neurogenic pathway. By sensory denervation as well as by capsaicin desensitization it is possible to determine the participation of the neural factor in the inflammatory response (JANCSÓ 1955, 1960, 1964, 1968; JANCSÓ et al. 1961, 1967, 1968; JANCSÓ-GÁBOR and SZOLCSÁNYI 1969, 1972; ARVIER et al. 1977).

No increase in vascular permeability was produced by capsaicin after sensory denervation (JANCSÓ 1960; JANCSÓ et al. 1967; LEMBECK et al. 1977); consequently mast cells might be involved only as a secondary step in the chain of events (ARVIER et al. 1977; LEMBECK and HOLZER 1979) and not as the primary site of action for capsaicin as proposed by KIERNAN (1977).

According to our hypothesis (JANCSÓ 1968; JANCSÓ et al. 1968) chemosensitive pain nerve endings – which correspond to the polymodal nociceptors (SZOLCSÁNYI 1976, unpublished results, 1977 a) – release a neurohumour when they are excited.

The efferent response manifests itself as neurogenic inflammation which includes the phenomenon of antidromic vasodilatation. The sensory and mediator-releasing functions of these receptors seem to be intimately related to each other at the level of the tetrodotoxin-resistant generative region (JANCSÓ-GÁBOR and SZOLCSÁNYI 1969; SZOLCSÁNYI 1975). It seems reasonable to assume that the mediator-releasing function of the capsaicin-sensitive sensory nerve endings has a functional significance by producing a local inflammatory response to accelerate the tissue-repairing reaction in the area where the pain-producing chemical agents invade or are released.

2. Internal Organs

New types of neural response characterized by their sensitivity to capsaicin have also been found recently in internal organs.

Stimulation of the peripheral stump of the cut vagal nerve of the rat pre-treated with atropine resulted in an increase in vascular permeability in the trachea, bronchi, oesophagus, and mediastinal connective tissue. The response was not inhibited by high doses of methysergide, promethazine, or indomethacin, but was completely absent in rats desensitized by capsaicin (SZOLCSÁNYI 1975; SZOLCSÁNYI et al. 1976).

Electrical stimulation of mesenteric nerves of the guinea-pig isolated ileum or taenia caeci resulted in contraction of the preparations pre-treated with adrenergic neurone blocking agents. The response was inhibited and abolished by capsaicin in an irreversible manner. The 50% reduction in size was achieved by a concentration of 1.5×10^{-8} g/ml (IC 50).

Smooth-muscle responses to electrical stimulation of parasympathetic preganglionic fibres, intramural cholinergic or purinergic fibres, mesenteric postganglionic adrenergic fibres, as well as the effect of nicotine were not inhibited, and the non-specific inhibition produced by higher concentrations of $10^{-5}-10^{-4}$ g/ml were always fully reversible after washing out the substance (SZOLCSÁNYI and BARTHÓ 1978, 1979; ANURAS et al. 1977; BARTHÓ and SZOLCSÁNYI 1978).

In this context it is wort mentioning that none of the authors who analysed the effect of capsaicin in different isolated tissues described any effect of the substance on autonomic nerve endings or neurotransmission (TOH et al. 1955; MOLNÁR ct al. 1969 a, b; FUKUDA and FUJIWARA 1969; TODA et al. 1972). Under in vivo conditions close arterial injection of capsaicin (5–50 µg) to the superior cervical ganglion of the cat was completely ineffective (MOLNÁR 1966) and the blood pressure of strongly desensitized rats did not differ from that of the controls (SZOLCSÁNYI 1975).

V. Concept of Sensory Neurone Blocking Effect of Pungent Acylamides

Ideas about the mechanism of capsaicin desensitization have developed step by step parallel with the accumulating experimental findings. It has been clear from the beginning that the site of action of capsaicin is peripheral in nature (JANCSÓ and JANCSÓ-GÁBOR 1949). The first hypothesis concerning the involvement of histamine in the desensitizing effect of capsaicin was discussed later as only one of the possibilities (Jancsó 1955). Afterwards a direct site of action on sensory nerve endings has been postulated (Jancsó and Jancsó-Gábor 1959; Pórszász and Jancsó 1959). It has been proposed that on the same nerve ending distinct receptive mechanisms are responsible for the initiation of impulses elicited by physical and chemical stimuli. According to this explanation the desensitized nerve ending is unresponsive to chemical stimuli but can still be excited by physical means (Jancsó et al. 1961; Keele 1962). The possibility was raised that after desensitization the impaired synthesis or storage of the mediator, which is released during excitation of the nerve ending, and produces neurogenic inflammation, "is responsible for the characteristic loss of chemosensitivity" (Jancsó 1964, 1968).

Further findings have formed the basis for concluding that "systemic desensitization affects the whole primary sensory neurone" and the loss of chemosensitivity is only one sign of the functional and ultrastructural impairment of the affected primary sensory neurones and their nerve endings. Therefore, capsaicin has been called a specific sensory neurone blocking agent (Szolcsányi et al. 1975; Szolcsányi 1975).

1. Neurone-Selective Site of Action

Sensory effects produced by pungent agents share many common characteristics (Table 4). These common properties and the following lines of evidence (details of which with the references are listed in other parts of Sect. H) favour the idea of dividing primary sensory neurones into two categories on the basis of their sensitivity to capsaicin-like pungent agents.

a) Electrophysiological Findings

α) *Exteroceptors.* In low doses the overwhelming majority of polymodal nociceptor units were excited without having any consistent effect on a wide range of other receptors. Warm-receptors and slowly adapting mechanoreceptors were not tested. After high doses no sign of gross activation of $A\alpha\beta$, $A\delta$ or fast-conducting C fibres was found. The dose range in which the specificity is valid for each type of receptor is not yet clarified, but preliminary findings suggest that most of them are completely insensitive to the stimulatory and long-lasting blocking effect of capsaicin. On the other hand, after higher doses indirect effects due to neurogenic inflammation should also be taken into account.

β) *Vagal Interoceptors.* Capsaicin-sensitive units resemble polymodal nociceptors in their slow conducting velocity, sparse or absent background activity, their responsiveness to high threshold mechanical stimuli besides their chemical sensitivity. None of the faster-conducting fibres were excited by the compound even if they were very highly sensitive to the veratrum alkaloids.

γ) *Preoptic Units.* Only warm-sensitive units were activated by capsaicin. The proportion of these units markedly decreased in desensitized rats.

b) Selective Loss of Sensory Function After Desensitization

Impaired regulation against overheating and failure in reaction to chemically induced pain stimuli of desensitized animals were accompanied by intact regulation

Table 4. Characteristics of the sensory effects produced by capsaicin and other pungent agents

	Chemogenic pain	Vagal chemoreflex	Heat loss response (warmth sensation)		
			Peripheral areas	Systemic application	Preoptic area
Activation					
Type of receptors (units)	Polymodal nociceptor	J type group	Warm-receptor?		Warm-sensors
Group of fibres	C	Mainly C	C		
Related to pungency	Yes	Yes	Yes	Yes	
Blocking effect after larger doses					
Systemic treatment	Irreversible	Long-lasting irreversible?	Irreversible	Irreversible	Irreversible
Local treatment	Long-lasting	Long-lasting	Long-lasting		Long-lasting irreversible?
Unaltered sensations	Mechanical pain, tactile, gustatory, slight change in heat-induced pain		Cold sensation induced by cooling or menthol		
Against biogenic substances, or to adequate stimulation of the sensors	Bradykinin, 5HT, histamine, acetylcholine etc.	5HT	Warming	Warming	Warming
Against other pungent agents	Yes	Yes		Yes	
Directly related to pungency	No	No		No	
Accompanied by similar neuromeselective ultrastructural changes	Small neurones in sensory ganglia and in nerve endings of the cornea	Small neurones in nodosal ganglia			Small PO/AH neurones

against cold and unchanged responsiveness to low-threshold or high-threshold mechanical stimuli. After desensitization of the human skin or tongue only sensitivity to warmth and chemogenic pain were impaired.

c) Lack of Effect on Efferent Nerves and Neurotransmission

Parasympathetic cholinergic, sympathetic preganglionic and postganglionic, as well as purinergic fibres and neural responses were resistant to the direct stimulatory or persistent blocking effect of capsaicin. The local anaesthesia induced by very high doses was fully reversible.

d) Pharmacological Findings

Structurally different pungent agents elicit not only pain and heat loss response but vagal chemoreflex as well in proportion to their pungency. None of the responses were evoked by non-pungent congeners.

e) Neurone-Selective Ultrastructural and Biochemical Changes After Desensitization

These events will be discussed in the forecoming section.

2. Mode of Action at the Neural Level

a) Site of Action on the Sensory Nerve Endings

It is impossible, for technical reasons, to detect whether a stimulus excites the generative terminal or regenerative axonal region of a cutaneous or mucosal free sensory nerve ending. In the case of capsaicin, however, the following findings favour a site of action on the generative, tetrodotoxin-resistant terminal region (Szolcsányi et al. 1975).

1) The development of local desensitization was not altered by pre-treatment of the area with local anaesthetics (Jancsó 1955).

2) One sign of excitation of these endings with pungent agents (the neurogenic inflammation) was inhibited neither by local anaesthetics (Jancsó et al. 1968), nor by tetrodotoxin (Jancsó-Gábor and Szolcsányi 1969; Szolcsányi 1975).

3) After local desensitization of the rat's eye, swollen mitochondria and a decrease in number of microvesicles in the naked portion of some fibres were observed. Axons ensheathed by Schwann cells were more resistant to the effect of capsaicin and the fine structure of non-neural elements remained unchanged (Szolcsányi et al. 1975).

The temperature-dependant excitatory effect of capsaicin and particularly its complete blockade by moderate cooling is a highly interesting phenomenon (Szolcsányi 1977a). Sensitization of cold-receptors by menthol is well known (Hensel and Zotterman 1952). It would appear that the excitatory effect of capsaicin on warm-receptors is due to a similar sensitization to the adequate stimulus of the receptor. How this thermodependence operates on polymodal nociceptors and how it is related to the stimulatory effect of capsaicin in general is a very interesting point.

The desensitizing effect is a graded response depending on the concentration of capsaicin used and on the time elapsed after the pre-treatment. After incomplete desensitization, excitation of polymodal nociceptor units to mechanical, noxious heat, and chemical stimuli was simultaneously diminished (unpublished observation). Another special feature of this stage is the rapid fatigue in response to repeated stimuli. This sign of impaired function which might be explained by an inhibition of the recovery process has been demonstrated on the basis of pain reaction to repeated non-desensitizing chemogenic pain stimuli (JANCSÓ 1968; SZOLCSÁNYI et al. 1975; JANCSÓ-GÁBOR 1976) and in the case of warm-sensitive preoptic units which retained their thermoresponsiveness after desensitization (HORI 1980).

b) Evidence for Impairment of the Whole Primary Sensory Neurone After Systemic Desensitization

α) Functional Findings. After systemic treatment the desensitizing effect is practically irreversible, while local desensitization lasts but a few days. Pre-treatment with inhibitors of axonal flow (colchicine, vinblastine) prolonged the local desensitizing effect of capsaicin, indicating that centrifugal axonal flow helps to restore the function of sensory receptors (SZOLCSÁNYI et al. 1975).

β) Ultrastructural Findings. Systemic capsaicin desensitization of adult rats induced selective mitochondrial swelling in the small B type of neurones of the trigeminal, spinal, and nodosal ganglia which was demonstrable even two months after the pre-treatment. No ultrastructural changes were observed in the large A type of primary sensory neurones, satellite cells, or neural elements of the sympathetic ganglia (JOÓ et al. 1969; SZOLCSÁNYI et al. 1975; SZOLCSÁNYI 1975). In 2-day-old newborn rats 30 min after capsaicin injection (50 mg/kg) more severe fine structural changes were present in sensory neurones of B type. Axonal degeneration of unmyelinated fibres in dorsal roots and in laminae I and II of the dorsal horn clearly shows that the capsaicin-sensitive neurones were completely damaged. Again, type A neurones and other cellular elements of sensory ganglia remained unimpaired (G. JANCSÓ et al. 1977, 1978; G. JANCSÓ 1978).

γ) Histochemical and Biochemical Findings. Fluoride-resistant acid phosphatase activity which is histochemically detectable in the small type of primary sensory neurones and their endings in the substantia gelatinosa of the dorsal horn disappeared in desensitized rats (G. JANCSÓ and KNYIHÁR 1975; JESSELL et al. 1978).

Substance P, an undecapeptide supposed to have a neurotransmitter role, is also highly concentrated in terminals of small-diameter primary sensory neurones. Substance P-like immunoreactivity in extracted dorsal horn samples as well as immunofluorescence in the substantia gelatinosa were markedly decreased in rats desensitized with capsaicin. Glutamic acid decarboxylase activity and opiate receptor binding sites in the dorsal horn did not change (GASPAROVIC et al. 1964; JESSELL et al. 1978). Intrathecal capsaicin also depleted substance P in the spinal cord of the rat (YAKSH et al. 1979). Degeneration of capsaicin-sensitive fibres following neonatal capsaicin pretreatment resulted in a reduction of the opiate binding sites in the dorsal horn (GAMSE et al. 1979 a). Thus, under in vivo conditions all fine structural and biochemical alterations induced by capsaicin desensitization seem

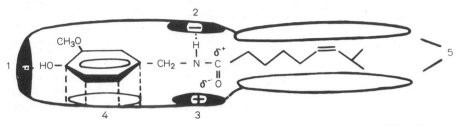

Fig. 4. Schematic representation of the hypothetical capsaicin receptor. 1: H-bonding site for the OH group; 2: Electronegative site for the H of the NH group and for the C^+ atom; 3: Electropositive site for the oxygen of the carbonyl group; 4, 5: Non-polar areas bound by van der Walls forces. (SZOLCSÁNYI and JANCSÓ-GÁBOR 1975)

to be restricted to a special class of primary sensory neurones. In accordance with this assumption capsaicin under in vitro conditions seems to release substance P from the primary sensory neurones only (GAMSE et al. 1979b; THERIAULT et al. 1979). Which of the described effects is of primary importance in the development of functional impairment is still unknown. The in vitro effects of capsaicin on isolated rat liver mitochondria (CHUDAPONGSE and JANTHASOOT 1976) or lysosomes (SMITH et al. 1970) seem to indicate that a selective uptake of the compound into these neurones might be responsible for its specificity under in vivo conditions. Prostaglandin biosynthesis in bull seminal homogenates was enhanced by capsaicin (COLLIER et al. 1975), while no change in corneal prostaglandin content was found after local desensitization (BARTHÓ et al. 1976). In the duodenal mucosa ultrastructural alterations with mitochondrial swelling were reported (NOPANITAYA and NYE 1974) in response to intraduodenal administration of capsaicin in high concentration (1.4×10^{-4} g/ml).

3. Structure-Activity Relationship

In order to get information about the possible molecular interactions involved in the excitation and sensory blockade caused by capsaicin, the pain-producing and desensitizing effects of about 50 capsaicin derivatives were analysed in the eye of rats (SZOLCSÁNYI and JANCSÓ-GÁBOR 1975b, 1976). It turned out that the presence of acylamide linkage and alkyl chain are not essential for pungency but are essential in the desensitizing effect. The desensitization potency was not parallel with the excitatory response. Strongly pungent homovanilloyl octylester (No. 23) failed to desensitize the receptors, while homovanilloyl dodecylamide (No. 10) proved to be a more potent desensitizing agent than capsaicin itself, although it was less pungent. A hypothetical multiple interaction with the receptive molecule has been presented (Fig. 4) according to which in respect of pungency site 2 is haptophoric and at site 5 only the non-polar nature of the molecule is necessary. All five moieties are critical for the desensitizing effect.

J. Concluding Remarks

A distinct group of primary sensory neurones including the warm-sensors of the preoptic area shares common biochemical properties, being highly susceptible to the excitatory and selective neurone blocking effects of capsaicin-like pungent agents. This loss of sensory function is responsible for the pyrexia and inability to regulate against overheating of animals pre-treated with pungent acylamides. Capsaicin seems to be a useful tool to analyse thermal homeostasis, since in contrast to thermal stimuli a one-sided asynchronous input from, and blockade of the warm-sensors can be achieved. Owing to the fact that central "thermosensitive units" can be identified only by analogy with the specific thermoreceptors of the skin (HENSEL 1973), the use of capsaicin has been, and I hope, will be a great help in this respect as well.

References

Alarie Y, Keller LW (1973) Sensory irritation by capsaicin. Environ Physiol Biochem 3:169–181

Anuras S, Christensen J, Templeman D (1977) Effect of capsaicin on electrical slow waves in the isolated cat colon. Gut 18:666–669

Arai S (1976) Effects of capsaicin on thermoregulatory center (in Japanese). Med J Osaka Univ 28:165–178

Armstrong DJ, Luck JC (1974) A comparative study of irritant and type J receptors in the cat. Respir Physiol 21:47–60

Arvier PT, Chahl LA, Ladd RJ (1977) Modification by capsaicin and compound 48/80 of dye leakage induced by irritants in the rat. Br J Pharmacol 59:61–68

Aschoff J (1970) Circadian rhythm of activity and body temperature. In: Hardy JD, Gagge AP, Stolwijk JAJ (eds) Physiological and behavioral temperature regulation. Thomas, Springfield, pp 905–919

Baraz LA, Khayutin VM, Molnár J (1968a) Analysis of the stimulatory action of capsaicin on receptors and sensory fibres of the small intestine in the cat. Acta Physiol Acad Sci Hung 33:225–235

Baraz LA, Khayutin VM, Molnár J (1968b) Effects of capsaicin upon the stimulatory action of potassium chloride in the visceral branches of spinal afferents of the cat. Acta Physiol Acad Sci Hung 33:237–246

Barthó L, Szolcsányi J (1978) The site of action of capsaicin on the guinea-pig isolated ileum. Naunyn-Schmiedeberg Arch Pharmacol 305:74–81

Barthó L, Pórszász J, Szolcsányi J (1976) Extraction of prostaglandin from corneae and irides of guinea-pigs pretreated with various drugs. In: Knoll J, Kelemen K (eds) Symposium on prostaglandins. Akadémiai Kiadó, Budapest, pp 107–110

Beckman AL (1970) Effect of intrahypothalamic norepinephrine on thermoregulatory responses in the rat. Am J Physiol 218:1596–1604

Benedek G, Obál F Jr, Jancsó-Gábor A, Obál F (1980) Effects of elevated ambient temperatures on the sleep-waking activity of rats with impaired warm reception. Waking Sleeping 4:87–94

Bessou P, Perl ER (1969) Response of cutaneous sensory units with unmyelinated fibers to noxious stimuli. J Neurophysiol 32:1025–1043

Bevan JA (1962) Action of lobeline and capsaicin on afferent endings in the pulmonary artery of the cat. Circ Res 10:792–797

Bligh J (1972) Neuronal models of mammalian temperature regulation. In: Bligh J, Moore R (eds) Essays on temperature regulation. North-Holland, Amsterdam, pp 105–120

Boulant JA (1974) The effect of firing rate on preoptic neuronal thermosensitivity. J Physiol (Lond) 240:661–669

Boulant JA, Bignall KE (1973) Hypothalamic neuronal responses to peripheral and deep-body temperatures. Am J Physiol 225:1371–1374

Boulant JA, Gonzales RR (1977) The effect of skin temperature on the hypothalamic control of heat loss and heat production. Brain Res 120:367–372

Boulant JA, Hardy JD (1974) The effect of spinal and skin temperatures on the firing rate and thermosensitivity of preoptic neurones. J Physiol (Lond) 240:639–660

Brender D, Webb-Peploe MM (1969) Vascular responses to stimulation of pulmonary and carotid baroreceptors by capsaicin. Am J Physiol 217:1837–1845

Burges PR, Perl ER (1973) Cutaneous mechanoreceptors and nociceptors. In: Iggo A (ed) Somatosensory system. (Handbook of sensory physiology, vol II). Springer, Berlin Heidelberg New York, pp 29–78

Cabanac M (1972) Thermoregulatory behavior. In: Bligh J, Moore R (eds) Essays on temperature regulation. North Holland, Amsterdam, pp 19–36

Cabanac M, Massonnett B (1974) Temperature regulation during fever: change of set point or change of gain? A tentative answer from a behavioural study in man. J Physiol (Lond) 238:561–568

Cabanac MJ, Stolwijk JAJ, Hardy JD (1968) Effect of temperature and pyrogens on single-unit activity in the rabbit's brain stem. J Appl Physiol 24:645–652

Cabanac M, Cormareche-Leydier M, Poirier LJ (1976) The effect of capsaicin on temperature regulation of the rat. Pfluegers Arch 366:217–221

Cabanac M, Cormareche-Leydier M, Poirier LJ (1977) The effect of capsaicin on temperature regulation of the rat. In: Cooper KE, Lomax P, Schönbaum E (eds) Drugs, biogenic amines and body temperature. Karger, Basel, pp 99–101

Chahl LA, Ladd RJ (1976) Local oedema and general excitation of cutaneous sensory receptors produced by electrical stimulation of the saphenous nerve in the rat. Pain 2:25–31

Chudapongse P, Jantasoot W (1976) Studies on the effect of capsaicin on metabolic reactions of isolated rat liver mitochondria. Toxicol Appl Pharmacol 37:263–270

Coleridge HM, Coleridge JCG (1972) Cardiovascular receptors. In: Downman CBB (ed) Modern trends in physiology, vol 1. Butterworths, London, pp 245–267

Coleridge HM, Coleridge JCG (1977) Impulse activity in afferent vagal C-fibres with endings in the intrapulmonary airways of dogs. Respir Phys 29:125–142

Coleridge HM, Coleridge JCG, Kidd C (1964a) Role of the pulmonary arterial baroreceptors in the effects produced by capsaicin in the dog. J Physiol (Lond) 170:272–285

Coleridge HM, Coleridge JCG, Kidd C (1964b) Cardiac receptors in the dog, with particular reference to two types of afferent ending in the ventricular wall. J Physiol (Lond) 174:323–339

Coleridge HM, Colerdige JCG, Luck JC (1965) Pulmonary afferent fibres of small diameter stimulated by capsaicin and by hyperinflation of the lungs. J Physiol (Lond) 179:248–262

Coleridge HM, Coleridge JCG, Dangel A, Kidd C, Luck JC, Sleight P (1973) Impulses in slowly conducting vagal fibres from afferent endings in the veins, atria and arteries of dogs and cats. Circ Res 33:87–97

Collier HO, McDonald-Gibson WJ, Saed SA (1975) Stimulation of prostaglandin biosynthesis by capsaicin, ethanol and tyramine. Lancet 1:702

Cooper KE (1972) Central mechanisms for the control of body temperature in health and febrile states. In: Downman CBB (ed) Modern trends in physiology. Butterworths, London, pp 33–54

Correa FMA, Graeff FG (1974) Central mechanisms of the hypertensive action of intraventricular bradykinin in the unanaesthetized rat. Neuropharmacology 13:65–75

Csillik B, Jancsó G, Tóth L, Kozma M, Kálmán G, Karcsu S (1971) Adrenergic innervation of hypothalamic blood vessels. A contribution to the problem of central thermodetectors. Acta Anat Acad Sci Hung 80:142–151

Dascombe MJ, Milton AS (1975) The effect of cyclic adenosine 3',5'-monophosphate and other adenine nucleotides on body temperature. J Physiol (Lond) 250:143–160

Dascombe MJ, Milton AS (1976) Cyclic adenosine 3',5'-monophosphate in cerebrospinal fluid during thermoregulation and fever. J Physiol (Lond) 263:441–463

Dirnhuber P, Green DM, Treagear RT (1965) Excitation of sensory neurones in the cat larynx by w-chloracetophenone and n-nonanoylvanillylamide. J Physiol (Lond) 178:41–42P

Douglas WW, Ritchie JM, Straub RW (1960) The role of nonmyelinated fibres in signalling cooling of the skin. J Physiol (Lond) 150:266–283

Eisenman JS (1969) Pyrogen-induced changes in the thermosensitivity of septal and preoptic neurons. Am J Physiol 216:330–334

Eisenman JS (1974) Depression of preoptic thermosensitivity by bacterial pyrogen in rabbits. Am J Physiol 227:1067–1073

Feldberg W, Lotti VJ (1967) Temperature responses to monoamines and on inhibitor of monoamine oxydase injected into the cerebral ventricles of rats. Br J Pharmacol 31:152–161

Foster RW, Ramage AG (1976) Evidence for a specific somatosensory receptor in the cat skin that responds to irritant chemicals. Br J Pharmacol 57:436–437P

Frens J (1976) Effect of capsaicin and pyrogen on thermoregulation in the goat. IRCS Med Sci Libr Compend 4:176

Frens J (1977) Pharmacological evidence for a set-point mechanism in thermoregulation. In: Cooper KE, Lomax P, Schönbaum E (eds) Drugs, biogenic amines and body temperature. Karger, Basel, pp 20–25

Frens J (1978) Is a "set-point" involved during fever. In: Houdas Y, Guieu JD (eds) New trends in thermal physiology. Masson, Paris, pp 47–49

Fukuda N, Fujiwara M (1969) Effect of capsaicin on the guinea-pig isolated atrium. J Pharm Pharmacol 21:622–623

Gamse R, Holzer P, Lembeck F (1979 a) Indirect evidence for presynaptic location of opiate receptors on chemosensitive primary sensory neurones. Naunyn-Schmiedeberg Arch Pharmacol 308:281–285

Gamse R, Molnár A, Lembeck F (1979 b) Substance P release from spinal cord slices by capsaicin. Life Sci 25:629–636

Gasparovic I, Hadvzovic S, Hukovic S, Stern P (1964) Contribution to the theory that substance P has a transmitter role in sensitive pathway. Med Exp 10:303–306

Giarman NJ, Tanaka C, Mooney J, Atkins E (1968) Serotonin, norepinephrine and fever. Adv Pharmacol 6A:307–317

Glatzel H (1968) Die Gewürze. Ihre Wirkungen auf den gesunden und kranken Menschen. Nicolaische Verlagsbuchhandlung, Herford

Göres E, Jung F (1959) Reizung von Gefäßrezeptoren durch Capsaicin. Acta Biol Med Ger 3:41–45

Govindarajan VS (1977) Pepper-chemistry, technology, and quality evaluation. CRC Crit Rev Food Sci Nutr 9:115–225

Gragg BG (1972) Plasticity of synapses. In: Bourne H (ed) The structure and function of nervous tissue, vol 4. Academic Press, New York, pp 2–60

Green DM, Tregear RT (1964) The action of sensory irritants on the cat's cornea. J Physiol (Lond) 175:37–38P

Guieu JD, Hardy JD (1970) Effects of heating and cooling of the spinal cord on preoptic unit activity. J Appl Physiol 29:675–683

Hegyes P, Földeák S (1974) Synthesis of homovanillic acid derivatives of capsaicin-like effect. Acta Phys Chim Szegediensis 20:115–120

Hellon RF (1970) The stimulation of hypothalamic neurones by changes in ambient temperature. Arch Gesamte Physiol Mens Tiere 321:56–66

Hellon RF (1975) Monoamines, pyrogens, and cations: their actions on central control of body temperature. Pharmacol Rev 26:289–321

Hensel H (1973) Neural processes in thermoregulation. Physiol Rev 53:948–1017

Hensel H, Zotterman Y (1952) The effect of menthol on the thermoreceptors. Acta Physiol Scand 24:27–34

Heubner W (1925) Zur Pharmakologie der Reizstoffe. Arch Exp Pathol Pharmakol 107:129–154

Heusner A (1956) Mise en évidence d'une variation nycthémérale de la calorification indépendante du cycle de l'activité chez le rat. CR Soc Biol (Paris) 150:1246–1248

Högyes A (1878) Beiträge zur physiologischen Wirkung der Bestandteile des Capsicum annuum. Arch Exp Pathol Pharmakol 9:117–130

Holzer P, Jurna I, Gamse R, Lembeck F (1979) Nociceptive threshold after neonatal capsaicin treatment. Eur J Pharmacol 58:511–514

Hori T (1980) The capsaicin desensitized rat: behavioral thermoregulation and thermosensitivity of hypothalamic neurons. In: Cox B, Lomax P, Milton AS, Schönbaum E (eds) Thermoregulatory mechanisms and their therapeuticum implications. Karger, Basel, pp 214–215

Hori T, Harada Y (1977) The effect of capsaicin on behavioral thermoregulation. J Physiol Soc Jpn 39:266–267

Hori T, Shinohara K (1978) Hypothalamic neurons responding to temperature in the newborn rat. In: Houdas Y, Guieu JD (eds) New trends in thermal physiology. Masson, Paris, pp 78–80

Hori T, Shinohara K (1979) Hypothalamic thermo-responsive neurones in the new-born rat. J Physiol (Lond) 294:541–560

Hori T, Tsuzuki S (1978a) Hypothermic responses to intrahypothalamic capsaicin in the new-born rat. Jpn J Biometeorol 15:8

Hori T, Tsuzuki S (1978b) Thermoregulation of rats desensitized by capsaicin in the early postnatal life. Jpn J Biometeorol 15:9

Horváth K, Jancsó G, Wollemann M (1979) The effect of calcium on the capsaicin activation of adenylate cyclase in rat brain. Brain Res 179:401–403

Iggo A, Ogawa H (1971) Primate cutaneous thermal nociceptors. J Physiol (Lond) 216:77–78 P

Issekutz B Jr, Lichtneckert I, Nagy H (1950a) Effect of capsaicin and histamine on heat regulation. Arch Int Pharmacodyn Ther 81:35–40

Issekutz B Jr, Lichtneckert I, Winter M (1950b) Effect of histamine, capsaicin, and procaine on heat-regulation. Arch Int Pharmacodyn Ther 83:319–326

Issekutz L, Hajdu P, Pórszász J (1955) Der Zusammenhang zwischen der brennenden Eigenschaft des Capsaicins und seiner Wirkung auf die Atmung und den Blutkreislauf. Acta Physiol Acad Sci Hung [Suppl] 6:107

Jancsó G (1978) Selective degeneration of chemosensitive primary sensory neurones induced by capsaicin glial changes. Cell Tissue Res 195:145–152

Jancsó G, Knyihár E (1975) Functional linkage between nociception and fluoride-resistant acid phosphatase activity in the Roland substance. Neurobiology 5:42–43

Jancsó G, Wollemann M (1977) The effect of capsaicin on the adenylate cyclase activity of rat brain. Brain Res 123:323–329

Jancsó G, Király E, Jancsó-Gábor A (1977) Pharmacologically induced selective degeneration of chemosensitive primary sensory neurones. Nature 270:741–743

Jancsó G, Sávay G, Király E (1978) Appearance of histochemically detectable ionic calcium in degenerating primary sensory neurons. Acta histochem (Jena) 52:165–169

Jancsó N (1947) Histamine as a physiological activator of the reticulo-endothelial system. Nature 160:227–228

Jancsó N (1955) Speicherung. Stoffanreicherung im Retikuloendothel und in der Niere. Akadémiai Kiadó, Budapest

Jancsó N (1960) Role of nerve terminals in the mechanism of inflammatory reactions. Bull Millard Fillmore Hosp 7:53–77

Jancsó N (1964) Neurogenic inflammatory responses. Acta Physiol Acad Sci Hung [Suppl] 24:3–4

Jancsó N (1965) Stimulation and desensitization of the heat-sensitive hypothalamic receptors by chemical agents. III. Hung. Conference on Therapy and Pharmacol. Res. 1964. Akadémiai Kiadó, Budapest, pp 23–39

Jancsó N (1968) Desensitization with capsaicin as a tool for studying the function of pain receptors. Proc Int Pharmacol Meet 9:33–55

Jancsó N, Jancsó-Gábor A (1949) Desensitization of sensory nerve endings (in Hungarian). Kisérl Orvostud [Suppl] 2:15

Jancsó N, Jancsó-Gábor A (1959) Dauerausschaltung der chemischen Schmerzempfindlichkeit durch Capsaicin. Naunyn-Schmiedeberg Arch Exp Pathol Pharmakol 236:142–145

Jancsó N, Jancsó-Gábor A (1965) Die Wirkungen des Capsaicins auf die hypothalamischen Thermoreceptoren. Naunyn-Schmiedeberg Arch Exp Pathol Pharmakol 251:136–137

Jancsó N, Jancsó-Gábor A, Takáts I (1961) Pain and inflammation induced by nicotine, acetylcholine and structurally-related compounds and their prevention by desensitizing agents. Acta Physiol Acad Sci Hung 19:113–132

Jancsó N, Jancsó-Gábor A, Szolcsányi J (1966) Effect of capsaicin on thermoregulation. Acta Physiol Acad Sci Hung 29:364

Jancsó N (the late), Jancsó-Gábor A, Szolcsányi J (1967) Direct evidence for neurogenic inflammation and its prevention by denervation and by pretreatment with capsaicin. Br J Pharmacol 31:138–151

Jancsó N (the late), Jancsó-Gábor A, Szolcsányi J (1968) The role of sensory nerve endings in neurogenic inflammation induced in human skin and in the eye and paw of the rat. Br J Pharmacol 33:32–41

Jancsó-Gábor A (1947) Some data to the pharmacology of histamine releasers (in Hungarian). D Pharm dissertation, Szeged

Jancsó-Gábor A (1976) Characteristics of the long-lasting "chemical analgesia" induced by capsaicin. In: Knoll J, Vizy E (eds) Symposium on analgesics. Akadémiai Kiadó, Budapest, pp 161–166

Jancsó-Gábor A (1980) Anaesthesia-like condition and/or potentiation of hexobarbital sleep produced by pungent agents in normal and capsaicin-desensitized rats. Acta Physiol Acad Sci Hung 55:57–62

Jancsó-Gábor A, Szolcsányi J (1969) The mechanism of neurogenic inflammation. In: Bertelli A, Houck JC (eds) Inflammation biochemistry and drug interaction. Excerpta Medica, Amsterdam, pp 210–217

Jancsó-Gábor A, Szolcsányi J (1970) Action of rare earth metal complexes on neurogenic as well as on bradykinin-induced inflammation. J Pharm Pharmacol 22:366–371

Jancsó-Gábor A, Szolcsányi J (1972) Neurogenic inflammatory responses. J Dent Res 41:264–269

Jancsó-Gábor A, Szolcsányi J, Jancsó N (the late) (1970) Irreversible impairment of thermoregulation induced by capsaicin and similar pungent substances in rats and guinea-pigs. J Physiol (Lond) 206:495–507

Jancsó-Gábor A, Szolcsányi J, Jancsó N (the late) (1970b) Stimulation and desensitization of the hypothalamic heat-sensitive structures by capsaicin in rats. J Physiol (Lond) 208:449–459

Jessell TM, Iversen LL, Cuello AC (1978) Capsaicin-induced depletion of substance P from primary sensory neurones. Brain Res 152:183–188

Joó F, Szolcsányi J, Jancsó-Gábor A (1969) Mitochondrial alterations in the spinal ganglion cells of the rat accompanying the long-lasting sensory disturbance induced by capsaicin. Life Sci 8:621–626

Keele CA (1962) The common chemical sense and its receptors. Arch Int Pharmacodyn Ther 139:547–557

Keele CA, Armstrong D (1964) Substances producing pain and itch. Arnold, London

Kiernan JA (1977) A study of chemically induced acute inflammation in the skin of the rat. QJ Exp Physiol 62:151–161

Lee TS (1954) Physiological gustatory sweating in a warm climate. J Physiol (Lond) 124:528–542

Lembeck F, Gamse R, Juan H (1977) Substance P and sensory nerve endings. In: Euler US, Pernow B (eds) Substance P. Raven, New York, pp 169–181

Lembeck F, Holzer P (1979) Substance P as neurogenic mediator of antidromic vasodilation and neurogenic plasma extravasation. Naunyn-Schmiedeberg Arch Pharmacol 310:175–183

Liebermeister C (1875) Handbuch der Pathologie und Therapie des Fiebers. Vogel, Leipzig

Lim RKS, Liu CN, Guzman F, Braun C (1962) Visceral receptors concerned in visceral pain and the pseudoaffective response to intraarterial injection of bradykinin and other algesic agents. J Comp Neurol 118:269–294

List PH, Hackenberger H (1973) Die scharf schmeckenden Stoffe von Lactarius vellereus Fries. Z Pilzkd 39:97–102

Luckner R, Toth L, Luckner M (1969) Vorschläge für den Drogenteil des DAB 7. 44. Mitt.: Fructus capsici. Pharm Zentralhalle 108:1–11

Lynn B (1977) Cutaneous hyperalgesia. Br Med Bull 33:103–108

Makara GB (1970) Superficial and deep chemonociception: differential inhibition by pretreatment with capsaicin. Acta Physiol Acad Sci Hung 38:393–399

Makara G, Csalay L, Frenkl R, Somfai ZS (1965) The effect of serotonin following desensitization with capsaicin. Acta Physiol Acad Sci Hung 27:21–25

Makara GB, György L, Molnár J (1967a) Circulatory and respiratory responses to capsaicin, 5-hydroxytryptamine in rats pretreated with capsaicin. Arch Int Pharmacodyn Ther 170:39–45

Makara GB, Stark E, Mihály K (1967b) Sites at which formalin and capsaicin act to stimulate corticotropin secretion. Can J Physiol 45:669–674

Martin HF III, Manning JW (1969) Rapid thermal cutaneous stimulation: peripheral nerve responses. Brain Res 16:524–526

Meeter E (1973) The functional significance of the cholinergic synapses responsible for carbachol hypothermia in the rat. In: Schönbaum E, Lomax P (eds) The pharmacology of thermoregulation. Basel, Karger, pp 492–498

Milton AS (1976) Modern views on the pathogenesis of fever and the mode of action of antipyretic drugs. J Pharm Pharmacol 28:393–399

Milton AS, Dascombe MJ (1977) Cyclic nucleotides in thermoregulation and fever. In: Cooper KE, Lomas P, Schönbaum E (eds) Drugs, biogenic amines and body temperature. Basel, Karger, pp 129–135

Milton AS, Wendlandt S (1971) Effects on body temperature of prostaglandins of the A, E, and F series on injection into the third ventricle of unanaesthetized cats and rabbits. J Physiol (Lond) 218:325–336

Mitchell JH, Gupta DN, Barnett SE (1967) Reflex cardiovascular responses elicited by stimulation of receptor sites with pharmacological agents. Circ Res 20:I-193–201

Mitchell D, Snellen JW, Atkins AR (1970) Thermoregulation during fever: change of set point or change of gain. Pfluegers Arch 321:292–302

Molnár J (1965) Die pharmakologischen Wirkungen des Capsaicins, des scharf schmeckenden Wirkstoffes im Paprika. Arzneim Forsch 15:718–727

Molnár J (1966) Effect of capsaicin on the cat's nictitating membrane. Acta Physiol Acad Sci Hung 30:183–192

Molnár J, György L (1967) Pulmonary hypertensive and other haemodynamic effects of capsaicin in the cat. Eur J Pharmacol 1:86–92

Molnár J, György L, Unyi G, Kenyeres J (1969) Effect of capsaicin on the isolated ileum and auricle of the guinea pig. Acta Physiol Acad Sci Hung 35:369–374

Molnár J, Makara G, György L, Unyi G (1969) The bronchoconstrictor action of capsaicin in the guinea pig. Acta Physiol Acad Sci Hung 36:413–420

Mrosovsky N (1974) Natural and experimental hypothalamic changes in hibernators. In: Lederis K, Cooper KE (eds) Recent studies of hypothalamic function. Karger, Basel, pp 251–267

Murakami N (1973) Effects of iontophoretic application of 5-hydroxytryptamine, noradrenaline and acetylcholine upon hypothalamic temperature-sensitive neurones in rats. Jpn J Physiol 23:435–446

Murakami N, Stolwijk JAJ, Hardy JD (1967) Responses of preoptic neurons to anesthetics and peripheral stimulation. Am J Physiol 213:1015–1024

Myers RD, Yaksh TL (1968) Feeding and temperature responses in the unrestrained rat after injections of cholinergic and aminergic substances into the cerebral ventricles. Physiol Behav 3:917–928

Nakayama T (1976) Hypothalamic and brainstem control of temperature regulation. In: Bhathia B, Chhina GS, Singh B (eds) Selected topics in environmental biology. Interprint, New Delhi, pp 37–40

Nakayama T, Suzuki M, Ishizuka N (1975) Action of progesterone on preoptic thermosensitive neurones. Nature 258:80

Nakayama T, Hori Y, Suzuki M, Yonezawa T, Yamamoto K (1978a) Thermo-sensitive neurons in preoptic and anterior hypothalamic tissue cultures in vitro. Neurosci Lett 9:23–26

Nakayama T, Suzuki M, Ishikawa Y Nishio A (1978b) Effects of capsaicin on hypothalamic thermo-sensitive neurons in the rat. Neurosci Lett 7:151–155

Nakayama T, Arai S, Yamamoto K (1979) Body temperature rhythm and its central mechanism. In: Suda M, Hayaishi O, Nakagawa H (eds) Biological rhythms and their central mechanism. Elsevier/North-Holland, Amsterdam, pp 395–403

Newman AA (1953a) Natural and synthetic pepper-flavoured substances (1). Chem Products (Lond) 16:343–345

Newman AA (1953 b) Natural and synthetic pepper-flavoured substances (2). Chemistry of the active principles of piper nigrum. Chem Products (Lond) 16:379–382

Newman AA (1953 c) Natural and synthetic pepper-flavoured substances (3). Chemistry of capsaicin, the pungen principle of the capsicum peppers. Chem Products (Lond) 16:413–417

Newman AA (1953 d) Natural and synthetic pepper-flavoured substances. (4). Synthetic substitutes. Chem Products (Lond) 16:467–471

Newman AA (1954 a) Natural and synthetic pepper-flavoured substances (5). Pungency and structure relationships. Chem Products (Lond) 17:14–18

Newman AA (1954 b) Natural and synthetic pepper-flavoured substances (6). Collective list. Chem Products (Lond) 17:102–106

Nopanitaya W Nye SW (1974) Duodenal mucosal response to the pungent principle of hot pepper (capsaicin) in the rat: light and electron microscopic study. Toxicol Appl Pharmacol 30:149–161

Obál F Jr, Benedek G, Jancsó-Gábor A, Obál F (1979) Salivary cooling, escape reaction and heat pain in capsaicin-desensitized rats. Pfluegers Arch 382:249–254

Osadchii LI, Balueva TV, Molnár J (1967) Reflex changes in systemic vascular resistance following intracoronary injection of capsaicin and veratrine in the cat. Acta Physiol Acad Sci Hung 32:215–219

Paintal AS (1977) Thoracic receptors connected with sensation. Br Med Bull 33:169–174

Perl ER (1976) Sensitization of nociceptors and its relation to sensation. Adv Pain Res Ther 1:17–28

Pórszász J, Jancsó N (1959) Studies on the action potentials of sensory nerves in animals desensitized with capsaicin. Acta Physiol Acad Sci Hung 16:229–306

Pórszász J, György L, Pórszász-Gibiszer K (1955) Cardiovascular and respiratory effects of capsaicin. Acta Physiol Acad Sci Hung 8:61–76

Pórszász J, Such GY, Pórszász-Gibiszer K (1957) Circulatory and respiratory chemoreflexes I. Analysis of the site of action and receptor types of capsaicin. Acta Physiol Acad Sci Hung 12:189–205

Reid WD, Volicer L, Smookler H, Beavan MA, Brodie BB (1968) Brain amines and temperature regulation. Pharmacology 1:329–344

Riccioppo Neto F, Corradi AP, Rocha e Silva M (1974) Apnea, bradycardia, hypothension and muscular contraction induced by intracarotid injection of bradykinin. J Pharmacol Exp Ther 190:316–326

Russell JA, Lai-Fook SJ (1979) Reflex bronchoconstriction induced by capsaicin in the dog J Appl Physiol 47:961–967

Sanoilenko AV (1970) Local responses of the resistance vessels during chemoreflexes from various parts of intestine. Fiziol Zh SSSR IM I M Sechenova 56:1227–1232

Schoener EP, Wang SC (1975) Leukocytic pyrogen and sodium acetylsalicylate on hypothalamic neurons in the cat. Am J Physiol 229:185–190

Smith JG Jr, Crounse RG, Spence D (1970) The effects of capsaicin on human skin, liver and epidermal lyososomes. J Invest Dermatol 54:170–173

Stary Z (1925) Über Erregung der Wärmenerven durch Pharmaka. Arch Exp Pathol Pharmakol 105:76–87

Sticher O, Soldati F, Joshi RK (1978) Hochleistungsflüssigkeitschromatographische Trennung und quantitative Bestimmung von Capsaicin, Dihydrocapsaicin, Nordihydrocapsaicin und Homodihydrocapsaicin in natürlichen Capsaicinoid-Gemischen und Fructus capsici. J Chromatogr 166:221–231

Szebeni A, Jancsó G, Wollemann M (1978) Capsaicin receptor binding. Acta Physiol Acad Sci Hung 60:193

Székely M, Szolcsányi J (1979) Endotoxin fever in capsaicin treated rats. Acta Physiol Acad Sci Hung 53:469–477

Széki T (1936) Vizsgálatok a füszerhatású vegyületek köréböl. Math Naturw Anzeiger Ung Akad Wissenschaft 54:807–814

Szolcsányi J (1967) Investigation on the metabolic rate in capsaicin desensitized rats. Acta Physiol Acad Sci Hung [Suppl] 32:108

Szolcsányi J (1975) Analysis of the mechanism of sensory and neuroregulatory functions by means of capsaicin and its congeners (in Hungarian). CSc thesis, Pécs

Szolcsányi J (1976) On the specificity of pain producing and sensory neuron blocking effect of capsaicin. In: Knoll J, Vizi E (eds) Symposium on analgesics. Akadémiai Kiadó, Budapest, pp 167–172

Szolcsányi J (1977a) A pharmacological approach to elucidation of the role of different nerve fibres and receptor endings in mediation of pain. J Physiol (Paris) 73:251–259

Szolcsányi J (1977b) The local efferent function of capsaicin-sensitive C-nociceptors. Proc IUPS Paris 13:736

Szolcsányi J (1978) Drug influences on behavioural thermoregulation in the rat. Acta Physiol Acad Sci Hung 51:199–200

Szolcsányi J, Barthó L (1978) New type of nerve-mediated cholinergic contractions of the guinea-pig small intestine and its selective blockade by capsaicin. Naunyn-Schmiedeberg Arch Pharmacol 305:83–90

Szolcsányi J, Barthó L (1979) Capsaicin-sensitive innervation of the guinea-pig taenia caeci. 309:77–82

Szolcsányi J, Jancsó-Gábor A (1973) Capsaicin and other pungent agents as pharmacological tools in studies on thermoregulation. In: Schönbaum E, Lomax P (eds) The pharmacology of thermoregulation. Basel, Karger, pp 395–409

Szolcsányi J, Jancsó-Gábor A (1975a) Analysis of the role of warmth detectors by means of capsaicin under different conditions. In: Lomax P, Schönbaum E, Jacob J (eds) Temperature regulation and drug action. Basel, Karger, pp 331–338

Szolcsányi J, Jancsó-Gábor A (1975b) Sensory effects of capsaicin congeners I. Relationship between chemical structure and pain producing potency of pungent agents. Arzneim Forsch 25:1877–1881

Szolcsányi J, Jancsó-Gábor A (1976) Sensory effects of capsaicin congeners II. Importance of chemical structure and pungency in desensitizing activity of capsaicin-type compounds. Arzneim Forsch 26:33–37

Szolcsányi J, Jánossy T (1971) Mechanism of the circulatory and respiratory reflexes evoked by pungent agents. Acta Physiol Acad Sci Hung 39:260–261

Szolcsányi J, Joó F, Jancsó-Gábor A (1971) Mitochondrial changes in preoptic neurones after capsaicin desensitization of the hypothalamic thermodetectors in rats. Nature 229:116–117

Szolcsányi J, Jancsó-Gábor A, Joó F (1975) Functional and fine structural characteristics of the sensory neuron blocking effect of capsaicin. Naunyn-Schmiedeberg Arch Exp Pharmacol 287:157–163

Szolcsányi J, Gábor JA, Salamon I (1976) Vascular permeability-increasing effect of electrical stimulation of peripheral nerves, sensory ganglia and spinal roots. Acta Physiol Acad Sci Hung 47:255

Theriault E, Otsuka M, Jessell T (1979) Capsaicin-evoked release of substance P from primary sensory neurons. Brain Res 170:209–213

Toda N, Usui H, Nishino H, Fujiwara M (1972) Cardiovascular effects of capsaicin in dogs and rabbits. J Pharmacol Exp Ther 181:512–521

Toh CC, Lee TS, Kiang AK (1955) The pharmacological actions of capsaicin and analogues. Br J Pharmacol 10:175–182

Torebjörk HE, Hallin RG (1974) Identification of afferent C units in intact human skin nerves. Brain Res 67:387–403

Van Zoeren JG, Stricker EM (1976) Thermal homeostasis in rats after intrahypothalamic injections of 6-hydroxydopamine. Am J Physiol 230:932–939

Virus RM, Gebhart GF (1979) Pharmacological actions of capsaicin: apparent involvement of substance P and serotonin. Life Sci 25:1273–1284

Webb-Peploe MM, Brender D, Shepherd JT (1972) Vascular responses to stimulation of receptors in muscle by capsaicin. Am J Physiol 222:189–195

Wit A, Wang SC (1968a) Temperature-sensitive neurons in preoptic/anterior hypothalamic region: effects of increasing ambient temperature. Am J Physiol 215:1151–1159

Wit A, Wang SC (1968b) Temperature-sensitive neurons in preoptic/anterior hypothalamic region: actions of pyrogen and acetylsalicylate. Am J Physiol 215:1160–1169

Yaksh TL, Farb DH, Leeman SE, Jessell TM (1979) Intrathecal capsaicin depletes substance P in the rat spinal cord and produces prolonged thermal analgesia. Science 206:481–483

CHAPTER 15

The Pathophysiology of Fever in the Neonate*

M. Székely and Z. Szelényi

A. Introduction

The development of a raised body temperature as a frequent accompaniment to many diseases has been known for a long time. The generally accepted view is that fever is a rise in deep-body temperature resulting from a change in its central control, which change can most conveniently be described as an upward re-setting of the so-called thermostat in the hypothalamus. This set-point elevation is thought to result from the action of some exogenous pyrogens, which release endogenous pyrogen from various cellular elements of the body. This in turn acts on structures of the central nervous system (CNS) responsible for the control of body temperature. It has been repeatedly shown that during fever body temperature is still *regulated* but at a higher level than normal, and various responses of the thermoregulatory effector mechanisms to thermal stimuli can still be observed in this state. In a recent volume of this series two reviews discussed several problems of fever genesis and antipyresis (FELDBERG and MILTON 1979; ROSENDORFF and WOOLF 1979).

For obvious reasons, most of the data available about the details of the mechanism of fever have come either from experience gained in adult humans with clinical fever or from studies on experimental fever reactions evoked in adults of various mammalian species. In both cases the characterization of the fever response has been based on the analysis of changes in body temperature and thermoregulatory functions developing during fever as compared with body temperature and the functioning of heat production/heat loss effector mechanisms observed under basal conditions (i.e. before the onset of disease or the injection of a pyrogen). Apparently, the development of the febrile rise in body temperature is the result of an increase in heat production and heat conservation, the changes in these two effector mechanisms mostly occurring simultaneously in the chill phase of fever. The extent of the contribution of increased heat production and decreased heat dissipation may vary depending on the environmental conditions and the species under study (STITT 1979).

The available evidence on the presence and nature of fever in the neonate of different species can be reviewed only if salient characteristics of temperature regulation of the newborn are also summarized briefly. Recent experimental results regarding the possible role of central mediators or modulators[1] in the development of fever in adult homeotherms are applicable to the neonate only to a limited ex-

---

* Manuscript closed: February 1979
1 For the sake of simplicity, the terms "mediator" and "modulator" will be used interchangably throughout this review without referring to a specific action at neuronal level

tent. Therefore, some new data on central effects of monoamines and other modulator substances in the newborn will be included in the following discussions. Data on febrile states occurring in human infants during infections and other pathological conditions will also be surveyed. Finally, a detailed analysis of recent results on experimental neonatal fever, its possible interpretations and relevance to pyrogen effects in the human neonate will be made.

B. Characteristics of Temperature Regulation in the Newborn

The essential feature of temperature regulation in homeothermic species is the fine balance of heat production and heat loss over a fairly large range of thermal environmental conditions. Information on the temperature of many, if not all, body sites including the skin, vital internal organs, and the CNS comes from thermoreceptors and is continuously being fed into thermointegrative structures residing mainly in the hypothalamus. Qualitatively and quantitatively appropriate output signals of central origin, reaching the peripheral thermoregulatory effectors, will evoke changes in heat production and heat dissipation in order to counterbalance the thermal load imposed on the body.

Stability of deep-body temperature is of prime importance in adult homeotherms, enabling them to perform the many complicated functions necessary to maintain life. Depending on the species, the ability to maintain the constancy of body temperature develops gradually during ontogenesis; examples ranging from the newborn lamb with a complete set of appropriate thermoregulatory mechanisms permitting homeothermy (DAWES and MOTT 1959; MERCER 1974; ALEXANDER 1975), to the newborn rat behaving almost like a poikilothermic animal (TAYLOR 1960), may be mentioned.

Detailed descriptions of current knowledge on thermoregulation of the newborn can be found in excellent recent reviews (HEY 1972; ALEXANDER 1975; BRÜCK 1978 a, b; MESTYÁN 1978). Accordingly, only those aspects of temperature regulation which are more closely related to the question of fever as it occurs in the neonate will be considered here.

I. Heat Production

Resting metabolic rate expressed on a body weight basis has been shown to be higher in the neonate than in adults of the same species, at least from the first week of extrauterine life onwards. Immediately after birth values of resting metabolic rate are reportedly lower than those measured later in the newborn period. Although no satisfactory explanation has been put forward for this early depression of metabolism or for its rapid rise, these phenomena may be linked to maturity, nutritional state, or other factors, such as post-partum cold-exposure (ANDREWS and SZÉKELY unpublished).

On exposure to an ambient temperature (T_a) below thermoneutrality, virtually all the species so far studied are already able to increase their metabolism well above the resting rate early in the newborn period. Metabolic responses to cold vary in extent in the newborn but may approach a level similar to that of the adults, at least in some species (ALEXANDER 1975; BRÜCK 1978a). While in adults the quantitatively most important mode of producing additional heat in a cold environment is held to be shivering, the newborn of many species produce thermoregulatory heat preferentially by non-shivering means. Non-shivering heat production is mediated by the sympathetic nervous system. This is evident from the finding that peripheral injection of noradrenaline (NA) evokes a large rise in oxygen consumption in the majority of species soon after birth without any measurable shivering activity (MOORE and UNDERWOOD 1960; KARLBERG et al. 1962; SCOPES and TIZARD 1963). The site of non-shivering thermogenesis has been localized to brown adipose tissue (see LINDBERG 1970), skeletal muscle (see JANSKY 1973), and some internal organs such as the brain (DONHOFFER and SZELÉNYI 1975; SZELÉNYI and DONHOFFER 1978). In addition, non-shivering thermogenesis is presumed to be more efficient than shivering, and this would appear to be favourable for the newborn with its relatively large surface/weight ratio. The latter feature promotes passive dissipation of heat to a greater extent, especially during cold-exposure.

II. Heat Loss

Defence against extreme thermal conditions may be assisted by appropriate modifications of heat dissipating mechanisms at both ends of the thermoneutral zone. In the human newborn vigorous vasomotor reactions have been shown to operate in reducing heat loss in cool environments and active vasodilatation is also available for increasing heat loss; vasodilatation has, however, a higher threshold core temperature for full activation during early extrauterine development than later in infancy (BRÜCK 1961). Local warming of the skin of human neonates (15 h old) evoked steep rises in skin blood flow (BRÜCK 1961). The presence and functioning of vasomotor regulation during thermoregulation may, however, be absent immediately after birth in very small animals such as the rabbit (JÁRAI 1969) and the rat (POCZOPKO 1961).

Although the human newborn exhibits very sensitive sweating responses on exposure to warm environments (SULYOK et al. 1973), the maximum amount of heat lost in this way may be considerably lower when compared with that lost by the adult human. The newborn seems less able to maintain constant body temperature during warm- and cold-exposure despite possessing virtually all the mechanisms for losing or conserving heat shortly after birth. In addition, the newborn can survive a much lower body temperature than adults; for hyperthermic tolerance no such difference has been reported (BRÜCK 1978a, b).

III. "Normal" Body Temperature

The preceding sections have mentioned the tendency of the newborn to develop hypothermia or hyperthermia on exposure to relatively mild cold or warm environments, respectively. The terms hypothermia and hyperthermia imply that there should also be some narrow range of deep-body temperature for the newborn, as for the adult, which would be most favourable for bodily functions and development. Immediately after birth body temperature of the newborn infant falls rapidly to values sometimes as low as 34.4°–35.0 °C in the usual thermal conditions of the delivery room, but in premature infants even lower values of body temperature may be encountered (Motil and Blackburn 1973). It has also been shown that, especially in premature infants, mortality rate is increased when the babies are kept at low T_a. This would mean that some low levels of body temperature present a definite disadvantage to the newborn.

Nevertheless, in comparison with adults, the range of normal body temperature may be larger in the newborn. Small and young premature infants may experience a fall in rectal temperature to a value approaching 35 °C without an increase in metabolic rate (Brück and Brück 1960). Furthermore, these babies spent quite a long time in quiet sleep without any sign of discomfort. The same authors also observed that during the first hours of life thermoregulatory heat production did not occur until rectal temperature fell below 34.5 °C. On the next day this rectal temperature threshold rose in the same babies. A similar extension of the "normal" body temperature towards higher values has not been observed in the human neonate.

In the adult guinea-pig the so-called interthreshold zone (i.e. the zone between threshold temperatures for shivering and for eliciting a rise in respiratory frequency) broadened markedly after adaptation to intermittent exposures to cold and warmth (Brück et al. 1970). By this analogy, it has been supposed by the same authors that in the newborn period there may be a transient state in thermoregulation resembling the phenomenon of adaptation, which would allow the infant to change its body temperature over a large range according to the thermal environment without the need to use thermoregulatory heat production or heat loss effectors.

The results obtained in neonates of other species exposed to cold are in keeping with the larger range of body temperature found in the human newborn. Newborn rats and rabbits, species known to be born at a rather immature state, have been shown to respond to cold-exposure with greater falls of colonic temperature immediately after birth than later in ontogenesis. More specifically, on exposure to mild cold, body temperature may fall considerably, a finding which might be explained by their small metabolic response at this T_a. When exposed to more severe cold they could, however, further increase their metabolism, indicating that the metabolic capacity had not been exhausted during exposure to mild cold (Várnai and Donhoffer 1970; Várnai et al. 1970). These findings may indicate that the relatively larger changes of body temperature may be manifestations of some regulation specific to the newborn period. In other words, it might be speculated that, for a given input of thermal stimuli, the thermoregulatory output may be lower than the one usually observed in homeothermic adults. This characteristic of the newborn is not limited to immaturity but can also be observed in more mature neonates such as the guinea-pig (Farkas et al. 1974). Some adult guinea-pigs have also been shown to exhibit this regulatory behaviour during exposure to various cold stimuli (Farkas et al. 1974).

In parallel with the reduced ability of the neonate to conserve heat at cold T_a, the efficiency of heat loss effectors at slightly warm T_a is also limited, and this may contribute to a higher incidence of hyperthermia. Indeed, even older children may run the risk of convulsions at body temperatures which would be easily tolerated by adults (see Chap. 18).

IV. Immaturity and Malnutrition

The lability of body temperature of premature human infants manifests itself mostly as hypothermia, although the tendency to develop a hyperthermic rise in body temperature at a T_a slightly above thermoneutrality has also been known for a long time (BLACKFAN and YAGLOU 1933).

Threshold body temperatures of premature human infants have been studied at both ends of the thermoneutral zone. Small infants (1–2 kg body weight) had a higher threshold for eliciting cutaneous heat dissipation than larger babies (HEY and KATZ 1970). Threshold body temperature for sweating was high in premature infants and decreased during the first few post-natal days (HEY and KATZ 1969). In a more recent investigation a slight but distinct rise of threshold oesophageal temperature was demonstrated for increased evaporative heat loss in small-for-dates and premature human infants when compared with full-term ones (SULYOK et al. 1973). In marasmic children exposure to a T_a of 38 °C at low humidity led to a marked rise in rectal temperature. After recovery no such rise in rectal temperature was observed in a similar warm environment (BROOKE and SALVOSA 1974).

The increased threshold for heat loss effector function and a decreased threshold for heat production effectors in immature and small infants might be interpreted as obvious signs of immaturity or deficiency of thermoregulatory mechanisms either centrally or peripherally or both. However, some data would allow an alternative explanation for the lability of body temperature found in the immature and malnourished newborn. In a study on human neonates it has been shown that hypothermic body temperatures may develop at low T_a without an increase or decrease in heat production. The former would imply that there was an inability to produce extra heat, the latter seems to show that this lack of metabolic response to cold may even be of an adaptive nature. Indeed, a further fall in body temperature below 33°–34 °C evoked a rise in oxygen consumption in these babies (HEY 1972). In marasmic Jamaican infants body temperatures at or below 35 °C were frequently encountered under moderately cool thermal conditions, suggesting that these infants might have developed hypothermia as a means of conserving calories (BROOKE 1972). BROOKE et al. (1973) demonstrated a further fall of body temperature at a T_a of 25 °C, which was due to the depletion of fat in brown adipose tissue in these marasmic children.

Under experimental conditions malnutrition has been shown to result in adaptive changes in thermoregulation. Adult semi-starved rats exposed to moderately cold T_a allowed their colonic temperature to fall with only a slight rise in metabolism. In more severe cold a larger rise in oxygen consumption led to stabilization of deep-body temperature at a lower level, demonstrating that the diminished increase in oxygen consumption at a T_a just below thermoneutrality was not due to an inability to produce heat (HEIM et al. 1964). Similar results have been obtained in 16- to 23-day-old rats semi-starved since birth and acutely exposed to cool T_a of 30° and 20 °C, except that in these young animals colonic temperature continued to fall at a T_a of 20 °C despite the rise in oxygen consumption being greater than at a T_a of 30 °C (HEIM and SZELÉNYI 1965). BIGNALL et al. (1974) observed a reduction of oxygen consumption in 5- to 12-day-old starved rats exposed to cold. They interpreted this finding as being the consequence of active suppression of metabolism by the CNS under the special conditions of starvation plus cold-exposure. In support of this hypothesis these authors argued that oxygen consumption was held constant and at a higher value in thermoneutrality than at a cold T_a.

While the fairly large range of body temperature observed in the newborn, particularly under conditions of immaturity and starvation, may suggest some kind of regulation, it does not tell us anything about the peripheral or central mechanisms responsible. Clinical experience indicates that extreme and long-term shifts of body temperature both in the hypothermic and in the hyperthermic range occurring shortly after birth will endanger life of the newborn infant. On the other hand, the opinion expressed by HEY may be quoted here, in that "a limited and controlled change in body temperature during thermal stress would help to conserve water and energy reserves, and it is just possible that a dampened response is a physiological adaptation of some value" (HEY 1972).

C. Central Mechanisms of Body Temperature Control

CNS structures play an important role in processing thermal signals coming from the periphery and also from CNS sites themselves such as the hypothalamus, spinal cord, and brain-stem. A wealth of literature is available on thermoregulatory responses evoked by monoamines and other modulators of CNS functions after central application (reviewed by HELLON 1975). When comparing temperature control of the newborn with that of the adult, it seems pertinent to gather the limited experimental evidence obtained so far on central mechanisms of temperature regulation in the newborn.

I. Central Thermosensitivity

Neonatal guinea-pigs have been shown to possess heat-sensitive structures in rostral hypothalamic sites, the stimulation of which leads to a depression of heat production evoked by acute cold-exposure. In young guinea-pigs spinal cord heating inhibited shivering, while hypothalamic heating preferentially blocked brown fat thermogenesis (ZEISBERGER and BRÜCK 1971).

Direct demonstration of thermosensitive elements in the CNS of newborn animals has so far been made in rabbits and rats. In rabbits aged more than 8 days some thermosensitive thalamic units were found, mainly with characteristics of interneurones (HENDERSON et al. 1971). In newborn rats HORI and SHINOHARA (1978) studied 332 hyothalamic units. Out of these, 59 units were found to be heat-sensitive and 7 other units showed a thermal sensitivity characteristic of the cold-sensitive units. In the same study, 3 warm-sensitive units exhibited an increased firing rate after a subcutaneous injection of capsaicin, and thereby provided evidence in support of hypothalamic thermosensitivity in a species which is born in a rather immature state.

This information is too limited to allow a comparison between the newborn and the adult regarding their central thermosensitivities.

II. Thermoregulatory Effects Evoked by Centrally Applied Monoamines

The presence of monoamines, such as NA and 5-hydroxytryptamine (5-HT), as well as the enzymes for their synthesis and breakdown has been demonstrated in the brains of neonates of different species. During development the concentrations of various monoamines – modulators of CNS functions – have been found to increase in the brains of cats (PSCHEIDT and HIMWICH 1966), rats (KARKI et al. 1962; LOIZOU and SALT 1970; LOIZOU 1972; COYLE and HENRY 1973), and rabbits (KARKI et al. 1962; MCCAMAN and APRISON 1964; PSCHEIDT and HIMWICH 1966), while in the brain of the newborn guinea-pig the amine levels are similar to those of the adults (KARKI et al. 1962). In the newborn rat the monoamine-containing neurones are differentiated biochemically before the completion of their morphological development (LOIZOU 1972). Despite the low level of NA in the rat and kitten hypothalami, the lower activity of enzymes degrading this amine may even result in a greater effectiveness of the locally released NA in the newborn than in the adult (TORDA 1977).

Thermoregulatory responses to centrally injected amines have been studied also in some newborn animals. The mammalian young so far investigated in some detail are the rabbit, rat, guinea-pig, kitten, and the lamb.

In the adult rabbit and guinea-pig intracerebroventricular (ICV) or hypothalamic injection of NA led to rises in heat production and/or body temperature at a thermoneutral T_a (see HELLON 1975). Neonates of these two species responded similarly to centrally applied NA, but in rabbits the extent of thermogenic responses declined with age (KOMÁROMI et al. 1969a). In the newborn guinea-pig hypothalamic injection of NA led to a thermogenic reaction only when the injection was made into a circumscribed area, a site different from the thermosensitive preoptic region (ZEISBERGER and BRÜCK 1971). In the same species there is evidence for a thermoregulatory connection between the lower brain-stem and this NA-sensitive hypothalamic area (SZELÉNYI et al. 1976). Several lines of evidence indicate that the thermogenic response to intrahypothalamic or ICV-injected NA is mediated by α-adrenoceptors in the neonatal guinea-pig (SZELÉNYI et al. 1977, KOMÁROMI 1977b) as in adults (ZEISBERGER and BRÜCK 1976).

Newborn rats exhibited a fall in oxygen consumption on central application of NA (TIRRI 1971), but the large dose of NA injected and the cold T_a applied may involve similar problems to those encountered in the case of the adult rat. Small doses of NA elicited a rise in body temperature in the adult rat; high doses led, however, to hypothermia (see HELLON 1975). In newborn lambs intrahypothalamic injection of NA evoked a fall in body temperature at a cold T_a but not at thermoneutrality (COOPER et al. 1976; PITTMAN et al. 1977). Newborn kittens (SZÉKELY 1979c), like adult cats (see HELLON 1975), responded to ICV-injected NA with a fall in colonic temperature.

In the newborn guinea-pig, injection of 5-HT into the lateral cerebral ventricle resulted in an initial fall of body temperature followed by a sustained rise (KOMÁROMI 1976), oxygen consumption showing parallel changes. The late rise in body temperature after 5-HT injection could be mediated by increased prostaglandin synthesis, since it was blocked by indomethacin pre-treatment (SZÉKELY 1978b). In the neonatal rabbit, ICV-injection of 5-HT caused a rapid and short-term fall in oxygen consumption from high values evoked by cold-exposure to levels corresponding to the resting metabolic rate, a response of the metabolic rate being seen only in rabbits older than 12–13 days. At a thermoneutral T_a no change in oxygen consumption could be observed in these neonatal rabbits (Szelényi and Moore 1980).

In the newborn lamb, ICV-injection of 5-HT affected body temperature only in the cold, i.e. heat loss increased and body temperature declined (Cooper et al. 1976).

It has been reported that the newborn rat responds with a fall of body temperature to an ICV-injection of 5-HT in a cold environment (Komáromi et al. 1969 b; Tirri 1971). Newborn kittens show rises of body temperature after ICV-injected 5-HT given at thermoneutrality (Székely 1978 b). The two latter responses are similar to those observed in the two species during adulthood (see Hellon 1975). In newborn kittens the hyperthermic response of body temperature to 5-HT developed in two phases interrupted by a transient decline up to the pre-injection level about 90 min after injection. The late, but not the first, rise in colonic temperature might have been mediated by an increased prostaglandin synthesis, since the late rise could be blocked by indomethacin pre-treatment (Székely 1978 b).

Central injection of cholinomimetic drugs decreases both body temperature and oxygen consumption in the neonatal guinea-pig exposed to cold (Zeisberger and Brück 1973; Komáromi 1976). γ-Aminobutyric acid when given into the lateral cerebral ventricle of the newborn rabbit and guinea-pig elicits rises in oxygen consumption and body temperature at a thermoneutral T_a (Komáromi et al. 1969 a; Komáromi 1976).

Taken collectively, the available evidence indicates that essentially the same thermoregulatory responses as observed later in ontogenesis can be evoked in newborn animals after central administration of the various modulator substances. If these modulators play an important role in central temperature control of the adult homeothermic mammals, this regulatory role seems to be already available at the very onset of extrauterine life, although its quantitative importance cannot be judged at present.

Since thermoregulatory effects of centrally injected prostaglandins are more closely related to the subject of experimental fever, they will be discussed in Sect. F.

D. Fever in the Human Neonate

On the basis of present day knowledge of neonatal temperature regulation, as summarized briefly in Sects. B and C, it is evident that at a quite early stage of extrauterine development central as well as peripheral mechanisms are already functioning in a more-or-less efficient way. In addition, complicating factors, such as immaturity and malnutrition can also affect thermoregulation but do not result in clear-cut deficiencies of body temperature control which would leave the newborn entirely helpless under the changing conditions of the environment.

Since body temperature of the healthy neonate may fluctuate within a somewhat larger range than usually encountered in homeothermic adults, it is difficult to define those high body temperatures which can be considered as hyperthermic or febrile levels.

I. Definition

The question of fever in the newborn is of utmost clinical interest for many reasons. First of all, fever in the newborn, as in adult patients, has always been regarded as one of the signs of many diseases, although it has been a general experience that fever may be frequently lacking in the early period of extrauterine life (EPSTEIN et al. 1951; MARZETTI et al. 1973; KORÁNYI 1978; DAUM and SMITH 1979). Another source of interest stems from the necessity to reduce febrile levels of body temperature in infants, since clinical complications of high body temperature have been frequently encountered both in fever and hyperthermia.

Reports on fever or pyrexia of the human neonate abound with differences or even uncertainties concerning the definition of fever either in qualitative or quantitative terms, or both. In many cases it is difficult to decide whether obviously high body temperatures in the neonate represent a fever in the classical sense of an increased set-point temperature brought about by changes in central regulation (i.e. primary disturbance of the CNS or the influence of pyrogens on CNS structures), or whether they are merely manifestations of hyperthermia resulting from changes in the peripheral mechanisms of heat loss and/or heat production or from extreme heat stress. Even when there is no question about the central origin of high body temperature, the evaluation of the actual level of body temperature may pose a problem.

As in adults, fever in the newborn is expected to develop as a result of bacterial or viral infections. Since infections, as judged by bacteraemia, can frequently occur from the very beginning of extrauterine life, the presence of bacterial or viral pyrogens may also be hypothesized. For obvious ethical reasons experimental investigations of fever reactions evoked by injecting or infusing standard doses of pyrogen or bacteria have not been carried out in otherwise healthy human infants. Data from two studies on the effect of pyrogen administered to phenylketonuric children are conflicting (BARTOLOZZI and CORVAGLIA 1967; BLATTEIS et al. 1973), and, furthermore, such studies are inappropriate to decide the question of what the reaction of the human neonate to pyrogen looks like.

Rises in deep body temperature can develop in the newborn during various diseases. A survey of the available literature on fever in the neonate reveals that there is no general agreement on the level of body temperature, which can unequivocally be called fever. Some workers regard rectal temperature over 37.4 °C as fever (CRAIG 1963), while others class as pyrexic only neonates with body temperatures higher than 39.0 °C (HARASHIMA and KURATA 1966).

Besides infections, dehydration has also been frequently reported to be the cause of high body temperature in the human neonate. In this case the mechanism of development of the febrile state is not completely understood, but it may either result from the inability of the neonate to sweat in a slightly warm environment, or it might be connected with a concomitant hypersalaemia in the CNS; the latter, when induced experimentally, results in a rise of body temperature in several species (MYERS and VEALE 1971). Quite a few cases have been described, in which the neonates showed no signs of pathological alteration, although high body temperatures sometimes lasting for several weeks could be observed (McCLUNG 1972; TEELE et al. 1975). Some of these "fevers" may have been caused by environmental

Table 1. Some findings on febrile human neonates

Source	Age group	Number of cases	Disease states	Lowest body temperature regarded as fever (°C)	Remarks
Craig (1963)	Newborn (40% younger than 3 days)	358	Various infections, dehydration, perinatal stress	37.4	77 immature babies
Bergström et al. (1972)	11–30 days	80	Bacteraemia (mostly E. coli)	38.0	High incidence of maternal infections
Harashima and Kurata (1966)	Newborn	106	Pneumonia	39.0	Data collected from clinical records from the years 1925–1935 (no sulpha drugs or antibiotics in use in Japan)
Teele et al. (1975)	Between 4 weeks and 2 years	600	Pneumonia, upper respiratory infections, unknown origin	38.9	Good correlation between fever, bacteraemia and white blood cell count
Roberts and Borzy (1977)	Younger than 7 weeks	61	Bacteraemia	37.9	Weak correlation between fever and bacteraemia, but better correlation between bacteraemia and white blood cell count
Nakamura et al. (1974)	Newborn	44	Septicaemia, purulent meningitis	38.0	All cases developing after maternal infections
Ladisch and Pizzo (1978)	Newborn	70 (episodes of fever)	Staphylococcus aureus sepsis		

or other factors not primarily connected with, or involved in, any known mechanisms of fever genesis.

Some features of neonatal fever are summarized in Table 1. Only those reports are included, in which the age or at least the age group of the febrile infants has been given. As can be seen, the various authors approached the question of neonatal fever from different angles, ranging from immaturity (CRAIG 1963) to the problem of the diagnostic value of fever and its coincidence with bacteraemia or a high white cell count (TEELE et al. 1975; ROBERTS and BORZY 1977).

It seems of interest to point out that immediately after birth neonates (including some premature babies) can exhibit fever during various infections that are also accompanied by fever in adults. Since nowadays early treatment may prevent or at least attenuate fever, it should be emphasized that at the time when antibacterial drugs were not yet in general use, fever used to be the most prominent and standard symptom of pneumonia in newborn babies (HARASHIMA and KURATA 1966). Two other reports (BERGSTRÖM et al. 1972; NAKAMURA et al. 1974) show that, in some newborn, fever can develop after maternal infections, and this has been taken as indirect evidence for the hypothesis that in these newborn infants infection and fever may have been connected with maternal infections developing at various stages of the perinatal period.

II. Occurrence of Fever and/or Changes in Body Temperature During Infections

The studies indicated in Table 1, involving the collection of clinical records in which neonatal fever had indeed occurred during disease states, do not answer the question of the frequency of fever in infected neonates. In trying to approach this problem, clinical studies have been sought in which changes of body temperature of newborn infants with various infections and/or bacteraemia have been discussed. Table 2 has been compiled from some of the clinical information which is most relevant to the nature of body temperature effects caused by pyrogens and/or bacterial invasion.

Neonatal infections may be signalled by higher body temperatures than normal, but a number of investigations undoubtedly show that fever may be completely absent in many cases, or at least in many phases, of neonatal infections, even when the presence of pyrogens or bacteria can be demonstrated (EPSTEIN et al. 1951; SMITH et al. 1956; LUBCHENCO 1961; SANFORD and GRULEE 1961; MARZETTI et al. 1973). While the lack of fever might be explained by the immaturity of thermoregulation or of some of its mechanisms, definitely hypothermic body temperatures have also been observed during infections (EPSTEIN et al. 1951; SMITH et al. 1956; SANFORD and GRULEE 1961). A hypothermic response to pyrogens or infections can, however, be a particular manifestation of a "response" to the pyrogenic agent, replacing the expected rise in body temperature. Even more interesting is the observation that large fluctuations of body temperature may also develop instead of fever in some infants in the course of infections (LUBCHENCO 1961; MARZETTI et al. 1973; NAKAMURA et al. 1974). This instability of body temperature, involving

Table 2. Occurrence of febrile rise or other change in body temperature during neonatal infections

Source	Age group	Number of cases	Types of change in body temperature				Remarks
			Increase (%)	Decrease (%)	No change (%)	Fluctuations (%)	
Epstein et al. (1951)	Newborn	26	58	42	0	0	9 hypothermic infants with shock
Marzetti et al. (1973)	Neonates (23 younger than 1 month)	43	Rectal temperature between 36° and 38.5 °C observed in different infants. No percentile distribution given				"Non-reactive" pattern in premature and full-term babies (lack of fever, poor antibody response, prolonged duration of fever observed in some cases)
Sanford and Grulee (1961)	Newborn		50	50	0	0	
Smith et al. (1956)	Younger than 30 days	102	57	2	41	0	In two cases hypothermia with fluctuations of body temperature
Lubchenco (1961)	Newborn (also prematures)		0	0	0	100	Instability of body temperature regarded as a sign for infection
Nakamura et al. (1974)	Newborn (3 younger than 2 days)	15	33	0	0	67	

both ends of the normal range under standard thermal conditions of the environment, may remind one of the well known "febris intermittens," a fever course frequently encountered in adults during septicaemia.

Obviously, it is very difficult to draw definite conclusions about the nature and frequency of neonatal fever from the above observations. To characterize changes in body temperature, especially in the newborn, several other circumstances should be known or standardized. One of these concerns the pyrogenic substance itself (i.e. the type of pathogenic bacteria or viruses, their "doses" during infection, changes in their concentration in plasma, etc.). It should be remembered that most of our knowledge on fever has come from experiments, in which a bolus injection or a standard infusion of the pyrogen was given by a particular route (intravenous, intraperitoneal, central administration). Other factors necessary to evaluate pyrogenic effects are: T_a during the course of infection, nutritional state of the patient, the time and nature of antibacterial or antipyretic treatment. A systematic analysis of various aspects of fever in the neonate seems to be, however, an almost hopeless task.

Some general conclusions can, nevertheless, be drawn from the above data on human neonatal fever:
1) Fever can develop in newborn infants even when immaturity and/or malnutrition coexist.
2) Neonatal infections cannot be characterized by the presence of fever (let alone the degree of fever!).
3) Hypothermia or fluctuations of body temperature may frequently occur during neonatal infections, which in other infants are accompanied by fever.

There is no reason to suppose that neonates are "unable" to respond with changes of body temperature to infections with various pathogenic agents containing pyrogenic substances. The response of the body temperature may sometimes be a fever in the usual sense, but in many cases "a sudden fall in body temperature without any change in environmental temperature may be a sign of the onset of one of the complications such as anoxia or infection" (BRIMBLECOMBE and BARLTROP 1978).

E. Experimental Fever in Newborn Animals

The relevant clinical studies are, understandably, usually concerned with changes in body temperature and cannot deal with the effector mechanisms that contribute to the particular change. As a consequence, in most cases it cannot be decided with certainty whether a rise in body temperature is equivalent to fever, in the sense of the definition used by BLIGH and JOHNSON (1973), or whether it is hyperthermia of another origin. Even less is known about the hypothermic reactions. Thus, the controversial reports published on the deviations of body temperature in infected human babies (Tables 1 and 2) are, indeed, difficult to interpret. For ethical reasons, in the human neonate the problem cannot be dealt with at the level it deserves. This would necessitate a penetrating, thorough analysis of neonatal fever, using more exactly defined experimental conditions.

I. Characteristics of Experimental Neonatal Fever

It was PITTMAN et al. (1973) who first investigated experimentally the effect of endotoxin in the newborn. They found that before the age of 60 h newborn lambs exhibited no change in body temperature in response to intravenous endotoxin, moreover, in older lambs fever developed only when they had already been in contact with some kind of pyrogen. BLATTEIS (1975) came to a similar conclusion from experiments on guinea-pigs: at thermoneutrality the temperature of the interscapular adipose tissue of guinea-pigs younger than 32 days was similar after recovery from light anaesthesia, irrespective of whether saline or endotoxin had been injected intravenously during this anaesthesia, although at cooler T_a fever was induced by endotoxin on some occasions in younger animals.

Both newborn guinea-pigs and lambs are relatively mature at birth – according to ALEXANDER (1975) they are "precocious" newborn. It was not surprising, therefore, that in the experiments of SATINOFF et al. (1976) on newborn rabbits, which are "immature" at birth, the autonomic thermoregulatory functions were unaltered after intraperitoneal (IP) pyrogen administration. It was rather unexpected, however, that in these rabbits fever still developed by behavioural means, i.e. if the animals were allowed to select a warmer environment, they did so after pyrogen administration. This was the first reported experimental observation not fully consistent with the previous data on newborn guinea-pigs and lambs.

SZÉKELY and SZELÉNYI (1977) tested the validity of neonatal unresponsiveness to pyrogenic substances in other species. Besides newborn guinea-pigs and rabbits they also studied newborn kittens and rats (i.e. four species born at widely different levels of maturity). These animals were injected IP with *Escherichia coli* endotoxin through a pre-implanted cannula, whilst they were maintained at about their individual thermoneutral environments (Fig. 1). A specific time course of body temperature changes was observed in each species following endotoxin administration; unresponsiveness to endotoxin could not be verified. The response varied with the species: it was a characteristic biphasic fever in 0- to 3-day-old guinea-pigs, a short-lasting monophasic fever in 0- to 3-day-old rabbits, a more sustained monophasic fever in 3- to 6-day-old kittens, while in 8- to 10-day-old rats a hypothermic period was observed 60–120 min after the endotoxin administration. These changes in body temperature could not have been brought about by behavioural means, since the animals were maintained at a standard T_a and had little opportunity for behavioural thermoregulation. Amongst the autonomic changes, the increase in brown fat thermogenesis is of particular interest. In adult rats the thermogenesis in interscapular brown adipose tissue has been shown to change proportionally with total heat production, and this relationship was similar, irrespective of whether cold or pyrogen was the factor evoking a rise in metabolism (SZÉKELY et al. 1973). Brown fat thermogenesis is more important in neonates than in adults, and it increased during the febrile response in newborn guinea-pigs (BLATTEIS 1976), rabbits (SZÉKELY and SZELÉNYI 1977), and probably also in febrile human babies (MATSANIOTIS et al. 1971). In 0- to 3-day-old rabbits no change in ear skin temperature or in respiratory frequency could be detected in the course of fever (Fig. 2), but heat loss effector functions when measured in a few experiments in response to external heat were also unchanged (SZÉKELY and SZELÉNYI 1979 b).

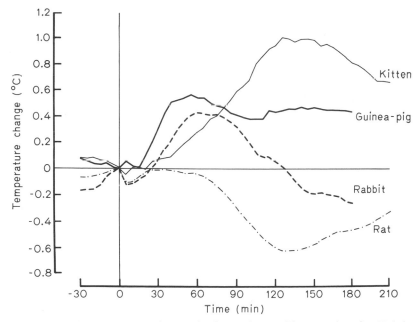

Fig. 1. Average body temperature changes in the newborn of four species after IP injection of 20 µg/kg *E. coli* endotoxin at the individual thermoneutral T_a. (Adapted from SZÉKELY and SZELÉNYI 1977)

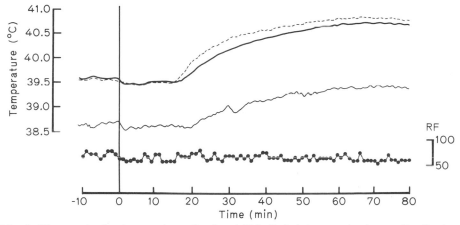

Fig. 2. Changes in the temperature of colon (*thick line*), interscapular brown fat (*broken line*), and ear skin (*thin line*) and in the respiratory frequency (RF) of a 2-day-old rabbit weighing 84 g, after IV injection of 20 µg/kg endotoxin, $T_a = 32.5$ °C. (SZÉKELY and SZELÉNYI 1979 b)

In 6- to 10-day-old rabbits the same endotoxin dose that had produced mono-phasic fever in 0- to 3-day-old animals, evoked a biphasic fever (Fig. 3), and the various heat producing and conserving mechanisms were activated in both phases (SZÉKELY 1978 a; SZÉKELY and SZELÉNYI 1979 b). With the same dose and route of administration, the latency and rate of the first rise observed in older rabbits coin-

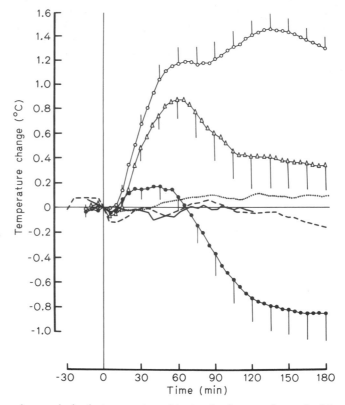

Fig. 3. Mean changes in body temperature ($\pm$ standard error of mean) of 0- to 3-day-old well-fed (*triangles*), 6- to 10-day-old well-fed (*open circles*), and 6- to 10-day-old starving (*solid circles*) rabbits, after IV injection of 20 µg/kg endotoxin at thermoneutrality. IV saline (*solid, dotted, and broken lines*) was ineffective in all groups. (Combined from Székely 1978a, 1979a)

cided with the monophasic fever of 0- to 3-day-old animals. The biphasic pattern of fever is well known for the adult rabbit (Grant 1949; Atkins and Bodel 1974; Szelényi and Székely 1979), and also for a number of other species (Bennett and Cluff 1957; Blatteis 1974) in response to larger doses of endotoxin or endogenous pyrogen (Atkins and Huang 1958a, b; King and Wood 1958; Bornstein et al. 1963; Snell 1971). This is not so, either in the adult cat (Bennett and Cluff 1957), or in the newborn kitten; 3- to 6-day-old as well as 6- to 10-day-old kittens responded with monophasic fever to IP or ICV endotoxin administration (Székely and Szelényi 1977; Székely 1978d, 1979c). In contrast, both adult (Blatteis 1974) and newborn (Székely 1978c) guinea-pigs responded to appropriate doses of endotoxin with biphasic fever. In adult rats IV endotoxin also elicits biphasic fever (Székely and Szelényi 1979a), and the temperature fall observed in the endotoxin response of newborn rats (Fig. 1) may correspond to the transient temperature decline between the two peaks of fever in the adult rat. In 6- to 10-day-old rabbits the two peaks were similar to those in adults, but they were more separated from each other, thus they become more pronounced.

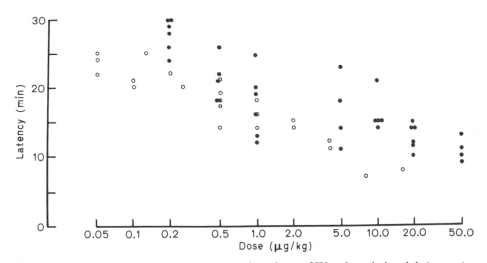

Fig. 4. Latency of temperature response to various doses of IV endotoxin in adult (*open circles*) and 6- to 10-day-old (*solid circles*) rabbits. T_a about thermoneutral. (SZÉKELY and SZELÉNYI 1979 b)

As in the adult rabbit (BENNETT and CLUFF 1957; ATKINS 1960; ATKINS and BODEL 1974) and in adults of other species (BLATTEIS 1974), in 6- to 10-day-old rabbits (SZÉKELY and SZELÉNYI 1979 b) as well as in 0- to 3-day-old guinea-pigs (SZÉKELY 1978 c) smaller doses of endotoxin evoke monophasic fever of long latency, and the biphasic fever of short latency was characteristic of larger doses only. The dose required to obtain biphasic fever was, however, larger in the newborn than in the adult. In the newborn the same endotoxin dose induced fever only after a longer delay than in adults (Fig. 4). Whether the endotoxin was given IP, IV, or ICV, with the same route of injection the extent of the maximum febrile temperature was independent of the dose in newborn guinea-pigs, kittens, and rabbits (SZÉKELY 1978 c, 1979 c; SZÉKELY and SZELÉNYI 1979 b), which is also in accordance with the data reported for the endotoxin response of adult animals. The maximum temperature rise after IV endotoxin injection was only slightly but statistically significantly smaller in 6- to 10-day-old than in adult rabbits (Fig. 5), while no difference was seen between the response of 0- to 3-day-old and 1-month-old guinea-pigs to ICV pyrogen (Fig. 6).

In more recent publications KLEITMAN and SATINOFF (1980) reported that at an ambient temperature of 32 °C autonomic means might contribute to the febrile response of 0- to 3-day-old rabbits, when the applied pyrogen dose was higher. This implies that the autonomic responses have a higher threshold of activation but, in the rabbit, the autonomic as well as the behavioural responses to pyrogens are present from birth. Even the higher dose of pyrogen could not, however, activate the autonomic responses in maternally neglected newborn rabbits, although a behavioural response was still possible.

From recent reports of KASTING et al. (1979 b) it appears that newborn lambs also can respond to endotoxin with some change of body temperature, although this change was a fall at the age of 5 h and a rise at the age of 32 h. These ex-

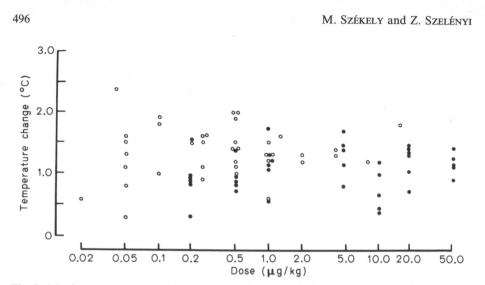

Fig. 5. Maximum temperature change in adult (*open circles*) and 6- to 10-day-old (*solid circles*) rabbits after various doses of IV endotoxin. Mean ($\pm$ standard error of mean) change was 1.38 ± 0.09 and 1.09 ± 0.07 °C ($p < 0.05$) for adult and newborn animals, respectively. T_a about thermoneutral. (SZÉKELY and SZELÉNYI 1979 b)

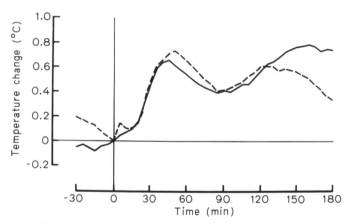

Fig. 6. Changes of body temperature in 0- to 3-day-old (*broken line*) and 1-month-old (*solid line*) guinea-pigs (average response of six animals in both groups) after ICV endotoxin injection at the individual thermoneutral T_a

periments were performed at an ambient temperature of 19 °C which is rather cold, since the "lower critical temperature" is about 35 °C and 25 °C in lambs aged 1–6 h and 29–36 h, respectively (MERCER et al. 1979).

BLATTEIS (1977) has also found that the unresponsiveness to endotoxin was relative, and higher doses given IV were more frequently followed by rises in body temperature exceeding 0.5 °C, and that intrahypothalamically administered pyrogen at a T_a of 27 °C (slightly lower than thermoneutral) evoked a febrile response in guinea-pigs immediately after birth, although in this series he also frequently observed hypothermic responses, particularly in "small-for-age" animals (BLATTEIS

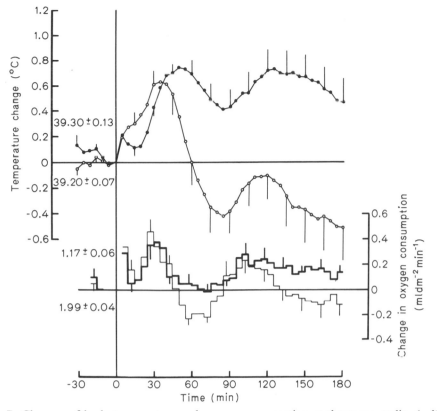

Fig. 7. Changes of body temperature and oxygen consumption at thermoneutrality (*solid circles, thick line*) or at $T_a = 20$ °C (*open circles, thin line*) in 0- to 3-day-old guinea-pigs after ICV injection of 0.2 µg endotoxin. (SZÉKELY and KOMÁROMI 1978)

and SMITH 1979). Similarly, in the experiments of SZÉKELY (1978 c) and SZÉKELY and KOMÁROMI (1978) 0- to 3-day-old guinea-pigs at a T_a of 20 °C became hypothermic after a dose of endotoxin that evoked a signicant biphasic febrile rise in body temperature in the thermoneutral environment (Fig. 7). At a T_a of 20 °C the course of the temperature change was also characteristically biphasic in the cold. The first-phase rise even reached a level approximating that seen at thermoneutrality. The fall in temperature occurring about 50–90 min after the endotoxin injection, between the two rising phases, was greatly enhanced in the cold. The rise during the second phase was also of the same magnitude as that seen at thermoneutrality (i.e. about 0.2°–0.3 °C), except that it started from a lower point so that even at its peak it failed to reach the pre-injection level. Thus, during the second and third hours of the endotoxin response widely different levels of body temperature were established, depending largely on T_a which also determined the extent of the preceding temperature fall; the temperature level reached by the end of this fall was only slightly modified (a temporary rise of 0.2°–0.3 °C) by the second-phase temperature rise. In other words this means that body temperature was more labile in the late periods of the endotoxin response than either during the first phase of the response or in animals treated with 0.9% NaCl. In 6- to 10-day-old rabbits that had been starved for 24 h before the experiment at thermoneutrality, the endotoxin injection was followed by a fall in body temperature 60–120 min after the endotoxin injection (Székely 1979 a) (Fig. 3). In newborn rats the only response to endotoxin was a reversible fall in body temperature following the injection by about 60–120 min (Fig. 1). In newborn guinea-pigs pre-treated with propranolol IP, body temperature also declined (Fig. 12) again about 60–100 min after the endotoxin administration (Székely 1979 b).

II. Differences Between Adult and Neonatal Febrile Responses

From these data it seems obvious that, in some respects, the febrile response of newborn animals is, indeed, different from that of adults. Besides differences in the peripheral effector functions such as the importance of brown fat thermogenesis there are also differences in the central thermoregulatory processes. These, however, do not prevent the genesis of fever, or at least some temperature change, in the neonate. The main differences between neonatal and adult responses to pyrogenic substances can be summarized as follows:

1. Even at T_a around thermoneutrality, the neonates may give a weaker hyperthermic response, no response, or a hypothermic response to endotoxins. The environmental temperature and nutritional factors have a strong influence on the thermal response to pyrogens.
2. A larger dose of endotoxin may be required in the neonate than in the adult to elicit the characteristic biphasic fever of short latency; administration of doses of endotoxin that in the adult induce short latency biphasic fever, frequently evoke monophasic fever in the neonate, and only after a long latency.
3. Some stages of the biphasic endotoxin response may be completely absent in the neonate, and appear later in ontogenesis, while other stages are present from birth.

It is not easy to interpret these differences. So far, there is no way of explaining all of them uniformly, but there have been numerous attempts to find out the mechanisms that could account for the defective febrile responsiveness of the newborn.

F. Reasons for Differences Between Neonatal and Adult Febrile Responses

I. Surface/Weight Ratio of the Body

It is generally assumed that the relative unresponsiveness and the hypothermic responses to pyrogens of neonates may be of peripheral origin, i.e. consequences of the relatively large surface area of the neonate. A similar explanation has also been given for the lack of response, or hypothermic response, frequently observed in the adults of small mammals after the administration of pyrogenic or other hyperthermia-inducing substances, particularly at T_a below thermoneutrality (Berry 1966; Van Miert and Frens 1968; Blatteis 1974, 1975).

As pointed out by Bligh (1973) and Baumann and Bligh (1975), the effect of T_a on the febrile response is usually explained by assuming that, because of the

large ratio of surface area to body mass, the endotoxin-induced rise in heat production cannot overcome or even compensate for the concurrent increase in heat loss
which, even in only moderately cool environments, results from the concomitant
shivering and gross body movements. This would imply that, owing to the enormous heat loss, heat production must increase even up to summit metabolism, but
it still cannot keep pace with the increased heat loss and thus, hypothermia develops. The naked body surface and poor vasomotor responses may, indeed, facilitate heat loss in the newborn and, although the newborn usually prefers non-
shivering thermogenesis to shivering (BRÜCK 1978 a, b), it also makes large body
movements when metabolic rate is increased, whether owing to cold or to pyrogenic substance.

The available data suggest that the explanation cannot be as simple as that.

First, because, by the same logic, almost any factor or substance eliciting an increase in metabolic rate should also result in hypothermia even in mild cold environments, and exposure to slightly cool T_a would, by itself, necessarily result in
severe irreversible hypothermia. However, this is not the case, either in the small
adult or in the neonate. Rats, mice, guinea-pigs, and other small adult mammals
are well known to respond with hyperthermia to a number of drugs at those T_a at
which pyrogens reportedly fail to elevate or induce a fall in body temperature
(BRECKENRIDGE and LISK 1969; FELDBERG and SAXENA 1971; SPLAWINSKI et al.
1974; BLÄSIG and HERZ 1978; MARTIN and MORRISON 1978). The neonates of various species have been reported to develop hyperthermia in response to central
(KOMÁROMI et al. 1969 a; ZEISBERGER and BRÜCK 1971; KOMÁROMI 1977 a, b), or peripheral (MOORE and UNDERWOOD 1960; KARLBERG et al. 1962; SCOPES and TIZARD
1963; KOMÁROMI 1977 a; BRÜCK 1978 a, b) administration of noradrenaline or to
central injection of γ-aminobutyric acid (KOMÁROMI et al. 1969 a; KOMÁROMI 1976).
Central injection of 5-HT (KOMÁROMI 1976; SZÉKELY 1978 b) or dopamine
(KOMÁROMI personal communication) is followed by an early fall and a later rise
in body temperature of newborn guinea-pigs, ICV injections of 5-HT elicit hyperthermia in the kitten (SZÉKELY 1978 b) and, although there are reports of neonatal
prostaglandin (PG) unresponsiveness (PITTMAN et al. 1975, 1977; BLATTEIS and
SMITH 1979), in other experiments centrally injected PGE$_1$ resulted in dose-dependent hyperthermia in newborn guinea-pigs, kittens, and rabbits (SZÉKELY and
KOMÁROMI 1978; SZÉKELY 1979 c; SZÉKELY and SZELÉNYI 1979 b). Furthermore, although in a moderately cool environment body temperature may be either unchanged or decreased to various levels both in small adults and in neonates of different maturity, it is obvious that in all cases, irrespective of the new, cold-induced
level of body temperature, this level can be maintained fairly stable without elevating heat production to a maximum. Summit metabolism can be induced by further
cooling.

Body temperature may even be increased in a cool environment. In his early
experiments BLATTEIS (1975) demonstrated that a greater percentage of young
guinea-pigs developed fever in a cool environment than at thermoneutrality. In the
experiments of SZÉKELY (1978 c) newborn guinea-pigs also showed a rise in body
temperature in response to endotoxin administration at a T_a much below thermoneutrality, although this rise was only temporary. Kittens in the same cool environment developed a sustained monophasic febrile rise in body temperature

(Székely 1979 c). In cool environments similar results have been reported for the endotoxin response of adult rats (Székely and Szelényi 1979 a) and newborn guinea-pigs.

Second, the hypothermia, if developed in response to endotoxin, did so in a particular way indicative of a coordinated physiological change rather than being a purely physical consequence of excessive heat loss. Hypothermic responses were usually observed in cool environments, and they were seen mainly in those species exhibiting biphasic fever. Kittens responded to endotoxin with a monophasic temperature rise both at 30° and 20 °C T_a, and a fall appeared only in the very cold environment of 10 °C (when the initial body temperature was also low), even then only 2–3 h after the endotoxin injection (Székely 1979 c and unpublished). At a T_a of 20 °C in studies of newborn guinea-pigs, which are almost the same size as kittens, but more mature, the net result after endotoxin injection was a temperature fall (Székely and Komáromi 1978). This hypothermia was, however, the consequence mainly of an enhancement of the "transient temperature fall" between the two phases of temperature rise. This "transient fall" was a coordinated reaction (Fig. 7): oxygen consumption decreased towards basal metabolic rate, to lower levels than those which had been initially required to maintain stable body temperature. Thus, the metabolic rate was certainly far from its peak value. In this situation, the relatively large surface area could have facilitated heat exchange with the environment. The final hypothermia was, however, the result mainly of the temperature fall in this circumscribed period, the first temperature rise being the same as in the thermoneutral environment, and the second phase also being of the same magnitude as at thermoneutrality but superimposed upon a lower temperature level. It seems to be a different problem why the low level of body temperature was maintained throughout the second and third hours of the endotoxin response. By the third hour body temperature also declined below baseline in kittens injected with endotoxin at a T_a of 10 °C.

It is interesting that in newborn rats, starving rabbits, and also in newborn guinea-pigs pre-treated IP with propranolol (Figs. 1, 3, and 12), the observed hypothermia in response to endotoxin developed in more-or-less the same period as the "transient fall" in normal guinea-pigs and rabbits. This suggests that, in all these cases, the underlying central regulatory mechanisms responsible for the various temperature declines may be identical. For some reason, the rising phases that in adult rats, 6- to 10-day-old well-fed rabbits, and 0- to 3-day-old guinea-pigs normally precede and follow this decline, could not develop in newborn rats, starving rabbits, and guinea-pigs pre-treated with propranolol. This reason may be different in each case, but clearly, the regulatory mechanisms responsible for the temperature rises cannot be identical with those responsible for the "transient fall."

The febrile response, at least in those species exhibiting biphasic fever is, therefore, not a homogenous thermoregulatory reaction, instead, it is a complex response consisting of different parts, some of which drive body temperature upwards, while others tend to depress body temperature. These parts follow each other in a definite order and it is the relationship between them that gives the net change in body temperature.

While the neonate's relatively large surface, by itself, cannot explain hypothermic responses to endotoxins, it certainly can increase the efficiency of a hypothermia-inducing drive in the period between the two rising phases. Thus, a net hypothermia is more easily observed in the newborn (and the small adult) than in larger adults with a relatively smaller surface area and a larger thermal inertia of the body. Cold T_a can augment the hypothermia; although in adult rabbits endotoxins usually elevate body temperature, if the environment is cold enough (0 °C), endotoxin also induces hypothermia in the shorn adult rabbit (GRANT 1949). In less severe cold (e.g. 25 °C), the hypothermia may be only marginal even in the newborn, thus, neither a significant temperature fall, nor temperature rise develops, and the "response" can appear in the form of no marked change in body temperature.

Thus, the relatively large surface of the newborn can be one factor, in addition to others, in explaining the hypothermic responses or, in less severe cold, the lack of responses to endotoxins. It cannot, however, explain per se either the hypothermia, or the differences between newborn and adult animals in the extent of the rising periods at thermoneutral T_a, or the differences in the latency of the response, or the lack of certain parts of the whole response. These require some other explanation.

II. Ability to Produce Endogenous Pyrogen

Inability or insufficient capacity of the newborn to produce endogenous pyrogens could be another possible explanation for the deficient febrile responsiveness of neonatal animals. The mere existence of a febrile response, whether achieved by autonomic or behavioural means, contradicts the idea that the endogenous pyrogen production may be totally absent. The blood of newborn as well as adult guinea-pigs, if mixed with endotoxin in vitro, has been shown to produce endogenous pyrogens that were effective in adult guinea-pigs (BLATTEIS 1977). The production of endogenous pyrogens in vivo may, however, be quantitatively different, i.e. it may be slower and/or weaker than in adults.

Although endogenous pyrogens are known to evoke a dose-related rise in body temperature (ATKINS 1960), the maximum temperature rise both in adult (BENNETT and CLUFF 1957; ATKINS 1960; SZELÉNYI and SZÉKELY 1979) and in newborn (SZÉKELY 1978c, 1979c; SZÉKELY and SZELÉNYI 1979b) animals was unaffected by wide-ranging differences in endotoxin dose. Thus, in vivo, even the smallest effective endotoxin doses seem to produce enough endogenous pyrogen to elevate body temperature to the same extent as larger endotoxin doses. This seems to imply that the dose of endotoxin influences the rate of production rather than the concentration of endogenous pyrogen. Therefore, it seems justified to suppose that, in the newborn treated with relatively large doses of endotoxin, the amount of endogenous pyrogen produced should be enough to bring about similar elevations in body temperature as in adults (at least at thermoneutrality), even if the endogenous pyrogen production is slower or weaker than in adults. At thermoneutrality endotoxins can evoke biphasic fever both in newborn guinea-pigs and rabbits. This fever course can be observed only if large amounts of endogenous pyrogen are present. Consequently, if the extent of the febrile rise in body temperature is different in neonatal and adult animals, the difference is unlikely to be explained by a deficient production of endogenous pyrogen.

The rate at which endogenous pyrogens are produced in response to an endotoxin stimulus may, however, influence the time lag between the endotoxin administration and the onset of fever, and this is what has been found in newborn rabbits (Fig. 4). In this respect, there was no difference between 0–3 and 6- to 10-day-old rabbits. The finding that the lowest endotoxin dose necessary to evoke the characteristic biphasic pattern of fever was higher in newborn rabbits than in adults (Székely and Szelényi 1979 b) is compatible with the idea of some kind of deficiency in the rate of endogenous pyrogen production. The lack of the second febrile "hump" in 0- to 3-day-old rabbits (Fig. 3) is unlikely to be the result of an insufficiency in endogenous pyrogen production, since the course of change in body temperature of 0- to 3-day-old rabbits was similar to the first febrile phase of 6- to 10-day-old rabbits (latency, rate of temperature rise, peak temperature). Therefore, the incomplete appearance of fever must have been due rather to some other deficiency in the central febrigenic process.

III. Role of Central Mediatory/Modulatory Substances

Some differences between newborn and adult animals in their cerebral metabolism of catecholamines, serotonin, and other substances, and also age-related differences in the thermoregulatory responses to central administration of these materials have been shown. Since many of these substances have been suspected of having a role in the pathogenesis of fever (for reviews see Bligh 1973; Feldberg 1975; Hellon 1975), it is tempting to suggest that the "immaturity" of the central aminergic systems and the differences in the amount and turnover of central transmitter or modulator substances might be responsible for differences in the febrile responses of newborn and adult animals.

Various centrally occurring substances, including prostaglandins (Milton and Wendlandt 1971), monoamines (Feldberg and Myers 1964), cations (Myers and Veale 1971), etc., have been suggested as the principal and ultimate central mediators of the febrile response. The biphasic character of fever does not, however, support the idea that any single substance could fulfil this role. Various parts of the endotoxin response can be influenced separately. For example, in newborn guinea-pigs neither the first nor the second rise, per se, was influenced by T_a, while the transient fall between them was enhanced in the cold (Fig. 7). Starvation, on the other hand, depressed only the rising phases in newborn rabbits (Fig. 3). This is suggestive of a mediatory sequence rather than any single "ultimate mediator."

1. Prostaglandins

Injections of prostaglandins (PGs) of the E series into the hypothalamus or ICV have been shown to produce a rise in body temperature in most of the species so far studied (Milton 1976), except the *Echidna* in which temperature fell after PG administration (Baird et al. 1974). Accordingly, the central PGs have been suggested to be the ultimate mediators in the pathogenesis of fever. Indirect evidence supports this postulate: the PG content of the cerebrospinal fluid increases during fever (Feldberg and Gupta 1973), aspirin-like antipyretics inhibit PG synthesis (Vane 1971), and decrease the febrile level of PGs in the cerebrospinal fluid (Feld-

BERG et al. 1973). Moreover, at least in the cat, the PGE-sensitive neurones of the rostral hypothalamus have been shown to respond to peripheral thermal stimuli or micro-iontophoretically applied biogenic amines (JELL and SWEATMAN 1977).

In lambs aged 4–168 h PGE_1 or PGE_2 injected into the cerebral ventricles or into the hypothalamus failed to influence body temperature (PITTMAN et al. 1975, 1977). This seemed to fit in with the lack of febrile response in newborn lambs. BLATTEIS and SMITH (1979) found that newborn guinea-pigs were also unable to respond to centrally applied PGs. However, the lambs remained unresponsive to PGs for longer than to pyrogens, and many of those lambs pre-sensitized by bacterial pyrogen and unable to react to PGE_1 experienced fever in response to endotoxin, which fever in turn, was successfully depressed by salicylates (PITTMAN et al. 1977). Furthermore, the PG-unresponsive lambs were able to maintain deep-body temperature in cold environments and to respond to hypothalamic injections of noradrenaline and 5-HT in the same manner as adults (COOPER et al. 1976). This has already challenged the postulated role of PGs in fever. The experiments of VEALE and COOPER (1975) – although not exactly in line with the findings of LIPTON and TRZCINKA (1976) – demonstrated that adult rabbits with massive destructions in the anterior hypothalamus respond with a slow-onset fever to IV endotoxin but not to centrally applied PGs. This indicated that beside the postulated hypothalamic PG-sensitive mechanism some other, non-PG-mediated, non-hypothalamic mechanism must also be important in the pathogenesis of fever, although under normal circumstances this (secondary) mechanism may be suppressed. The same conclusion can be drawn from the experiments in which fever was evoked in the *Echidna* (BAIRD et al. 1974). Drugs antagonizing the action of exogenous PGs did not antagonize the pyrogen-induced fever (CRANSTON et al. 1975 a, b, 1976, 1978; LABURN et al. 1977).

On the other hand, exogenous PGE may not act on exactly the same structures as PGs liberated endogenously in the course of fever. Conversely, the endogenous substances may reach a higher concentration at their point of action than is the case with exogenous PG administration. (This could be an explanation for the antipyretic action of salicylates in lambs, which were PG resistant but pyrogen sensitive.) It is also possible that some other arachidonic acid metabolite influences temperature regulation and not PGE_1 itself. Moreover, exogenous PGs might modify the endogenous metabolism of endoperoxides.

None of the evidence to the contrary, all of which is indirect, rules out a role of PGs in fever; this role, however, cannot be exclusive.

In contrast to the finding of BLATTEIS and SMITH (1979), SZÉKELY and KOMÁROMI (1978) reported that newborn guinea-pigs responded to ICV administration of 10 ng PGE_1 with a monophasic rise in body temperature in thermoneutral and moderately cold environments. It was concluded that, while the finding allows for the PGs having a role in the endotoxin response, the whole of the fever course with its characteristic biphasic pattern could not be explained solely by a central PGE_1 mechanism. This experiment did not prove, but did not exclude either, the possible involvement of PGs in the central mediation of fever.

In addition to newborn guinea-pigs, 6- to 10-day-old rabbits (SZÉKELY and SZELÉNYI 1979 b) and kittens (SZÉKELY 1979 c) also exhibited a dose-dependent rise in body temperature following central administration of PGE_1. This response may possibly be quantitatively different from that of adult guinea-pigs, rabbits, and cats after similar PG injections, but data comparing responses to the same PG in adult and newborn animals under similar circumstances are lacking.

A difference in PG susceptibility in the newborn as compared with the adult would not be easily explained. A selective, total insensitivity of the nervous system to PGs, when the sensitivity to other substances is good (as reported for the lamb: PITTMAN et al. 1975, 1977; COOPER et al. 1976) is difficult to visualize. It is more likely that the amount of PG reaching the sensitive targets is smaller, either because of lower synthesis of PGs or PG-like substances, or because of faster elimination of these substances. Though the details of PG synthesis in the brain have not been clarified, PGs are certainly synthesized in brain tissue (PACE-ASCIAK and NASHAT 1976; PACE-ASCIAK and RANGARAJ 1976). We know somewhat more about PG catabolism. In the lamb brain the level of 15-prostaglandin-hydroxy-dehydrogenase, which is held to be the main PG-catabolizing enzyme during foetal life, has been shown virtually to disappear in the foetus at term and in the newborn lamb (PACE-ASCIAK and RANGARAJ 1976). This disappearance raises the question of some alternative, perhaps non-enzymatic route (or routes) of inactivation or elimination occurring in the brain at these stages of ontogenesis. Thus, the low levels of 15-prostaglandin-hydroxy-dehydrogenase do not support, but neither do they preclude the possibility that the elimination of PG-like substances may be faster in the newborn. Enhanced PG catabolism would not be a unique mechanism. It has been shown to take place at critical periods of ontogenesis (at different stages, depending on the organ and the species), in order to prevent noxious effects of excessive PG activity (PACE-ASCIAK and MILLER 1973; PACE-ASCIAK 1977). The large-scale changes in PG metabolism in connection with the processes of parturition (LIGGINS and GRIEVES 1971; SHARMA et al. 1973; WILLMAN and COLLINS 1976; WILLMAN et al. 1977; EDQVIST et al. 1978) may not be desirable in every organ, e.g. it may adversely affect cerebral blood flow and metabolism (WELCH et al. 1974; PICKARD et al. 1977), therefore a more effective elimination of cerebral PGs may be brought into play both in the foetus and the mother around birth. This reasoning seems, however, to be rather teleological.

Not incompatible with the presumption of rapid inactivation or antagonization of PGs is the idea put forward by KASTING et al. (1978 a, b) of an endogenous antipyretic factor preventing fever in both the neonatal lamb and the ewe in the period preceding delivery by a few days and following it by a few hours. More recently this phenomenon has been attributed to the function of vasopressin which, after central application in moderate or large doses, respectively, prevented the first phase or the whole course of fever in the ewe (KASTING et al. 1979 a). Since in some organs (e.g. kidney), there appears to be a certain antagonism between the action of PG and vasopressin (GRANTHAM and ORLOFF 1968; ANDERSON et al. 1975), this finding may be extremely interesting.

Pregnant rabbits have also been shown to give only weak responses to pyrogens (KULLANDER 1977), although they were found to react to centrally injected PGE_1 (NACCARATO and HUNTER 1979). Nevertheless, it should be pointed out that unresponsiveness to pyrogens at term cannot be extended to every species: while it is, perhaps, debatable, whether or not the human neonate can experience fever immediately after birth, women can certainly become febrile owing to infections, within hours after giving birth to their child, and there are also reports (see Sect. D.I) demonstrating simultaneous febrile events in mother and baby due to maternal infection. There are also data showing that even ewes at term may develop fever in some instances (ABRAMS 1978; SILVER, personal communication). On the other hand, it seems that not only the febrile responsiveness, but also the ability to withstand heat and cold stress is impaired around term in some species (rabbit) (VAUGHN et al. 1978).

If PGs or similar substances are really involved in the pathomechanism of fever, their increased catabolism could, perhaps, account for the smaller extent of the rise in body temperature or for its complete lack in various neonates, e.g. in lambs or in rats after pyrogen administration.

The positive thermoregulatory reactions observed in response to PGE_1 in newborn guinea-pigs, rabbits, and kittens do not necessarily imply that PGs are involved in the febrile response. An increasing number of data indicate that it is not a PG itself, but rather some other derivative or derivatives of arachidonic acid that may be important in the febrile response (CRANSTON et al. 1975 b, 1978; LABURN et al. 1977). It appears that exogenous PGE may have a hyperthermic action of its own, and PGs can be liberated during the course of fever, together with other metabolites of arachidonic acid, some of which may also have a hyperthermic action (MILTON et al. 1980). According to the attractive idea of DASCOMBE and MILTON (1979), it is also possible that some arachidonic acid derivatives of peripheral origin cross the blood–brain barrier and enter the CNS from the cerebral circulation during the action of endotoxin.

Another way to investigate the possible role of endogenous PGs and/or other arachidonic acid breakdown products in fever is to study the fever response after blocking arachidonic acid metabolism.

In newborn guinea-pigs pre-treatment with indomethacin, an agent known to inhibit arachidonic acid breakdown (VANE 1971), prevented the development of the first-phase rise and the subsequent fall in body temperature characteristic of the biphasic response to endotoxins, but a rise in body temperature coinciding in time with the second fever phase still persisted (Fig. 8). Since indomethacin has a long-lasting effect, this rise probably cannot be explained by PG action. For the first rise, however, products of arachidonic acid metabolism seem to be indispensable (SZÉKELY 1978 c).

From the original figures of VAN MIERT and VAN DUIN (1977) it is obvious that moderate doses of the PG-synthesis blocker, flurbiprofen, mainly inhibited the first phase of fever in adult rabbits, though larger doses reduced the temperature rise of the second phase, too.

Almost identical results have been reported for the effect of centrally applied vasopressin on the febrile response of the ewe: moderate doses prevented the first phase, larger doses abolished the whole response (KASTING et al. 1979 a).

The finding of MILTON et al. (1977) is relevant here: the PG content of the cerebrospinal fluid was elevated only in those cats in which a fever started within about 30 min of the pyrogen injection. The slowly responding cats, in which fever commenced after a latency of about 90 min, exhibited no change in the PG level of their cerebrospinal fluid.

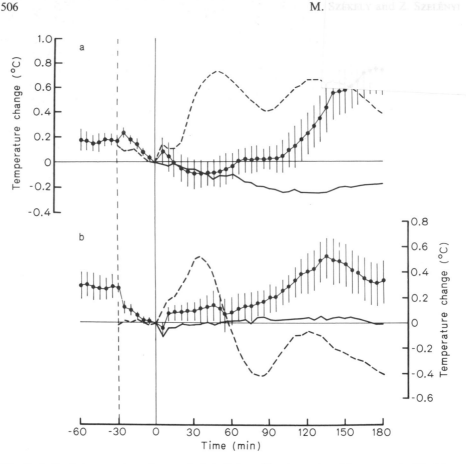

Fig. 8a, b. Body temperature changes in 0- to 3-day-old guinea-pigs at thermoneutrality (**a**) or at $T_a = 20\,°C$ (**b**). Animals pre-treated with indomethacin received a second dose of indomethacin IP 30 min before the ICV injection of endotoxin (*solid circles*) or saline (*solid line*). Endotoxin response of control animals (*broken line*). (Adapted from Székely 1978c)

In newborn kittens indomethacin pre-treatment, similar to that given to newborn guinea-pigs, strongly reduced not only the early parts but also the late rise of the febrile response (Székely 1979c). Besides, the transient temperature fall separating the two rising phases appears to involve central serotonergic processes (see Sect. F.III.2) which, in turn, have been shown to enhance endogenous PG-like activity in the CNS (Székely 1978b). Therefore, an increase in central PG-like activity may also be among the factors which participate in the second phase of febrile temperature rise.

The lack of rise in body temperature in the corresponding period (first 60 min) of the endotoxin response of newborn rats, and perhaps also of starving rabbits, could be taken as an indication of either a decreased synthesis or increased catabolism of hyperthermia-inducing arachidonic acid metabolites. This mechanism, however, cannot account for the apparent fall in body temperature in subsequent periods.

2. Serotonin

Like the coordinated rise in body temperature during the first phase of fever in those species exhibiting biphasic fever, the temperature fall between the two phases also seems to involve active coordination by the central thermoregulatory apparatus. There exist some observations in support of this opinion. In the newborn guinea-pig (Fig. 7), and also in the adult rat (SZÉKELY and SZELÉNYI 1979 a) and the adult rabbit (GRANT 1949) during this period the metabolic rate fell to (at thermoneutrality) or below (in the cold) the values that had been seen before the start of fever. According to data from adult rats (SZÉKELY and SZELÉNYI 1979 a; SZÉKELY and SZOLCSÁNYI 1979) and rabbits (GRANT 1949; SZELÉNYI and SZÉKELY 1979), heat loss also increases in this period.

This fall in body temperature is not simply a rebound phenomenon. Its appearance is not dependent on the preceding first-phase rise in body temperature. It starts at a rather well-defined time after the endotoxin administration, quite independently of the actual temperature reached during the first phase, and even irrespective of whether it has been preceded by any rise in body temperature (SZÉKELY 1978 c; SZÉKELY and SZELÉNYI 1979 a). For example, in starving rabbits and also in newborn rats, and in newborn guinea-pigs pre-treated IP with propranolol, no rise preceded the fall which started at the same time as the transient fall in well-nourished rabbits and guinea-pigs. Conversely, in adult rats pre-treated with capsaicin (SZÉKELY and SZOLCSÁNYI 1979), which showed an enormous rise in temperature during the first phase, the transient fall still commenced at the same time as in control rats. This uniformity suggests that the time elapsing before the onset of the temperature fall is perhaps required to produce and accumulate a hypothermia-inducing substance, in much the same way as the shorter interval between the endotoxin injection and the first temperature rise is needed to produce and accumulate some hyperthermia-inducing substance.

So far, no hypothermia-inducing PG-like material has been found which could account for this coordinated decline in body temperature. Therefore, the presence of some hypothermia-inducing central substance, other than PG, has to be postulated as an important factor in this particular stage of the febrile response. Various substances might be considered for this role; first of all those other than PGs, that had long been thought to play a principal role in the pathogenesis of fever (serotonin, noradrenaline, acetylcholine, cations, etc.), but many of which proved to cause hypothermia in one species or the other. A survey of all the relevant substances is impossible, partly because of their great number and partly because only a few of them have been assayed for basic thermoregulatory effects in neonates. The striking variability in the temperature responses to the administration of these compounds has also been a great obstacle in studies on adult animals.

Although it was 5-HT that, from experiments on adult cats, had first been suggested as "the" central mediator of fever (FELDBERG and MYERS 1964), the species differences observed both in adult (BLIGH 1973; FELDBERG 1975; HELLON 1975), and in newborn (SZÉKELY 1978 b) animals in response to central application of 5-HT did not support this idea. Moreover, ICV administration of 5-HT has been shown to depress fever induced by typhoid–paratyphoid A and B (TAB) vaccine in the sheep (BLIGH and MASKREY 1970).

Attempts to study the effect on febrigenesis of blocking endogenous 5-HT synthesis in adult animals yielded equivocal results. Mainly because of the ease with
which fever can be induced in the rabbit, this has been the species most thoroughly
studied for the possible role of serotonergic processes in the febrile response. As
a result of an IP pre-treatment with the 5-HT-synthesis blocking agent (KOE and
WEISSMAN 1966) p-chlorophenylalanine (pCPA), the subsequent febrile response
was either enhanced (GIARMAN et al. 1968; TEDDY 1971) or unchanged (DES PREZ
and OATES 1968; CARRUBA and BÄCHTOLD 1976), while monoamine oxidase inhibitors which increase 5-HT availability also augmented the febrile response
(COOPER and CRANSTON 1966). However, these differences may only reflect our insufficient knowledge of the precise action of central 5-HT in this species: centrally
injected 5-HT has been reported to elicit hypothermia (BLIGH et al. 1971), hyperthermia, or no change (PEINDARIES and JACOB 1971; JACOB and PEINDARIES 1973)
in body temperature of rabbits, depending on dose, T_a, route or location of injection, and probably some other unknown experimental factors.

In the cat, in which species central 5-HT is unanimously held to elicit a rise in
body temperature, pCPA pre-treatment has been reported to reduce the extent of
a subsequent febrile response (HARVEY and MILTON 1974 b). In adult mice centrally
injected 5-HT is known to evoke hypothermia (BRITTAIN and HANDLEY 1967), and
the hypothermic response to endotoxin is augmented by tryptophan and diminished by cyproheptadine pre-treatment (MOON and BERRY 1968).

In newborn animals, as in adults, the febrile response ought to be compared
with the particular thermoregulatory responses evoked by centrally injected monoamines within the same species.

In the newborn guinea-pig injections of 5-HT into the cerebral ventricles elicit
primary hypothermia (KOMÁROMI 1976; SZÉKELY 1978 b). Intraperitoneal pre-
treatment with pCPA modified endotoxin fever in that the hypothermic period between the two rising phases was greatly attenuated or virtually absent, even in a
cold environment (SZÉKELY 1978 c, d). The periods of temperature rise, by themselves, were hardly influenced except that the first rise was slightly enhanced
(Fig. 9). Minute doses of pCPA given ICV led to similar results, suggesting that
central and not peripheral serotonergic processes were involved in the changes observed.

The effect of centrally administered 5-HT in the newborn rat is hypothermic
(TIRRI 1971), in accord with the adult rat, in which central serotonergic mechanisms may also be thermolytic (LIN 1978). In 8- to 10-day-old rats pre-treated
with pCPA an endotoxin injection caused no change in body temperature (SZÉ-
KELY unpublished), in contrast to the usual fall 60–120 min after injection. This
suggests the participation of 5-HT in the endotoxin-induced temperature fall, and
supports the idea mentioned earlier (Sect. F.I) that the transient temperature decline of newborn guinea-pigs and the temperature fall in the corresponding period
of the endotoxin response of newborn rats may have more-or-less the same underlying central regulatory mechanism. It is most likely that the same applies also to
the rabbit.

In the kitten, in which fever is usually monophasic (SZÉKELY and SZELÉNYI
1977; SZÉKELY 1979 c), central administration of 5-HT has been reported to evoke
primary hyperthermia (SZÉKELY 1978 b). In kittens pre-treated with pCPA (Fig. 10)

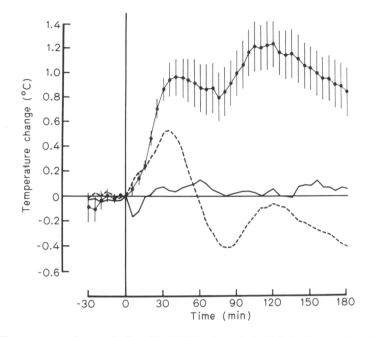

Fig. 9. Temperature changes induced by ICV endotoxin (*solid circles*) or saline (*solid line*) in 0- to 3-day-old guinea-pigs pre-treated IP with pCPA. $T_a = 20$ °C. Endotoxin response in control animals at the same T_a (*broken line*). (SZÉKELY 1978c)

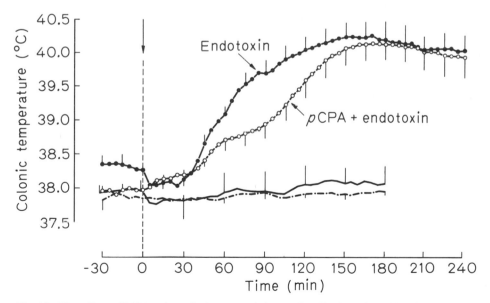

Fig. 10. The effect of ICV endotoxin (*open circles*) or saline (*broken dotted line*) in newborn kittens pretreated IP with pCPA and in control kittens injected with endotoxin (*solid circles*) or with saline (*solid line*). T_a about thermoneutral. (SZÉKELY 1978d)

the monophasic febrile temperature rise is temporarily halted within the interval 60–90 min after endotoxin injection (Székely 1978 d), i.e. during a period roughly coinciding with the pCPA-sensitive period in guinea-pigs and rats. Thus, serotonergic mechanisms may also be involved in the kitten's febrile response, and while their action is again confined to a circumscribed period of the whole response, these mechanisms result, in this species, in a temperature rise.

Measurements of hypothalamic content of 5-HT revealed no dramatic changes in the course of the endotoxin response of either newborn guinea-pigs or kittens, the levels of 5-hydroxyindoleacetic acid were, however, significantly increased in both species during a strictly defined period of the response, coincident with that in which pCPA modified fever in other experiments (Hahn and Székely 1979). These data are in accordance with the finding of Mašek et al. (1973) that, in adult rats, the hypothalamic serotonin turnover increased one hour after IV injection of streptococcal mucopeptide, but not earlier and not later.

All these data are very much in favour of the idea that central serotonergic mechanisms operate at a more-or-less identical stage of the febrile response in all these species, the actual form of participation and the net effect on body temperature depends mainly on the species. This finding reconciles the species specificity of the 5-HT action with the apparent involvement of 5-HT in the febrile response, and offers one explanation of why fever is biphasic in one species and monophasic in another, why a dominant temperature fall is observed in guinea-pigs in response to endotoxin at a T_a of 20 °C, while in kittens the response at that T_a is still a temperature rise.

Thus, the central mediation of fever seems to take place in a sequence of steps: in the first step arachidonic acid derivatives lead to a temperature rise, next, mechanisms involving hypothalamic serotonin induce a transient fall in some species and a further rise in others, and this, in turn, is followed by a temperature rise of some different mediation. The various steps can be influenced separately, and they appear to be quite distinct. The sequence is probably similar in adult animals, but the larger body and consequently the larger thermal inertia tends to decrease the rate of change in body temperature, therefore the specific fever course cannot be analysed with the same precision as in the newborn.

The fact that in the guinea-pigs pre-treatment with indomethacin also prevented the "transient temperature decline" suggests that the presence of those arachidonic acid metabolites responsible for the first rise, or the presence of this rise itself, is necessary to evoke the serotonergic mechanism. The former version seems more likely, since – as discussed in Sect. F.III.2 – the decline or definite fall is independent of the first-phase temperature rise.

The ensuing second-phase rise in temperature after endotoxin injection cannot be explained by these mechanisms.

3. Noradrenaline

With regard to the second rise of body temperature in the course of fever, the possible role of NA has to be considered, particularly since several reports have confirmed that the activation of central noradrenergic mechanisms elicits hyperthermia in the guinea-pig (Zeisberger and Brück 1971; Komáromi 1977a) and in the

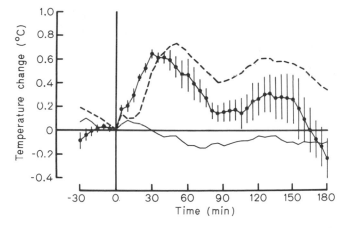

Fig. 11. Temperature response to ICV injection of saline (*solid line*) or endotoxin (*solid circles*) in 0- to 3-day-old guinea-pigs pretreated with ICV α-methyl-*p*-tyrosine. T_a about thermoneutrality. The fever response of control guinea-pigs (*broken line*). (SZÉKELY 1979 b)

rabbit (KOMÁROMI et al. 1969 a). However, since in kittens centrally applied NA leads to hypothermia, whereas their body temperature rises in the period of the febrile response corresponding to the second phase in guinea-pigs (SZÉKELY 1978 d, 1979 c), and since there is no reason why the central mediation of this particular phase should be different from that in other species when the mediation of the previous parts of fever is similar, the role of central noradrenergic mechanisms in the development of the second phase of fever seems to be debatable.

Data suggesting an involvement of catecholamines in the fever response are:
a) A diminution of the febrile response has been shown by GIARMAN et al. (1968) and TEDDY (1971) in adult rabbits pre-treated IP with the catecholamine-depleting drug α-methyl-p-tyrosine (SPECTOR et al. 1965).
b) Pretreatment of cats with 6-hydroxydopamine injections ICV, which causes selective destruction of catecholaminergic neurones, resulted in an enhancement of the febrile response (HARVEY and MILTON 1974a). This is in accordance with the hypothermic response observed upon central administration of NA to cats.

While the experiments using 6-hydroxydopamine indicated the involvement of central catecholaminergic receptors in cat fever, the experiments on rabbits can also be interpreted as the depletion of peripheral catecholamine stores, and therefore do not prove unequivocally the role of central nonadrenergic processes in the pathomechanism of fever.

Newborn guinea-pigs that have been pre-treated with α-methyl-p-tyrosine injections ICV exhibited a fall in hypothalamic NA content by about 50%, from 1.33 ± 0.08 to 0.66 ± 0.05 µg/mg (standard errors are quoted). The subsequent fever course was, however, not much affected by this (Fig. 11), except perhaps for a slight decline in body temperature starting with the transient fall; this trend might have been a consequence of relative 5-HT excess due to 5-HT liberation during the transient fall (SZÉKELY 1979 b).

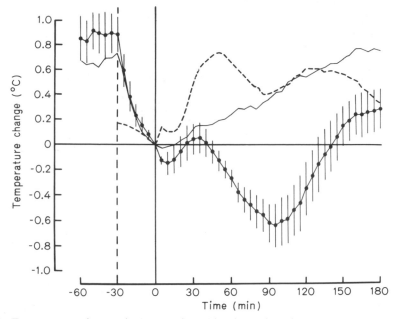

Fig. 12. Temperature changes in 0- to 3-day-old guinea-pigs after ICV injection of saline (*solid line*) or endotoxin (*solid circles*) preceded by an IP injection of propranolol 30 min earlier. T_a about thermoneutral. The normal febrile response is also demonstrated (*broken line*) (SZÉKELY 1979 b)

The hypothalamic NA content did not differ between newborn guinea-pigs treated with 0.9% NaCl and with endotoxin, and similar findings have also been reported for kittens (HAHN and SZÉKELY 1979).

In newborn guinea-pigs centrally applied α-adrenoceptor blockers, in doses which reportedly prevent the effect of centrally applied NA, did not influence the subsequent fever course, neither did centrally applied β-adrenoceptor blockers (SZÉKELY 1979 b). In kittens the findings were similar (SZÉKELY 1979 c).

Peripherally injected propranolol (β-blocker) did, however, influence the fever course in guinea-pigs (Fig. 12): both the first and the second rise were strikingly diminished or abolished, while the temperature fall still developed at the time of its usual occurrence. Peripheral administration of α-adrenoceptor blockers was without effect (SZÉKELY 1979 b).

This suggests that in the guinea-pig, and probably also in other species, peripheral β-receptor integrity rather than the function of central adrenergic mechanisms is a basic-requirement for the development of the usual fever course.

4. Other Factors

Our knowledge of the role in fever of cholinergic factors, histamine, taurine, cations, cyclic nucleotides, or other mediatory or modulatory substances is too sparse for a useful discussion, especially as far as the newborn are concerned. It is likely, however, that many of those substances not mentioned in this survey are also involved in endotoxin-induced thermoregulatory changes.

5. Similarities of Fever Mediation in Newborn and Adult Animals

In the newborn, all the substances mentioned (PG, 5-HT, NA) initiated thermoregulatory responses that were principally similar to those seen in the adults of the same species (see also Sect. C.II). Quantitative differences, although possible (as discussed for PGs), are very difficult either to prove or to refute. These substances have been shown to participate in only circumscribed periods of the complex fever course (if at all), and not in the whole febrile response. Consequently, possible age-related differences in their turnover might modify one or other part of the fever course and not affect the whole febrile response. The role of these substances may be quite similar in adults as in the newborn, while the temperature changes may yet be somewhat different because of differences in surface/weight ratio.

Disturbances in the central (or peripheral) metabolism of the putative mediators (PG, 5-HT, NA) can modify the fever response. The modification may, however, be very similar in newborn and adult animals. For instance, the PG-synthesis blocker indomethacin in newborn guinea-pigs, and flurbiprofen in adult rabbits, reduced only the first phase of fever (Sect. F.III.1). On the other hand, pCPA diminished some part or the whole of the fever response in kittens and in adult cats, respectively (Sect. F.III.2). In addition, peripheral NA depletion reduced fever in adult rabbits, while in newborn guinea-pigs, which rely to a greater extent on non-shivering thermogenesis, the peripheral β-blocker propranolol abolished the rising phases of fever (Sect. F.III.3).

Data from this pharmacological analysis provide a basis for better understanding of the hypothalamic response to endotoxin in a cold environment. There is, again, a similarity between newborn and adult animals: the endotoxin response of newborn guinea-pigs at a T_a of 20 °C (SZÉKELY 1978c) was very similar to that of adult rabbits (GRANT 1949) and rats (SZÉKELY and SZELÉNYI 1979a) at values of T_a around 0° and 20 °C, respectively.

It is quite possible that starvation may also influence the febrile response in adult animals similarly as it did in newborn rabbits, i.e. by depressing the periods of temperature rise. There are, however, no experimental data to support this.

It appears, therefore, that the information regarding the role of mediatory or modulatory substances in fever is not specific to the neonate, but refers to mechanisms common to newborn and adult animals. The only exception, perhaps, is the lack of the second phase of fever in 0- to 3-day-old rabbits.

From the above data, taken collectively, it is obvious that these mechanisms could give a sufficient explanation neither for the differences between adult and newborn animals in the latency of fever after injections of identical doses of the pyrogens, nor for the need of higher pyrogen doses in the neonate to produce the characteristic biphasic course of fever. Also, a difference between adult and newborn animals in the metabolism of some of these substances could not easily explain, by itself, the differences in fever height, although an enhanced PG catabolism could contribute to the mechanisms which diminish the febrile temperature rise in some newborn. To develop a hypothermic response to pyrogens, the presence of some of these central substances (5-HT) is necessary but not sufficient: the simultaneous presence of other factors (large surface, cool environment) is also indispensable. To give a satisfactory explanation for all the characteristics of the neonatal febrile response, other possibilities must also be taken into account, beside the role of central modulatory substances.

IV. Fever as an Abnormal Drive

In adult animals the repertoire of effector mechanisms used in fever is practically identical to that used in defence to cold. Newborn lambs failed to respond to IV endotoxin despite appropriate responses to thermal stress. From this, COOPER and VEALE (1974) concluded that "the maturation necessary in the nervous system to respond to leucocyte pyrogen appears not to be the same development as is necessary for induction of shivering in response to cold," and that the fever-inducing central mechanism produces an abnormal drive, from a source outside the basic thermoregulatory pathways, to the heat conserving and producing mechanisms. An initial suggestion that this drive may be of PGE origin was, however, not substantiated, since even those lambs responding with fever to endotoxin were unresponsive to centrally applied PGE (PITTMAN et al. 1975, 1977).

BLATTEIS (1977) came to much the same conclusion with newborn guinea-pigs, in which temperature regulation was also competent at birth, but IV-administered endotoxin did not evoke fever. Injections of leucocyte pyrogen into the preoptic area immediately after birth often resulted in fever, but the number of reactive animals increased with advancing age. Increasing the volume of the same dilution of pyrogen, thus administering a larger total amount, also increased the number of reactive guinea-pigs. The existence of specific leucocyte pyrogen-sensitive units in the preoptic area was therefore postulated (BLATTEIS and SMITH 1979), and it was also assumed that many of these leucocyte pyrogen-sensitive units are morphologically or biochemically immature at birth, but the density of mature units increases with age. A larger volume of the injectate would suffuse a wider area and reach sufficient leucocyte pyrogen-sensitive loci to evoke a febrile response while, with advancing age, a smaller area would contain enough mature units, and this could account for the age-dependent increase in reactive animals.

Furthermore, in accordance with recent opinions that various independent networks may be involved in the central regulation of body temperature (CABANAC 1975; SATINOFF and HENDERSEN 1977; SATINOFF 1978), BLATTEIS and SMITH (1979) have speculated that two separate pathways may project from the proposed leucocyte pyrogen-sensitive sites: one to autonomic integrators, which may be immature, and another to behavioural integrators, which may be functional at birth. This reasoning, at the same time, indicates that postulating the immaturity or even the existence of some specific leucocyte pyrogen-sensitive loci is not essential.

Indisputably, the experiments of SATINOFF et al. (1976) and KLEITMAN and SATINOFF (1980) indicate that more than one integrating circuit may be involved in the febrile response and that these start functioning at different stages of ontogenesis, their sensitivity being unequal at birth. These data do not, however, suggest any integratory leucocyte pyrogen-receptive mechanism distinct from the main thermoregulatory circuits and specific to fever. On the contrary, under nonfebrile conditions both adult and newborn animals usually prefer to use behavioural means of temperature regulation seeking warmth or cold, huddling, etc., rather than autonomic means. This preference appears to be already operational at birth, and this is reflected in the higher threshold of signals needed to activate autonomic than behavioural functions. Thus, the uneven responsiveness of various (autonomic and behavioural) functions to pyrogens seems to be rather closely paralleled by their uneven responsiveness to thermal stimuli.

This, however, does not preclude the existence in certain species of a central pyretogenic mechanism separate from the basic central thermointegrative mechanisms, but this is pure conjecture, even indirect evidence is lacking. Even if it existed, an "immaturity" of this postulated pyretogenic mechanism could explain only differences in the heights of neonatal and adult fevers, and furthermore, the differences in fever height might have some other, more appropriate or more conceivable explanation. The rest of the differences are inexplicable in this way. This "immature pyretogenic mechanism" could not account for a hypothermic response to endotoxin, and probably not for the longer latency of fever in the newborn, nor for the need of larger endotoxin doses to get a biphasic fever. All these features require some other explanation.

While it seems unnecessary to postulate some separate central mechanisms specific for febrigenesis, it is possible or even likely that more than one site of endogenous pyrogen action exists – hypothalamus, brain-stem, etc. (ROSENDORFF and MOONEY 1971; LIPTON and TRZCINKA 1976). This could explain fevers of completely different latency, course, and height. The slow-onset fever of rabbits with ablated hypothalami (VEALE and COOPER 1975) supports this possibility. LIPTON and KIRKPATRICK (1980) even demonstrated a case of a human baby with completely destroyed hypothalamic tissue, who was unable to thermoregulate in cold and warm environments, but was still able to develop fever in the course of a virus infection.

V. Relation Between Responsiveness to Thermal and Pyrogenic Stimuli

There is still another alternative way to explain some of the discrepancies between the neonatal and adult responses to pyrogenic substances. This is to connect the neonate's "defective" responsiveness to pyrogens to its "defective" responsiveness to thermal stimuli.

In a particular animal some thermal input (deep-body temperature, mean skin temperature, etc.) may elicit weaker activation of thermoregulatory effector (output) mechanisms than in other animals. It is conceivable that, in this animal, the activation of thermoregulatory effector mechanisms may also be proportionally weaker following non-thermal (e.g. pyrogenic) stimuli converging on the central thermoregulatory pathways, provided that they do converge on these pathways, as shown in most models of temperature regulation. This means that the relative unresponsiveness of neonates to pyrogens derives directly from the peculiarities of the neonatal thermoregulation, thus, postulating any special pyretogenic central mechanism separate from the general thermoregulatory circuitry becomes unnecessary.

In fact, there is no direct experimental evidence of this proportionality between the general thermoregulatory and the febrile responses. If, however, this proportionality exists, then the deviation in thermoregulatory input/output ratio (see

Sect. B.III) observed in the newborn could result in a reduction of the febrile rise in body temperature. The inter-species differences in the endotoxin reactions of various neonates do show a certain parallelism with their ability to maintain deep-body temperature in moderately cold environments, which ability, in turn reflects their thermoregulatory input/output ratio.

Although newborn guinea-pigs are usually good thermoregulators, the body temperature at a T_a of 20 °C was slightly but significantly lower than at a T_a of 30 °C, even in those animals responding with biphasic fever to endotoxin (SZÉKELY 1978c) and in which the fever height was of the same order as in older guinea-pigs (Fig. 6). In smaller (possibly underfed) or small-for-age guinea-pigs the temperature is more labile (FARKAS et al. 1974), indicating a disproportionality between their thermoregulatory input and output functions; this could explain greater variations in endotoxin responses, particularly at T_a below thermoneutrality, which seems to be in line with the findings reported by BLATTEIS (1977) and BLATTEIS and SMITH (1979). Newborn rabbits, when exposed to cold, allow a fall in body temperature (VÁRNAI et al. 1970; ALEXANDER 1975), and the maximum rise in their body temperature to endotoxin challenge was somewhat smaller than in adult rabbits (Fig. 5). The newborn rat is even less able to maintain homeothermy when exposed to cold (VÁRNAI and DONHOFFER 1970; ALEXANDER 1975), and in this species there were no periods of the endotoxin response in which a temperature rise was observed (Fig. 1).

It is interesting that starvation, which can modify the responsiveness to thermal influences (see Sect. B.IV), i.e. can decrease responsiveness to both cold and warm environmental stimuli (ANDREWS et al. 1974), also depressed the rising phases of fever in newborn rabbits. To some extent, the maternally neglected newborn rabbits from the experiments of KLEITMAN and SATINOFF (1980), the small-for-age guinea-pigs from the experiments of BLATTEIS and SMITH (1979), and the starved newborn rabbits of SZÉKELY (1979a) may be considered similar in this respect.

During exposure to moderate cold, the metabolic rate of warm-acclimatized adult rats often fails to reach a level that would be necessary to maintain the initial body temperature, despite the fact that metabolic rate could be further elevated by more severe cold. Thus, in moderate cold, body temperature declines with only moderate elevation of metabolism (DONHOFFER and SZELÉNYI 1967). In this connection it may be of interest that the maximum febrile rise in body temperature after IV endotoxin injection was slightly larger in cold-acclimatized than in warm-acclimatized rats (SZÉKELY and SZELÉNYI, unpublished).

Recent data demonstrate that the febrile hyporesponsiveness at term in pregnant ewes (KASTING et al. 1978a, b) and rabbits (KULLANDER 1977) may also be accompanied by decreased responsiveness to cold or warm stimuli, at least in the rabbit (VAUGHN et al. 1978).

These data seem to lend indirect support to the suggestion that the decreased responsiveness to pyrogens and to thermal stimuli may be interconnected. The point or points in the thermoregulatory circuitry, which are responsible for the decreased responsiveness, cannot be located precisely. They may be either on the thermoreceptive side or, more likely, somewhere in the central thermointegrative mechanisms. Considering more than one such point would be in accordance with the postulate of SATINOFF and HENDERSEN (1977) and SATINOFF (1978) on multiple integrative circuits. The responsiveness of some of these points may be different in neonates and adults, which could account for a relative unresponsiveness of the autonomic functions in the presence of good behavioural responses to endotoxin in the newborn rabbit.

Even if the decreased thermal responsiveness of the newborn could account for a decreased pyrogenic response, it could, at most, explain variations in the height of the rising phases of fever, but could not account for a hypothermic response, nor could it account for the lack of fever in the newborn lamb, which is an excellent thermoregulator (DAWES and MOTT 1959; ALEXANDER 1975; MERCER et al. 1979). It would also be difficult to explain exclusively by this mechanism such differences as the longer latency or the monophasic response after endotoxin doses that evoke biphasic fever of short latency in adults. Therefore, to explain the whole spectrum of peculiarities of neonatal fever, the role of other factors must also be considered.

VI. Relationship of Factors Influencing Neonatal Febrile Response

In summing up the possible explanations of the deviant febrile responsiveness in the neonatal period, it seems obvious that none of the suggested mechanisms could alone account for all the differences between neonatal and adult responses to pyrogenic substances. The fever response is a complicated sequence of thermoregulatory events, each part of which utilizes the centrally coordinated function of thermoregulatory effectors. No single factor or substance could fulfil the role of a link between the endogenous pyrogen and all the various thermoregulatory changes evoked by pyrogens, instead, various factors must be postulated, all of which may act in different integrating circuits or on different structures (hypothalamus, brainstem, etc.).

Most of the differences between neonatal and adult fever responses appear to be of a quantitative nature. The production of endogenous pyrogens as well as the involvement of central mediatory or modulatory substances in the febrile reaction seems to be only quantitatively different in newborn and adult animals of the same species. Possible quantitative differences can, however, modify or modulate the fever response in such a way that the whole reaction becomes qualitatively different in the neonate. Thus, each part of the sequence of the characteristic febrile thermoregulatory changes can already be present in the newborn, but the temperature manifestation of the various parts may be widely different.

The *first rise* may be smaller in the newborn, partly because of a quicker degradation of the arachidonic acid derivatives that are indispensable for this part of the fever, and partly because any response to a given thermal or non-thermal stimulus is smaller since the thermoregulatory input/output ratio is different for neonates and adults. In fact, the temperature rise in this period can vary between zero (e.g. newborn rat) and values that are similar to those observed in the adults of the same species (e.g. newborn guinea-pig). This phase of fever is particularly sensitive to nutritional changes and requires the integrity of peripheral β-adrenoceptors.

The extent of the *subsequent fall* in body temperature, which involves central serotonergic mechanisms, may again vary, depending on the actual conditions. The relatively large surface area of the newborn facilitates heat loss and makes heat exchange easier, particularly in the cold, thus, the net temperature change after endotoxin may be a fall even in the presence of otherwise intact temperature elevating periods (e.g. newborn guinea-pigs at a T_a of 20 °C). If the preceding temperature rise is too small or is inhibited, then this fall is the first and usually the only change in body temperature in response to pyrogens (e.g. newborn rats, starving rabbits, guinea-pigs pre-treated with IP propranolol). If T_a is not low, the fall in temperature may be negligible. So, depending on T_a, large differences in body temperature may occur, to some extent accounting for the greater temperature lability observed in later stages of fever. In some species, in which 5-HT results in hyperthermia, body temperature increases in this period also, thus, monophasic fever develops.

The *second rise* is the least constant part, both in adult, and in newborn animals. It does not require the activation of CNS prostaglandins. The temperature level established by the end of the previous periods is only slightly modified by the second-phase rise in body temperature – hypo- and hyperthermic levels are equally possible. Depending mainly on T_a, body temperature may vary over a wider range without adequate effort to compensate, thus the animal shows an enhanced *thermal lability*. Thermal lability in the late stages of the endotoxin effect can be demonstrated in those species, too, in which fever is characteristically monophasic.

Looked at in this way, those differences which, at first sight seem to suggest a qualitatively different regulatory mechanism in the newborn, can be explained in most cases simply on a quantitative basis. This sort of explanation utilizes the particular features of neonatal thermoregulation (surface/weight ratio, input/output ratio, etc.) in explaining the peculiarities of the neonatal fever response, instead of seeking some basically new form of regulation specific for fever.

G. Concluding Remarks

I. Human Applications

Special care must be taken when data obtained on experimental animals are extrapolated to human beings. Besides the species difference, there are, as a rule, differences in the conditions accompanying the fevers which develop under clinical and experimental circumstances. Infected human babies can be flooded with unknown amounts of pyrogens from the invading bacteria, in a way which resembles a continuous slow infusion, while in experimental animals a single known dose of endotoxin is given. Further, in most experiments, healthy well-fed animals are injected with pyrogens and maintained throughout the experiment under strictly defined experimental conditions. In contrast, in the course of naturally occurring infections of human babies the environmental conditions are usually variable and, often as a first sign of their illness, these babies frequently have disturbances in their normal feeding pattern.

Some conclusions applicable to paediatric medicine may still be drawn from the experimental studies. In the infected neonates, fever may be absent, or there may even be hypothermia. This may be expected to occur more readily in slightly cool environments, particularly in very small babies and if the feeding of the baby is disturbed in any way. Even mild nutritional deficits can lead to serious thermoregulatory consequences, including the diminution of the active rise in temperature during fever, the relative enhancement of a regulated fall in certain periods of a febrile reaction, and the enhancement of passive shifts in body temperature with a swing either upwards or, more frequently, downwards, depending on T_a. Such shifts (if any) are less extreme in healthy well-fed babies.

Thus, the animal studies provide an experimental background for the usual clinical findings (see Sect. D). It must, therefore, be emphasized once again, that it is not necessarily a febrile temperature rise that should be looked for if the possibility of infection arises in a neonate; hypothermia or merely greater thermal lability instead of fever is also of diagnostic value. However, under certain circumstances, fever may also develop in the neonate.

II. Definition of Fever

Theoretical considerations also arise from the experimental data discussed. Some of these refer to the definition of fever. The definition used by BLIGH and JOHNSON (1973) is excellent, since it puts an emphasis on the central regulatory mechanisms which, in a coordinated manner, can push body temperature to a higher level. From the present discussion, however, it appears that it is exactly the same central thermoregulatory process that leads to biphasic fever in some instances and results in hypothermia in other cases. This reveals the discrepancy between the central regulatory process and the net result on body temperature, i.e. an animal can be in a febrile state from the point of view of central regulations whilst not being febrile from the point of view of its body temperature. While the pyrogen-induced hypothermia can hardly be called fever, it should be identified as an equivalent of fever, both for clinical and for experimental purposes, at least as regards central regulation (and after all, this is what matters and makes fever different from other hyperthermias).

III. Set-Point Change in Fever

Finally, this discussion leads to the problem of the hypothesized upward displacement of the thermoregulatory set-point mechanism which is generally assumed to take place during fever. Since in the newborn of some species fever height may approximate that of adults, while in the newborn of other species fever height is smaller than in adults or hypothermia may even develop, it would seem that various forms of re-setting can occur in different neonates. A more thorough analysis, however, indicates that this is not an exact description of what happens. Namely, all parts of the sequential events in fever are centrally regulated, but the regulation is not uniform: not only the strength but also the direction of the central thermoregulatory drive changes sequentially, in order to produce the biphasic fever, and the sequence is probably similar in those species exhibiting monophasic fever. The sequential pattern of thermoregulatory changes does not support the idea that a uniform re-adjustment of the central thermoregulatory mechanisms could account for the whole fever course. Thus, if a set-point exists, the biphasic fever implies that it is continuously changing.

On the other hand, as it has been described earlier, in Sect. F.VI irrespective of whether the endotoxin elicits biphasic or monophasic fever in a species, during the endotoxin action body temperature becames more dependent on T_a. This thermal lability conflicts with the classic idea of a change of set-point (reviewed by HAMMEL 1972) which is presumed to be independent of T_a. The thermal lability during endotoxin action can be more easily reconciled with the idea of MITCHELL et al. (1970) that a change in gain or sensitivity of the thermoregulatory control system occurs during fever. This could also fit in with the greater thermal lability of the newborn upon exposure to thermal influences of the environment.

It appears therefore that, at least in the first part of the febrile response to pyrogens, there may be some factors which, indeed, result in a re-adjustment of thermoregulatory set-point mechanisms, all of which cause specific unidirectional changes, if any, in the central thermoregulatory drive, within any one species. Thus, among those factors participating in the fever response, PGs cause a drive to elevate body temperature at all environmental temperatures, 5-HT results in a drive to depress body temperature in some species and to elevate it in others at any T_a. These factors are also functioning in small and newborn animals; their manifestation depends, in part, on T_a and conditions of peripheral effector functions, and on hypothalamic temperature (ANDERSEN et al. 1963; LIPTON and KENNEDY 1979). Besides these factors other factors may exist, at least in some (later) periods of the febrile response, which can change the gain or sensitivity of the thermoregulatory control system and lead to a greater lability of body temperature.

Acknowledgements. We acknowledge with thanks the continuous interest shown by Professor Sz. DONHOFFER and Professor J. MESTYÁN. The generous help of Dr. ANN SILVER in correcting the manuscript and the technical assistance given by Mrs. M. SZELÉNYI is also acknowledged. We are very grateful to Dr. IBOLYA KOMÁROMI and to Dr. ANN SILVER for allowing us to refer to their unpublished observations.

Figures 1, 2, 3, 4, 5, 7, 11, and 12 are reproduced (some of them in a modified version) by the permission of Acta physiol. Acad. Sci. hung. from various papers which appeared in this journal. By permission, Figs. 8 and 9 are reproduced (Fig. 8 with slight modifications) from J. Physiol. (Lond.) *281* (1978). Figure 10 is reprinted with permission from Life Sciences *22* (1978): Székely, M.: "Endotoxin fever in para-chlorophenylalanine (PCPA) treated newborn guinea pigs and kittens," copyright: Pergamon Press, Ltd.

This work was supported, in part, by the Scientific Research Council, Hungarian Ministry of Health (3-06-0302-03-2/A).

References

Abrams RM (1978) Thermal physiology of the fetus. In: Sinclair JC (ed) Temperature regulation and energy metabolism in the newborn. Grune and Stratton, New York, pp 75–89
Alexander G (1975) Body temperature control in mammalian young. Br Med Bull 31:62–68
Andersen HT, Hammel HT, Hardy JD (1963) Modifications of the febrile response to pyrogen by hypothalamic heating and cooling in the unanesthetized dog. In: Hardy JD (ed) Temperature: its measurement and control in science and industry, vol III, part 3. Biology and medicine. Reinhold, New York, pp 597–601
Anderson RJ, Berl T, McDonald KM, Schrier RW (1975) Evidence for an in vivo antagonism between vasopressin and prostaglandin in the mammalian kidney. J Clin Invest 56:420–426
Andrews JF, Mercer JB, Ryan EM, Székely M (1974) The metabolic effect of starvation related to ambient temperatures in new-born lambs. Ir J Med Sci 143:357–358
Atkins E (1960) Pathogenesis of fever. Physiol Rev 40:580–646
Atkins E, Bodel P (1974) Fever. In: Zweifach BW, Grant L, McCluskey RT (eds) The inflammatory process. Academic Press, New York, pp 467–513

Atkins E, Huang WC (1958 a) Studies on the pathogenesis of fever with influenzal viruses. II. The effects of endogenous pyrogen in normal and virus-tolerant recipients. J Exp Med 107:403–414

Atkins E, Huang WC (1958 b) Studies on the pathogenesis of fever with influenzal viruses III. The relation of tolerance to the production of endogenous pyrogen. J Exp Med 107:415–435

Baird JA, Hales JRS, Lang WJ (1974) Thermoregulatory responses to the injection of monoamines, acetylcholine, and prostaglandins into a lateral cerebral ventricle of the echidna. J Physiol (Lond) 236:539–548

Bartolozzi G, Corvaglia E (1967) Effect of pyrexia on the blood phenylalanine level in patients with phelylketonuria undergoing treatment (in Italian). Clin Pediatr 19:1577–1578

Baumann IR, Bligh J (1975) The influence of ambient temperature on drug-induced disturbances of body temperature. In: Lomax P, Schönbaum E, Jacob J (eds) Temperature regulation and drug action. Karger, Basel, pp 241–251

Bennett IL, Cluff LE (1957) Bacterial pyrogens. Pharmacol Rev 9:427–475

Bergström T, Larson H, Lincoln K, Winberg J (1972) Studies on urinary tract infections in infancy and childhood. Eighty consecutive patients with neonatal infections. J Pediatr 80:858–866

Berry LJ, (1966) Effect of environmental temperature on lethality of endotoxin and its effect on body temperature in mice. Fed Proc 25:1264–1270

Bignall KE, Heggeness FW, Palmer JE (1974) Effects of acute starvation on cold-induced thermogenesis in the preweanling rat. Am J Physiol 227:1088–1093

Blackfan KD, Yaglou CP (1933) The premature infant; a study of the effects of atmospheric conditions on growth and on development. Am J Dis Child 46:1175–1236

Blatteis CM (1974) Influence of body weight and temperature on the pyrogenic effect of endotoxins in guinea pigs. Toxicol Appl Pharmacol 29:249–258

Blatteis CM (1975) Postnatal development of pyrogenic sensitivity in guinea pigs. J Appl Physiol 39:251–257

Blatteis CM (1976) Effect of propanolol on endotoxin-induced pyrogenesis in newborn and adult guinea pigs. J Appl Physiol 40:35–39

Blatteis CM (1977) Comparison of endotoxin and leukocytic pyrogen pyrogenicity in newborn guinea pigs. J Appl Physiol Respir Environ Exercise Physiol 42:355–361

Blatteis CM, Smith KA (1979) Hypothalamic sensitivity to leukocytic pyrogen of adult and newborn guinea pigs. J Physiol (Lond) 296:177–192

Blatteis CM, Billmeier G, Gilbert T (1973) Thermoregulation of phenylketonuric children. Fed Proc 32/31:1056

Bläsig J, Herz A (1978) Evidence of a role of endorphines in emotional hyperthermia. Naunyn-Schmiedeberg Arch Pharmacol 302:R 61

Bligh J (1973) Temperature regulation in mammals and other vertebrates. Elsevier/North Holland, Amsterdam Oxford New York

Bligh J, Johnson KG (1973) Glossary of terms for thermal physiology. J Appl Physiol 35:941–961

Bligh J, Maskrey M (1970) The interaction between the effects on thermoregulation of TAB vaccine injected intravenously and monoamines injected into a lateral cerebral ventricle of the Welsh Mountain sheep. J Physiol (Lond) 213:60–62 P

Bligh J, Cottle WH, Maskrey M (1971) Influence of ambient temperature on thermoregulatory responses to 5-hydroxytryptamine, noradrenaline and acetylcholine injected into the lateral cerebral ventricles of sheep, goats and rabbits. J Physiol (Lond) 212:377–392

Bornstein DL, Brendenberg C, Wood WB Jr (1963) Studies on the pathogenesis of fever XI. Quantitative features of the febrile response to leucocytic pyrogen. J Exp Med 117:349–364

Breckenridge BMcL, Lisk RD (1969) Cyclic adenylate and hypothalamic regulatory functions. Proc Soc Exp Biol Med 131:934–935

Brimblecombe F, Barltrop D (1978) Children in health and disease. Bailliere Tindall, London, p 136

Brittain RT, Handley SL (1967) Temperature changes produced by the injection of catechol-amines and 5-hydroxytryptamine into the cerebral ventricle of the conscious mouse. J Physiol (Lond) 192:805–814

Brooke OG (1972) Influence of malnutrition on body temperature of children. Br Med J 1972:331–333

Brooke OG, Salvosa CB (1974) Response of malnourished babies to heat. Arch Dis Child 49:123–127

Brooke OG, Harris M, Salvosa CB (1973) The response of malnourished babies to cold. J Physiol (Lond) 233:75–91

Brück K (1961) Temperature regulation in the newborn infant. Biol Neonate 3:65–119

Brück K (1978a) Heat production and temperature regulation. In: Stave U (ed) Perinatal physiology. Plenum, New York, pp 445–498

Brück K (1978b) Thermoregulation: control mechanisms and neural processes. In: Sinclair JC (ed) Temperature regulation and energy metabolism in the newborn. Grune and Stratton, New York, pp 157–185

Brück K, Brück M (1960) Der Energieumsatz hypothermer Frühgeborener. Klin Wochenschr 38:1125–1130

Brück K, Wünnenberg W, Gallmeier H, Ziehm B (1970) Shift of threshold temperature for shivering and heat polypnea as a mode of thermal adaptation. Pfluegers Arch 321:159–172

Cabanac M (1975) Temperature regulation. Annu Rev Physiol 37:415–439

Carruba Mo, Bächtold HP (1976) Pyrogen fever in rabbits penetrated with p-chlorophenyl-alanine or 5,6-dihydroxy-tryptamine. Experientia 32:729–730

Cooper KE, Cranston WI (1966) Pyrogens and monoamine oxidase inhibitors. Nature 210:203–204

Cooper KE, Veale WL (1974) Fever, an abnormal drive to heat-conserving and -producing mechanisms? In: Ledris K, Cooper KE (eds) Recent studies of hypothalamic function. Karger, Basel, pp 391–398

Cooper KE, Pittman QJ, Veale WL (1976) The effect of noradrenaline and 5-hydroxytrypt-amine injected into a lateral cerebral ventricle, on thermoregulation in the new-born lamb. J Physiol (Lond) 261:223–234

Coyle JT, Henry D (1973) Catecholamines in fetal and newborn rat brain. J Neurochem 21:61–67

Craig WS (1963) The early detection of pyrexia in the newborn. Arch Dis Child 38:29–39

Cranston WI, Hellon RF, Mitchell D (1975a) Fever and brain prostaglandin release. J Physiol (Lond) 248:27P–29P

Cranston WI, Hellon RF, Mitchell D (1975b) A dissociation between fever and prostaglan-din concentration in cerebrospinal fluid. J Physiol (Lond) 253:583–592

Cranston WI, Duff GW, Hellon RF, Mitchell D, Townsend Y (1976) Evidence that brain prostaglandin synthesis is not essential in fever. J Physiol (Lond) 259:239–249

Cranston WI, Dawson NJ, Hellon RF, Townsend Y (1978) Contrasting actions of cyclohe-ximide on fever caused by arachidonic acid and by pyrogen. J Physiol (Lond) 285:35P

Dascombe MJ, Milton AS (1979) Study on the possible entry of bacterial endotoxin and prostaglandin E_2 into the central nervous system from the blood. Br J Pharmacol 66:565–572

Daum RS, Smith AL (1979) Bacterial sepsis in the newborn. Clin Obstet Gynecol 22:385–408

Dawes GS, Mott JC (1959) The increase in oxygen consumption of the lamb after birth. J Physiol (Lond) 146:295–315

Des Prez RM, Oates JA (1968) Lack of relationship of febrile response to endotoxin and brain stem 5-hydroxytryptamine. Proc Soc Exp Biol Med 127:793–794

Donhoffer SZ, Szelényi Z (1967) The role of brown adipose tissue in thermoregulatory heat production in the warm- and cold-adapted adult rat. Acta Physiol Acad Sci Hung 32:53–60

Donhoffer SZ, Szelényi Z (1975) The homeothermia of the brain: thermoregulatory heat production. In: Jansky L (ed) Proceedings of the satellite symposium on thermoregula-tion. XXVI. International Congress of Physiological Sciences, Prague, 1974. Academia, Prague, pp 73–78

Edqvist L-E, Kindahl H, Stabenfeldt G (1978) Release of prostaglandin $F_{2\alpha}$ during the bovine peripartal period. Prostaglandins 16:111–119

Epstein HC, Hochwald A, Ashe R (1951) Salmonella infections of the newborn infant. J Pediatr 38:723–731

Farkas M, Várnai I, Donhoffer SZ, (1974) Thermoregulatory heat production and the regulation of body temperature in the new-born and adult guinea-pig. Acta Physiol Acad Sci Hung 45:23–35

Feldberg W (1975) Body temperature and fever: changes in our views during the last decade. The Ferrier Lecture 1974. Proc R Soc Lond [Biol] 191:199–229

Feldberg W, Gupta KP (1973) Pyrogen fever and prostaglandin activity in cerebrospinal fluid. J Physiol (Lond) 228:41–53

Feldberg W, Milton AS (1979) Prostaglandins and body temperature. In: Vane JR, Ferreira SH (eds) Inflammation. (Handbook of experimental pharmacology, vol 50/1) Springer, Berlin Heidelberg New York, pp 617–656

Feldberg W, Myers RD (1964) Effects on temperature of amines injected into the cerebral ventricles. A new concept of temperature regulation. J Physiol (Lond) 173:226–236

Feldberg W, Saxena PN (1971) Fever produced by prostaglandin E_1. J Physiol (Lond) 217:547–556

Feldberg W, Gupta KP, Milton AS, Wendlandt S (1973) Effect of pyrogen and antipyretics on prostaglandin activity in cisternal c.s.f. of unanaesthetized cats. J Physiol (Lond) 234:279–303

Giarman NJ, Tanaka C, Mooney J, Atkins E (1968) Serotonin, norepinephrine and fever. Adv Pharmacol 6/A:307–317

Grant R (1949) Nature of pyrogen fever: effect of environmental temperature on response to typhoid-paratyphoid vaccine. Am J Physiol 159:511–524

Grantham JJ, Orloff J (1968) Effect of prostaglandin E_1 on the permeability response of the isolated collecting tubule to vasopressin, adenosine 3'-5'-monophosphate, and theophylline. J Clin Invest 47:1154–1161

Hahn Z, Székely M (1979) Hypothalamic monoamine contents in endotoxin fever of newborn guinea-pigs and kittens. Neurosci Lett 11:279–282

Hammel HT (1972) The set-point in temperature regulation: analogy or reality. In: Bligh J, Moore RE (eds) Essays on temperature regulation. North Holland, Amsterdam Oxford New York, pp 121–137

Harashima S, Kurata M (1966) Temperature regulation in the neonate and the infant. Fed Proc 25:1321–1323

Harvey CA, Milton AS (1974a) The effect of intraventricular 6-hydroxydopamine on the response of the conscious cat to pyrogen. Br J Pharmacol 52:134–135P

Harvey CA, Milton AS (1974b) The effect of para-chlorophenylalanine on the response of the conscious cat to intravenous and intraventricular bacterial pyrogen and to intraventricular prostaglandin E_1. J Physiol (Lond) 236:14–15P

Heim T, Szelényi Z (1965) Temperature regulation in rats semistarved since birth. Acta Physiol Acad Sci Hung 17:247–255

Heim T, Mestyán GY, Szelényi Z (1964) Effect of semi-starvation on temperature regulation in the rat (in Hungarian). Kisérletes Orvostudomány 16:239–246

Hellon RF (1975) Monoamines, pyrogens and cations: their actions on central control of body temperature. Pharmacol Rev 26:289–321

Henderson TC, Luckwill RG, Nayernouri T (1971) Single unit responses to temperature change in the brain of newborn rabbits. Int J Biometeor 15:309–312

Hey EN (1972) Thermal regulation in the newborn. Br J Hosp Med 1972:51–64

Hey EN, Katz G (1969) Evaporative water loss in the new-born baby. J Physiol (Lond) 200:605–619

Hey EN, Katz G (1970) The range of thermal insulation in the tissues of the new-born baby. J Physiol (Lond) 207:667–681

Hori T, Shinohara K (1978) Hypothalamic neurons responding to temperature in the newborn rat. In: Houdas Y, Guien JD (eds) New trends in thermal physiology. Masson, Paris, pp 78–80

Jacob J, Peindaries R (1973) Central effects of monoamines on temperature of the conscious rabbit. In: Schönbaum E, Lomax P (eds) The pharmacology of thermoregulation. Karger, Basel, pp 202–216

Jansky L (1973) Non-shivering thermogenesis and its thermoregulatory significance. Biol Rev 48:85–132

Járai I (1969) The redistribution of cardiac output on cold exposure in new-born rabbits. J Physiol (Lond) 202:559–567

Jell RM, Sweatman P (1977) Prostaglandin-sensitive neurones in cat hypothalamus: relation to thermoregulation and to biogenic amines. Can J Physiol Pharmacol 55:560–567

Karki N, Kuntzman R, Brodie BB (1962) Storage, synthesis and metabolism of monoamines in the developing brain. J Neurochem 9:53–58

Karlberg P, Moore RE, Oliver TK (1962) The thermogenic response of the newborn infant to noradrenaline. Acta Paediatr Scand 51:284–292

Kasting NW, Veale WL, Cooper KE (1978a) Suppression of fever at term pregnancy. Nature 271:245–246

Kasting NW, Veale WL, Cooper KE (1978b) Evidence for a centrally active, endogenous antipyretic near parturition. In: Veale WL, Ledris K (eds) Current studies of hypothalamic function 1978, vol 2. Karger, Basel, pp 63–71

Kasting NW, Cooper KE, Veale WL (1979a) Antipyresis following perfusion of brain sites with vasopressin. Experientia 35:208–209

Kasting NW, Veale WL, Cooper KE (1979b) Development of fever in the newborn lamb. Am J Physiol 236:R184–R187

King MK, Wood WB (1958) Studies on the pathogenesis of fever V. The relation of circulating endogenous pyrogen to the fever of acute bacterial infections. J Exp Med 107:305–317

Kleitman N, Satinoff E (1980) Febrile responses in normal and maternally-neglected newborn rabbits. In: Cox B, Lomax P, Milton AS, Schönbaum E (eds) Thermoregulatory mechanisms and their therapeutic implications. Karger, Basel, pp 102–184

Koe BK, Weissman A (1966) p-Chlorophenylalanine: a specific depletor of brain serotonin. J Pharmacol Exp Ther 154:499–516

Komáromi I (1976) The central effect of 5-hydroxytryptamine, gamma-amino-butyric acid and carbachol on thermoregulation in the neonatal guinea-pig. Acta Physiol Acad Sci Hung 47:15–27

Komáromi I (1977a) Effects of alpha- and beta-adrenergic blockers on the actions of noradrenaline on body body temperature in the newborn guinea-pig. Experientia 33:1083–1084

Komáromi I (1977b) Effect of alpha and beta blockers on body temperature and heat production in the newborn guinea-pig. Acta Physiol Acad Sci Hung 50:299–306

Komáromi I, Moore RE, Sinanan K (1969a) Central effects of noradrenaline and GABA on thermogenesis in the neonatal rabbit. J Physiol (Lond) 202:118P

Komáromi I, Moore RE, Sinanan K (1969b) Central effects of 5-hydroxytryptamine, tranylcypromine a monoamino oxidase inhibitor and gamma-aminobutyric acid on thermogenesis in the neonatal rat. J Physiol (Lond) 205:7P–8P

Korányi G (1978) Neonatal infections. In: Kerpel-Fronius E, Véghelyi PV, Rosta J (eds) Perinatal medicine. Akadémiai Kiadó, Budapest, pp 1069–1093

Kullander S (1977) Fever and parturition. An experimental study in rabbits. Acta Obstet Gynecol Scand [Suppl] 66:77–85

Laburn H, Mitchell D, Rosendorff C (1977) Effects of prostaglandin antagonism on sodium arachidonate fever in rabbits. J Physiol (Lond) 267:559–570

Ladisch S, Pizzo PA (1978) Staphylococcus aureus sepsis in children with cancer. Pediatrics 61:231–234

Liggins GC, Grieves S (1971) Possible role for prostaglandin F_2 in parturition in sheep. Nature 232:629–631

Lin MT (1978) Effects of specific inhibitors of 5-hydroxytryptamine uptake on thermoregulation in rats. J Physiol (Lond) 284:147–154

Lindberg O (ed) (1970) Brown adipose tissue. Elsevier, Amsterdam Oxford New York

Lipton JM, Kennedy JI (1979) Central thermosensitivity during fever produced by intra-PO/AH and intravenous injections of pyrogen. Brain Res Bull 4:23–34

Lipton JM, Kirkpatrick J (1980) Fever capacity after brain lesions. In: Cox B, Lomax P, Milton AS, Schönbaum E (eds) Thermoregulatory mechanisms and their therapeutic implications. Karger, Basel, pp 71–74

Lipton JM, Trzcinka GP (1976) Persistence of febrile response to pyrogens after PO/AH lesions in squirrel monkeys. Am J Physiol 231:1638–1648

Loizou LA (1972) The postnatal ontogeny of monoamine-containing neurons in the central nervous system of the albino rat. Brain Res 40:395–418

Loizou LA, Salt P (1970) Regional changes in monoamines of the rat brain during postnatal development. Brain Res 20:467–470

Lubchenco LO (1961) Watching the newborn for disease. Pediatr Clin North Am 8:476–478

Martin GE, Morrison JE (1978) Hyperthermia evoked by the intracerebral injections of morphine sulphate in the rat: the effect of restraint. Brain Res 145:127–140

Marzetti G, Laurenti F, Caro MD, Conca L, Orzalesi M (1973) *Salmonella München* infections in newborns and small infants. Clin Pediatr 12:93–97

Mašek K, Kadlecová O, Rašková H (1973) Brain amines in fever and sleep cycles changes caused by streptococcal mucopeptide. Neuropharmacology 12:1039–1047

Matsaniotis N, Pastelis V, Agathopoulos A, Constantsas N (1971) Fever and biochemical thermogenesis. Pediatrics 47:571–576

McCaman RE, Aprison MH (1964) The synthetic and catabolic enzyme systems for acetylcholine and serotonin in several discrete areas of the developing brain. Brain Res 9:220–233

McClung HJ (1972) Prolonged fever of unknown origin in children. Am J Dis Child 124:544–550

Mercer JB (1974) Thermoregulation in the new-born lamb. PhD thesis, T.C.D. Dublin

Mercer JB, Andrews JF, Székely M (1979) Thermoregulatory responses in new-born lambs during the first thirty-six hours of life. J Therm Biol 4:239–245

Mestyán J (1978) Energy metabolism and substrate utilization in the newborn. In: Sinclair JC (ed) Temperature regulation and energy metabolism in the newborn. Grune and Stratton, New York, pp 39–74

Milton AS (1976) Modern views on the pathogenesis of fever and the mode of action of antipyretic drugs. J Pharm Pharmacol 28:393–399

Milton AS, Wendlandt S (1971) Effects on body temperature of prostaglandins of the A, E and F series on injection into the third ventricle of unanaesthetized cats and rabbits. J Physiol (Lond) 218:325–336

Milton AS, Smith S, Tomkins KB (1977) Levels of prostaglandin F and E in cerebrospinal fluid of cats during pyrogen induced fever. Br J Pharmacol 59:447–448 P

Milton AS, Cremades-Campos A, Sawhney VK, Bichard A (1980) Effects of prostacyclin, 6-oxo-PGE$_1$ and endoperoxide analogues on the body temperature of cats and rabbits. In: Cox B, Lomax P, Milton AS, Schönbaum E (eds) Thermoregulatory mechanisms and their therapeutic implications. Karger, Basel, pp 87–92

Mitchell D, Snellen JW, Atkins AR (1970) Thermoregulation during fever: Change of set-point or change of gain. Pfluegers Arch 321:293–302

Moon RJ, Berry LJ (1968) Effect of tryptophan and selected analogues on body temperature of endotoxin-poisoned mice. J Bacteriol 95:764–770

Moore RE, Underwood MC (1960) Possible role of noradrenaline in control of heat production in the newborn mammal. Lancet 1:1277–1278

Motil KJ, Blackburn MG (1973) Temperature regulation in the neonate. A survey of the pathophysiology of thermal dynamics and of the principles of environmental control. Clin Pediatr 12:634–639

Myers RD, Veale WL (1971) The role of sodium and calcium ions in the hypothalamus in the control of body temperature of the unanaesthetized cat. J Physiol (Lond) 212:411–430

Naccarato EF, Hunter WS (1979) Febrile response to prostaglandin E$_1$ in pregnant rabbit. Fed Proc 38:1054

Nakamura T, Tada H, Ushijima H (1974) A clinical study of neonatal septicemia and meningitis. A correlation between maternal peripartum fever and perinatal infections (in Japanese). Acta Neonate Jpn 10:182–192

Pace-Asciak CR (1977) Prostaglandin biosynthesis and catabolism in the developing fetal sheep lung. Prostaglandins 13:649–660

Pace-Asciak C, Miller D (1973) Prostaglandins during development. I. Age-dependent activity profiles of prostaglandin 15-hydroxy dehydrogenase and 13,14-reductase in lung tissue from late prenatal, early postnatal and adult rats. Prostaglandins 4:351–362

Pace-Asciak C, Nashat M (1976) Catabolism of prostaglandin endoperoxides into prostaglandin E_2 and $F_{2\alpha}$ by the rat brain. J Neurochem 27:551–556

Pace-Asciak CR, Rangaraj G (1976) Prostaglandin biosynthesis and catabolism in the developing fetal sheep brain. J Biol Chem 251:3381–3385

Peindaries R, Jacob J (1971) Interactions between 5-hydroxytryptamine and a purified bacterial pyrogen when injected into the lateral cerebral ventricle of the wake rabbit. Eur J Pharmacol 13:347–355

Pickard JD, MacDonell LA, MacKenzie ET, Harper AM (1977) Prostaglandin-induced effects in the primate cerebral circulation. Eur J Pharmacol 43:343–351

Pittman QJ, Cooper KE, Veale WL, Van Petten GR (1973) Fever in newborn lambs. Can J Physiol Pharmacol 51:868–872

Pittman QJ, Veale WL, Cooper KE (1975) Temperature responses of lambs after centrally injected prostaglandins and pyrogens. Am J Physiol 228:1034–1038

Pittman QJ, Veale WL, Cooper KE (1977) Effect of prostaglandin, pyrogen and noradrenaline, injected into the hypothalamus, on thermoregulation in newborn lambs. Brain Res 128:473–483

Poczopko P (1961) A contribution to the studies on changes of energy metabolism during postnatal development. I. Development of mechanisms of body temperature regulation in rats. J Cell Comp Physiol 57:175–184

Pscheidt GR, Himwich HE (1966) Biogenic amines in various brain regions of growing cats. Brain Res 1:363–368

Roberts KB, Borzy MS (1977) Fever in first eight weeks of life. Johns Hopkins Med J 141:9–13

Rosendorff C, Mooney JJ (1971) Central nervous system sites of action of a purified leucocyte pyrogen. Am J Physiol 220:597–603

Rosendorff C, Woolf CJ (1979) Inhibition of fever. In: Vane JR, Ferreira SH (eds) Anti-inflammatory drugs. (Handbook of experimental pharmacology, vol 50/2.) Springer, Berlin Heidelberg New York, pp 255–279

Sanford HN, Grulee CG (1961) In: Kelley VC (ed) Brennemann's practice of pediatrics, vol I, chap 42. Hoeber, Scranton, Pa

Satinoff E (1978) Neural organization and evolution of thermal regulation in mammals. Science 201:16–22

Satinoff E, Hendersen R (1977) Thermoregulatory behavior. In: Honig WK, Staddon JER (eds) Handbook of operant behavior. Prentice-Hall, Englewood Cliffs, pp 153–173

Satinoff E, McEwen GN, Williams BA (1976) Behavioral fever in newborn rabbits. Science 193:1139–1140

Scopes JW, Tizard JPM (1963) The effect of intravenous noradrenaline on the oxygen consumption of new-born mammals. J Physiol (Lond) 165:305–326

Sharma SC, Hibbard BM, Hamlett JD, Fitzpatrick RJ (1973) Prostaglandin $F_{2\alpha}$ concentrations in peripheral blood during the first stage of normal labour. Br Med J 1:709–711

Smith RT, Platou ES, Good RA (1956) Septicemia of the newborn. Current status of the problem. Pediatrics 17:549–575

Snell ES (1971) Endotoxin and the pathogenesis of fever. In: Kadis S, Weinbaum G, Ajl SJ (eds) Microbial toxins, vol V. Bacterial endotoxins. Academic Press, New York London, pp 277–340

Spector S, Sjoerdsma A, Udenfriend S (1965) Blockade of endogenous norepinephrine synthesis by α-methyl-p-tyrosine, an inhibitor of tyrosine hydroxylase. J Pharmacol Exp Ther 147:86–95

Spławiński JA, Reichenberg K, Vetulani J, Marchaj J, Kaluza J (1974) Hyperthermic effect of intraventricular injections of arachidonic acid and prostaglandin E_2 in the rat. Pol J Pharmacol Pharm 26:101–107

Stitt JT (1979) Fever versus hyperthermia. Fed Proc 38:39–43

Sulyok E, Jéquier E, Prod'hom LS (1973) Thermal balance of the newborn infant in a heat-gaining environment. Pediatr Res 7:888–900

Székely M (1978a) Biphasic endotoxin fever in the newborn rabbit. Acta Physiol Acad Sci Hung 51:389–392

Székely M (1978b) 5-hydroxytryptamine induced changes in body temperature of newborn kittens and guinea-pigs and the effect of indomethacin thereon. Experientia 34:58–59

Székely M (1978c) Endotoxin fever in the new-born guinea-pig and the modulating effects of indomethacin and p-chlorophenylalanine. J Physiol (Lond) 281:467–476

Székely M (1978d) Endotoxin fever in para-chlorophenylalanine (PCPA) treated newborn guinea-pigs and kittens. Life Sci 22:1585–1588

Székely M (1979a) Nutritional state and the endotoxin fever of newborn rabbits. Acta Physiol Acad Sci Hung 53:279–283

Székely M (1979b) Central and peripheral noradrenergic mechanisms in endotoxin fever of newborn guinea pigs. Acta Physiol Acad Sci Hung 54:257–263

Székely M (1979c) Endotoxin fever in the kitten. The role of prostaglandins and mono-amines. Acta Physiol Acad Sci Hung 54:265–276

Székely M, Komáromi I (1978) Endotoxin and prostagladin fevers of newborn guinea pigs at different ambient temperatures. Acta Physiol Acad Sci Hung 51:293–298

Székely M, Szelényi Z (1977) The effect of E. coli endotoxin on body temperature in the new-born rabbit, cat, guinea pig and rat. Acta Physiol Acad Sci Hung 50:293–298

Székely M, Szelényi Z (1979a) Endotoxin fever in the rat. Acta Physiol Acad Sci Hung 53:265–277

Székely M, Szelényi Z (1979b) Age-related differences in thermoregulatory responses to endotoxin in rabbits. Acta Physiol Acad Sci Hung 54:389–399

Székely M, Szelényi Z (to be published) Thermal adaptation and endotoxin fever in the rat. Acta Physiol Acad Sci Hung

Székely M, Szolcsányi J (1979) Endotoxin fever in capsaicin treated rats. Acta Physiol Acad Sci Hung 53:469–477

Székely M, Szelényi Z, Sümegi I (1973) Brown adipose tissue as a source of heat during pyrogen-induced fever. Acta Physiol Acad Sci Hung 43:85–88

Szelényi Z, Donhoffer SZ (1978) The effect of cold exposure on cerebral blood flow and cerebral available oxygen (aO_2) in the rat and rabbit. Thermoregulatory heat production by the brain and the possible role of neuroglia. Acta Physiol Acad Sci Hung 52:391–402

Szelényi Z, Moore RE (1980) Thermal neutrality and the effect of intraventricular 5-hydroxytryptamine on oxygen consumption in the conscious neonatal rabbit. Acta Physiol Acad Sci Hung 55:135–147

Szelényi Z, Székely M (1979) Comparison of the effector mechanisms during endotoxin fever in the adult rabbit. Acta Physiol Acad Sci Hung 54:33–41

Szelényi Z, Zeisberger E, Brück K (1976) Effects of electrical stimulation in the lower brainstem on temperature regulation in the unanaesthetized guinea-pig. Pfluegers Arch 364:123–127

Szelényi Z, Zeisberger E, Brück K (1977) A hypothalamic alpha-adrenergic mechanism mediating the thermogenic response to electrical stimulation of the lower brainstem in the guinea-pig. Pfluegers Arch 370:19–23

Taylor PM (1960) Oxygen consumption in newborn rats. J Physiol (Lond) 154:153–168

Teddy PJ (1971) Discussion after W. Feldberg's paper "On the mechanism of action of pyrogens." In: Wolstenholme GEW, Birch J (eds) Pyrogens and fever. A Ciba Foundation Symposium. Churchill Livingstone, Edinburgh London, pp 124–129

Teele DW, Pelton SI, Grant MJA et al. (1975) Bacteremia in febrile children under 2 years of age: results of cultures of blood of 600 consecutive febrile children seen in a "walk-in" clinic. J Pediatr 87:227–230

Tirri R (1971) Central effects of 5-hydroxytryptamine and noradrenaline on body temperature and oxygen consumption in infant rats. Experientia 27:274–276

Torda C (1977) Release of hypothalamic catecholamines during activity and rest newborn kitten. Gen Pharmacol 8:47–50

Vane JR (1971) Inhibition of prostaglandin synthesis as a mechanism of action of aspirin-like drugs. Nature New Biol 231:232–235

Van Miert ASJPAM, Frens J (1968) The reaction of different animal species to bacterial pyrogens. Zentralbl Vet Med 15/A:532–543

Van Miert ASJPAM, Van Duin CTM (1977) The antipyretic effect of flurbiprofen. Eur J Pharmacol 44:197–204

Várnai I, Donhoffer SZ (1970) Thermoregulatory heat production and body temperature in the new-born rat. Acta Physiol Acad Sci Hung 37:35–49

Várnai I, Farkas M, Donhoffer SZ (1970) Thermoregulatory heat production and the regulation of body temperature in the new-born rabbit. Acta Physiol Acad Sci Hung 38:299–315

Vaughn LK, Veale WL, Cooper KE (1978) Impaired thermoregulation in pregnant rabbits at term. Pfluegers Arch 378:185–187

Veale WL, Cooper KE (1975) Comparison of sites of action of prostaglandin E and leucocyte pyrogen in brain. In: Lomax P, Schönbaum E, Jacob J (eds) Temperature regulation and drug action. Karger, Basel, pp 218–226

Welch KMA, Spira PJ, Knowles L, Lance JW (1974) Effects of prostaglandins on the internal and external carotid blood flow in the monkey. Neurology 24:705–710

Willman EA, Collins WP (1976) The concentrations of prostaglandin E_2 and prostaglandin F_{2alpha} in tissues within the fetoplacental unit after spontaneous or induced labour. Br J Obstet Gynaecol 83:786–789

Willman EA, Rodock CH, Collins WP, Clayton SG (1977) The relation between umbilical cord tissue prostaglandin E_2 levels, mode of onset of labour, fetal distress and method of delivery. Br J Obstet Gynaecol 84:605–607

Zeisenberger E, Brück K (1971) Central effects of noradrenaline on the control of body temperature in the guinea pig. Pfluegers Arch 322:152–166

Zeisberger E, Brück K (1973) Effects of intrahypothalamically injected noradrenergic and cholinergic agents on thermoregulatory responses. In: Schönbaum E, Lomax P (eds) The pharmacology of thermoregulation. Karger, Basel, pp 232–243

Zeisberger E, Brück K (1976) Alteration of shivering threshold in cold- and warm-adapted guinea-pigs following intrahypothalamic injections of noradrenaline and of an adrenergic alpha-receptor blocking agent. Pfluegers Arch 362:113–119

CHAPTER 16

The Treatment of Fever from a Clinical Viewpoint

C. A. DINARELLO

A. Introduction

In most clinical settings, the reduction of elevated body temperature is a routine procedure. During the past 200 years, increasingly more sophisticated pharmacological agents have expanded our ability to reduce body temperature, while several physical methods have been available for over 25 centuries. Despite the variety of procedures which can lower body temperature, treatment should be appropriate for the particular clinical problem. For example, the physician who is treating a patient with a febrile illness considers whether reducing the fever will obscure information concerning the progress of the disease or the effectiveness of a particular drug. Other aspects which should be considered include the physical status of the patient, the cause of the temperature elevation, and whether the elevation of body temperature is harmful to the patient.

Although the vast majority of patients with elevation of body temperature have fever, a few may be experiencing hyperthermia. In distinguishing fever from hyperthermia it is helpful to consider the thermostatic "set-point" model for hypothalamic thermoregulation. In this sense fever is elevated core temperature which results from an elevated set-point. Humans use physiological as well as behavioural methods for conserving body heat until internal body temperature matches that of the hypothalamic set-point. In addition, thermogenesis, as manifested by shivering, can also increase core temperature. Both heat production and heat conservation will continue until the temperature of the blood bathing the hypothalamus reaches that of the elevated thermostatic setting. On the other hand, hyperthermia is elevated core temperature at a time when the set-point is a normal temperature level. Humans can experience hyperthermia from excessive heat exposure, increased heat production, or inability to dissipate body heat. The treatment of fever is often different from that of hyperthermia and thus it is important to make the proper diagnosis. In some cases, using certain pharmacological agents for reducing fever can adversely affect a patient with hyperthermia.

B. The Treatment of Uncomplicated Fever

Fever occurs in several uncomplicated infections due to viruses and there is little question that viral infections account for the majority of self-limited human illnesses. In the physically healthy individual, whether to treat the fever due to a viral upper respiratory tract infection, an influenzal illness, or a systemic viral disease is a personal preference. Certain accompanying symptoms include malaise, headache, and myalgias which can be alleviated by the same agents which reduce fever. Thus, the treatment of fever, per se, is seldom an isolated procedure in these illnesses. For the majority of viral diseases, no specific anti-infective therapy is available; therefore, the use of antipyretics does not inferfere with the clinical assessment of treatment. Some viruses, notably the agents which cause hepatitis, and other viruses which affect the liver, reduce the ability to conjugate antipyretics and thus their use in these patients may lead to further hepatocellular damage or result in toxic blood levels of the drugs. Some rare viral infections which produce encephalitis, meningitis, or localized brain lesions such as herpes encephalitis may be associated with high fevers and in these patients, elevated core temperature aggravates the ill-effects of brain swelling (discussed in Sect. E.II).

In the pre-antibiotic era, fevers due to infections such as typhoid, typhus, and pneumococcal pneumonia rarely were in excess of 41.1 °C (106 °F) (DuBois 1949). The observation led to the concept that humans have a set-point protective "ceiling" in most febrile diseases. However, this is not always the case and some bacterial infections, particularly Gram-negative organisms, are a common cause of hyperpyrexia (over 41.1 °C, 106 °F) (SIMON 1976). A documented bacterial infection with or without fever as a prominent symptom requires treatment with appropriate antibiotics. However, in certain circumstances the patient has been treated with antibiotics prior to obtaining proper cultures and the choice of antibiotic is made on an empirical basis. In other cases, even when the proper cultures have been taken, antibiotic resistance is a potential danger, particularly in infections due to Gram-negative organisms where resistance transfer factor may reverse the antibiotic sensitivity during appropriate therapy. In either situation, the physician may rely on the presence or absence of fever as an important indicator that treatment is effective. Thus, in these circumstances, it may be more judicious to withhold antipyretic therapy than to reduce fever.

Several clinicians have investigated the possible benefit of fever in the final outcome of common infectious diseases in humans. These have been reviewed (BENNETT and NICASTRI 1960; KLASTERSKY and KASS 1970) and it is clear that there is no convincing evidence that fever is helpful to humans who are infected with either viruses or bacteria. There is no increase in antibody with fever (JUNG 1935) and fever does not increase the anamnestic response to bacterial or influenzal antigens (KOOMEN and MORGAN 1954). In fact, fever seems to be detrimental to the survival of patients with pneumococcal pneumonia (BENNETT and NICASTRI 1960). Although there is the notable case that *Neisseria gonorrhoeae* and *Treponema pallidum* do not grow at elevated temperatures and that infections caused by these agents were often treated in the pre-antibiotic era with hyperthermia, specific antibiotic therapy for infectious diseases assures the best method of eliminating the disease.

The choice of an antipyretic should be based on consideration of its effectiveness in reducing fever as well as its potential side effects. Some antipyretics can produce significant side effects and are not used routinely; these include phenacetin, which can cause methaemoglobinaemia and indomethacin, which can cause bone marrow suppression (LOVEJOY 1978). Aspirin has the longest record of routine use by humans and hence many of its adverse side effects are known. Nevertheless, aspirin has one of the most favorable risk/benefit ratios of any drug. Acetaminophen (paracetamol) has been available for a relatively short period and the spectrum of its side effects is less known. Several studies have evaluated which agent is better in reducing body temperature; aspirin or acetaminophen. The paediatric age group provides the best data because fevers in children tend to be higher than in adults and are most often due to uncomplicated viral or bacterial infections. When aspirin or acetaminophen were compared with a placebo, a significant reduction of body temperature was observed (COLGAN and MINTZ 1957; EDEN and KAUFMAN 1967; STEELE et al. 1972; TARLIN et al. 1972); when compared with each other, no difference was observed. There is a drop in body temperature within 30–60 min following a single dose and this reaches a maximum of 1.5–2.25 °C (2.7–4.0 °F) by 3 h (LOVEJOY 1978). Thereafter, the temperature begins to rise. The combination of aspirin and acetaminophen at the same dosage level for each is more effective in the rapidity at which temperature falls as well as the duration of effect than for each individual drug (STEELE et al. 1972).

In most clinical settings, the use of antipyretics alone suffices to reduce fever. There is no evidence that salicylates or acetaminophen lower body temperature in afebrile humans (RAWLINS et al. 1971; SNELL and ATKINS 1968; WOODBURY and FINGL 1975) and this supports several animal studies which demonstrate that antipyretics only reduce the elevated hypothalamic set-point of pyrogen-induced fever. In febrile adults humans with fever secondary to myocardial infarction, a single oral dose of acetaminophen of 1.5 g reduced body temperature to normal levels in 3–6 h (HANSON et al. 1975). Peak plasma levels of the drug varied between 0.8 and 3.0 mg/100 ml and the time of peak drug concentration also varied considerably between 1 and 5 h following oral administration. In patients with levels of 0.5 mg or less per 100 ml, no antipyretics effect was noted.

Acetaminophen and aspirin in oral doses of 500–650 mg have approximately the same ability to lower body temperature of febrile adult patients (BEAVER 1966). The need to repeat the dose of antipyretics may be related to continued synthesis and release of endogenous pyrogen (ADLER et al. 1969) and the short duration of action of antipyretics (KOCH-WESER 1976; LEVY 1978). In adults, the total daily dose of acetaminophen should not exceed 3 g under ordinary circumstances and this should be lower in patients with impaired hepatic function. The dose limits in children are related to body surface or weight considerations.

There can be little doubt that acetaminophen should be used as an antipyretic in patients allergic to salicylates or who have gastrointestinal intolerance to aspirin. In addition, acetaminophen is preferable to aspirin in patients with haemophilia, von Willebrand's disease, other diseases of blood coagulation, or who are being treated with oral anticoagulants. Aspirin is contraindicated in patients with hyperuricaemia, gouty arthritis, peptic ulcer, or asthma. However, with the exceptions cited above, there is no advantage or benefit of using acetaminophen rather than aspirin for the treatment of uncomplicated fevers.

Several physical methods can also be used to reduce body temperature. The most common is water or alcohol sponging. Ice-water sponging reduces body temperature more rapidly than tepid water or a mixture of alcohol and water (STEELE et al. 1970). The use of air-conditioned rooms, fans, and cooling blankets will also reduce core temperature by facilitating air and surface heat conduction from the skin. These latter methods, like any physical method in which heat is removed from the body, can place a considerable physiological demand on the individual. For example, if physical methods are used at a time when the hypothalamic set-point remains elevated, shivering and vasoconstriction will occur as the hypothalamic drive to raise core temperature competes with the removal of heat peripherally. Thus, the ideal circumstance for reducing body temperature during fever combines the use of an antipyretic which lowers the hypothalamic set-point with physical methods which promote heat dissipation (STEELE et al. 1970; STERN 1977). In some circumstances, overzealous methods to reduce a fever can lead to hypothermia. This is often the case in the paediatric age group where phenobarbitone is administered in conjunction with antipyretics and sponging. Barbiturates have been shown to have a central effect on thermoregulation and to induce hypothermia in human subjects exposed to cold (HIROVONEN 1975). Generally speaking, humans have a greater tolerance to hypothermia than hyperthermia. Some of the electrocardiographic abnormalities observed in patients with hypothermias (34.5 °C, 94 °F) induced with ice-mattresses to combat high fevers are reversible (MARTINEZ-LOPEZ 1976).

C. The Treatment of Hyperpyrexia

Any patient with fever in excess of 41.1 °C (106 °F) (hyperpyrexia) requires emergency medical care. For some patients with pre-existing cardiovascular, pulmonary or central nervous system (CNS) diseases, mental disorders, or in children who have had a febrile seizure, the temperature at which the individual is a risk may be considerably lower. It is important to consider first the clinical setting and the prior medical status of the patient. Efforts to reduce hyperpyrexia should be instituted with rapidity before physiological changes secondary to the effects of high temperature produce significant morbidity.

The acute hyperpyretic episode can be caused by several disease processes. Infection still ranks as the most common cause of fever and also of hyperpyrexia (SIMON 1976; DINARELLO and WOLFF 1979 a, b). Infections of the CNS such as meningitis or encephalitis are associated with high fevers. CNS haemorrhages, especially into the ventricular system or near the hypothalamus, are commonly accompanied by hyperpyrexia (reviewed by PLUM and VAN UITERT 1978; MIYASAKI et al. 1972). Hyperpyrexia may also be a presenting sign in neonates who sustain an intraventricular haemorrhage (reviewed in POMERANCE and RICHARSON 1973). The mechanism for these abnormally high fevers is thought to be due to the fact that the third ventricle is only millimetres from the location of the thermoregulatory centre in the anterior hypothalamus. Haemorrhage secondary to necrosis is also thought to be due to the hyperpyrexia occasionally seen in patients with CNS tumours in the vicinity of the hypothalamus (PLUM and VAN UITERT 1978). There is an excellent animal model in the cat and rat for producing hyperpyrexia secondary to CNS trauma and haemorrhage in the region of the hypothalamus (RUDY et al. 1977, 1978). The pathogenesis of the fever in experimental animals suggests that the extravasated blood, rich in platelets, is a source of prostaglandins which raise the hypothalamic set-point. Endogenous pyrogen may also be produced as a result of the inflammatory process in the haemorrhaged area. The ability of antipyretics to inhibit prostaglandin synthesis in platelets as well as brain tissue has been proposed as the mechanism (RUDY et al. 1978). In humans with hyperpyrexia secondary to a CNS haemorrhage, aspirin, and acetaminophen are effective in reducing the fever (SIMON 1976).

Whether produced by systemic infection or a CNS haemorrhage, hyperpyrexia places significant demands on the cardiovascular and pulmonary system because of the dramatic increase in oxygen consumption at high temperatures. There is a 13% increase in the metabolic rate per °C (7% per °F) in human subjects experiencing fever (DUBOIS 1936). These studies were carried out on human patients with high fevers secondary to typhoid, malaria, and tuberculosis as well as with experimental fevers produced by typhoid vaccine (reviewed by HARDY 1976). This increase in oxygen consumption is an anticipated value for a $Q_{10} = 2.3$ which is observed for many biochemical reaction rates. For patients with coronary arteriosclerosis, the increased demand for oxygen may lead to myocardial ischaemia or even infarction. The cardiac output and pulse rate increase and peripheral resistance is elevated because of the vasoconstriction (CRANSTON 1959). There is also marked hyperventilation in humans with high fevers and this leads to low pCO_2 and increased pH of the blood (reviewed in ALTSCHULE and FREEDBERG 1945). At the same time, humans with fever have abnormally high serum levels of pyruvate and lactate which fall with defervescence (GILBERT 1968). Patients with restrictive lung disease clearly are at risk during high fever. Other physiological changes which have been documented in patients with high fevers due to infectious diseases or induced experimentally in human volunteers using typhoid vaccine include depression of the T-wave of electrocardiograms, haemoconcentration, hepatocellular damage, and decreased cerebral blood flow (reviewed in ALTSCHULE and FREEDBERG 1945). At temperatures of 41.7 °C (107 °F), liver damage is manifested by increased serum transaminase (BULL et al. 1979) and electroencephalographic tracings are depressed with increasing fever (CABRAL et al. 1977).

Many of these physiological alterations in hyperpyrexia are due to tissue hypoxia and acidosis. It is now advisable to monitor arterial blood gases and pH when treating these patients. This is particularly helpful in the management of patients with septicaemia due to either Gram-positive or Gram-negative organisms since respiratory alkalosis is often seen as a consequence of the tachypnoea. The patient with hyperpyrexia due to septicaemia also requires monitoring of the central venous pressure or pulmonary wedge using a Swan-Ganz catheter. Fluid is given to maintain the vascular volume in order to counter extravasation which occurs with vasoactive kinins. Evaporative water losses at high temperatures also contribute to decreased vascular volume and decreased venous pressure. In severe hyperpyrexia associated with septicaemia, hypotension develops along with decreasing blood pH. The latter is treated with intravenous infusions of sodium bicarbonate. The mechanism of hypotension in sepsis is thought to be due to many factors including volume depletion, pooling of blood, and myocardial pump failure. The use of α-adrenoceptor blocking drugs (i.e. dopamine) is often instituted in patients whose hypotension is unresponsive to increased fluids. Chlorpromazine also acts as an α-blocker as well as an antipyretic and is often successful in increasing blood pressure in these situations (WEINBERG 1978).

It is not advisable to give excessive amounts of aspirin to these patients since this may worsen the acidosis. Acetaminophen given rectally (1,200 mg) every 2–4 h until core temperature is reduced is usually effective in hyperpyrexia. Cooling blankets or ice-baths are frequently necessary. Although iced gastric lavage and cold intravenous fluids have been used, they may not be significantly more effective than peripheral cooling methods for patients with hyperpyrexia (SIMON 1976). If cooling blankets and ice-baths are instituted to help reduce temperature, it is necessary to block shivering with agents like chlorpromazine in order to prevent increased metabolic heat. Chlorpromazine has been successful in preventing shivering during rapid cooling and has the added advantage of increasing the seizure threshold during hyperpyrexia (SHIBOLET et al. 1967, 1976; NOE and ABER 1973). Chlorpromazine can also be considered an antipyretic apart from its ability to block muscle shivering. The hypothermic action of chlorpromazine has been well documented and there is evidence that its effect on lowering body temperature is due to α-adrenergic blockade, decreased utilization of glucose and free fatty acids and, most importantly, a direct effect on the central nervous system (CHAI et al. 1976; POLK and LIPTON 1975). In women who receive prostaglandins to induce mid-trimester abortions, chlorpromazine has been used to treat the hyperpyrexia which accompanies the use of these agents (GRUBER et al. 1976) and in some instances it has also caused hypothermia. Chlorpromazine has also been used to treat periodic hypothalamic discharge syndrome, a rare febrile disease of central origin (WOLFF et al. 1964). In general, however, chlorpromazine as an antipyretic is less effective than aspirin or acetaminophen in the treatment of hyperpyrexia. Chlorpromazine also causes peripheral vasodilatation and exposes more surface area to the cooling blankets. Recently, nitroprusside infusions ($0.5~\mu g~kg^{-1}~min^{-1}$) have been used to induce vasodilatation and increased contact with cooling blankets when chlorpromazine was ineffective (KATLIC et al. 1978).

Corticosteroids are frequently given in large doses to patients with severe septic shock. Recent evidence suggest that this practice significantly reduces mortality (SCHUMER 1976; GILL et al. 1978). Doses of dexamethasone, 3 mg/kg or 2 g Solumedrol can produce rapid hypothermia (1.7 °C, 3.4 °F in 4 h) and it is likely that the steroids are acting centrally (GILL et al. 1978). There is evidence that corticosteroids inhibit prostaglandin synthesis in a manner similar to that of non-steroidal antipyretics (GREAVES and MCDONALD-GIBSON 1972). This may be the most likely mechanism for steroid hypothermia since the doses used are very large. Corticosteroids could also prevent the release of endogenous pyrogen since phagocytic function is reduced in the presence of large amounts of steroids (DINARELLO and WOLFF 1978). There is little doubt that high-dose steroids are indicated in treating patients with hyperpyrexia due to sepsis but their benefit in non-septic hyperpyrexia is unknown.

D. The Treatment of Prolonged Fevers

In most patients with fever lasting one or two weeks, the underlying cause is soon discovered or the patient recovers spontaneously. In the case of spontaneous recovery, a protracted viral illness is usually presumed to be the source of fever. In other patients, however, fever continues for two or three weeks during which time physical examination, chest X-ray, blood tests, and routine cultures do not reveal the cause of fever. In these patients a provisional diagnosis of fever of unknown origin

(FUO) is made (DINARELLO and WOLFF 1979 a). Although a diagnosis of FUO is used after three weeks of fever, many patients with FUO have fever for months and some for more than a year. In either circumstance, the fever itself, and not necessarily the cause of fever, can result in significant calorific, metabolic, and physiological imbalances. In patients with FUO for several weeks significant anaemia and weight loss can occur. There is hardly a human system which is not adversely affected by prolonged fever. Drug metabolism is impaired (ELIN et al. 1975); human sperm production is reduced (LAZARUS and ZORGNIOTTI 1975), hypoferraemia and anaemia are present (ELIN et al. 1975); nitrogen wasting occurs (ROE 1966) and several other systems show signs of reduced function. In addition to the easily correctable changes like salt and water losses, there may be discomfort due to headache, general malaise, and muscle aches. Thus, it is not uncommon for the physician caring for a patient with FUO to consider some form of treatment despite the inability to uncover the cause of the prolonged fever.

Non-specific therapy for those patients with persistent fever in combination with debilitating nutritional and physiological imbalances may be instituted with caution. The approach to empirical therapy in an FUO patient must first consider whether the risk of the therapy outweighs the potential benefit. Thus, there are few, if any indications for empirical antibiotic or cytotoxic chemotherapy (DINARELLO and WOLFF 1979 b). The approach is first to employ antipyretics such as acetylsalicylic acid or acetaminophen. These are given in maximum dosages and if the patient improves, they are continued for varying periods of time. If these drugs fail then other prostaglandin synthetase inhibitors such as indomethacin or ibuprofen are tried. If these agents prove ineffective and the patient continues to be ill, adrenal corticosteroid therapy should be considered if the physician is convinced that the underlying cause of the FUO is not infectious. Initially, prednisone is given around the clock and at reasonable anti-inflammatory dosage (e.g. 10 mg every 6 h). If improvement occurs and signs of inflammation recede then the patient is switched to a single daily dose and eventually to alternate day therapy. The latter is done to minimize undesirable side effects. Most empirical therapy is non-specific and the patient may relapse when treatment is discontinued. With such patients or with therapeutic failures it may be necessary to perform another complete evaluation as often as every four to six months since in rare patients abnormalities may become apparent only after prolonged periods of time.

E. The Treatment of Fever in High-Risk Patients

Although there is general agreement that hyperpyrexia requires treatment, moderate fevers of 38.8°–40 °C (102°–104 °F) are not necessarily life-threatening. More often moderate fevers are treated because the accompanying consitutional symptoms like headache and myalgias are not well tolerated. There is, however, a group of patients in whom moderate fever can be detrimental (Table 1). We identify these individuals because of certain concomitant illness which are worsened by even mild temperature elevations. These include: (1) children with febrile seizures; (2) patients with head injury; (3) patients with severe mental disorders; (4) patients with compromised cardiovascular system, and (5) pregnant women.

Table 1. Risk groups for moderate fever

Clinical situation	Complication of fever
Infantile febrile seizures	Lowers seizure threshold
Head injury or CNS disease	Increases cerebral oedema and intracranial pressure
Mental disorders	Increased hallucinations
Cardiovascular disease	Increased oxygen demands
Pregnancy	Teratogenic for developing foetus

I. Children with Febrile Seizures

The mechanisms for the production of febrile seizures are still unclear but the two major predisposing factors are clearly antecedent brain injury and familial incidence (OUELLETTE 1974). Febrile seizures are true epileptic events and prolonged seizures lead to brain anoxia (MELDRUM 1976). Therefore, a child with a history of recurrent febrile seizures or even a child with a single prior febrile convulsion should be prevented from experiencing further seizures. The difficulty arises in devising an effective prophylatic regimen. There is no argument that the child who experiences prolonged or focal febrile seizures or the child who has an epileptic lesion and convulses with temperature elevations should be treated with daily anticonvulsant drugs. Phenobarbitone still remains the drug of choice. There is controversy whether the child who has a simple, single, generalized febrile seizure needs to be treated with daily anticonvulsants. Some clinicians prefer intermittent anticonvulsants while others use daily therapy. A large number of paediatricians recommend no anticonvulsants. Both schools of thought agree, however, that prevention of significant fever is paramount in preventing the recurrence of a febrile seizure in children between 6 months and 6 years.

Under most clinical settings, children who are susceptible to a febrile seizure are at risk when temperature rises above 38.8 °C (102 °F). There is no evidence that a rapid rise in temperature is more likely to result in a febrile seizure than the absolute height of fever, although this view is held by many. The important point to make is that a susceptible child who is ill and begins to develop fever should be promptly treated with antipyretics or sponging as well as examined and treated appropriately for the cause of the fever. Nevertheless, these children will develop fever even under the watchful eye of the parent. The emergency treatment for a child who is actively having a febrile seizure is first focused on the seizure. The child should be placed in a semi-prone position to minimize aspiration of pharyngeal contents. Adequate oxygenation should be provided. Most paediatric neurologists recommended treating the seizures with intravenous diazepam, 0.3 mg/kg at a rate of 1 mg/min. Also recommended is phenobarbitone, 3–6 mg/kg intravenously. The danger is using both these drugs to suppress the seizure in status epilepticus is respiratory arrest. It is better to repeat the diazepam dose in these cases. For small children in whom difficulty is experienced in giving intravenous medication, rectal paraldehyde is effective, 1 ml/year of age diluted 1:1 with mineral oil.

Once seizure activity is subsiding, fever must be reduced. Tepid water sponges and rectal acetaminophen or aspirin (120 mg/year of age). This can be repeated orally or rectally in 3–4 h if the fever is not below 38.3 °C (101 °F). Tepid water sponges seem to lessen shivering in children and are as effective as, but preferable to, ice-baths. Body temperature must be monitored carefully over the next few hours since in many cases, fever spikes continue to occur. The diagnosis of the fever procedes next, followed by appropriate treatment.

II. Patients with Head Injury

Patients who sustain head injuries or who have had a recent neurosurgical procedure within the cranial vault are in great danger of increasing cerebral oedema as body temperature rises. There are animal experiments which demonstrate that brain oedema increases 40% with a rise of 2 °C (4 °F) (CLASEN et al. 1974). In addition, the hypertensive component in patients with closed head injuries worsens the cerebral oedema but is itself not the cause. The precise mechanism for elevated body temperature increasing cerebral oedema is not entirely clear but it seems to occur in both white and grey matter. Prolonged periods of cerebral oedema reduce the change of neurological recovery and hence fever must be prevented in these cases. The difficulty lies in the fact that a significant number of these patients are febrile because of their brain injury; for example, high fever occurs in meningitis, encephalitis, brain abscess, and CNS haemorrhage. The primary treatment for these fevers is specific anti-infective therapy, and antipyretics. Antipyretics are very useful in reducing the hyperpyrexia of strokes and other CNS lesions (SIMON 1976). There is also experimental evidence that indomethacin is effective (RUDY et al. 1977). When these drugs are ineffective in preventing temperature elevations, cooling blankets are used. These can be very effective but shivering is often induced. The use of chlorpromazine to combat shivering is sometimes contraindicated because the drug clouds the evaluation of mental status.

III. Patients with Severe Mental Disorder

In this risk group mildly elevated temperature from colds or similar infections can disorient the patient. Although such situations are not irreversible, such patients are sometimes placed on increasing doses of antipsychotic drugs because of mental decompensation when, in fact, they require treatment for their infection and antipyretics for their fever. Fever-induced hallucinations can occur in schizophrenic patients but also in normal patients without prior history of psychosis or mental disease. This is often recognized as toxic psychosis and was often seen in the pre-antibiotic era. The treatment for both groups should be lowering the fever and not antipsychotic drugs.

IV. Patients with a Compromised Cardiovascular System

Several studies in humans have demonstrated that cardiac output during fever is only slightly elevated (reviewed in ROE 1966). The reason for this is that there is a considerable reduction in the peripheral blood flow and a compensation in the blood flow to the muscles. Nevertheless, patients with coronary artery disease or myocardial diseases are at risk because of increased pulse rate and oxygen consumption (DUBOIS 1936). At high temperatures seen in hyperpyrexia (41.2 °C, 106 °F), oxygen demands of the myocardium can increase up to 100% and exceed the limitation of coronary perfusion. The treatment of persons with fever and known or poor coronary artery perfusion should include ample oxygen and sufficient antipyretics. In older patients with sepsis, fever and the infection produce metabolic acidosis and increase the risk of myocardial infarction.

V. Pregnant Women

Certain viruses or bacteria during pregnancy (notably rubella and *Treponema*) will infect and cause severe damage to the foetus. Other maternal infections which are not known to invade the foetus may cause damage primarily because of maternal fever. The foetus is a thermal sink and cannot thermoregulate separately from its mother; hence, maternal fever causes increased foetal temperature. There is considerable evidence that maternal fever secondary to localized infection as well as hyperthermia due to sauna bathing can cause anencephaly, microphthalmia, seizures, leucoencephalopathy, mental retardation, and distal limb malformations (MILLER et al. 1978; SMITH et al. 1978; FRASER and SKELTON 1978; LEVITON and GILLES 1979). These are retrospective studies but nevertheless suggest a causal relation. Animal studies, however, confirm the findings in humans. Brain growth, learning disabilities, exencephaly, and encephaloceles have been produced in animal models with brief exposures to hyperthermia (3°–4 °C, 6°–8 °F) (FERM and KILHAM 1977; EDWARDS et al. 1974a, b). There are no prospective studies to date for humans. However, in view of the animal data and retrospective reports, fever in a pregnant woman may put the foetus at risk and should be promptly treated.

The treatment of fever in pregnant women is not without risk itself. Acetaminophen has been shown to form toxic metabolite by oxidation reactions present in microsomes of human foetal liver cells (ROLLINS et al. 1979). The ability of the foetal liver to conjugate acetaminophen protects against the build-up of these toxic metabolites. The foetus uses glutathione and sulphation for conjugation while glucuronidation, the method used by adult liver, has not been detected in foetal liver (ROLLINS et al. 1979). If the amount of acetaminophen crossing the placental barrier is large enough to deplete glutathione stores and saturate sulphate conjugation, it is likely that the toxic metabolites will impart severe damage. There is no evidence as yet that acetaminophen is unsafe during pregnancy when ingested in therapeutic doses for short periods of time. However, the ability of human foetal liver cells to oxidize acetaminophen into toxic metabolites is a potential danger with prolonged use or high doses of this antipyretic.

F. The Treatment of Hyperthermias

Human beings have several ways to thermoregulate. Besides the ability of the hypothalamic thermoregulatory centre to control peripheral heat loss or induce thermogenesis through shivering, behavioural methods which include clothing and shelters have permitted humans to survive environmental temperatures from the Antartic continent to the equatorial deserts. Nevertheless, humans are subject to hyperthermia. Dangerously high levels of core temperature can result from over-insulation, exercise, dehydration, overheating, metabolic derangements, or certain drugs. Generally, the mechanism for causing hyperthermia is the inability to dissipate the necessary amount of heat from the body surface in order to maintain normal body temperature. In heat stroke and the overheating which occurs from sauna baths, hot environments, newborn incubators, or heating tables, the source of heat is exogenous. In the hyperthermias which occur with overinsulation, dehydration, exercise, metabolic disorders, or from certain drugs, the source of heat is endogenous, i.e. the metabolic heat produced by the consumption of calories.

I. Overinsulation

Overinsulation is observed in paediatric patients, usually under two years of age, although older children and some adults are also susceptible. It is most commonly seen in the physician's office or emergency room during the winter months when the patient, dressed in several layers of clothes, is brought to medical attention because of an upper respiratory tract infection (BACON et al. 1979). Temperatures as high as 39.5 °C (103 °F) have been recorded. Clinically, it is important to recognize this situation before embarking on laboratory investigations such as blood cultures and radiographic studies. The removal of excessive insulation and placing the patient in a neutral thermal environment usually results in a reduction of body temperature to a level commensurate with the illness. This form of hyperthermia is rarely seen in children who are well.

II. Metabolic Disorders

Mild elevations in body temperature are commonly associated with phaeochromocytoma (SMITHWICK et al. 1950) but temperatures as high as 41.5 °C (106.7 °F) have been recorded in some patients with this tumour (BELT and POWELL 1934; HOWARD and BARKER 1937; HARRIN 1962). There seems to be a relationship between the ability of these tumours to secrete adrenaline and whether the clinical symptoms include high fever (FRED et al. 1967). Most tumours secrete both adrenaline and noradrenaline. It has been proposed that the adrenaline has a direct effect on body temperature by increasing cellular metabolism and decreasing heat dissipation through its cutaneous vasoconstrictive properties (ENGEL et al. 1942). Patients with acute crises of these adrenosecreting tumours often present with shock and leucocytosis accompanying their elevated temperatures which suggests infection; but these individuals are not infected (FRED et al. 1967). Patients with hyperthermic crises due to phaeochromocytomas have been treated with both aspirin and wet sponges with a rapid fall in temperature.

Hyperthermia due to thyroid thermogenesis is perhaps the most common and best example of overproduction of metabolic heat. Some patients with hyperthyroidism seek medical attention because of elevated temperature, intolerance to heat, and increased sweating. The mechanism for thyroid thermogenesis is related to increased activity of the sodium pump (EDELMAN 1974). It has also been speculated that the hyperthermia of dehydration and hypernatraemia are also due to this mechanism. The importance of the sodium pump for non-shivering thermogenesis

Table 2. Drugs which can induce hyperthermia

Amphetamines	Monoamine oxidase inhibitors
Aspirin	Phencyclidine
Atropine	Prostaglandin E_2
Chlorpromazine	Tricyclic antidepressants
D-Lysergic acid diethylamide	

has been supported by laboratory experiments in which ouabain prevents the increased metabolism induced by hypernatraemia and excess thyroid hormone (NISSAN et al. 1966). Treatment of acute thyrotoxicosis, and hence the elevated body temperature, is best accomplished with propranolol. Treatment of dehydration and hypernatraemia is hydration. Aspirin and other prostaglandin synthetase inhibitors are not effected in these hyperthermias and may contribute to acidosis.

III. Drug-Induced Hyperthermia

Table 2 lists drugs which can induce hyperthermia. Patients with atropine poisoning can have hyperthermia before other anticholinergic symptoms become apparent. Besides the accidental overdosage with drugs which contain atropine-like compounds (CHAPMAN and BEAN 1956), acute mushroom poisoning with *Amanita* species can lead to hyperthermia. The mechanism for sweating is prevented in these subjects and despite the massive peripheral vasodilatation and tachycardia, body temperature is invariably elevated. Treatment with cooling blankets is recommended while antipyretics are of no use.

Aspirin overdosage can also be a cause of hyperthermia. High levels of salicylates induce several metabolic and biochemical alterations, but the impairment of oxidative phosphorylation and the resultant increase in heat production in various body tissues leads to temperatures as high as 42.4 °C (108 °F) (SEGAR and HOLLIDAY 1958). Toxic levels of salicylates also appear to interfere with normal cooling mechanisms and there is also an accompanying dehydration which worsens the hyperthermia (TEMPLE 1978). These cases of hyperthermia induced by large doses of aspirin underscore the clinical observation that aspirin does not lower body temperature when the hypothalamic set-point is at normothermic levels. The hyperthermia of aspirin overdose must be differentiated from the fever observed in patients who develop hepatitis secondary to aspirin toxicity (SCHALLER 1978).

Despite the fact that phenothiazines and particularly chlorpromazine are used as antipyretics, there is a well-known syndrome of hyperthermia in patients receiving these drugs when exposed to warm environments or exercise (GREENLAND and SOUTHWICK 1978; MCALLISTER 1978; OPPENHEIM 1973; WISE 1973). Hyperthermia is associated almost exclusively with heat exposure or exercise and chronic use of the drug. In some cases temperatures of 41.1 °C (106 °F) have been recorded and fatalities are not uncommon (ZELMAN and GUILLAN 1970). The mechanism is apparently central and may be related to dopamine function in the hypothalamus (MCALLISTER 1978). It may als be due to the anticholinergic property of phenothiazines (POLK and LIPTON 1975). There is data that chlorpromazine inhibits prostaglandin synthesis (KRUPP and WESP 1975) but how this property results in hyperthermia is still unclear. Other experiments have shown that phenothiazines increase prostaglandin synthesis (VOGEL et al. 1976) and this effect could explain both the vasodilation and the hyperthermia seen in patients receiving this drug. The treatment of these hyperthermias is rapid physical cooling and withdrawal of the drug. Aspirin is not used.

With increasing use of psychotomimetic drugs like D-lysergic acid diethylamide (LSD) and phencyclidine (PCP) there have been reports of hyperthermia as high as 42.4 °C (108 °F) secondary to overdoses of these drugs (KLOCK et al. 1975; JAN et al. 1978; GALT et al. 1974). LSD is capable of many biochemical effects and most are thought to be due to LSD's ability to block 5-hydroxytryptamine receptors. The treatment for these fevers is cooling blankets for moderately elevated temperatures or ice-bath immersion for severe hyperthermia (41.6 °C, 107 °F) (KLOCK et al. 1975). If shivering occurs, it is advisable to give parenteral phenothiazines since these will combat both thermogenesis from muscle contraction and the psychotic episodes. There are animal models in which LSD has been shown to be a powerful agent in raising body temperature through non-shivering thermogenesis and its antagonism by phenothiazines (ROSZELL and HORITA 1975).

Both classes of antidepressants, tricyclics, and monoamine oxidase inhibitors, produce hyperthermia in humans under various clinical situations such as mild exercise, heat stress, or overdosage (JORI and GARATINI 1965). Amphetamines and related compounds will also produce hyperthermia when taken in large quantities (GINSBERG et al. 1970). In some cases, the acute toxicity is accompanied by hypotension but there is a contraindication to the use of sympathomimetics in these situations since they worsen the hyperthermia. Cooling blankets, ice-baths, and corticosteroids are helpful in controlling the acute toxic reaction to overdoses of these agents. No data exist for the efficacy of phenothiazines or aspirin in these cases.

The dangers of hypertonic saline infusions to induce mid-trimester abortion have been significant and they are now being replaced by prostaglandins. Prostaglandin E_2 (PGE_2) administered in vaginal suppositories (LIPPES and HURD 1975; PHELAN et al. 1978) and intra-amniotic $PGF_{2\alpha}$ (HOROWITZ 1978) have been highly successful in inducing mid-trimester abortion. Because prostaglandins are rapidly destroyed by certain enzymes, analogues which are less susceptible to degradation have been developed and used clinically. The most successful have been 15(S)-15-methyl PGE_2 and $PGF_{2\alpha}$ for both intravaginal and intramuscular administration (GRUBER et al. 1976; BIENARZ et al. 1974; BRENNER et al. 1974; BRENNER et al. 1975, LAUERSEN et al. 1975). The major side effects are hyperthermia and gastrointestinal symptoms. The incidence of significant hyperthermia varies in each study but is between 50% and 90% of patients receiving either the native prostaglandins or the new analogues. The route of administration does not seem to contribute to the likelihood of inducing elevated temperatures. Generally, patients do not raise body temperature more than 1 °C (2 °F) and there is no change in the white blood cell count or acute-phase reactants. No infectious cause has been implicated and the mechanism of elevated temperature in these women is apparently a direct effect of prostaglandin on the central thermoregulatory centre. These patients represent the human experience of the hyperthermic effect of prostaglandins which has been well characterized in animal models. Because these patients feel cold and occasionally

Table 3. Hypersensitivity to drugs which cause fever in the absence of other clinical signs

Antihistamines	Mercaptopurine
Barbiturates	Methyldopa
Chlorambucil	Nitrofurantoin
Cimetidine	p-Aminosalicylic acid
Dilantin	Penicillins
Hydralazine	Procaine amide
Ibuprofen	Quinidine
Iodides	Salicylates
Isoiazid	Thiouracil

shiver, these temperature elevations may be more similar to fever than to hyperthermia. Nevertheless, aspirin is ineffective.

The treatment of choice for temperature elevations in women receiving these agents has been chlorpromazine. In one study (Gruber et al. 1976) pre-treatment with prochlorperazine prevented the pyrexia and had no effect on the progress of the abortion. In only one study (Lippes and Hurd 1975) was chlorpromazine ineffective in reducing the temperature of patients receiving PGE_2 vaginal suppositories.

IV. Drug Hypersensitivity

Recently increased body temperature has been reported with the use of cimetidine in patients with peptic ulcers (Ramboer 1978). However, the cause of temperature elevation is more likely due to a hypersensitivity to the drug than a direct effect of cimetidine on temperature regulation. Patients who have elevated temperatures while on this drug also have elevated liver enzymes and mild eosinophilia (McLoughlin et al. 1978; Corbett and Holdsworth 1978). Although there is a report that cimetidine causes hyperthermia when injected into the third ventricle by nature of its ability to block H_2 receptors (Nistico et al. 1978), there is no evidence that this is the mechanism in humans. There is a considerable list of drugs which cause fever because of the development to hypersensitivity to the drug and not because of the direct effect on thermoregulation. Many of these drugs produce only fever and no other signs or symptoms; therefore, it is often difficult to make a diagnosis of drug-induced fever. Withdrawal of the offending drug is usually sufficient to reduce and end the fevers. Table 3 lists the common drugs which have been reported to cause fever in the absence of rashes, liver enzyme elevations, or white blood cell changes.

V. Heat Stroke Syndromes

Overheating syndromes are often a common problem in hospital emergency-rooms, especially during hot, humid weather. The morbidity and mortality from these cases can be significant and various studies have revealed how young, healthy persons succumb to severe hyperthermia due to overheating (reviewed in Shibolet et al. 1976). The cause of heat stroke is the accumulation of body heat leading to temperatures which are harmful or even incompatible with life. For humans this seems to begin at 42 °C (107.5 °F). Therefore, emergency treatment is first aimed at reducing the temperature and the second priority is correction of the imbalances which accompany heat stroke. The latter include severe acidosis, cellular hypoxia, hypotension, brain swelling, hypernatraemia, and coagulopathies.

Rapid cooling can be achieved with ice-water-baths, ice-packs over the groin and axilla, ice-water–alcohol sponges with high-speed fan, and air-conditioned rooms. Cooling blankets do not offer enough direct surface area for rapid cooling. Other methods such as ice-saline infusions and cold peritoneal dialysis have been used. At the same time, it is important to make blood gas and blood pH determinations. A large intravenous catheter should be inserted to treat shock but if the tip is near the heart no iced solutions should be used. Rapid cooling leads to shivering and further thermogenesis. Intramuscular chlorpromazine, 25–50 mg, is indicated to prevent this. Oxygen is given and urine output monitored. There is no indication for aspirin or similar compounds in the treatment of these hyerthermias. Often these patients will mimic acute sepsis and fever and so they will receive antibiotics and antipyretics. These may not be as harmful as the delay in the diagnosis of heat stroke.

References

Adler RD, Rawlins M, Rosendorff C, Cranston WI (1969) The effects of salicylate on pyrogen-induced fever in man. Clin Sci 37:91 97

Altschule MD, Freedberg AS (1945) Circulation and respiration in fever. Medicine (Baltimore) 24:403–440

Bacon C, Scott D, Jones P (1979) Heatstroke in well-wrapped infants. Lancet 1:422–425

Beaver WT (1966) Mild analgesics: a review of their clinical pharmacology. Am J Med Sci 250:577–604

Belt AE, Powell TO (1934) Clinical manifestations of the chromaffin cell tumors arising from the suprarenal sympathetic syndrome. Surg Gynecol Obstet 59:9–15

Bennett I Jr, Nicastri A (1960) Fever as a mechanism of resistance. Bacteriol Rev 24:16–34

Bieniarz J, Hunter G, Scommegna A et al. (1974) Efficacy and acceptability of 15(S)-15-methyl-prostaglandin E_2-methyl ester for midtrimester pregnancy termination. Am J Obstet Gynecol 120:840–843

Brenner WE, Dingfelder JR, Staurovsky LG (1974) Intramuscular administration of 15(S)-15-methyl-prostaglandin E_2-methyl ester for induction of abortion. Am J Obstet Gynecol 120:833–836

Brenner WE, Dingfelder JR, Staurovsky LG (1975) The efficacy and safety of intramuscularly administered 15(S)-15-methyl-prostaglandin-E_2-methyl ester for induction of artificial abortion. Am J Obstet Gynecol 123:17–31

Bull JM, Lees D, Schuette W et al. (1979) Whole body hyperthermia: a phase I trial of a potential adjuvant to chemotherapy. Ann Intern Med 90:317–323

Cabral R, Prior PF, Scott DF, Brierley JB (1977) Reversible profound depression of cerebral electrical activity in hyperthermia. Electroencephalogr Clin Neurophysiol 42:697–701

Chai CY, Fann YD, Lin MT (1976) Hypothermic action of chlorpromazine in monkeys. Br J Pharmacol 57:43–49

Chapman J, Bean WB (1956) Iatrogenic heatstroke. JAMA 161:1375–1377

Clasen RA, Pandolfi S, Laing I, Casey D Jr (1974) Experimental study of relation of fever to cerebral edema. J Neurosurg 41:576–581

Colgan MT, Mintz AA (1957) The comparative antipyretic effect of n-acetyl-p-aminophenol and acetylsalicylic acid. J Pediatr 50:552–561

Corbett CL, Holdsworth CD (1978) Cimetidine-fever. Br Med J 1:753

Cranston WI (1959) Fever, pathogenesis and circulatory changes. Circulation 20:1133–1142

Dinarello CA, Wolff SM (1978) Pathogenesis of fever in man. N Eng J Med 298:607–612

Dinarello CA, Wolff SM (1979 a) Fever of unknown origin. In: Mandell GL, Douglas RG Jr, Bennett JE (eds) Principles and practices of infectious diseases. Wiley and Sons, New York, pp 421–428

Dinarello CA, Wolff SM (1979 b) Approach to the patient with fever of unknown origin. In: Mandell GL, Douglas RG, Bennett JE (eds) Principles and practices of infectious diseases. Wiley and Sons, New York, pp 407–421

Dubois EE (1936) Basal metabolism in health and disease, 3 rd edn. Lea Febiger, Philadelphia

Dubois EE (1949) Why are fever temperatures over 106 °F rare? Am J Med Sci 17:361–368

Edelman IS (1974) Thyroid thermogenesis. N Eng J Med 290:1303–1308

Eden AN, Kaufman A (1967) Clinical comparison of three antipyretic agents. Am J Dis Child 114:284–290

Edwards MJ, Penny RH, Lyle J, Jonson K (1974 a) Brain growth and learning behaviour of the guinea-pig following prenatal hyperthermia. Experientia 30:406–407

Edwards MJ, Lyle JG, Jonson KM, Penny RH (1974 b) Prenatal retardation of brain growth by hyperthermia and the learning capacity of mature guinea-pigs. Dev Psychobiol 7:579–584

Elin RJ, Vesell ES, Wolff SM (1975) Effects of etiocholanolone-induced fever on plasma anti-pyrene half-lives and metabolic clearance. Clin Pharmacol Ther 17:447–457

Engel FL, Mencher WH, Engel GL (1942) Epinephrine shock as a manifestation of pheochromocytoma of the adrenal medulla. Report of a case with successful removal of the tumor. Am J Med Sci 204:649–653

Ferm VH, Kilham J (1977) Synergistic teratogenic effects of arsenic and hyperthermia in hamsters. Environ Res 14:483–486

Fraser FC, Skelton J (1978) Possible teratogenicity of maternal fever (letter). Lancet 2:634

Fred HL, Allred DP, Garber HE, Retiene K, Lipscomb H (1967) Pheochromocytoma masquerading as overwhelming infection. Am Heart J 73:149–154

Galt JM, Ludgate CM, Pettigrew RT (1974) Circulatory and electrolyte changes during hyperthermia to 42 degrees. Can J Physiol 72:30–31

Gilbert VE (1968) Blood pyruvate and lactate during febrile human infections. Metabolism 32:943–951

Gill W, Wilson S, Long WB (1978) Steroid hypothermia. Surg Gynecol Obstet 146:944–946

Ginsberg MD, Hertzman M, Schmidt-Nowara WW (1970) Amphetamine intoxication with coagulopathy, hyperthermia and reversible renal failure. Ann Intern Med 73:81–85

Greaves MW, McDonald-Gibson W (1972) Inhibition of prostaglandin biosynthesis by corticosteroids. Br Med J 2:83–84

Greenland P, Southwick WH (1978) Hyperthermia associated with chlorpromazine and full-sheet restraint. Am J Psychiatry 135:1234–1235

Gruber W, Brenner WE, Staurovsky CNM, Dingfelder JR, Wells JS (1976) Evaluation of intramuscular 15(S)-15-methyl prostaglandin $F_{2\alpha}$ thromethamine salt for induction of abortion, medications to attenuate side effects and intracervical laminaria tents. Fertil Steril 27:1009–10023

Hanson A, Johansson BW, Malmquist J, Tonnesson M (1975) The effect of paracetamol on fever in various non-infectious diseases. In: Lomax P, Schönbaum E, Jacob G (eds) Temperature regulation and drug action. Karger, Basel, pp 227–232

Hardy JD (1976) Fever and thermogenesis. Isr J Med Sci 12:942–950

Harrin B (1962) Sustained hypotension and shock due to an adrenaline-secreting phaeochromocytoma. Lancet 2:123–124

Hirovenen J (1975) Effects of ethanol, barbituates, phenothiazines and biogenic amines on man during exposure to cold. In: Lomax P, Schönbaum E, Jacob G (eds) Temperature regulation and drug action. Karger, Basel, pp 252–256

Horowitz AJ (1978) Midtrimester abortion utilizing intraamniotic prostaglandin F_2 alpha, laminaria and oxytocin. J Reprod Med 21:236–240

Howard JE, Barker WH (1937) Paroxysmal hypertension and other clinical manifestations associated with benign chromaffin cell tumors. Bull Johns Hopkins Hosp 61:271–377

Jan K, Dorsey S, Bornstein A (1978) Hyperthermia from phencyclidine. N Engl J Med 299:722

Jori A, Garatini S (1965) Interaction between imipramine-like agents and catecholamine-induced hyperthermia. J Pharm Pharmacol 17:480–482

Jung RW (1935) Immunologic studies in hyperpyrexia. Arch Phys Ther 16:397–404

Katlic MR, Ramos LG, Zinner MJ (1978) Sodium nitroprusside in the treatment of extreme pyrexia. N Eng J Med 299:154

Klastersky J, Kass EH (1970) Is supression of fever or hypothermia useful in experimental and clinical infectious diseases? J Infect Dis 121:81–85

Klock JC, Boerner U, Becker CE (1975) Coma, hyperthermia, and bleeding associated with massive LSD overdose, a report of eight cases. Clin Toxicol 8:191–203

Koch-Weser J (1976) Acetaminophen. N Engl J Med 295:1297–1300

Koomen T Jr, Morgan HR (1954) An evaluation of the anamnestic serum reaction in certain febrile illnesses. Am J Sci 228:520–524

Krupp P, Wesp M (1975) Inhibition of prostaglandin synthetase by psychotropic drugs. Experientia 31:330–331

Lauersen NH, Secher NJ, Wilson KH (1975) Midtrimester abortion induced by serial intramuscular injections of 15(S)-15-methyl-prostaglandin E_2 methyl ester. Am J Obstet Gynecol 123:665–670

Lazarus BA, Zorgniotti AW (1975) Thermoregulation of the human testis. Fertil Steril 26:757–759

Leviton A, Gilles F (1979) Maternal urinary tract infections and fetal leukoencephalopathy. N Engl J Med 301:661

Levy G (1978) Clinical pharmacokinetics of aspirin. Pediatrics 62:867–872

Lippes J, Hurd M (1975) The use of chlorpromazine and lomotil to prevent and/or reduce the side effects of prostaglandin E_2 used for abortion. Contraception 12:569–577

Lovejoy FH Jr (1978) Aspirin and acetaminophen: a comparative view of their antipyretic and analgesic activity. Pediatrics 62:904–909

Martinez-Lopez JI (1976) Induced hypothermia: electrocardiographic abnormalities. South Med J 69:1548–1550

McAllister RG Jr (1978) Fever, tachycardia, and hypertension with acute catatonic schizophrenia. Arch Intern Med 138:1154–1156

McLoughlin JC, Callender ME, Love AHG (1978) Drug-fever with cimetidine. Lancet 1:499–500

Meldrum BS (1976) Secondary pathology of febrile and experimental convulsions. In: Brazier HAB, Coceani F (eds) Brain dysfunctions and infantile febrile convulsions. Raven, New York, pp 213–222

Miller P, Smith DW, Shepard TH (1978) Maternal hyperthermia as a possible cause of anencephaly. Lancet 1:671–672

Miyasaki K, Miyachi Y, Armimitsu K, Kita E, Yoshida M (1972) Post-traumatic hypothalamic obesity – an autopsy case. Acta Pathol Jpn 22:779–802

Nissan S, Aviram A, Czaczkes JW (1966) Increased O_2 consumption of the rat diaphragm by elevated NaCl concentrations. Am J Physiol 210:1222–1224

Nistico G, Rotiroti D, De Sarro A, Maccar E (1978) Mechanisms of cimetidine-induced fever. Lancet 2:265–266

Noe JM, Aber RC (1973) Treatment of fever in burned children. Clin Pediatr (Phila) 12:376–378

Oppenheim G (1973) Nutism and hyperthermia in a patient treated with neuroleptics. Med J Aust 2:228–229

Ouellette EM (1974) The child who convulses with fever. Pediatr Clin North Am 21:467–481

Phelan JP, Meguiar RV, Matey D, Newman C (1978) Dramatic pyrexic and cardiovascular response to intravaginal prostaglandin E_2. Am J Obstet Gynecol 132:28–32

Plum F, Van Uitert R (1978) Nonendocrine diseases and disorders of the hypothalamus. Res Publ Assoc Res Nerv Ment Dis 56:415–473

Polk DL, Lipton JM (1975) Effects of sodium salicylate, aminopyrine and chlorpromazine in behavioral temperature regulation. Pharmacol Biochem Behav 3:167–172

Pomerance JJ, Richardson CJ (1973) Hyperpyrexia as a sign of intraventricular hemorrhage in the neonate. Am J Dis Child 126:854–855

Ramboer C (1978) Cimetidene fever. Lancet 1:330–331

Rawlins MD, Rosendorff C, Cranston WI (1971) The mechanisms of action of antipyretics. In: Wolstenholme GEW, Birch J (eds) Pyrogens and fever. CIBA Foundation Symposium. Churchill Livingstone, Edinburg London, pp 175–190

Roe CF (1966) Fever and energy metabolism in surgical diseases. Monogr Surg Sci 3:85–132

Rollins DE, Bahr C, Glaumann H, Moldeus P, Rane A (1979) Acetaminophen: potentially toxic metabolite formed by human fetal and adult liver microsomes and isolated fetal liver cells. Science 205:1414–1416

Roszell DK, Horita A (1975) The effects of haloperidoland thioridazine on apomorphine and LSD induced hyperthermia in the rabbit. J Psychiatr Res 12:117–123

Rudy TA, Williams JW, Yakash TL (1977) Antagonism by indomethacin of neurogenic hyperthermia produced by unilateral puncture of the anterior hypothalamic/preoptic region. J Physiol (Lond) 272:721–735

Rudy TA, Westergaard JL, Yakash TL (1978) Hyperthermia produced by simulated intraventricular hemorrhage in the cat. Exp Neurol 58:296–310

Schaller JG (1978) Chronic salicylate administration in juvenile rheumatoid arthritis: aspirin "hepatitis" and its clinical significance. Pediatrics 62:904–909

Schumer W (1976) Steroids in the treatment of clinical septic shock. Ann Surg 184:333–346

Segar WE, Holliday MA (1958) Physiologic abnormalities of salicylate intoxication. N Engl J Med 259:1191–1193

Shibolet S, Coll R, Gilat T (1967) Heatstroke: its clinical picture and mechanism in 36 cases. Q J Med 36:525–548

Shibolet S, Lancaster MC, Danon Y (1976) Heatstroke: a review. Aviat Space Environ Med 47:280–301

Simon HB (1976) Extreme pyrexia. JAMA 236:2419–2421

Smith DW, Clarren SK, Harvey MA (1978) Hyperthermia as a possible teratogenic agent. J Pediatr 92:878–883

Smithwick RH, Greer WER, Robertson CW, Wilkins RW (1950) Pheochromocytoma. A discussion of symptoms, signs and procedures of diagnostic value. N Engl J Med 242:252–256

Snell ES, Atkins E (1968) The mechanisms of fever. In: Bittar EE, Bittar N (eds) The biological basis of medicine, vol 2. Academic Press, New York, pp 397–419

Steele RW, Tanaka PT, Lara RP (1970) Evaluation of sponging and oral antipyretic therapy to reduce fever. J Pediatr 123:824

Steele RW, Young FSH, Bass JW (1972) Oral antipyretic therapy. Am J Dis Child 123:204

Stern RC (1977) Pathophysiologic basis for symptomatic treatment of fever. Pediatrics 59:92–98

Tarlin L, Landrigan Babineau R (1972) A comparison of the antipyretic effect of actaminophen and aspirin. Am J Dis Child 124:889–892

Temple AR (1978) Pathophysiology of aspirin overdosage toxicity, with implications for management. Pediatrics 62:873–876

Vogel EL, Giessler AJ, Bekemeir H (1976) Influence of psychoactive and other drugs on prostaglandin biosynthesis and prostaglandin action. Acta Biol Med Ger 35:1051–1052

Weinberg AN (1978) Infectious disease emergencies. In: Gardner L (ed) Handbook of medical emergencies. Medical Examination Publishing, Garden City, pp 178–189

Wise TN (1973) Heatstroke in three chronic schizophrenics: case reports and clinical considerations. Compr Psychiatry 14:263–267

Wolff SM, Adler RC, Buskirk ER, Thompson RH (1964) A syndrome of periodic hypothalamic discharge. Am J Med 36:956–967

Woodbury DM, Fingl E (1975) Analgesics and antipyretics. In: Goodmann LS, Gilman A (ed) Pharmacological basis of therapeutics, 5th edn. Macmillan, New York, pp 325–350

Zelman S, Guillan R (1970) Heatstroke in phenothiazine-treated patients: a report of three fatalities. Am J Psychiatry 126:1787–1790

CHAPTER 17

Malignant Hyperthermia: A Review

B. A. BRITT

A. Introduction

Malignant hyperthermia (MH) has been extensively reviewed in the medical literature (BRITT 1973, 1976; FURNISS 1971). In spite of the wealth of readily available
information, the condition unfortunately remains largely unknown to the majority
of physicians. This may be because although information about MH in medical
journals has been extensive, that in basic medical textbooks has been scanty. It is
hoped that this review will help to bridge this gap.

Malignant hyperthermia is a hereditary trait characterized by hypercatabolic
reactions induced by anaesthetic drugs or by physical or emotional stress. These
reactions are characterized by:
1. Tachycardia
2. Arrhythmias
3. Unstable blood pressure
4. Skeletal Muscle Stiffness
5. Hyperventilation
6. Cyanosis
7. Hypoxia
8. Respiratory and metabolic acidosis
9. Myglobinuria
10. Elevation in the serum of muscle enzymes
11. Various electrolyte derangements.

Prior to a reaction, a susceptible individual may exhibit a number of minor
skeletal and cardiac muscle abnormalities, for example excessive muscularity, joint
hypermobility, skeletal muscle cramps and mitral valve prolapse. Diagnosis of the
trait can be made by detection in isolated skeletal muscle of greater than normal
rises in resting tension in the presence of caffeine and/or halothane.

B. History

Reports of unexpected fever during anaesthesia have been described since the beginning of the twentieth century (TUTTLE 1900; BURFORD 1940). GUEDEL in 1937
reported that during 20 years of practice he had seen six cases of post-operative hyperthermia which he thought might have been due to diethyl ether. In all instances
the temperature rose within a few hours to between 108 °F and 110 °F and all
patients died. Necroscopy showed only cerebral oedema. LEE, in his 1953 edition
of *A Synopsis of Anaesthesia* noted that "ether convulsions" associated with exces-

sive rises in temperature had been reported with increasing frequency since 1926 and that many of the "convulsions" occurred in children and young adults. HEWER in the sixth edition (1948) of *Recent Advances in Anaesthesia and Analgesia* discussed a series of 22 patients afflicted with "late ether convulsions" which were associated with intense muscle activity and followed by high temperatures. CULLEN, in the third edition (1951) of *Anaesthesia in General Practice* described "ether convulsions" and high fevers in adolescents and robust young adults. He listed as contributory factors high endogenous or exogenous temperatures, retention of carbon dioxide and hypoxia. Finally, the author has discovered in ancestors of present day MH patients evidence of fulminant fevers during anaesthetics administered as early as 1922 (BRITT, unpublished work).

The first case report in which the genetic nature of MH was recognized was published by DENBOROUGH and LOVELL, first in the July 2nd, 1960 issue of *Lancet* and later in more detail in the June 1962 issue of the *British Journal of Anaesthesia*. DENBOROUGH described a successfully treated case of MH in a young, previously healthy male who had been anaesthetized with halothane. This man had been very apprehensive prior to induction because ten of his relatives had died during anaesthesia. During anaesthesia the patient rapidly developed pallor, cyanosis, tachycardia and a hot, sweaty skin. He remained comatose for 30 min following anaesthesia. Dr. Denborough subsequently investigated this proband's family and found that ten relatives had died during anaesthesia. For all ten, the anaesthetic agents used were ethyl chloride and ether. In the three best documented cases the deaths were preceded by convulsions and fulminant fevers. The pattern of inheritance was compatible with a dominant gene or genes.

From that time onward similar families began to be reported with progressively increasing frequency. For instance, in 1969 BRITT et al. described a family of 138 individuals at risk, 21 of whom had MH reactions during anaesthesia. Eight of these had died during or shortly after completion of the surgery.

It was not until the late 1960s that MH was recognized to be due not to a primary disturbance of the central hypothalamic temperature regulating centre but rather to a peripheral effect located in the skeletal muscle. The 170s witnessed a blossoming of research into the genetic and biochemical nature of MH and into its diagnosis and clinical management. Research into MH, in turn, has contributed to an improved understanding of the function of the muscle cell. In this review we have included data obtained from analysis of 678 human cases of MH.

C. Epidemiology

I. Previous Anaesthetics

Almost half of all human MH reactions have been preceded by one or more previous apparently uneventful general anaesthetics (BRITT et al. 1977b). PUSCHEL et al. (1978) have described a MH crisis in a man who had thirteen prior normal general anaesthetics! The reasons for the failure of malignant hyperthermic susceptible (MHS) individuals to always develop a reaction during anaesthesia appear to be multiple. Thus, a reaction appears to be more likely to occur:

1. If the premedication has included a belladonna alkaloid
2. If a potent inhalational anaesthetic has been used in combination with succinylcholine (BRITT et al. 1977b)
3. If the duration of the anaesthetic has been long (and, therefore, the dose of the triggering agents has been large)
4. If immediately prior to the anaesthetic the patient has been exercising violently, has sustained extensive muscle trauma or has been feverish or very apprehensive
5. If during induction errors of anaesthetic technique have permitted the development of hypercarbia, hypotension or hypoxia with attendant lactacidosis.

Many actual cases of MH go unrecognized, either because they are so mild as to be undetectable without the aid of a temperature monitor or because they are misdiagnosed – for instance, as cerebral or pulmonary embolus, infection, myocardial infarction, mismatched blood transfusion or insufficiently frequent changing of the soda lime cannister.

II. Incidence

In North America and Europe the incidence of recognized human MH reactions is about 1:15,000 anaesthetics and in middle-aged adults is about 1:50,000 to 1:100,000 anaesthetics (BRITT and KALOW 1970b). In Japan, the incidence varies from 1:7,000 to 1:110,000 anaesthetics in different hospitals (KIKUCHI et al. 1978). Higher incidences may be reported in paediatric hospitals, not only because of a truly higher occurrence in young than in old patients but also because of the much greater use of inhalational anasthetic agents and succinylcholine in paediatric than in adult hospitals. In the latter institutions, anaesthetics are much more often maintained with some combination of drugs known to be safe for MHS patients, such as barbiturates, narcotics, tranquillizers, nitrous oxide or pancuronium. The true incidence of the MH myophathy is, therefore, undoubtedly much higher than has been reported previously.

III. Sex and Age

Although MH is not a sex-linked trait, sex influence is present. Thus, males are more commonly affected than females (BRITT et al. 1977b) (Table 1). In both sexes with the onset of puberty, i.e. at about age 15, the incidence declines slightly. After the age of 30 years the decline becomes more precipitious in both sexes. By old age the condition is almost unknown, only one case in the entire world having been reported over the age of 75 years.

Malignant hyperthermia is also very rare, but not completely unknown in pregnant females. We are aware of at least 12 cases of MH occurring during or after spinal or epidural anaesthesia for vaginal or Caesarian deliveries (BRITT, unpublished work). LUCKE (1977) has experienced a case of MH developing during a Caesarian section in a pig. Nevertheless, MH reactions are much less common in pregnant than in non-pregnant females. Thus, some factor, possibly hormonal, appears to protect pregnant females from MH reactions but seems to put males at increased risk for MH crises.

Table 1. Relationships between sex and age in MH cases

Age (years)	Number of patients		Male/female ratio
	Males	Females	
0–14	165	102	1.70
15–29	166	59	2.80
30–44	57	33	1.75
45–59	23	10	2.30
60	5	1	5.00

Statistics	df	χ^2	P
χ^2 due to regression	1	2.00	N. S.
χ^2 due to deviation from linearity	3	7.32	N. S.
Total χ^2	4	9.32	N. S.

Abbreviations: N. S., not significant probability (P); df, degrees of freedom; χ^2, chi square

Table 2. Mortality from MH reactions in various geopolitical areas

	Number of patients		Percentage of patients surviving	Statistics		
	Died	Survived		df	χ^2	P
Canada	47	102	68.5			
United States	112	203	64.9	1	0.56	N.S.
Japan	30	31	50.8	1	5.06	*
South Africa, Australia and New Zealand	19	16	45.7	1	5.42	*
Continental Europe	41	29	41.3	1	13.37	***
United Kingdom and Ireland	31	8	21.0	1	27.33	***
Other	1	3	75.0	1	I.D.	

Abbreviations: I.D., insufficient data; N.S., not significant probability (P); *, probability of <0.05; ***, probability of <0.001; df, degrees of freedom; χ^2, chi squares are for Canada versus other geopolitical areas

MH reactions may occur in newborns. Not only have we observed several such instances in piglets but one human case has also been reported from Maine by Sewall (personal communication).

IV. Geographical Distribution and Racial Incidence

The geographical and racial distribution of MH is widespread but not entirely world-wide (Tables 2 and 3). Human cases have been reported from across Canada and the United States, throughout Europe, including the USSR, and the United Kingdom and Ireland. Cases have also occurred in South Africa, Australia, New Zealand, and Japan and other parts of Asia. On the other hand no cases have been described so far in Africa north of South Africa. It is not yet known whether these

Table 3. Racial distribution of MH cases

Race	Number of patients
Caucasian	388
Negro	35
Oriental	66
East Indian	2
Other	16

omissions are due to racial differences or to environmental (climatic or dietary) factors. At least two cases of MH reactions have occurred in temperate climates in black patients who have immigrated from African countries (Sudan and Zaire). A mixture of caucasian genes in these individuals is very unlikely. MH reactions have been reported not infrequently in black patients from North America and in "coloured" patients from South Africa. Admixture of caucasian genes in both these groups of patients is highly probable.

V. Species

Malignant hyperthermia has been described in species other than humans. Sporadic cases have occurred in dogs such as racing greyhounds (BAGSHAW et al. 1978), in cats (DE JONG et al. 1974), race horses (KLEIN 1975), and cattle (BRADLEY 1976). While occurrence in these species is relatively rare, occurrence in pigs is quite common (CAMPION and TOPEL 1975; BERMAN and KENCH 1973; LUCKE et al. 1977; HARRISON 1979). MH in pigs is also known as Pork Stress Syndrome (PSS) or Pale Soft Exudative Pork (PSEP). PSS was first described in Denmark in 1953 (LUDVIGSEN). Incidence in the pig varies according to breed, being most frequent and severe in Pietrain swine, of intermediate frequency and severity in Landrace hogs and least frequent and most mild in Poland-China pigs. MHS families have been rarely detected in other breeds such as the York. Within each pig strain the incidence and severity of MH susceptibility is increased by the attempts of breeders to produce lean and heavily muscled animals with rapid growth rates and high feed efficiencies (HARRISON 1979; NELSON 1973). Although the absolute identity of porcine and human MH has been questioned (BERMAN and KENCH 1973), the PSS pig has been an extremely useful experimental model for the investigation of MH (HARRISON 1979; NELSON 1976). Although unlike humans most hypercatabolic reactions in pigs are induced by stress rather than anaesthesia, this difference is probably not due to an aetiological dissimilarity but rather to the economic impracticality of anaesthetizing sick pigs.

VI. Heredity

The hereditary aspects of MH have been widely reported (DENBOROUGH et al. 1962; KALOW and BRITT 1973; JAFFE and WEDLEY 1972). Denborough considered MH to be due to an autosomal dominant gene or genes (Fig. 1). A second even larger

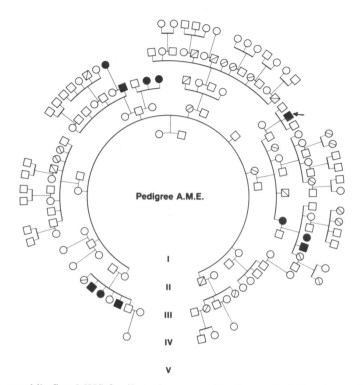

Pedigree A.M.E.

I

II

III

IV

V

Fig. 1. The world's first MHS family to be reported in the medical literature. This family is of Welsh descent. (Adapted from DENBOROUGH et al. 1962)

family detected by W. G. LOCHER in Wisconsin (personal communication) and reported by BRITT et al. (1976c) (Fig. 2) in 1968 appeared to possess a single autosomal dominant gene, since:
1. There was transmission through three successive generations
2. About half the offspring of each affected parent were afflicted
3. Both males and females were affected
4. Direct transmission of the trait from fathers to sons occurred.
Unfortunately the only method of detecting the trait at that time was the observation of a MH reaction during or following anaesthesia. Thus a number of susceptible individuals in these families probably escaped detection.

With the advent of the caffeine contracture test accurate diagnosis of individuals who had never been subjected to anaesthesia has become possible. As the result of assessment of large numbers of these in vitro muscle tests along with associated clinical investigations of the patients and their families it has become evident that a single autosomal dominant gene can account for the observed human data in some families (Fig. 3) but not in others (Fig. 4) (KALOW et al. 1979; WILLIAMS et al. 1978). Thus, not infrequently both parents of a proband are MHS, more than 50% of the offspring of a MHS parent are also MHS, the offsprings' MH characteristics tend to resemble the means of their parents and more than three MH phenotypes can be distinguished. Investigation of MHS families has demonstrated

Malignant Hyperthermia Pedigree "CW"

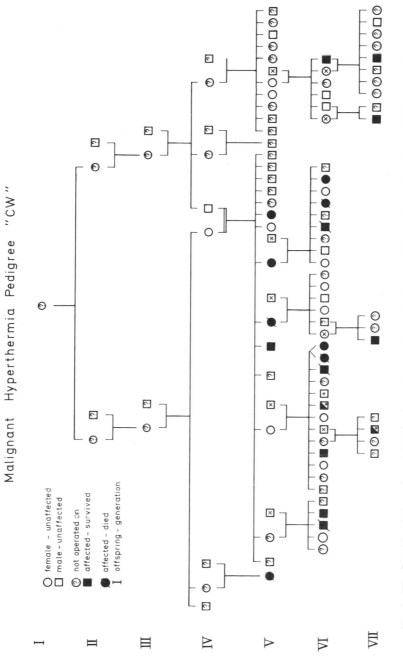
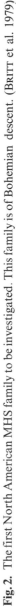

Fig. 2. The first North American MHS family to be investigated. This family is of Bohemian descent. (Britt et al. 1979)

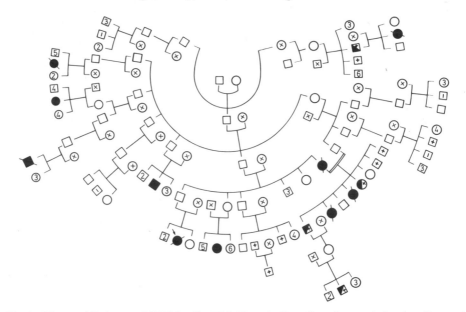

Fig. 3. The world's largest MHS family. This French-Canadian clan, a skeletal pedigree of which is shown above, contains over 4,000 individuals

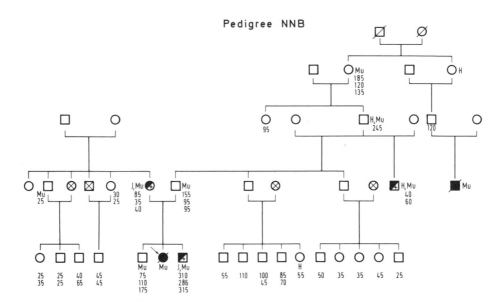

Fig. 4. Both parents of the MHS proband are also MHS. A single dominant gene, therefore, may not account for the MH defect in the proband and for two siblings. Some but not all MHS individuals in this family have elevated serum CKs. Clinical skeletal muscle anomalies and elevated serum CKs are not perfectly correlated

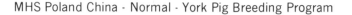

MHS Poland China - Normal - York Pig Breeding Program

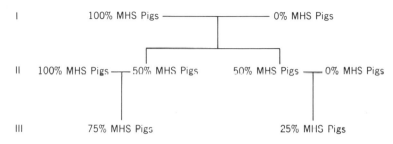

Fig. 5. In generation I pigs, all of whose ancestors for many preceding generations were MHS (100% MHS), were bred with pigs all of whose ancestors for many preceding generations were normal (0% MHS). In generation II the offspring (50% MHS) of the generation I breeding were bred with other 100% MHS or 0% MHS pigs to produce generation III offspring which were either 75% MHS or 25% MHS

that within given families there is often dissociation between clinical muscle abnormalities characteristic of MH and elevated serum creatine kinases (CKs) (ELLIS et al. 1978 b). In human families, therefore, at least two different non-allelic genes are probably present. Presently available evidence would indicate that one of these genes is autosomal dominant and rare while the other may be autosomal recessive and fairly common.

Genetic studies of MHS swine by BRITT et al. (1978 a) and by WILLIAMS et al. (1978) suggest that the inheritance of porcine MH is also determined by more than one gene. Thus a controlled three generation mating of MHS with normal pigs has shown that in this species the inheritance is also due to more than one gene. In the first generation normal (0% MHS) pigs were mated with pigs which had been bred for many generations to have MH (100% MHS pigs). Half of the offspring (50% MHS pigs) of the second generation were bred with 0% MHS pigs and the other half with 100% MHS pigs to produce 25% and 75% pigs, respectively, in the third generation (Fig. 5). The severity of the MH trait in each animal was assessed by determination of clinical responses (heart rate, skin colour, muscle tone and skin, nasal and rectal temperatures) during in vivo halothane anaesthesia and pharmacological responses (contracture amplitudes) of skeletal muscle fascicles during in vitro equilibration with caffeine and/or halothane.

The results showed that for both the in vivo and the in vitro studies: (1) the trait was observed phenotypically in all animals of the second generation; (2) the offspring in each generation tended to behave like the mean of their parents, i.e. they did not segregate as expected into one parental type of the other; and (3) rather than the expected three phenotypes (Fig. 6a), five phenotypes could be distinguished. The claim of EIKELENBOOM et al. (1978) that MH in Dutch Landrace pigs is due to a single autosomal recessive gene is not valid. This is because this investigation, like the early human studies, diagnosed MH by means of a single halothane anaesthetic, thus ensuring that some MHS animals would escape detection. Additionally, the study made no attempt to distinguish varying degrees of severity of the syndrome and did not ensure the purity (MHS or normal) of the ancestry of the parent animals.

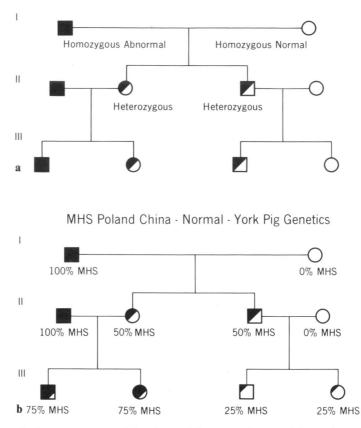

Fig. 6. a In a single gene autosomal dominant defect a maximum of three phenotypes was possible: homozygous normal, homozygous MHS and heterozygous MHS. In generation III, the offspring segregated into one or other parental type. **b** In our strain of MHS Poland China-York pigs at least five phenotypes were observed. In generation III, the MH characteristics of the offspring resembled the mean of their parent's MH characteristics. The MH defect in these animals, therefore, must have been due to more than one gene pair

VII. Triggering Factors

Acute hypercatabolic reactions can be triggered in genetically predisposed MHS individuals by drugs or stress and possibly by other environmental factors.

1. Drugs

Triggering drugs are, unfortunately for anaesthetists, those that are mainly confined to anaesthetic practice. For instance, several skeletal muscle relaxants (succinylcholine chloride, decamethonium, gallamine, d-tubocurarine, and n-allyl nortoxiferine) have been shown to be capable of inducing or aggravating MH reactions (BRITT et al. 1977b; BRITT and KALOW 1970b; BRITT et al. 1974b) (Table 4). In human patients succinylcholine is a potent precipitator of early and

Table 4. Relationships between individual anaesthetics and skeletal muscle rigidity during MH reactions

Anaesthetics[a]	Number of patients		% Rigid	Statistics		
	Rigid	Non-rigid		df	χ^2	P
Halothane	209	49	81.0			
Methoxyflurane	14	2	87.5	1	0.1	N.S.
Enflurane	11	6	64.7	1	1.73	N.S.
Trichloroethylene	1 ⎫	1 ⎫	50.0			
Diethyl Ether	5 ⎬ 7	2 ⎬ 8	71.4	1	8.15	**
Cyclopropane	1 ⎭	5 ⎭	16.7			
Ketamine	1	0	∞		I.D.	
Local Anaesthetics	7	3	70.0	1	0.21	N.S.
Succinylcholine	20 ⎫ 23	7 ⎫ 8	74.7	1	0.44	N.S.
d-tubocurarine	3 ⎭	1 ⎭	75.0			

Abbreviations: I.D., insufficient data; N.S., not significant probability (*P*); **, probability of <0.01; df, degrees of freedom; χ^2, chi squares are for halothane versus other anaesthetic agent
[a] Anaesthetics listed are in each case the sole anaesthetic agent used

intense, but nevertheless transient, rigidity but is a weak inducer of fever and biochemical dearrangements and by itself is not lethal. In MHS swine succinylcholine can aggravate reactions triggered by halothane. Without halothane succinylcholine can usually, but not always, induce reactions in MHS swine (NELSON et al. 1973; LUCKE et al. 1976 b). These succinylcholine reactions are associated with a greater rise in aerobic but a lesser rise in anaerobic metabolism than are MH reactions induced in susceptible hogs by halothane (GRONERT and THEYE 1976).

D-tubocurarine alone can occasionally cause a non-fatal fever in MHS humans (Table 4) and in conjunction with inhalational agents can aggravate already established reactions (BRITT and KALOW 1970 b). On the other hand, pancuronium, a non-depolarizing muscle relaxant with a steroidal structure, appears to be safe for MHS patients (personal observation). Whether or not its safety is related to its steroid molecule has not yet been established, but it is of interest that Althesin, the only intravenous induction anaesthetic which appears to be capable of significantly delaying the onset of MH reactions (HARRISON 1973), also has a steroidal structure.

All the potent inhalational anaesthetics are capable of inducing MH reactions (BRITT et al. 1977 b; BRITT and KALOW 1970 b; OJIMA et al. 1971) (Table 4). Implicated agents include:
1. Halothane
2. Enflurane isoflurane
3. Methoxyflurane
4. Diethyl Ether
5. Divinyl ether
6. Fluroxene
7. Trichloroethylene
8. Ethyl chloride
9. Cyclopropane.

Table 5. Frequency of early signs of MH reactions

Signs present in first 30 min of anaesthesia	Number of patients		Percentage of patients with sign present	Statistics		
	Sign not present	Sign present		df	χ^2	P
Tachycardia	39	370	90.5	χ	χ	χ
Tachypnoea	36	173	82.8	1	6.97	**
Rigidity	93	355	79.2	1	19.82	***
Altered blood pressure	57	197	77.6	1	20.05	***
Fever	55	146	72.6	1	31.51	***
Cyanosis	84	189	69.2	1	48.51	***

Abbreviations: **, probability (P) of <0.01; ***, probability of <0.001; df, degrees of freedom; χ^2s are for tachycardia versus other signs of MH

The reactions triggered by these volatile agents tend to be slower in onset and development than are the reactions caused by succinylcholine. Eventually, however, in untreated cases inhalational anaesthetics so severely damage the muscle cells as to kill a considerable portion of patients.

Even nitrous oxide has been claimed by ELLIS et al. (1974) to be capable of precipitating MH in a single patient; this report has been questioned (LUCKE et al. 1975; LACK 1975). No case similar to Ellis' has ever been discovered subsequently in spite of the extensive use of nitrous oxide for elective anaesthesia of MHS patients.

Lidocaine, mepivacaine, bupivacaine, and other amide local anaesthetics occasionally cause MH crises in severely afflicted individuals (Table 4) and frequently worsen crises triggered by other agents (KLIMANEK et al. 1976) or by stress. Conversely, ester local anaesthetics may be effective in the treatment of acute MH reactions. These opposing actions of amide and ester local anaesthetics may be due to their different MH-triggering potentials at physiological pHs (ester local anaesthetics have higher peaks) less hydrogen bonding between the carbonyl oxygen and tertiary amine group of the ester than the amide local anaesthetics (in the former these two groups are separated by a two carbon chain and in the latter by only one carbon) and the absence of any obstructing methyl groups in the ortho position of the phenyl ring of the ester local anaesthetics as opposed to their presence in the amide local anaesthetics (BIANCHI and BOLTON 1967). Ketamine, a narcotic which even in normal patients increases skeletal muscle tone, has caused MH reactions in both humans (unpublished work) and in pigs (Table 5).

The role of ethanol in triggering MH reactions is uncertain. The author has observed that the same MHS muscle which exhibits halothane-induced contractures in the absence of caffeine also develops contractures in the presence of ethanol. These responses are not seen with normal muscle. On the other hand many MHS patients drink alcohol without developing any evidence of MH reactions. A few, however, do complain of muscle cramps, palpitations and flushing after injection of small quantities of alcohol. HALEVY and MARX (1971) have reported a MH reaction occurring during a thiopentone, nitrous oxide, oxygen-succinylcholine and halothane anaesthetic in a woman who was inebriated at the time of induction.

Whether alcohol played a role in triggering this reaction is unknown, but it should be noted that she had had a previous uneventful anaesthetic while sober.

Caffeine, a methylxanthine which depletes the sarcoplasmic reticulum (SR) of calcium and thereby elevating myoplasmic calcium (JOHNSON and INESI 1969), induces anxiety, tremors and cyanosis in MHS pigs but not in normal hogs (JAMES 1978). The role of caffeine in inducing or aggravating MH reactions in susceptible humans is not known. The amount of caffeine in a day's coffee ration is a tiny fraction of that in the smallest dose of caffeine used in the caffeine contracture test. Nevertheless, some severely afflicted MHS patients state that they never or rarely drink coffee because it induces in them anxiety, palpitations, flushing, hyperventilation, and muscle cramps. Other MHS patients drink coffee without any ill effects. Caffeine plus halothane, but not caffeine plus pentobarbital, induces in rabbits a syndrome strongly resembling MH (fever, rigidity, acidosis, and hyperkalaemia) (DURBIN and ROSENBERG 1979).

Parasympatholytics (atropine and scopolamine), sympathomimetics (vasopressors and isoproterenol), cardiac glycosides (digoxin), quinidine analogues and calcium salts aggravate MH reactions (BARLOW and ISAACS 1970) and rarely may by themselves precipitate crises (BRITT et al. 1977b; BRITT 1980). Other agents which have been postulated to play a role in triggering MH reactions on the basis of isolated case reports include vitamin E.

2. Stress

Malignant hyperthermia crises may be induced in susceptible individuals by stress, for instance by high environmental temperatures, sudden change from very high to very low environmental temperatures (diving into cold water on a very hot day), mild infections, extreme emotional excitement, and extensive muscle injury or violent muscle exercise (BRITT 1980; EIKELENBOOM et al. 1976). A combination of two or more of the above is especially apt to precipitate a stress reaction, for example playing strenuous competitive sports during hot weather. MHS pigs are prone to stress-induced reactions to an even greater extent than are humans (BALL et al. 1973; EIKELENBOOM et al. 1976). Stress immediately preceding surgery (exercise, trauma, and apprehension) appears to increase the incidence of anaesthetic-induced reactions (LUCKE and DENNY 1978). The commencement of pain in the recovery room following anaesthesia may also induce MH reactions even when anaesthesia has been conducted with non-triggering agents. Similarly, drug-induced reactions may be aggravated after the partial return of consciousness by the stress of pain, physical manipulation, loud noises or glaring lights.

3. Diet

Some substance in the diet of MHS patients may predispose them to anaesthetic- or stress-induced MH reactions (HORSEY 1968). As will be discussed in a later section of this paper, the MH defect may be characterized by excessive unsaturation of structural phospholipids. Thus, a diet high in such lipids could conceivably increase the incidence of reactions in MHS individuals.

4. Climate

MH reactions are more common in temperate and cold climates than in tropical areas. This greater frequency in cold environments may be related to adaptive changes in lipid and catecholamine metabolism in cold-acclimated individuals (Masoro 1976; Mount 1976).

5. Elevated Serum Calcium

Rises in extracellular fluid calcium play such an important role in the pathogenesis of MH that rarely reactions may be triggered in patients with no inherited susceptibility to MH, if serum calcium is sufficiently elevated at the time of induction of anaesthesia, e.g. in patients with malignant parathormone-producing tumours (Schweizer et al. 1971; Borden et al. 1976).

D. The Acute Reactions

I. Clinical Appearance

The most unique, although not the most consistent, early feature of a MH crisis is skeletal muscle rigidity (Tables 4 and 5). Most typically the rigidity commences shortly after the infusion of succinylcholine (Britt 1980; Yoh et al. 1974; Wolfe et al. 1973; Waltomath 1973; Stovner 1968). Fasciculations are either grossly exaggerated or paradoxically may be entirely absent (James 1970). Then instead of the expected paralysis, a rigor-mortis-like muscle stiffness begins. This stiffness is due to an increase in the resting tension of the muscles and presents as a hardness of the muscle bellies on palpation rather than as cyclical spasms. In pigs rigidity usually begins in the rear limbs. In humans, muscle stiffness most commonly commences in the jaw muscles, making intubation or insertion of an airway or mouth gag difficult or impossible (Britt et al. 1977 b; Britt and Kalow 1970 b; Howat et al. 1973). Repeated doses of succinylcholine worsen rather than relieve the stiffness. Rigidity spreads to the remainder of the skeletal muscles after a variable time.

In those who have not received succinylcholine, the onset of the muscle stiffness may be delayed, its development more insidious and the sites of first detection may be the muscles of the extremities or of the chest. The rigidity induced by inhalational agents is ultimately more intense and less reversible than is that due to succinylcholine. Rigidity precipitated by a combination of inhalational agents and muscle relaxants, for instance halothane and succinylcholine, is particularly intractable.

About 18% of patients never manifest any perceptible increase in muscle tone (Furniss 1971; Jago and Payne 1977). While some of these individuals may have a different (and as yet unknown) skeletal muscle defect, some other cases appear to be aetiologically similar to those displaying rigidity. They rather have had very mild inherent defects, have received neither belladonna alkaloids nor succinylcholine; have had anaesthesia with weak triggering agents such as cyclopropane (Table 4) and have not undergone muscle exercise or injury immediately prior to anaesthesia nor had their anaesthetics administered by techniques which permit the development of hypoxia, hypercarbia, hypotension or other stress-creating disturbances.

The most consistent early feature of a MH crisis is a tachycardia (Table 5). Tachycardia is observed within the first 30 min of anaesthesia in 90% of all MH reactions (Table 5) (BRITT 1980) and is eventually present in nearly all cases (NICHOLSON 1971; WOLFE et al. 1973; WILLIAMS 1976). Tachycardia usually occurs prior to the detection of fever and occasionally even before the onset of muscle rigidity (BRITT 1980). Thus, unless there is some other obvious explanation, tachycardia during anaesthesia should be considered to be due to MH until proven otherwise. Confusion of the tachycardia of MH with the tachycardia of too light anaesthesia can only have the most unfortunate consequences for the patient.

Rapid multifocal ventricular arrhythmias frequently occur in conjunction with or shortly after the onset of the tachycardia. Such arrhythmias may take the form of frequent multifocal ventricular extrasystoles, trigeminal or bigeminal rhythms or runs of ventricular tachycardia (TONOGAI et al. 1978; KONDO 1971; DILLON 1968). These arrythmias and the preceding sinus tachycardia appear to be due, at least in part, to a primary defect in the heart muscle similar to that in the skeletal muscle. Later arrhythmias due to electrolyte abnormalities may occur; for instance, tall peaked T waves may be induced by hyperkalaemia. An early cause of death may be conversion of an arrhythmia into ventricular fibrillation. Such conversion is especially apt to be precipitated by physical stimulation of the patient, for instance moving the patient from the operating table to a transport trolley.

Another common early sign of MH is instability of the systolic blood pressure (BRITT 1980; KATZ 1970) (Table 5). The levels vary more than usual from one reading to the next, generally with an overall moderate rise until shortly before cardiac arrest when profound hypotension and bradycardia supervene. The early hypertension seems to be due to a combination of increased cardiac output – itself a result of increased heart rate and myocardial contractility – and to intense arteriolar spasm (GRONERT and THEYE 1976 b).

If the patient is breathing spontaneously, rapid and deep respirations (WINCKLER et al. 1971; RYAN and PAPPER 1970) and excessive heat and discolouration of the soda lime cannister may be observed (Table 5). These changes represent an attempt of the body to excrete the excess carbon dioxide and heat being produced by the hypercatabolizing muscles and other tissues. The skin often acquires a red flushing of the anterior surface of the neck and upper chest (BRITT et al. 1974). A similar flushing is regularly observed in MHS pigs before or during induction of anaesthesia (BRITT 1980). The cause of this flushing is not certain but may be secondary to hypercarbia or to transient instability of the musculature of the peripheral blood vessels. Flushing is usually followed by a peculiar mottled cyanosis (BRITT 1980; KIKUCHI et al. 1977; JAMES 1970) of ominous prognostic import which is partly secondary to arteriolar spasm and partly to hypoxaemia arising from increased oxygen consumption by the muscles. Rigidity of the chest wall muscles makes ventilation of the lungs difficult and may, thereby, contribute to the cyanosis (WILSON et al. 1967; BERGERA and FRITZ 1971).

The fever of a MH reaction is due both to decreased heat loss secondary to peripheral vasospasm and to increased heat production in the muscles. Since the fever is a result, not a cause, of the various biochemical dearrangements which occur in the muscles during a MH reaction (LUCKE et al. 1976 a), it tends to be of relatively late onset (WINCKLER et al. 1971). Seventy-three percent of patients exhibit detect-

Table 6. Relationship between mortality and maximum temperature attained during MH reaction

Maximum temperature °F	Number of patients		Percentage of patients surviving
	Died	Survived	
99–100.9	2	55	96.49
101–102.9	7	72	91.14
103–104.9	17	86	83.50
105–106.9	38	61	61.62
107–108.9	106	53	33.33
109–110.9	49	8	14.04
>111	18	1	5.26

Statistics	df	χ^2	P
χ^2 due to regression	1	194.04	***
χ^2 due to deviation from linearity	5	11.69	*
Total χ^2	6	205.73	***

Abbreviations: *, probability of <0.05; ***, probability of <0.001; df, degrees of freedom; χ^2, chi square

able rises in temperature during the first 30 min of anaesthesia (BRITT 1980) (Table 5). Thus, by the time detectable rises in body temperature have been observed, the patient's future may already have been seriously compromised. It must be remembered, however, that the low incidence of early fever recognition compared to early recognition of techycardia is, at least partly, due to failure by many anaesthetists to monitor temperature during *every* anaesthetic. If routine temperature recording were to become invariable during all anaesthetics the mortality from inadvertent MH reactions undoubtedly would decline dramatically (BRITT et al. 1977 b; BRITT 1980; WILSON 1971; HALL 1978; SHIBATA et al. 1971). Actually, early recognition of fever in 73% of cases is a considerable improvement over the 35% recognition of fever reported by the author in 1974. This increase appears to be mainly due to more frequent routine temperature monitoring. It is gratifying that during the same period mortality from MH reactions has correspondingly declined.

The maximum temperature level attained is quite variable. As a rule, however, the higher the maximum temperature, the higher is the mortality rate (BRITT 1980; BRITT and KALOW 1970 b) (Table 6). Death has, however, occurred in patients whose maximum temperature elevations have been relatively low (Table 6), while on the other hand survival has occurred after fevers of 44 °C (Table 6).

In general, higher temperatures are recorded following the use of skeletal muscle relaxants alone than during anaesthesia with inhalational agents alone (Table 7). No significant differences among the various inhalational agents with regard to their influence on maximum temperature attained have been observed.

A few patients develop a mumps-like swelling of the parotid glands during MH reactions (MARX 1969). The cause of this swelling is not known.

Table 7. Relationships among individual agents and maximum temperatures attained during MH reactions

Maximum temperature °F		Inhalational agent + succinylcholine + curare	Inhalational agent	Inhalational agent + curare	Inhalational agent + succinylcholine	Succinylcholine + curare	Succinylcholine	Curare
< 106.9		31	22	7	183	13	17	6
> 107.0		36	20	6	116	1	0	0
Ratio								
< 106.9/> 107.0		0.86	1.10	1.17	1.58	13.00	∞	∞
χ^2 Inhalational agents+succinylcholine+curare vs. other combinations	df	–	1	1	1	1	1	1
	χ^2	–	0.18	0.04	4.43	8.34	13.87	4.39
	P	–	N.S.	N.S.	*	**	***	*

Abbreviations: χ^2s are for inhalational agent + succinylcholine plus curare versus other combinations; N.S., not significant probability (*P*); *, probability of < 0.05; **, probability of < 0.01; ***, probability of < 0.001; df, degrees of freedom

II. Laboratory Changes

The effect of halothane on the blood composition of MHS individuals is better described in swine than in humans. Thus, in humans MH reactions occur unexpectedly and blood sampling is usually not commenced for some time after the crisis has begun. In pigs, on the other hand, MH reactions can be induced at will and under controlled conditions (BERMAN and KENCH 1973; WILLIAMS et al. 1971; GRONERT and THEYE 1976a; R. A. POLLOCK et al. 1974). Malignant hyperthermia following enflurane (Ethrane): a case report, unpublished work). They have shown that within minutes (between 3 and 21 min) of commencing administration of halothane to MHS pigs rises occur in serum magnesium, sodium, potassium, calcium, and phosphate and in blood glucose, lactate and pyruvate with corresponding falls in arterial pH and increases in base deficits. Hypercarbia and hypoxaemia also occurred at this time (BRITT 1980; GRONERT et al. 1977). At 30 min blood epinephrine and norepinephrine values become substantially elevated (GRONERT and THEYE 1976a).

Later (at 80 min) serum calcium (STANEC et al. 1978) and potassium values become depressed to below pre-halothane levels (BRITT 1980). In human patients substantially similar changes are recorded (BRITT 1980; KIKUCHI 1977), although the very early elevations of serum calcium, potassium and magnesium may often be missed because of failure to sample early. The marked rises in blood glucose are accompanied by only slight elevations of blood insulin and cortisol. This may be because of the inhibitory α-adrenergic effects of the increased circulating catecholamines on insulin and cortisol secretions (HALL et al. 1976b). The decline in serum calcium usually precedes that of potassium. The low serum potassium and calcium levels may persist for several days.

After several hours in both swine and humans large molecules begin to leak out of the muscles across the by now damaged and leaky sarcolemma to the blood, first myoglobin (Britt 1980) and then the even larger enzymes such as creatine kinase (CK) (Denborough et al. 1970a, Woolf et al. 1970; Kacinec et al. 1974; Blume et al. 1978; K. Venugopal and H. Konchigeri successful management of malignant hyperthermia: a case report, unpublished work), lactic dehydrogenase (LDH), hydroxy butyric dehydrogenase (HBDH), glutamic oxalic transaminase (GPT), and aldolase (Denborough et al. 1970b). These enzymes reach their maximal blood levels 24–96 h after the beginning of a MH reaction. The low mortality rates reported for patients exhibiting myoglobinuria or elevated serum CK levels are probably artifactual, being due to the unfortunate fact that patients whose muscle is so damaged as to allow these molecules to escape often die before they can be detected outside the muscle.

The above laboratory abnormalities may be found in all or part during the more fulminant crises. At the other extreme many mild reactions may be accompanied only by moderate metabolic acidosis, and most by rises in serum CK.

III. Late Complications

Because of its smaller molecular size compared with haemoglobin, myoglobin readily traverses the glomerular membrane and obstructs the renal tubules (Yana et al. 1977; Bernhardt and Hoerder 1977). Unlike haemoglobin, the myoglobin molecule can penetrate into the renal parenchymal cells. Oliguria and a rising blood urea nitrogen (BUN) follow (Thomford et al. 1969; Satnick 1969). Acute renal failure is a not uncommon finding in the more stormy reactions (Britt 1980). Occasionally renal failure, rather than being oliguric, is polyuric (Lieberman et al. 1978).

Platelets, fibrinogen and other clotting factors may become depleted, leading to multiple haematomata and intractable bleeding from body orifices and wound and needle sites (Sage and Hall 1972; Daniels et al. 1969). This acute consumption coagulopathy appears to be induced by a primary defect of the platelets. Since platelets are in essence floating muscle cells, containing many components and functions similar, if not identical, to those of muscle cells, such a MH defect of the platelets is not surprising. The acute disseminated intravascular coagulopathy is usually a fatal complication of MH reactions (Purkis et al. 1967).

Another late complication of ominous prognostic import is acute pulmonary oedema characterized by loud moist rales in both lung fields and copious amounts of pink frothy sputum surging up through the endotracheal tube (Gibson and Gardiner 1969; Satnik 1969). Pulmonary oedema is at least partly secondary to rigor of the left ventricle which prevents blood from exiting from the pulmonary vasculature. Acute left heart failure may also be partially secondary to increased tone of the pulmonary microcirculation arising either because of a primary MH defect in the vascular smooth muscle or because of the vasoconstricting action of the elevated blood catecholamine concentrations and carbon dioxide tensions and the low blood oxygen tensions.

Some patients with the aid of heroic treatment linger on for several hours or days before finally dying, never regaining consciousness, with fixed and dilated pupils, absent deep tendon reflexes, upgoing plantar reflexes and perhaps intermit-

Table 8. Relationships between mortality and neurological abnormalities during and after MH reactions

Sign	Number of patients		Statistics		
	Died	Survived	df	χ^2	P
Coma					
Present	94	75			
			1	43.12	***
Not present	6	64			
Convulsions					
Present	44	28			
			1	27.23	***
Not present	16	68			
Reflexes					
Decreased	20	15			
Normal	9 ⎫ 15	66 ⎫ 73	1	17.86	***
Increased	6 ⎭	7 ⎭			
Pupils fixed and dilated					
Yes	70	29			
			1	57.51	***
No	10	69			

Abbreviations: ***, probability (P) of <0.001; df, degrees of freedom; χ^2, chi square

tent, generalized or localized convulsions (PURKIS et al. 1967; BRITT and KALOW 1970a; STEPHEN 1967) (see Table 8). Whether such brain death is caused by a primary MH brain defect or is secondary to the many biochemical and physiological disturbances to which the brain is subjected during a MH crisis has not yet been determined.

IV. Post Mortem Examination

Routine post mortem examinations often show little other than minor changes consistent with acute terminal hypoxia, for instance congestion and oedema of brain, lung, liver, and kidney cells. Meticulous examination of microscopic sections of skeletal muscle, however, reveal acute rhabdomyolysis with necrosis (GULLOTTA and HELPAP 1976).

V. Prognosis

Survival from MH reactions has steadily been improving since study of this condition was commenced in 1966. At that time the survival rate was less than 20%. By 1979 survival had risen to 91%. This increase has been mainly due to cases being successfully treated in North America and not to cases reported from other geopolitical areas. The higher survival rates in North America appear to be a result: in part of more frequent and better educational programs within hospitals; more consistent use of monitoring, for example of temperature and blood gases during

Table 9. Relationship between the use of anaesthetics or relaxants and mortality during MH reactions

Anaesthetic	Number of patients		Percentage of patients surviving	Statistics		
	Died	Survived		df	χ^2	P
Halothane	310	454	60.21	X	X	X
Methoxyflurane	11	9	45.00	1	1.13	N. S.
Enflurane	9	13	59.09	1	0.04	N. S.
Trichloroethylene	1	0		1	I. D.	X
Chloroform	1	0		1	I. D.	X
Diethyl Ether	10	2	16.67	1	7.24	**
Cyclopropane	4	7	63.64	1	0.00	N. S.
Ketamine	0	1		1	I. D.	X
Local Anaesthetics	2	8	80.00	1	0.99	N. S.
Succinylcholine	0	32	∞	1	19.59	***
d-tubocurarine	0	5	∞	1	1.92	N. S.

Abbreviations: χ^2s are for halothane versus other anaesthetics. N. S., not significant probability; **, probability (P) of <0.01; ***, probability (P) of <0.001; I. D., insufficient data for analysis; df, degrees of freedom

anaesthesia; greater use of and familiarity with MH protocols and MH emergency trolleys; earlier cessation of triggering drugs with consequent lower maximum temperatures and serum potassium; and the early administration of dantrolene sodium.

Mortality varies considerably according to geopolitical location, being low in North America and significantly higher in Australia, New Zealand, the United Kingdom, Ireland, and Europe. This data may, however, be somewhat biased because of the more faithful reporting of North American MH cases to our Central Registry. Furthermore very recent data (not included in this statistical study) from Japan suggests that intensive per anaesthetic monitoring of their patients has begun to pay dividends in the form of sharply improved survival rates.

In anaesthetic-induced reactions mortality is entirely associated with the use of inhalational agents and not muscle relaxants (Table 9). Mortality is slightly worse in patients who have had no previous anaesthetics.

Mortality considered according to type of operation appears to be more closely related to the general risk associated with that type of operation than with concurrent presence of a MH reaction, with the possible exception of gynaecological procedures. Survival surprisingly appears to be no better in academic than in non-academic hospitals.

The immediate cause of death in individuals dying early – usually during the anaesthetic itself – seems to be a ventricular fibrillation arising out of a preceding multifocal ventricular arrhythmia. Patients expiring several hours after the commencement of anaesthesia die of acute pulmonary oedema or consumption coagulopathy. Those dying several days after anaesthesia generally have suffered irreversible central neurological deterioration (WOLFE et al. 1969; STEPHEN 1967; PURKIS et al. 1967). A few years ago a number of patients died from acute renal failure, but with the advent of efficient dialysis techniques this cause of death has been sharply reduced.

In surviving patients permanent neurological damage (decreased intelligence, blindness, deafness, paralysis, inco-ordination, and convulsions) is much more common in individuals who have sustained a cardiac arrest than in those who have not.

VI. Differential Diagnosis

Malignant hyperthermic reactions must be differentiated from other conditions that may produce fever during anaesthesia, for example:
1. Decreased heat loss due to immersion of patients in a super-abundance of heavy drapes (LEE et al. 1979)
2. Increased external heating by a too hot K thermia blanket (TANABE et al. 1971), or by a malfunctioning ventilator (FIVEHOUSE and WATSON 1968)
3. Increased internal heat production due to:
   a) Excessive shivering in response to cold or struggling (NICHOLSON 1969)
   b) Endocrinopathies such as thyrotoxicosis and pheochromocytoma (NICHOLSON 1969)
   c) Oesteogenesis inperfecta (DE PINNA 1978; SOLOMONS and MYERS 1973)
   d) Infection, either pre-existing or induced by infusion of infected blood, by intravenous fluids or by contamination of the wound site (HESS et al. 1974; MODELL 1966)
   e) Mismatched blood transfusion (BRITT unpublished work).
4. Combined decreased heat loss and increased heat production due to:
   a) An abnormality of the central temperature regulating mechanism in the hypothalamus secondary to an intracranial lesion, e.g. head injury, or exposure of the hypothalamus to prostaglandin E or 5-hydroxytryptamine (MILTON and WENDLANDT 1971; FELDBERG and MYERS 1964)
   b) Idiosyncratic response to psychoactive drugs, e.g. glutethimide, monoamine oxidase inhibitors, amphetamines, butyrophenones, tricyclics, and phenothiazines (LEWIS 1965; GREENBLATT et al. 1978; STANLEY and PAL 1964).

E. Aetiology and Pathophysiology of Rigid MH

I. Aetiology

The aetiology of MH has not yet been entirely clarified in spite of a number of years of intensive investigation. Nevertheless, the most likely immediate cause of the acute hypercatabolism of rigid MH appears to be a sudden rise in the concentration of myoplasmic calcium (DENBOROUGH 1979). This hypothesis is supported by the observation that drugs which raise myoplasmic calcium, for example lidocaine, cardiac glycosides, caffeine, and calcium salts, worsen the prognosis of in vivo MH reactions (BRITT et al. 1977 b; BRITT 1980). Caffeine in vitro causes contractures that are larger in susceptible than in normal skeletal muscle fascicles (BRITT et al. 1976 b; ELLIS et al. 1978 b). These contractures are further enhanced by calcium

(MOULDS and DENBOROUGH 1974a; NELSON 1978). On the other hand, drugs which lower myoplasmic calcium, for instance procaine amide (HARRISON 1973; JOHNSON and INESI 1969), dantrolene (ELLIS and BRYANT 1972; ELLIS and CARPENTER 1972), and verapamil (FLECKENSTEIN 1971), improve survival from in vivo crises (BRITT 1980). In vitro these agents along with diltazem, a benzothiazepine derivative that also lowers myoplasmic calcium (NAKAJIMA et al. 1976; UCHIDA 1976), and calcium-free Krebs Ringer solution attenuate caffeine-induced contractures of MHS skeletal muscle fascicles (ANDERSON and JONES 1978).

The abnormality that could account for the sudden and rapid rise of myoplasmic calcium during a MH reaction has yet to be firmly established.

Some reasonable possibilities based on known muscle physiology are:
1. Abnormally low accumulation of calcium by the sarcoplasmic reticulum SR.
2. Defective accumulation of calcium by the mitochondria
3. Excessively fragile sarcolemma with, therefore, passive diffusion of calcium into the myoplasm from the extracellular fluid
4. Exaggeration of adrenergic innervation with resulting multiple indirect effects.
These possibilities are not necessarily mutually exclusive since MH may well be a widespread membrane disease involving not only membranes of different cell types but also different membranes with a given cell type.

1. Defective Calcium Uptake into, Binding by and/or Release from the Sarcoplasmic Reticulum

The SR normally takes up and binds calcium during muscle relaxation and then releases calcium during muscle contraction (SANDOW 1970; HUXLEY 1965). The uptake of calcium is against a concentration gradient, the energy for which is obtained through coupling of calcium uptake to hydrolysis of ATP by SR ATPase. Binding of calcium is to calsequestrin, a protein component of the SR membrane (MACLENNAN 1973; BOWERS 1974). Release of calcium from the SR being with the concentration gradient, it is a passive phenomenon. Evidence for a primary defect in one or more of these functions is considerable.

The greater than normal contractures induced in MHS skeletal muscle by caffeine and the reversal of these excessive contractures by dantrolene and by procainamide suggest an inability of the SR to accumulate calcium. There may, therefore, be possibly a less than normal total calcium content of the muscle. The evidence for this latter postulation is, however, controversial (BRITT et al. 1975b; BENNETT et al. 1977).

It might be argued that the excessive caffeine contractures of MHS skeletal muscle are due solely to an effect of caffeine on a site other than the SR, for instance the sarcolemma. This postulation is, however, disproved by the studies of WOOD (1978) and other workers (TAKAGI 1977; ROSENBERG 1978). Thus WOOD, using chemically skinned, single, skeletal muscle fibres (devoid of sarcolemma, transverse tubules and mitochondria but containing SR and contractile elements) has presented data showing that the percentage of fibres with lower than normal thresholds for caffeine contracture are higher in MHS than in normal skeletal muscle samples. This work has been confirmed by TAKAGI (1977). Finally, ROSENBERG (1978) has observed that chemical skinning of normal rat skeletal muscle fi-

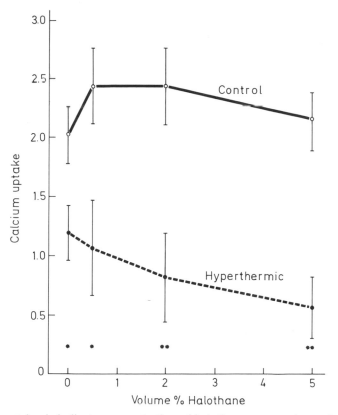

Fig. 7. Horizontal axis indicates concentration of halothane expressed as volume percent added to a homogenate of sarcoplasmic reticulum. Vertical axis indicates uptake into sarcoplasmic reticulum of $Ca^{45}Cl$ in mM/mg protein during 5 min. (BRITT et al. 1973, p 453)

bres has no diminishing effect on caffeine contractures in either the presence or the absence of halothane.

Other indirect evidence supporting a SR defect in MHS muscle is the report of BRYANT and ANDERSON (1977) that in muscle fibres from MHS pigs a threshold contraction occurs when the interior of the muscle has been depolarized only slightly, i.e. to -85 mV. In muscle fibres from normal pigs, on the other hand, depolarization to -60 mV is necessary to initiate a visible contraction. The addition of dantrolene to the MHS fibres shifts the threshold potential toward that of the normal fibres.

In some human MHS patients calcium accumulation by isolated SR is less than normal (BRITT 1971; BRITT et al. 1973) and this difference is potentiated by in vitro halothane (Fig. 7). HEFFRON and MITCHELL (1976) have reported in SR isolated from MHS pigs a moderate reduction in the rate of: (1) calcium uptake, (2) calcium binding, and (3) calcium binding capacity. Two to six percent halothane moderately inhibits these parameters equally in both MH-susceptible and MH-resistant porcine SR. HEFFRON and MITCHELL postulate that halothane exerts its effect on the SR and MHS swine skeletal muscle by inhibiting their SR ATPase activity.

On the other hand, several other reports have described calcium uptake into porcine MHS SR as being normal or slightly increased (NELSON et al. 1972; STEWARD and THOMAS 1973). This hyper-efficient response is further improved by in vitro halothane. Pretreatment of MHS swine, however, with in vivo halothane does inhibit markedly calcium uptake into their SR (BRITT et al. 1975c). These observations suggest a secondary rather than a primary defect in porcine SR. Thus, in the presence of halothane, the calcium-accumulating or -retaining abilities of in situ MHS SR may be impaired by a low myoplasmic pH (NAKAMURA and SCHWARTZ 1972) or by a deficiency in an impure SR preparation – one containing substances capable of impairing the calcium–accumulating and/or -retaining capacities of the SR. For instance, the preparation might be contaminated with fragments of abnormal mitochondria, sarcolemma or catecholamine receptors.

2. Defective Calcium Uptake into, Binding by, and/or Release from the Mitochondria

A primary defect in the skeletal muscle mitochondria of MHS patients has been postulated (BRITT et al. 1973b, 1975a; HULL et al. 1971; WILSON et al. 1966). The mitochondria in addition to being the site of cell respiration are also storage vesicles for calcium. They function as long-term repositories for excess calcium which is beyond the capacity of the SR to take up during each relaxation cycle. Some evidence for a defect in calcium accumulation by MHS mitochondria does exist (POPINIGIS 1973).

On microscopic examination the mitochondria are not infrequently abnormal. The structural changes in the mitochondria may, however, all be secondary to their enforced residence in an environment excessively high in calcium.

Halothane has been claimed to have no influence on succinate oxidation in mitochondria isolated from the skeletal muscle of MHS swine. Halothane does stimulate succinate oxidation in mitochondria isolated from the skeletal muscle of normal swine. The stimulating effect is prevented when $CaCl_2$ (9.4–2.0 mM) is added to the mitochondrial suspension before halothane. In both MHS and normal mitochondria low (less than 2.0 vol-%) doses of halothane reversibly inhibit oxidation of $NADH_1$-linked substrates (HARRIS et al. 1971; COHEN and MARSHALL 1968; HALL et al. 1973).

In MHS swine calcium uptake into and binding by isolated skeletal muscle mitochondria is less than normal (BRITT et al. 1975a; DENBOROUGH et al. 1973b; GRONERT and HEFFRON 1979). CHEAH and CHEAH (1976, 1978) have observed in MHS Pietrain pigs a greater than normal rate of calcium efflux from skeletal muscle mitochondria. This accelerated efflux is inhibited by bovine serum albumin (BSA) in the MHS mitochondria. BSA has no effect on calcium efflux from the normal Pietrain skeletal muscle mitochondria. Whether these various deviant actions of calcium on the MHS mitochondria are due to a primary defect within the MHS mitochondria or whether they are a defence mechanism against a superabundance of calcium being presented to the mitochondria by the bathing myoplasm is not yet known. It is also of interest that a low pH (less than 6.0) in the bathing medium (state known to exist in the myoplasm during MH reactions) causes a rapid fall in the ADP/O_2 ratio and thereby increases heat production (MITCHELSON and HIRD 1973).

3. Passive Diffusion of Extracellular Fluid Calcium
Across a Defective Sarcolemma into the Myoplasm or Release of Bound Calcium from the Sarcolemma to the Myoplasm

What evidence exists for a defect in the ability of the sarcolemma to keep calcium out of the muscle cell? MCINTOSCH and BERMAN (1974) have shown that the phospholipids of MHS porcine sarcolemma and SR contain fatty acids which are more unsaturated than normal. They and others have postulated that this abnormality may be associated with an increased permeability of the sarcolemma to calcium. This hypothesis is supported by the report that halothane unsaturates fatty acid components of cell membranes and that MH is more common in cold-acclimated than in warm-acclimated humans (BRITT unpublished work).

Since the normal concentration of calcium in the ECF is about $2.5 \times 10^{-3}\ M$, while that in the myoplasm is only about $5 \times 10^{-7}\ M$, calcium would, when the sarcolemma is incompetent, be expected to flow from the ECF into the myoplasm. Even prior to anaesthesia MHS sarcolemma may be somewhat leakier than normal since in many susceptible human (BARLOW and ISAACS 1970; SOLOMONS and MYERS 1973; LARARD et al. 1972) and porcine (BERMAN and KENCH 1973; LARARD et al. 1972) subjects serum CK concentrations are elevated – the elevations apparently being due to outward seepage of the enzyme across the super-fragile sarcolemma.

The sarcolemma, as well as controlling calcium flux, binds calcium. During contraction some of the bound calcium is released into the myoplasm in the vicinity of the SR where it acts as a trigger for the release of still more calcium from the SR (ENDO et al. 1970; THORPE and SEEMAN 1973; THORENS and ENDO 1975). It may be that in MH patients reactions are triggered, at least in part, by the release of excessive amounts of "trigger" calcium from the SR or by increased sensitivity of the SR to trigger calcium.

4. Exaggerated Catecholamine Innervation

The depletion of SR calcium induced by triggering drugs or stresses may be secondary to an exaggerated sensitivity of sarcolemmal adenyl cyclase to catecholamines (WILLIAMS et al. 1978; WINGARD 1977, 1978). AHERN et al. (1976) have observed that treating susceptible Pietrain pigs with haloperidol retards the onset of severity of halothane–induced MH reactions. Similarly, HALL et al. (1975), LISTER et al. (1975, 1976), SHORT (1978), and SHORT et al. (1976) have pretreated MHS hogs with other drugs which reduce the availability of catecholamines to the skeletal muscle adrenergic receptor sites, for example with reserpine and phentolamine. These animals when subsequently challenged with halothane have not developed MH crises. LUCKE and DENNY (1977) and LUCKE et al. (1978) have found that combined adrenalectomy and bretyllium infusion prevents the induction by halothane of MH reactors in susceptible pigs. As a corrollary of the above the same group have reported that noradrenaline plus propranolol or phenylephrine infusions induce fatal MH reactions in susceptible Pietrain pigs (HALL et al. 1977). The inability of other workers to reproduce these results in other strains of MHS swine, for instance in Poland China pigs (BRITT unpublished work), may be simply a reflection of the lesser severity of the MH defect in the latter breed of pigs.

KERR et al. (1975) have claimed that epidural anaesthesia of MHS Poland China pigs prevents MH reactions in the blocked area but not in the unblocked part of the body. GRONERT et al. (1977), however, have found that tetracaine epidural anaesthesia of MHS Poland China pigs does not prevent MH induced by halothane and succinylcholine but does prevent the expected increase in epinephrine and norepinephrine. They have also found that pre-treatment of the pigs with dantrolene not only prevents the occurrence of MH during halothane challenge (GRONERT et al. 1976) but also inhibits rises in blood catecholamines due to stress, combined respiratory and metabolic acidosis, or haemorrhagic hypotension.

GRONERT and THEYE (1970 a) have also noted that during halothane-induced MH reactions in pigs significant elevations of blood epinephrine and norepinephrine occur much later than did rises of other parameters, e.g. lactate, potassium and oxygen consumption. GRONERT et al. (1977) claim, therefore, that increased release of catecholamines play only a secondary role in the pathophysiology of MH reactions. Their report does not, however, consider the possibility that the muscle catecholamine receptors (e.g. sarcolemmal adenyl cyclase) or the cAMP–protein-kinase pathway might be abnormally sensitive to catecholamine stimulation. In another publication, GRONERT et al. (1978 b) do present data which does support this possibility. This latter data demonstrate that in MHS pigs the ability of halothane and succinylcholine to raise myocardial oxygen consumption is blocked by prior administration of propranolol, a β-adrenoceptor blocking drug.

In humans hypersensitivity of the muscle catecholamine receptors also appears to play a role in the pathogenesis of MH reactions. Thus, in humans administration of catecholamine-like vasopressors, for instance phenylephrine and methamphetamine, markedly increases mortality while administration of drugs which have some antisympathetic action, for example chlorpromazine and propranolol, improves survival (BRITT et al. 1977).

The stress-induced reactions which occur in both MHS pigs and in MHS humans may be, therefore, triggered by an uncontrolled activation of the adrenergic pathway within the muscle cell. The findings of WILLNER et al. (1979) support this concept since they have found that in skeletal muscle excised from MHS humans adenyl cyclase is more active than in skeletal muscle removed from normal humans. They have also observed that in this same MHS skeletal muscle the levels of cAMP are elevated. It has not been established whether this hyperactive adenyl cyclase is solely responsible for MH crises or whether it merely activates another defect lying in a more distal part of the excitation-contraction coupling system.

It is known that the skeletal muscle β-adrenergic receptor (BOWMAN and NOTT 1969) consists of two components. An outer part facing the synaptic cleft is a key hole which receives the catecholamine key. The inner component facing the myoplasm is the enzyme adenyl cyclase. This enzyme in the absence of the catecholamine transmitter is kept inactive through the presence on it of two calcium ions. When the catecholamine combines with the receptor the two calcium ions are extruded – not to the myoplasm as might be expected, but rather to the extracellular fluid (Fig. 8). The loss of the two calcium ions activates the adenyl cyclase so that

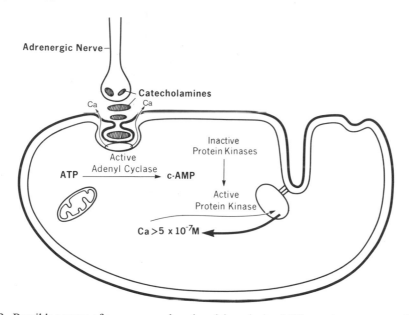

Fig. 8. Possible source of excess myoplasmic calcium during MH reaction: super sensitivity of adenyl cyclase to catecholamines

ATP is converted to cAMP (SUTHERLAND et al. 1962). The cAMP in turn activates a number of protein kinases. These have the capacity to reinforce acetylcholine-induced muscle contraction and its several support systems. For example, a protein kinase increases the uptake of calcium into the SR, but since the extra calcium taken up is not bound within the SR, more calcium is available for release during the next cholinergic-induced action potential. The net effect, therefore, of this protein kinase is to increase release of calcium from the SR during each contraction (RABINOWITZ et al. 1965). cAMP may also increase myocardial contractility by accelerating calcium influx through the calcium-conducting pores of the sarcolemma during the plateau phase of the action potential (OPIE 1978).

II. Pathophysiology

The elevated myoplasmic calcium has a number of heat producing effects that markedly elevate the metabolic rate (WILLIAMS et al. 1975). Increases of myoplasmic calcium activate phosphorylase a (WILLNER et al., to be published), thereby increasing catabolism of glycogen to lactate, carbon dioxide and heat. Oxygen consumption is correspondingly increased. The activation of phosphorylase a drives electron transport in the mitochondria. Excess heat production resulting from the activation of phosphorylase a is, therefore, both anaerobic and aerobic (HALL et al. 1976a). Activation of phosphorylase a is further reinforced by another cAMP-stimulated protein kinase via phosphorylase kinase (KREBS et al. 1966; SUTHERLAND and RALL 1960).

The excess lactate is transported to and taken up by the liver (HALL et al. 1978) where it is converted to glucose or catabolized to carbon dioxide and water. DI-

Marco et al. (1976) have reported that in the liver of MHS pigs slaughtered immediately after stress the rate of incorporation of lactate into glucose is 43% less and the oxidation of lactate to carbon dioxide is 38% less than in the livers of normal pigs anaesthetized with halothane; lactate uptake by their livers is accelerated substantially, but that increase is inadequate to deal with the vastly increased amounts of lactate being brought to the liver from the hypercatabolizing muscle. The insufficient ability of MHS livers to metabolize lactate during halothane anaesthesia may be partially due to the reduction in hepatic blood flow which occurs with the onset of hyperthermia.

Certainly no substantial evidence in favour of a primary defect in the liver exists. Thus liver function tests such as serum bilirubin and BSP retention remain normal or only slightly elevated during and after a MH crisis. Furthermore, measurements of temperatures, oxygen, carbon dioxide, and lactate levels in halothane-containing blood entering and leaving isolated MHS and normal pig livers reveal no differences in these parameters between the two categories of hogs (Britt et al. 1978 b).

High concentrations of myoplasmic calcium have several other effects that further raise heat production and also induce muscle contracture. The elevated myoplasmic calcium combines with troponin, a filament of globular proteins with long and thread-like tropomyosin which lies within the helixes of actin. The calcium induces a conformational change and a rotation of the troponin, which in turn causes a movement of the tropomyosin in such a way as to reveal the receptor sites on the actin to the myosin cross-bridges. During stress another of the cAMP-activated protein kinases potentiates the formation of this calcium-troponin complex (Britt 1977).

The elevated myoplasmic calcium causes excessive activation of myosin ATPase during MH crises (Krzywicki 1971). Hydrolysis by myosin ATPase of ATP to ADP plus phosphate heat is therefore accelerated. The ATP hydrolysis induces formation of actomyosin (Perry 1965) intermittently in normal muscle and permanently during reactions in MHS muscle. During relaxation the myosin cross-bridges are negatively charged because of the presence on them of ATP. They, therefore, project away from the shank of the myosin filament since it is also negatively charged. During contraction the addition of calcium to the ATP on the myosin cross-bridges (now combined with actin receptors) neutralizes their negativity. The bridges now bend inward toward the myosin shank pulling the myosin along the axis of the actin filament. The calcium-induced ATPase activity of the myosin head splits the ATP to ADP and phosphate, thus breaking the calcium-linked connection between the myosin bridge and actin receptor. Almost immediately a similar reaction sequence occurs at the next myosin cross-bridge so that the myosin is pulled along yet another step. In this way the myosin slides over the actin in a ratchet-like fashion forming short and rigid actomyosin (Wakabayashi and Ebashi 1968; Ebashi et al. 1967).

As the muscle temperature rises the above events become self-sustaining since the increased temperature eliminates the calcium requirement for myosin-actin interaction (Fuchs 1975). This thermal inactivation of the Ca^{2+}-regulating mechanism of actomyosin is potentiated by the decline in ATP levels. Thus two key events in the MH reaction, namely rise in muscle temperature and fall in muscle ATP, can perpetuate a muscle rigor independent of the intracellular calcium concentration (WALTEMATH 1973).

In normal muscle, once the acetylcholine-induced muscle action potential ceases, calcium is taken back into the SR and the muscle returns to its resting, relaxed state. During a MH crisis, however, the myoplasmic calcium remains permanently elevated so that muscle contracture, heat, carbon dioxide and lactic acid production and oxygen consumption continue unabated.

Some of the excess calcium is absorbed by the mitochondria. Within the mitochondria, the resulting toxic calcium concentration uncouples oxidative phosphorylation from electron transport, thereby decreasing ATP production but further accelerating oxygen consumption and output of lactate, carbon dioxide and heat. This effect is aggravated by lipid soluble volatile anaesthetics (HALL 1973).

Early in the reaction, ATP levels in the muscle are reasonably well maintained through conversion of creatine phosphate and ADP to creatine and ATP (LOHMANN 1934). Once, however, the muscle's store of high energy creatine phosphate has been exhausted, muscle ATP declines rapidly (NELSON et al. 1974). The fall is particularly marked in red muscle. This ATP decline may be exacerbated by the lack of complete availability of another source of ATP replacement, namely adenylate kinase

$$2\,ADP \rightarrow ATP + AMP.$$

This is because, for reasons not fully understood, MHS skeletal muscle may suffer from a deficiency of adenylate kinase (K. SCHMIDT et al. 1979; a new approach to the molecular pathology of malignant hyperpyrexia, unpublished work; SCHMITT et al. 1974).

When depletion of ATP occurs the MHS crisis becomes irreversibly fatal. First, ATP (though not ATP hydrolysis) is necessary for muscle relaxation. There is, however, not sufficient ATP to separate actin from myosin. Rigor mortis, therefore, develops even before death has occurred (BRITT 1979a). Second, there is not enough ATP to serve as substrate for SR ATPase. Calcium is, consequently, not retaken into the SR. This effect is independent of and in addition to any primary defect that might exist in the SR membrane. Third, the sarcolemmal ATPases fail through lack of their substrate ATP. Ions and molecules, therefore, simply follow their natural concentration gradients. Thus, potassium, magnesium, phosphate, and, somewhat later, large molecules such as myoglobin and then the even larger enzyme such as CK leak outward.

The myoglobin obstructs the renal tubules, thereby inducing acute renal failure. Calcium, because its concentration gradient is in the reverse direction, flows into the myoplasm, thus exacerbating the already existing calcium-dependent biochemical dearangements.

Another reason for the fulminant fever of MH may be decreased heat loss (OPIE 1978). WILLIAMS et al. (1978) have observed that in MHS pigs during the early phases of a reaction, and in spite of the increased temperature of the perfusing blood, the peripheral blood vessels undergo intense spasm. Thus the exposed muscles at the operative site appear gelantinous and bloodless even though the driving pressure in the large central vessels is still well maintained (BRITT 1979a). This spasm may be secondary to catecholamine stimulation or may be due to a primary MH defect of the vascular smooth muscle.

III. Malignant Hyperthermia – Widespread Membrane Defect

Malignant hyperthermia appears to be a widespread membrane defect, involving both different membranes within the same cell type, as indicated in the preceding pages, and membranes of different cell types. Thus in the skeletal muscle there is evidence for calcium-related defects in the sarcoplasmic reticulum, the mitochondria and the sarcolemma, in particular the catecholamine receptor area of the sarcolemma. This defect may be a molecular abnormality common to all three membranes. The work of McINTOSCH and BERMAN (1974) and DRABIKOWSKI et al. (1972) suggests that the defect may lie in the structural lipids of these membranes. There is also evidence that similar calcium-related biochemical defects are present in other types of cells, for example nerve (BRITT et al. 1977 a) and brain cells, bone (BRITT et al. 1979), platelets (SOLOMONS et al. 1978), red blood cells (KELSTRUP et al. 1973), cardiac muscle and hormone-producing and -secreting cells. Hence the severe neurological deterioration, consumption coagulopathy, haemolysis, bizarre arrhythmias, depletion of thyroxin and elevation of blood glucose that are characteristic features of fulminant MH reactions may be initiated by primary defects in tissues other than skeletal muscle rather than by the secondary effects of electrolyte, acid-base and temperature disturbances. Additionally, the intramuscular nerve abnormalities (BRITT et al. 1979; LACOUR et al. 1971), platelet and red blood cell abnormalities, atypical glucose tolerance curves (DENBOROUGH et al. 1974) and abnormal thyroid function (LISTER 1973) which can sometimes be detected in MHS patients undergoing elective investigation may also be primary anomalies.

It is uncertain whether the myopathy of MH is secondary to a primary neurogenic lesion or is a widespread abnormality involving membranes of many different cell types and different membranes within given cell types. The work of MOULDS (1978) would suggest that MHS muscle is not denervated. He has shown that in denervated muscle electrical stimulation induces a greatly increased twitch tension, a decreased frequency of stimulation is required to produce a tetanus and a tetanus is followed by an increased time to relaxation. These abnormalities of contraction and relaxation are all absent in MHS muscle. HARRIMAN et al. (1978) in a microscopic examination of 75 MHS families, never encountered the classical features of a denervated muscle, i.e. collateral reinnervation, type grouping or group atrophy have always been absent.

The role of brown fat and prostaglandins in heat generation during MH crises has yet to be investigated (OKUMURA and KURO 1975). Perfusion of isolated MHS and normal pig livers with halothane has revealed no differences in temperatures, blood gases, electrolytes or enzymes in the blood leaving the livers (BRITT et al. 1978 b). This organ, therefore, is probably not abnormal in MHS pigs. This may be because it is of epithelial origin while muscle, brain, nerve, bone, red blood cells, and platelets are all of connective tissue origin.

IV. Miscellaneous Observations on the Aetiology of MH

HARRIMAN et al. (1978) have found that tissue culture of human skeletal muscle shows no significant differences between MHS and normal muscle with respect to rate of growth, progress of differentiation and cell morphology. Similarly, LIEW and OKU (unpublished work) have not detected any differences between normal and MHS muscle protein separated by two dimensional SDS acrylamide electrophoresis. These results suggest that either the genetic defect does not involve the muscle fibre directly, that the defect is only revealed when susceptible muscle is exposed to anaesthetic agents or that the techniques employed have not been sufficiently discriminating. Evidence in support of the latter postulation is some more recent work of LIEW and OKU (unpublished work) on platelets. As with muscle they found that two-dimensional electrophoresis of MHS platelets revealed no consistent abnormalities. Treatment of the platelets with radioactive ATP prior to electrophoresis and with autoradiography after electrophoresis has demonstrated, however, that the phosphorylating proteins of the MHS platelets are markedly different from the normal platelets.

F. Preanaesthetic Diagnosis of MH

Identification prior to anaesthesia of individuals carrying the MH trait is of major importance. This step alone can greatly reduce mortality from MH reactions. To date no single test has been devised that is sufficiently inexpensive and non-invasive to permit application to the general population. Nevertheless, some relatively simple investigations can be performed on patients who require anaesthesia, for example searching for clinical muscle anomalies, ascertaining previous untoward anaesthetic history and, when indicated, measuring serum creatine kinase (CK). Persons who exhibit deviations from normal of several of these parameters and relatives of known MHS probands should be asked to undergo more intensive studies of their skeletal and heart muscle, motor nerves, bones, and platelets (BRITT 1979 b). These studies are described in the following sections.

I. Skeletal Muscle Studies

1. Signs and Symptoms of Musculoskeletal System

Muscle and other connective tissue anomalies are present in about two-thirds of all MHS patients and in approximately one-third of first degree relatives (BRITT et al. 1977b; BRITT 1980; ODA et al. 1977). Muscle volume and strength are often, but not always, greater than normal (BRITT 1980; WINCKLER et al. 1971). The muscle bellies are shorter and thicker than usual so that they appear rounded and bulging rather than fusiform (THOMPSON and TALLACK 1973). The muscle bellies may not be always bilaterally symmetrical. Intervening areas of muscle atrophy are usually so small as to be at least partially obscured by the hypertrophied muscle (THOMPSON and TALLACK 1973). In a few patients, however, the atrophied muscle groups are predominant. These latter individuals may exhibit frank arthrogryposis (ITOHDA et al. 1976) or weakness and wasting of the distal parts of the limbs. The atrophy may occur at an early age, usually as soon as the child attempts to walk. More commonly, atrophy occurs late in life and not infrequently develops in individuals who when younger were muscular athletes.

While muscle strength for short bursts of activity is often greater than normal, this super-strength may not be sustained during prolonged exercise in some individuals. A few may become weaker than normal during and after an extended period of muscular work (POLLOCK and TURNER 1974). The muscles, although strong, are sometimes not well co-ordinated (SNOW et al. 1972): opposing muscle group do not seem to be well balanced. The patients, therefore, while active in sports, are generally not very proficient unless the sport requires great physical strength but minimal coordination and duration, for example weight lifting. Because of the lack of motor coordination, some MHS children experience difficulty in learning to write (BRITT 1979a) and are diagnosed as having dyslexia.

Some patients complain of skeletal muscle cramps, aches, and pains which occur with variable frequency, either spontaneously, during and after exercise, emotional stress and infectious illness or after anaesthesia (BRITT 1979a; BRITT et al. 1977b). These may occur in the muscles of the limbs, back, chest or abdominal walls. When present, they may occasionally be so severe as to be almost incapacitating. These muscle cramps can be at least partially relieved with a combination of gentle heat, muscle vibrations, and oral dantrolene. A change of life style to a less stressful (both physically and emotionally) way of life may also be necessary.

Some other musculoskeletal abnormalities that are common in MHS patients are:

1. Stocky, short stature
2. Joint hypermobility with frequent joint dislocation [e.g. of patella (HAUSMAN et al. 1970) and shoulder] occurring after little or no trauma
3. Joint dislocations
4. Ptosis and strabismus – often both present in the same person (BRITT 1980; MURRAY and WILLIAMS 1969)
5. Thoracic kyphosis
6. Kyphoscoliosis (MAYER et al. 1978)
7. Lumbar Lordosis (LENARD and KETTLER 1975)
8. Hernias (usually congenital inguinal hernias but also umbilical and hiatus hernias (BRITT 1980)
9. Webbed neck (PINSKY and LEVY 1973)
10. Various types of club foot
11. Chronic muscular low backache and herniation of the nucleus pulposus induced by relatively minor trauma (WILSON et al. 1967)
12. Pectus carinatum
13. Hypoplasia of the mandible
14. Poor dental enamel
15. Crowded, mis-shaped lower teeth.

A very few patients have an associated hypokalaemic familial periodic paralysis with attacks of muscle weakness being induced by violent exercise or a high carbohydrate meal and relieved by rest, by a low carbohydrate diet and by potassium intake. Diagnoses of myotonia congenita, muscular dystrophy or polymyositis have occasionally been made in MHS patients. In all the patients displaying polymyositis, evidence of MH in relatives has been lacking. Rigid MH reactions in polymyositis patients may, therefore, represent an acquired form of MH.

2. Electromyography

Electromyography changes occur in about half of all MHS patients (KONNO 1974, 1976). The abnormality most frequently observed is an increased incidence of poly-

Table 10. Serum enzyme levels in a survivor from malignant hyperpyrexia and three of his first degree relatives. Normal values are shown in parentheses

Subject	Age	Examination of muscles	Creatine phospho-kinase CPK (0–70 I.U./litre)	Glutamic oxaloacetic transaminase SGOT (5–30 I.U./litre)	Lactate dehydro-genase LDH (100–250 I.U./litre)	Ornithine carbamyl transferase (0–2.5 I.U./litre)
Propositus	31	Normal	1,405	124	332	0.7
Father	64	Myopathy	372	74	320	0.9
Paternal aunt	66	Myopathy	408	72	285	1.1
Female sibling	28	Normal	393	44	284	0.7

Source: DENBOROUGH MA, FORSTER JFA, HUDSON MD, CARTER NG, ZAPF P (1970) Malignant hyperpyrexia – a serious, preventable complication of general anaesthesia. In: Australasian Congress of Anaesthesiology, Melbourne, Australia. Butterworths, London, p 167

phasic action potentials. Fibrillation potentials have also been detected occasionally (LACOUR et al. 1970).

3. Serum Creatine Kinase Elevations

High serum CK concentrations in MHS patients and their relatives were first described by DENBOROUGH et al. (1970a) (Table 10) and by ISAACS and his associates (see ISAACS 1973). Somewhat conflicting CK studies of MHS families have since been reported by other workers (BARLOW and ISAACS 1970; ZSIGMOND et al. 1972b; ELLIS et al. 1972, 1975). The author has encountered many problems in attempting to use CK elevation as a marker of MH. Mean values are higher in MHS probands than in control patients, but the standard errors are larger and many false positive and false negative values occur. The use of the Antonik rather than the Rosalki technique of measurement slightly but not substantially improves discrimination between normal and MHS subjects (BRITT et al. 1978). Values may be falsely low if the sample is exposed to light or is not promptly frozen in dry ice or liquid nitrogen. Normal subjects may have elevated serum CK levels for many reasons other than MH (BRITT et al. 1976a).

Substantial increases in serum CK can be caused by errors of sampling such as excessive tourniquet pressure, forcible suction of blood through the sampling needle or squirting of blood against the wall of the syringe. Many muscle damaging conditions can also raise the serum CK, for example:
1. A recent myocardial infarction (HESS et al. 1964)
2. Muscular dystrophy and other myopathies (MCCRIMMON and LEWIN 1967)
3. Paranoid schizophrenia (MELTZER 1969)
4. Various neurological disorders (WILLIAMS and BRUFORD 1967)
5. Hypothyroidism (FLEISHER and MCCONAHEY 1964)
6. Acute and chronic alcoholism (NYGREN 1965)
7. A recent intramuscular injection
8. Skeletal muscle trauma or exercise (BRITT unpublished work).

In spite of these problems, in some human families the serum CK is higher than normal in at least some of the patients who have had reactions and in some of their relatives. In a study reported by the author several years ago (BRITT et al. 1976a) values were consistently elevated in affected persons in 45% of families. In 35% of MHS families serum CKs were elevated in some individuals but the elevations tended to be small and not always reproducible and did not always occur in the patients who had reactions. In the remaining 20% of MHS families, serum CK values were within normal limits in all individuals including the probands. Thus with respect to CK investigations we have found two types of MHS families: those in which affected subjects have elevated serum CK levels and those in which these levels are normal. Unfortunately, between these two distinctive categories are a substantial number of families with inconsistent data. For the whole population, MH families with and without elevated serum CK values represent the two tails of a distribution curve and not merely the choice between two alternatives. Under these circumstances, one should not be surprised that the pattern of inheritance of CK values in families may be ambiguous.

In members of MHS families a significant positive relationship exists between high serum CKs and clinical muscle abnormalities. Thus, the combined presence of both a high CK and a muscle abnormality in the same individual is a much better marker of the MH trait than is the presence of either alone. Highly significant positive relationships are also present among skeletal muscle abnormalities in patients or relatives, elevated serum CK levels in patients or relatives and histories of MH reactions in relatives (BRITT et al. 1976a).

In MHS humans the serum CK varies with age much more than it does in normal people. In MHS patients, therefore, values tend to be higher in early and middle adulthood than in childhood or in old age. In normal persons little relationship between age and serum CK is observed. On the other hand, for healthy control subjects serum CK levels are significantly higher in males than in females, while for MHS probands CK values of males are statistically similar to those of females.

In both MHS and normal swine age is also an important factor in determining CK levels. Values peak at 19 weeks of age, an age correlating well with the period of maximum growth of skeletal muscles (HEFFRON and MITCHELL 1975a, b). Like humans, some but not all MHS pigs have elevated serum CK concentrations. There is much variation among animals within families and even greater variation among breeds, with the highest levels being recorded in MHS Pietrain pigs (ELIZONDO et al. 1976) followed by MHS Landrace swine (WOOLF et al. 1970), which in turn are followed by Poland China hogs (GRONERT and THEYE 1976a; JONES et al. 1972; ANDERSON and JONES 1976b). The difference in serum CK levels between normal and MHS pigs is increased by pretreating the animals with caffeine.

Serum CK values rise during exercise, e.g. labour (ISHERWOOD et al. 1975), more in MHS patients than in normal individuals. Bed rest reduces the differences between MHS and normal persons. Thus in individuals hospitalized for 24 h prior to diagnostic muscle biopsy the CK is elevated in only 40% of probands. Values are also elevated in 9% of control patients. CK measurement, therefore, has only a limited role to play in the diagnosis of individuals belonging to known or suspected MHS families. In such kindreds CK measurement in conjunction with skeletal muscle abnormalities is of value mainly in identifying branches of the clan most likely to be affected and, therefore, most in need of skeletal muscle biopsies. In random populations CK screening is of little use in the identification of MHS patients (KALOW et al. 1979).

ZSIGMOND et al. (ZSIGMOND 1975; ZSIGMOND et al. 1972 a, b) and ANIDO (1976) have claimed that the brain bands of CK isoenzyme of isolated MHS serum and skeletal muscle are elevated. HEFFRON and ISAACS (1976) and HASSAN et al. (1978), however, have not been able to reproduce ZSIGMOND's findings. CK isoenzyme measurement, either by electrophoresis or by column chromatography, has not, therefore, proved to be useful in the diagnosis of MH.

4. Serum Pyrophosphate

SOLOMONS and MYERS (1973), VAN WORMER et al. (1975), and TAN et al. (1978) have reported that serum pyrophosphate is higher in MHS patients than in normal subjects. This elevation may be secondary to increased conversion of ATP to cAMP and pyrophosphate by an overactive adenyl cyclase in MHS muscle.

5. Skeletal Muscle Biopsy

Skeletal muscle biopsy is required to make a definitive diagnosis of MH (MOULDS and DENBOROUGH 1974b). Several tests are available to examine the excised muscle. These may be employed separately, but diagnostic accuracy is enhanced when they are utilized in combination on the same muscle sample.

6. Caffeine and Halothane Contracture Tests

The caffeine and halothane contracture tests are now performed in many laboratories throughout the world. Using this method from the log caffeine and log caffeine plus halothane response curves, the concentration of caffeine in mM required to raise the resting tension of the isometric skeletal muscle fascicles by one gram is calculated. This value is defined as the "caffeine-specific concentration."

Caffeine induces in rigid MHS muscle a greater than normal contracture (i.e. decreases the caffeine-specific concentration) (MOULDS and DENBOROUGH 1974a; BRITT et al. 1980a; NELSON et al. 1975) (Fig. 9 and Table 11). In non-rigid MHS muscle caffeine induces a less than normal contracture (i.e. increases the caffeine-specific concentration). Indeed most of the muscle strips removed from non-rigid probands exhibit no contracture at all at even the highest dose of caffeine. In some but not all rigid and non-rigid MHS muscle, halothane alone precipitates a contracture (MOULDS and DENBOROUGH 1974a; MOULDS et al. 1974), which it rarely does with normal muscle.

The addition of both caffeine and halothane further increases the contractures of both rigid MHS and normal muscle. The increases are slightly greater for the MHS than for the normal muscle. Thus the discrimination between the normal and the rigid MHS patients is better in the presence than in the absence of halothane. In fact the muscle fascicles of some mildly afflicted rigid MHS patients exhibit normal contractures in the presence of caffeine alone but greater than normal contractures in the presence of caffeine with halothane. Much less often the reverse is

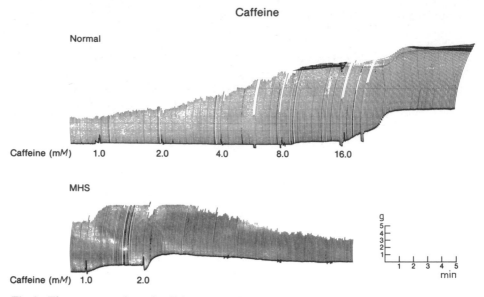

Fig. 9. The concentration of caffeine required to raise the resting tension of a MHS skeletal muscle fascicle by 1.0 g is less than the concentration of caffeine required to raise the resting tension of a normal skeletal muscle fascicle by 1.0 g

true (BRITT 1979, unpublished work). In non-rigid MHS muscle caffeine in the presence of halothane usually precipitates a normal contracture but may in some instances induce a greater than normal contracture.

These data obtained in the presence of caffeine alone, of halothane alone and of halothane plus caffeine support the concept that non-rigid and rigid MH are different aetiological conditions. It also confirms that MH without rigidity is very much less common than the rigid variety. Probably less than one in ten MHS probands has non-rigid MH, as evidenced by less than normal or even no contractures in the presence of caffeine.

Rigid MHS patients whose muscles exhibit contractures in the presence of halothane alone are those who have sustained extremely fulminant MH reactions. Those whose muscles do not develop contractures in the presence of halothane but do manifest greater than normal contractures in the presence of caffeine alone usually have MH reactions of intermediate severity. Finally, those patients whose muscles have not produced contractures in the presence of halothane alone nor have exhibited greater than normal contractures in the presence of caffeine alone but have developed greater than normal contractures in the combined presence of caffeine plus halothane have for the most part had very mild reactions (BRITT et al. 1980 a).

We see, therefore, that the caffeine, the halothane and the caffeine plus halothane tests are not measuring the same phenomenon. The tests may not be entirely independent, but they nevertheless indicate at least two factors which are separately variable. This means genetically that there are often, or always, two different kinds of genes contributing to the predisposition of MH. Whether these genes are

Table 11. Relationship between caffeine-specific concentrations (CSC) and temperature in normal and MHS patients

MH status	CSC in absence of halothane		Ratio 22/37	Statistics	
	22 °C	37 °C		t (22 vs 37)	P
Rigid MHS	4.778[a] (0.404) 15	2.919 (0.259) 15	1.637	3.87	**
Normal	16.847 (1.87) 13	7.331 (0.593) 13	2.298	4.85	***
Non-rigid MHS	22.88 (2.03) 12				
Statistics					
t (Rigid MHS vs normal)	6.74	7.15			
P (Rigid MHS vs normal)	***	***			
t (Non-rigid MHS vs normal)	2.19	–			
P (Non-rigid MHS vs normal)	*	–			

Abbreviations: CSC, caffeine specific concentration, i.e. dose of caffeine required to raise the resting tension of the skeletal muscle fascicle by 1.0 in absence of halothane; **, probability (*P*) of <0.01; ***, probability of <0.001; t, Student's *t*-test
[a] First figure=CSC; second figure (in brackets)=standard error; third figure=number of patients

allelic or occur in different loci remains to be investigated. In any case according to the caffeine tests, we are not dealing with a simple dominant inheritance of MH predisposition; the situation is more complicated and not yet clear (KALOW et al. 1979).

Persons with normal values for caffeine but abnormal or borderline values in the caffeine-halothane tests have been observed also in a few healthy control subjects. In a previously reported series (KALOW et al. 1977, 1979), one such deviant value was found among 35 controls. There are four such values in a second and independent series of 34 controls. Thus, the chances are that one is dealing with a genetic variant which may affect as much as 3% to 10% of the population. It could be that a rare, possibly dominant variant in addition to this common and probably recessive factor is causing the predisposition to rigid MH.

Caffeine contracture test results have been reported at both 22 °C and at 37 °C (BRITT et al. 1980a). The authors have found that caffeine alone induces a greater contracture at 37 °C than at 22 °C. On the other hand caffeine in the presence of halothane induces contractures at 37 °C which are slightly (although not significantly) less than those observed at 22 °C. Contractures induced by halothane are significantly less at 37 °C than at 22 °C. Diagnostic discrimination between the normal and the MHS halothane contractures is greater at 22 °C than at 37 °C.

The temperature of transporting the muscle from the operating theatre to the laboratory is of some importance. Muscle transported at 4 °C remains suboptimally reactive for some hours. On the other hand, muscle transported at 37 °C is immediately optimally reactive but fatigues more rapidly than does muscle transported at 22 °C. MHS (but not normal) muscle transported at 22 °C but measured at 37 °C may develop a spontaneous contracture when first lowered into the 37 °C Krebs Ringer bath (Moulds and Denborough 1974a). This initial spontaneous contracture does not occur in muscle transported at 37 °C (Britt et al. 1979a, 1980b).

Increasing the concentration of calcium in the bathing solution increases the contractures of both the MHS and the normal skeletal muscle fascicles with a greater effect evident on the MHS muscle (Moulds et al. 1974). In MHS but not in normal muscle raising the concentration of potassium in the bathing solution (to 80 mM CKl) induces (without other additives) a large contracture but eliminates twitch tension of MHS muscle but not of normal muscle (Moulds et al. 1974).

MHS but not normal muscle sometimes but not always responds to succinylcholine with a large and sustained contracture. Anderson and Jones (1978) and Moulds and Denborough (1974a) have found that the introduction of procaine or dantrolene to the bath relieves caffeine- or halothane-induced contractures.

Britt et al. (1980b) have compared the effects of halothane, enflurane, isoflurane, and methoxyflurane on MHS and normal muscle fascicles. Halothane shows the greatest ability to potentiate caffeine contractures, with enflurane following and methoxyflurane showing the least ability. The greatest diagnostic discrimination between the MHS and the normal muscles is provided by halothane.

Ryanodine, an alkaloid extracted from Ryania Speciosa, has been suggested as an alternate to caffeine as a test drug for the diagnosis of MH (Casson and Downes 1978). As ryanodine is freer than caffeine of actions on structures other than the SR and since its effect on the SR is more potent than that of caffeine, ryanodine should be preferred as a test drug to caffeine. Unfortunately, secure commercial supplies of ryanodine are not available in Canada at the present time.

To conclude, over 10 years of experience has shown the caffeine contracture test to be a sensitive and accurate means of diagnosing MH since:
1. It provides several parameters in which MHS muscle differs from normal muscle
2. These changes are not seen in other myopathies
3. There is little overlapping between the MHS and the normal muscle
4. It reveals the non-rigid as well as the rigid muscle to be different from the normal muscle (Britt 1973a, 1979b, 1980a).

7. Skinned Fibre Test

Recently an exciting new tool has become available to MH researchers. By the method of Wood, a muscle fascicle secured to an applicator stick is placed in a solution of 5.0 mM ethylene diamine tetra acid (EDTA), 2.5 mM adenosine triphosphate (ATP) and 170 mM potassium propionate. After 24 h the muscle fascicle is transferred to a second solution identical to the first except for the addition of 50% glycerol. Over a period of several days this solution chemically skins off the outer sarcolemma, transverse tubules and mitochondria leaving only the SR and myofibrillar system. When skinning is complete, a single cell is dissected from the fascicle and mounted between a clamp and a force transducer. The skinned fibre is viewed through an inverted microscope.

The fibre, suspended between its two clamps, lies in a bathing chamber. Two studies are performed. In the first the chamber is initially filled with a solution which induces movement of free calcium into the SR and then with a solution which contains caffeine but no ionized calcium. If, in the presence of caffeine and the absence of free calcium, an increase in tension of the skinned fibre occurs, the tension increase must be due to release of calcium from the SR since no cytoplasmic calcium is present. This procedure is repeated several times using progressively larger concentrations of caffeine on each addition so that a dose-response curve is obtained. In the second study the chamber is initially filled with a solution which induces movement of free calcium out of the SR (thus depleting the SR of their calcium) and then with a solution which contains no caffeine but which does contain ionized calcium. This procedure is also repeated several times using progressively larger concentrations of calcium so that a dose-response curve is obtained. If, in the absence of caffeine and the presence of free calcium, an increase in tension of the skinned fibre occurs, the increase must be due to the direct action of the free calcium in the bathing solution on the myofibrils, since no calcium is available in the SR for release.

The author has, in fact, found that the mean tension rise induced by caffeine is greater in rigid MHS than in normal fibres. Additionally, the mean threshold for caffeine induced tension rise is lower in MHS than in normal fibres. This rigid MHS SR, when challenged with caffeine must be less able than are normal SR to retain their calcium. On the other hand, the mean tension rise induced by exogenous calcium in the rigid MHS fibres does not differ significantly from the mean tension rise induced by exogenous calcium in normal fibres. Moreover, the mean threshold for calcium induced tension rise of MHS fibres is similar to that observed for normal fibres. Thus rigid MHS myofibrils must be normally sensitive to calcium. In other words the defect of rigid MH cannot be accounted for by an abnormal response of some part of the myofibrillar apparatus to calcium.

The tension increases produced by caffeine in these skinned single fibres correlate reasonably well with the contractures induced by caffeine plus halothane in whole muscle fascicles. Several (at least eight) fibres must be measured, since not all exhibit super-contracture in the presence of caffeine. The percentage of hyperreactive fibres from a given muscle fascicle appears to give yet another measure of the severity of the MH defect and also provides further evidence that more than one different and non-allelic gene contributes to the defect. Whether the fibres that exhibit excessive tension on the skinned fibre test are the same fibres which appear hypertrophied on microscopic sections has not yet been determined.

This test is important aetiologically because it demonstrates that the calcium inducing the contracture must be coming from the SR, since no sarcolemma or transverse tubules are present, since in the rigid fibres the myofibrils respond normally to exogenous calcium and since in the rigid fibres the SR release excessive quantities of calcium in the presence of caffeine. It is also important diagnostically since it has several advantages over the whole muscle caffeine contracture test. For instance, a much smaller volume of muscle is required. The muscle fascicle can be stored in the freezer for long periods of time. The test can be repeated on one sample many times (for each experiment a single cell is dissected free from the main fascicle; the latter is then returned to cold storage). The disadvantages of this test compared with the caffeine contracture test are that considerably more skill is required, more expensive equipment is necessary, the test as performed by Wood's technique cannot be begun until several days after excision of the muscle from the patient and, finally, the test is time consuming since many fibres must be measured as not all are abnormal and each fibre must be measured sequentially by direct visualization through a microscope throughout the entire test is necessary.

TAKAGI (1977) and ENDO and BLINKS (1973) have reported that the threshold for halothane contracture of single mechanically skinned fibres prepared from MHS humans is less than normal. Mechanically skinned MHS fibres have also been prepared by HAHN and GODT (1977). This technique will probably not play a major role in the diagnosis of MH since the technical skill required to skin fibres mechanically is much greater than to skin fibres chemically and since very fresh specimens are essential to maintain viability of the muscle cells during mechanical skinning.

8. Halothane-Induced Contracture of Thin Muscle Sections

This technique developed by MABUCHI and SRETER (1977) and RYAN (1977) has been adapted by RYAN (1979) for use in the diagnosis of MH. Thirty-μm thick sections of skeletal muscle are placed on a cover slip after washing in a sucrose medium. Halothane (0.1 ml) is placed in a well 1.0 cm below the cover slip. Contractures of the muscle induced by halothane are observed through a binocular light microscope. The time to initial contracture is graded. The speed of onset of contracture and the percentage of fibres contracting at 15 min are significantly greater for MHS than for normal fibres.

This test has so far had limited use. Numbers of probands compared with normal controls have been small. Correlations of this test with the caffeine contracture test have not been reported so far. Nevertheless, if these unknowns can be answered satisfactorily this test has considerable potential since it requires very small amounts of muscle and equipment readily available in every hospital.

9. ATP Depletion Test

Malignant hyperthermic susceptible skeletal muscle contains slightly less than the normal amount of ATP and when exposed in vitro to halothane loses its ATP at a faster rate than normal muscle (HARRISON et al. 1969; GRONERT 1979). Thus, for muscle equilibrated at 37 °C in Krebs Ringer solution at pH 7.4 bubbled with carbogen for 30 min, the ratio of ATP in muscle equilibrated with 4.0 vol-% halothane to ATP in muscle equilibrated without halothane is significantly less for rigid

MHS than for normal skeletal muscle. In non-rigid MHS muscle the ATP depletion ratio is also significantly reduced. The decrease, however, is not as great as that observed in rigid MHS muscle. ATP ratios tend to decline with advancing age and this factor must be considered when interpreting results (BRITT et al. 1976b). This test, while therefore useful, is not quite as valuable as is the caffeine contracture test.

II. Microscopy

Many, but not all, patients exhibit minor, non-specific and inconsistent microscopic abnormalities of their skeletal muscle (HARRIMAN and ELLIS 1978, ISAACS et al. 1973; GULLOTTA and HELPAP 1975; BRITT et al. 1976b; RESKE-NIELSEN 1978). The most common finding is a greater than normal variation in fibre diameter. Both small angular fibres and large fibres may be seen on structural stains such as haematoxylin and eosin and on enzyme stains such as for ATPase. The small, sharply angulated fibres may be faintly basophilic. HARRIMAN (1979) feels that these are derived from splitting of large fibres. The angulated fibres are both type I and type II. The type I to type II fibre ratio may be normal, decreased or increased (BRITT et al. 1973). Rarely, frankly atrophic (RESKE-NIELSEN 1978) and even necrotic fibres are seen that may or may not be accompanied by regenerating fibres or lymphocytic infiltration. Necrosis of fibres increased markedly during acute reactions (FABER et al. 1975).

The atrophic fibres contain dark staining pyknotic nuclei. The large rounded fibres, on the other hand, contain excessive numbers of centrally situated nuclei unlike normal nuclei that have all, except about 1%, the nuclei lying in close proximity to the sarcolemma. The central nuclei are fairly diffusely distributed throughout the fibres.

On NADase stains evidence of localized foci containing reduced numbers of and/or disorganized mitochondria may be seen in both type I and type II fibres excised from a few (4.0%) of the more severely afflicted individuals. These may occur as either ill-defined multiple foci termed "moth-eaten" or as only one or two larger and more sharply circumscribed foci of mitochondrial loss called "targetoid fibres". KING and DENBOROUGH (1973) and ISAACS and BARLOW (1974) have described much more extensive areas of mitochondrial loss and disorganization which have been defined as "central cores". Electron microscopy demonstrate increased numbers of degenerating giant mitochondria of variable shape with crystalline inclusions. The mitochondria may be swollen and contain only remnants of cristae.

Cytoplasmic bodies have been reported (HARRIMAN 1979; RESKE-NIELSEN et al. 1975) consisting of a central homogenous mass that is deeply eosinophilic with a lighter peripheral halo on haematoxylin and eosin stains. On electron microscopy the central mass is osmiophilic and homogeneous. Filaments radiate from it into the halo.

Rarely tubular aggregates occur. On haematoxylin and eosin these consist of basophilic granules. These granules are observed on NADase stains to occur in type II fibres, and ultrastructurally they are seen to correspond to foci of transverse tubule proliferation. Frank tubular aggregates have been observed by GULLOTTA et al. (1976), by HARRIMAN and ELLIS (1978) and by RESKE-NIELSEN (1978).

On electron microscopy there may be areas of expansion of the cisterns of the SR and proliferation of the sarcolemma (GULLOTTA and HELPAP 1975). Myofibrillar disarray with streaming of the Z-lines may be observed (RESKE-NIELSEN 1973, 1978; RESKE-NIELSEN et al. 1975). Ring fibres have been detected in 5% of the author's MHS patients.

LaCOUR et al. (1971) and RESKE-NIELSEN et al. (1978) have reported that in some of their MHS patients silver stains reveal bead-like degeneration of intramuscular neurones with regeneration and sprouting of many new and abnormal endings in other parts of the same sample. HARRIMAN and ELLIS (1978) have observed that the motor nerves are normal except that in the more severely myopathic muscle the motor end plates are often unusually large or extended and may show distal and ultra-terminal sprouting. In electron micrographs, non-specific changes occur in terminal expansions including dense "mulberry" bodies and numerous cisternae. HARRIMAN and ELLIS note though that they have not observed patients who have shown classical evidence of denervation in the form of collateral reinnervation of muscles.

III. Heart Muscle Studies

Heart muscle abnormalities characteristic of a cardiomyopathy are present in a considerable number of MHS patients (HUCKELL et al. 1978a, b; Teiglin et al. 1981).

1. Clinical Features

Healthy muscular MHS individuals not infrequently complain of palpitations, transient episodes of tachycardia and pain localized to the left anterior chest. On physical examination there may be precordial systolic murmurs and mid-systolic clicks. MHS patients exhibiting such findings may have episodes of cardiac standstill or ventricular fibrillation (HUCKELL et al. 1978a, b), usually precipitated by physical exercise, emotional excitement or sudden changes in environmental temperature. Young and previously healthy relatives of known MHS patients have occasionally died unexpectedly during mild exercise. Post mortem examinations have not been helpful in identifying the cause. One must consider the possibility that some of these deaths may also have been due to cardiac standstill or ventricular fibrillation of cardiomyopathic hearts.

2. Electrocardiograms

More than one third of MHS patients have abnormal electrocardiograms. The most commonly observed findings are ventricular and/or atrial hypertrophy and myocardial ischaemia (HUCKELL et al. 1977).

3. Echocardiograms

About 40% of MHS individuals exhibit abnormal echocardiograms. Most commonly found is mitral valve prolapse. Thickening of the ventricular and atrial walls and asynchronous septal motion have also been recorded (BRITT, unpublished work).

4. Myocardial Scanning with Thallium-201 (Rest and Exercise)

Individuals with dead areas of muscle due to myopathy exhibit cold spots (areas of reduced thallium uptake) on both rest and exercise. Those with ischaemic (but not dead) areas of muscle display cold spots on exercise but not on resting scans.

HUCKELL et al. (1978 a, b) and Feiglin et al. (1981) have performed rest and exercise scans on known MHS patients. The procedure is that after completion of a graded exercise 12 lead ECG on a treadmill, 1.5 mCi of thallium-201 is injected intravenously. The patient is exercised for a further 2 min and then rested for 15 min. Photographs of the heart muscle are then made with a gamma ray camera. Imaging is discontinued when 300 000–400 000 counts have been collected. The patient is rested for 2 h and imaging with the gamma ray camera is repeated. The first set of photographs constitute the exercise portion of the study. Patients exhibiting equivocal results have the rest portion repeated 2 weeks later.

The data indicate that this technique provides a method of diagnosing hitherto unsuspected cardiomyopathies in some MHS patients. Eighteen of thirty MHS patients have been shown to have myocardial perfusion defects. Since the amount of radiation received by each patient is small (about half that sustained during an intravenous pyelogram), the risk benefit ratio for this procedure is low.

Diagnosis of cardiomyopathies in MHS patients is important since paroxysmal arrhythmias have occasionally led to their deaths. These arrhythmias can be treated by prophylactic or therapeutic therapy with one or more of verapamil (NAYLOR and SZETO 1972), procaine amide (JOHNSON and INESI 1969; HARRISON 1973a), diltiazem (SAIKAWA et al. 1977) or propranolol (BRITT, unpublished work) as indicated for the individual patient.

5. Cardiac Catheterization and Angiography

Eight of the other MHS patients have had cardiac catheterization studies performed. These have revealed increased left ventricular end diastolic pressures, dilatation of the left ventricle, abnormal contraction patterns (delayed contraction of some areas) and decreased ejection fractions [1]. All eight patients had normal coronary arteries (HUCKELL et al. 1978a, b).

6. Heart Muscle Biopsy

Light and electron microscopic examination of heart muscle obtained from nine MHS patients has revealed minor non-specific abnormalities (MAMBO 1981).

IV. Extramuscular Nerves

BRITT et al. (1977a) have shown that motor neurone counts are statistically less in the motor nerves supplying one or more of four skeletal muscles (extensor digitorum brevis, soleus, thenar and hypothenar) of MHS patients than of normal individuals. This test forms a very useful complement to the caffeine contracture test,

---

1   Ejection Fraction $= SV/EDV = ESV + SV$, where $SV =$ stroke volume, $EDV =$ end diastolic volume and $ESV =$ end systolic volume

but because of some overlapping between the normal and the MHS subjects, it would be unwise to rely upon it as a sole diagnostic criterion.

ROBERTS et al. (to be published) measured in normal and MHS patients twitch height of muscle contractions (thumb adduction) induced by intermittent electrical stimulation of the ulnar nerve before and after 5 min of tourniquet compression of the upper humerus. They have found that in normal individuals a post-ischaemic depression of twitch height occurred, while in MHS patients a transient rise in twitch height occurs 2 min after release of the cuff. This test is simple, rapid and non-invasive and so is worthy to future investigation.

V. Platelets

The contractile mechanism of platelets is very similar to that of muscle (JOHNSON et al. 1966). Thus it is not surprising that abnormalities have been observed in MHS platelets. SOLOMONS et al. (1978) have detected by means of thin layer chromatography that halothane reduces the ATP + ADP/AMP ratio of MHS platelets. ZSIGMOND et al. (1978) have stated that platelets removed from some but not all MHS relatives exhibit abnormal aggregation in the presence of epinephrine and collagen. This has been confirmed by ISAACS (1981). GLYNN (unpublished work) has noted that pretreatment with caffeine inhibits collagen-induced aggregation of most MHS fresh platelet samples. This effect usually is not seen in normal platelet samples. OKU (unpublished work) has discovered that the dose of ADP required to initiate change of shape of platelets from discoid to irregularly round is greater in MHS than normal platelets. Thus a primary rather than a secondary platelet defect may be responsible for the acute consumption coagulopathy that is a feature of some fulminant MH reactions.

VI. Red Blood Cells

Similarly, the haemolysis of red blood cells which occurs during MH crises and during sampling of MHS blood may be triggered by a primary abnormality in these cells. The data about this is, however, conflicting. HARRISON and VERBURG (1973) several years ago reported that red blood cells isolated from MHS Landrace swine exhibited greater than normal fragility. ZSIGMOND et al. (1978), however, have described normal fragility in red blood cells isolated from MHS humans. KELSTRUP et al. (1973) have claimed that relatives of MHS patients exhibit a less than normal oubain-sensitive ATPase activity of their red blood cells. Their data, however, do not indicate whether these individuals are themselves susceptible, since no skeletal muscle biopsies were performed on their patients. The author has found Na^+K^+ ATPase activity of human and porcine red blood cells to be normal. SCHANUS et al. (1981) have observed that MHS Pietrain pigs have a severe deficiency of red blood cell glutathione peroxidase. Such a deficiency would be expected to lead to increased susceptibility of the red blood cells to stress.

VII. Endocrines

DENBOROUGH et al. (1974) have described increased glucose-induced insulin responses in MHS individuals. Release of insulin from the B cells of the Islets of Langerhans is a calcium-mediated phenomenon.

The incidence of mild hypothyroid function (low serum thyroxin and high serum thyroid stimulating hormone) is moderately greater in MHS patients than in individuals chosen at random from the general population. EIGHMY et al. (1978) have described normal mean serum T_3 and T_4 values for MHS human patients.

VIII. Bone and Appendages

The calcium content of MHS bones and teeth may be moderately lower than normal. This is expressed clinically as poor dental enamel with many cavities and a greater than expected incidence of fractures. The low bone calcium may be measured quantitatively by means of neutron activation analysis (HARRISON et al. 1979).

IX. Miscellaneous

Failure of descent of the testicle (LENARD and KETTLER 1975; PINSKY and LEVY 1973), spontaneous retinal detachment (SNOW 1970a) and hypertelorism (BRITT, unpublished work) have been noted in a few patients. Many MHS individuals have hyperactive personalities (WINGARD 1977). Some but not all MHS patients exhibit moderately low plasma cholinesterase fluoride numbers (ELLIS et al. 1978a).

G. Management of Inadvertent Fulminant Malignant Hyperthermia Reactions

In spite of intensive diagnostic efforts within MHS families, and in spite of careful pre-anaesthetic evaluation of all patients for a family history of MH and for skeletal and other connective tissue abnormalities, unexpected acute and severe MH reactions will continue to occur until such time as a rapid, cheap, reliable and non-invasive test has been developed for the diagnosis of MH in all patients in the general population presenting for anaesthesia.

I. Stop Triggering Agents

The single most important factors in the successful management of such cases are early diagnosis and cessation of triggering drugs (WILSON 1978; WADE 1973; SNOW 1970a, b). Therapy must be carried out with the same urgency as therapy of a cardiac arrest. Thus no human MHS patients suffering crises in which the triggering agents have been withdrawn within 10 min of induction have died (Table 12). On the other hand, over 56% of MH reactions in which the offending drugs have been administered for over 1 h have had fatal terminations (BRITT et al. 1977b; BRITT 1980). Any case in which the diagnosis is uncertain should be treated as MH until proven otherwise beyond all doubt. It is essential not only to turn off the inhalational agent vaporizor but also to renew the soda lime and to change the rubber parts of the gas machine to new rubber tubing, reservoir bags and ventilator bellows. These changes are vital because of the high lipid solubility of potent inhalational anaesthetics. The rubber:gas solubility coefficient of halothane is 121

Table 12. Relationship between duration of anaesthesia and mortality from MH reactions

Duration of anaesthesia in minutes	Number of patients		% of patients surviving
	Died	Survived	
1–9	0	41	100
10–29	13	59	81.94
30–59	32	43	57.33
60–89	36	31	46.27
90–119	31 ⎫	29 ⎫	
120–149	28 ⎬ 94	12 ⎬ 71	43.03
150–179	14	11	
>180	21 ⎭	19 ⎭	

while that of methoxyflurane is 724. This means that 3.5% of all halothane and 25% of all methoxyflurane leaving the vaporizor goes not into the patients lungs, but rather into the rubber tubing. When the vaporizor is turned off the anaesthetic slowly re-emerges from the rubber and re-enters the inspired gas over a period of several hours.

II. Lower Body Temperature

Reduction of the temperature is vital, since mortality is proportional to the maximum temperature attained. In order to achieve significant temperature reduction in fulminant cases, drastic and rapid cooling must be not only by external methods such as ice water baths (GRUHL 1971), but also by internal techniques, for example, gastric, rectal and wound cooling and peritoneal dialysis. Although cooling should be prompt and vigorous, it must not be continued too long; otherwise the malignant hyperthermia may be succeeded by an equally malignant hypothermia, during which the patient appears to lose all control over central temperature regulation so that the temperature passively follows the environmental temperature. It is, therefore, advisable to discontinue cooling when the temperature has fallen to about 37.5° or 38 °C. Secondary temperature rises may again recur over the next several hours or even days, but these tend to be milder and more easily managed by further applications of external cooling without internal cooling. Complicated techniques such as extracorporeal cooling are recommended only when a highly qualified cardiovascular team is immediately available. Extracorporeal cooling should never be attempted to the exclusion of simpler and more rapidly applicable cooling methods.

Cooling can be accelerated through the use of tranquillizers such as chlorpromazine. Chlorpromazine inhibits both shivering and non-shivering thermogenesis by depressing electron transport at the first phosphorylation site. Chlorpromazine also accelerates heat loss by dilating the previously constricted superficial blood vessels. Finally, chlorpromazine has an anti-adrenergic action. Mortality is significantly lowered in MHS patients who have received chlorpromazine during their reactions (BRITT et al. 1977c; BRITT 1980).

The not infrequent lack of success of cooling is probably due to one or more of:

a) Cooling without chlorpromazine with, therefore, stimulation of catecholamine release

b) Insufficient cooling with, therefore, continued rise in temperature and consequent continued hyperactivity of enzyme reactions

III. Correct Blood Gases

1. Oxygen and Carbon Dioxide Tensions

To bring the arterial oxygen and carbon dioxide tensions into the normal ranges, the inspired oxygen concentration should be enriched but not raised to 100%, and artificial ventilation should be increased so that the minute volume approximates three times the Radford nomogram, that is, about 15–20 cc oxygen/kg body wt, 15–20 times per minute – or about 20 litres/min in a 70-kg man.

2. Base Deficit

The metabolic acidosis is best treated with sodium bicarbonate, the dose being sufficient, as determined by the base deficit to return the pH half way to normal. Complete correction of the base deficit seems to worsen survival statistically. This may be because the higher pH reduces the ionization of some treatment drugs such as procaine that depend on being in the ionized state for their effect. It might be thought that THAM would be the buffer of choice since THAM, unlike $NaHCO_3$, is distributed within the muscle cell and since THAM does not overload the circulation with sodium. Clinical experience, however, does not bear out this theory. Survival is slightly worse after THAM than after $NaHCO_3$ (BRITT 1980), so on an empirical basis, $NaHCO_3$ is the buffer of choice.

IV. Lower Myoplasmic Calcium

1. Dantrolene

Dantrolene sodium (Dantrium, Norwich Eaton Pharmaceuticals) is a diphenylhydantoin analogue (Fig. 10). An oral preparation has been used for some years to relieve muscle spasms (GELENBERG and POSKANZER 1973; CHYATTE et al. 1973). More recently, an intravenous preparation has become available and is presently

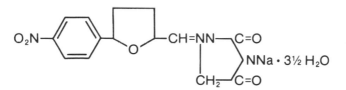

Fig. 10. Dantrolene Na (Dantrium) is a benzathiazepine derivative which, by inhibiting release of calcium from the sarcoplasmic reticulum, decreases contraction and heat production in skeletal muscle during MH reactions

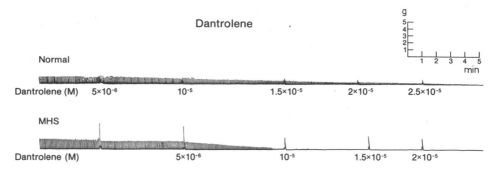

Fig. 11. Dantrolene inhibits electrically induced twitch tensions of both normal and MHS skeletal muscle fascicles

the drug of choice in the treatment of acute MH reactions. Its efficacy in the therapy of MH was first discovered by HARRISON (1975). He has reported that dantrolene relieves halothane-induced reactions of MHS swine. In other publications HARRISON (1977) and also KERR et al. (1978) have observed that pretreatment with dantrolene preventes the induction of an MH reaction in MHS pigs. NELSON and FLEWELLEN (1979) have shown that in vivo dantrolene attenuates halothane-induced contractures and potentiations of indirect twitches of MHS pigs. The efficacy of dantrolene sodium in humans has been confirmed by a number of case reports (BRITT, personal observations).

Extensive in vitro studies on the site and mode of action of dantrolene have been performed. Dantrolene has no significant action on smooth or heart muscle. Rather its effects are on skeletal muscle. ELLIS et al. (1973) have demonstrated by performing crossover circulation experiments on vascularly isolated, but neurally intact, hind limbs of dogs that the site of action of dantrolene is peripheral and not central. Dantrolene attenuates contractions in skeletal muscle that are being stimulated either directly or indirectly via its nerve. The action of D-tubocurarine (a non-depolarizing neuromuscular blocker) or of edrophonium (an anticholinesterase agent) on twitch tension is not altered by dantrolene. These various actions indicate, therefore, that dantrolene must act at some point distal to the motor nerves.

Microelectrode studies show that a dose of dantrolene that reduces the twitch response of skeletal muscle has no effect on either resting or on action potentials of the muscle membrane. EMGs are not altered by dantrolene. Dantrolene also does not alter total membrane capacitance or membrane resistance (ELLIS and BRYANT 1972). Since, therefore, dantrolene does not affect electrical excitability of the muscle membrane and does not disrupt the transverse tubules, it cannot act by decreasing electrical conduction between the postsynaptic junctions and the SR.

Dantrolene has no influence on the resting influx of Ca^{++45} from the extracellular fluid to the myoplasm (DESMEDT and HAINAUT 1977). Dantrolene does inhibit Ca^{++45} influx into skeletal muscle myoplasm from the SR which is induced by either electrical stimulation or by chloride. Dantrolene inhibits potassium-induced contractures. Dantrolene antagonizes caffeine-induced twitch tensions and also electrically induced twitch tensions (Fig. 11) in normal and MHS skeletal muscle.

EDTA increases and calcium reduces sensitivity of skeletal muscle contraction to dantrolene (ELLIS and BRYANT 1972). The above effects are unaltered by curare. These several results suggest that dantrolene in some way prevents release of calcium from the SR to the myoplasm, either by a direct action or by inhibition of release of trigger calcium from the sarcolemma – probably at the level of the transverse tubules (MOULDS 1977). The former postulation has been confirmed by studies utilizing the photoprotein aequorin (DESMEDT and HAINAUT 1977).

Evidence for the ability of dantrolene to accelerate calcium uptake into the SR is less clear cut. Some workers have found that dantrolene has no effect on caffeine-induced contractures (ELLIS and BRYANT 1972) while others, on the contrary, have found that dantrolene does inhibit caffeine-induced contractures. ANDERSON and JONES (1976a, 1978) have reported that in MHS porcine muscle dantrolene inhibits halothane-induced contractures.

The beneficial effect of dantrolene during MH reactions thus appears to be due to both inhibition of release of calcium from the SR and to increase in uptake of calcium into the SR. Because the former effect may well be the more important, it is essential to commence dantrolene therapy early. If dantrolene is given late, after the SR have been depleted of all their calcium, it may be ineffective.

Prior to the approval of intravenous dantrolene sodium by the Health Protection Branch of the Canadian Government, and the Food and Drug Administration of the U.S.A., several different home-made formulations of dantrolene were devised. For example, dantrolene was first prepared for intravenous use in the treatment of porcine MH by HARRISON (1975). His formulation consisted of dantrolene sodium 300 mg, mannitol 26.64 g, sodium hydroxide 48 mg and water ad 600 ml. The disadvantage of this formulation was that several hours of stirring was required to achieve solubilization of the dantrolene.

In order to achieve a preparation which would dissolve rapidly and also in order to remove the starch, talc, magnesium stearate and lactose that are present as binding agents in dantrolene capsules, GRONERT et al. (1978a) recommended placing thirty-two 100-mg capsules in 4 litres of sterile water and stirring for 30 min. He then filtered the resulting liquid through a 201 grade filter paper. The clear orange filtrate was sterilized by passing through a 0.45 mM Millipore filter. Eighty millilitres of 10% citric acid was added to the sterile filtrate to lower its pH to 3.0 and thereby induced precipitation of dantrolene crystals. The crystals were collected by vacuum filtration and dried overnight in a laminar flow hood. The crystals were weighed aseptically into 500-mg lots and placed in sterile 100-ml vials. When desired the crystals were reconstituted with 100 ml of a sterile aqueous solution containing 88 mg NaOH. The suspension was immediately added to a sterile 900 ml solution containing 44.5 g mannitol to make the solution isotonic. The dantrolene dissolved within 2–3 min.

A more simple technique was to place five 100-mg capsules of dantrolene in a bottle of warm 15% or 20% mannitol and shake. The resulting solution was run through a Millipore blood filter placed in the intravenous line. Since no sodium hydroxide was used in this formulation, the common ion effect of Gronert's and Harrison's formulations were avoided, and so the amount of dissolved dantrolene was greater (about 0.5 mg-%) (ELLIS, personal communication).

A rather different formulation is that of FUKUCHI et al. (1979), who prepared dantrolene by sealing 1 400 mg crystalline dantrolene in an ampule. This was then heat sterilized at 105 °C for 60 min, and 350 ml aqueous solution of 1.0 *M* nicotinamide was placed in a separate vial and subjected to autoclave sterilization. When needed these two vials were mixed to give 0.4 W/V% dantrolene at pH 9.0–9.3.

Fortunately, these tedious "moonshine" efforts are now past history. Intravenous dantrolene has finally been approved for use in North American hospitals. The commercial preparation is manufactured in a lyophilized formulation in combination with sodium hydroxide and mannitol. Thus a vial which is to be reconstituted with 50 ml water contains 20 mg dantrolene, 3,0 g mannitol and enough sodium hydroxide to raise the pH to 9.5. The reconstituted drug should be administered at the rate of 1.0 mg (2.5 cc)/kg per minute until the temperature begins to fall and/or muscle stiffness starts to subside. A maximum of 10 mg/kg may be given over a 15-min period. This dosage may be repeated in 4 h if the reaction recurs. The initial loading dose of dantrolene may be followed by a maintenance infusion in an IV bag of 250 cc 5% glucose of 1.0 mg/kg over a 1- to 4-h period until all evidence of an active MH crisis has disappeared. As soon as possible i.v. dantrolene should be replaced with oral dantrolene. If therapy continues over a several-day period, liver function studies should be performed since reductions in liver function have been reported after prolonged administration of high doses of dantrolene to debilitated patients (EBERLEIN 1979).

2. Procaine HCl and Procaine Amide

Procaine, chlorprocaine and procaine amide substantially reduce mortality from human MH reactions. Their use in porcine MH reactions is less clear cut and may even be ineffective. These agents, when ionized, i.e. under physiological conditions, reverse the myocardial hypercatabolism by increasing the movement of calcium into the SR. Release of calcium from the SR is prevented. Procaine amide may also exert its beneficial effect because of its ability to inhibit secretion of catecholamines from the adrenal medulla and from sympathetic nerve endings.

We no longer recommend procaine HCl or procaine amide as the sole means of relieving skeletal muscle stiffness. This is because the doses required to achieve effective concentrations in the region of the skeletal muscle SR are so large as to depress, perhaps fatally, the myocardium. Rather these agents, in small quantities, have their present use in the treatment of the rigor and the hypercatabolism of the heart muscle.

Not more than 1.0 mg/kg per minute should be infused, under continuous EKG control, until some improvement in the arrhythmia occurs or until a maximum of 7.0 mg/kg has been administered. Since the arrhythmia is caused, at least initially, by a MH defect of the heart muscle similar to that of the skeletal muscle, relief of the arrhythmia signals that the drug has penetrated to the region of the myocardial SR.

When using procaine HCl a pure preparation should be used since GRIST et al. (1973) have discovered that chlorocresol present in some commercial formulations precipitates a calcium-induced loss of respiratory mitochondria. It may be that the procaine-induced muscle contractures observed by CLARKE and ELLIS (1975) were due to such impurities in their procaine preparation rather than to the procaine itself.

3. Verapamil

Verapamil (Isoptin), a papaverine analogue, is a new drug which has just become available in oral and intravenous formulations for general use in Canada. It inhibits influx of calcium into the myocardial sarcoplasm by blocking the calcium-conducting channels of the sarcolemma. In vitro, in MHS and normal skeletal muscle verapamil partially but not completely inhibits caffeine-induced contractures but increases moderately electrically induced twitch tensions. It may, therefore, actually increase release of calcium from the SR.

Verapamil has been used successfully in Germany in the management of at least one human MH reaction by CSONGRADY (1976). In Canada, in one human MHS patient afflicted with stress-induced ventricular tachycardia, verapamil provided complete relief (WAXMAN, personal communication). Apart from these isolated examples, however, verapamil has not undergone in vivo testing in human MHS patients. Its apparent ability to increase twitch tensions in skeletal muscle fascicles may render it not as satisfactory as dantrolene in the therapy of MH crises.

4. Diltiazem

Diltiazem, a benzothiazepine derivative, has a profound effect in relaxing vascular smooth muscle. In isolated MHS and normal skeletal muscle doses of diltiazem in the range of 1×10^{-7} M to 1×10^{-3} M inhibit both caffeine-induced contractures and also electrically induced twitch tensions. The role of this drug in the in vivo management of MH reactions remains to be determined.

V. Correct Abnormal Serum Potassium Levels

Early hyperkalaemia has usually been treated with insulin. Fifty units of regular insulin in 50 cc 50% glucose is the recommended dose for a 70-kg man (TOBIAS and MILLER 1970). Serum potassium should be measured frequently since once the serum potassium starts to decline, it falls very rapidly through the normal range to sometimes excessively low levels. Insulin therapy must then be discontinued and replaced with infusions of potassium chloride. Since the hypokalaemia represents a profound total body depletion of potassium, it may be necessary to maintain the potassium chloride infusions for several days. Insulin and potassium therapy of potassium disturbances during MH reactions have not infrequently been unsuccessful because of too late and too little application.

VI. Control Arrhythmias

Sinus tachycardia and other rapid arrhythmias should be treated with one or more of: propranolol, verapamil or procaine amide. The heart rate should be kept below

100/min in adults and 120/min in small children. Failure to do so leads to early on-set of myocardial exhaustion with associated clinical signs of heart failure, particularly acute pulmonary oedema.

VII. Stabilize Membranes

Attempts have been made to treat MH reactions with large (pharmacological) doses of hydrocortisone (2–4 g in an adult patient) (RAITT and MERRIFIELD 1974). The recommendation for steroid therapy has been based on the observation of EL-LIS that in one patient whose MH reaction was claimed to have been induced by nitrous oxide, hydrocortisone in vitro depressed halothane-induced contractures of the skeletal muscle fascicles. In another publication CAIN and ELLIS (1977) achieved similar results using methylprednisolone on fascicles excised from 12 MHS patients. Retrospective statistical data is, however, less sanguine. The data shows that survival is significantly lower for patients who have received steroids during their MH reactions than for patients who have not. This data may, however, be biased in that only those suffering especially fulminant reactions tend to receive steroids. Steroids may exert a beneficial effect by stabilizing cell membranes and thereby by preventing oedema of brain and muscle cells. Steroids, not only glucocorticoids but also drugs such as pancuronium and Althesin, may also be of benefit during MH reactions because of their ability to improve the binding of calcium by cell membranes.

VIII. Administer Drugs Which Exert Osmotic Force

Infusion of mannitol by pulling fluid from brain cells and interstitial spaces helps to reverse cerebral oedema. Furosemide prevents tubular reabsorption of sodium and so correct the hypernatraemia induced by large doses of sodium bicarbonate. Furosemide also slows influx of sodium and water into the muscle, thus inhibiting oedema of the muscle cells. Both mannitol and furosemide, through their diuretic action, dislodge myoglobin from the renal tubules, thereby preventing acute renal failure. The dose of mannitol should be about 100 cc 20% mannitol/kg body wt., while that of furosemide should be about 1.0 mg/kg body wt.

Once persistent anuria and a rising BUN develop, however, diuretics are harmful. Haemodialysis then becomes the treatment of choice and has been successful in a number of instances.

Use of diuretics with or without dialysis during and after MH reactions has not been followed by improved survival. This is, however, probably due to the fact that these therapies have tended to have been used mainly in only very fulminant MH reactions and only after renal failure has already developed.

IX. Use Drugs of Supportive Value in the Therapy of MH Reactions: Narcotics, Barbiturates and Antipyretics

Statistical studies have shown that narcotics, barbiturates and antipyretics slightly improve survival from already established MH reactions. Narcotics probably exert their effect by blocking conduction across cell membranes. Barbiturates may act by inhibiting mitochondrial electron transport or by antagonizing the stimulatory effect of calcium on cell membrane conduction. The mode of action of antipyretics may be by their inhibitory effect on prostaglandin synthesis by the platelets (SMITH and WILLIS 1971). When used as pretreatment, none of these agents are able to prevent MH reactions.

X. Treat Acute Consumption Coagulopathy

A large variety of drugs have been employed to treat the acute consumption coagulopathy that complicates fulminant MH reactions. These have included: heparin, coumarin, dicoumerol, warfarin, phenindione, protamine sulphate, aminocaproic acid, vitamin K, antihaemophilic factor, factor IX, thrombin, fresh frozen plasma and platelet concentrates. Neither the coagulant agents nor the anticoagulants appear to be statistically beneficial in the therapy of MH reactions.

XI. Avoid Drugs Contraindicated During MH Reactions

1. Lidocaine

Lidocaine has no role to play in the treatment of MH. This drug has the opposite action to procaine and procainamide on the SR. Thus it accelerates calcium loss from the SR and prevents re-uptake of calcium into the SR. Its use significantly increases mortality. The opposing effects of two such closely related drugs as procaine and lidocain, on the SR are probably a reflection of differences in receptor binding and affinity. The carbonyl oxygen and tertiary amine are separated by one carbon in the lidocaine molecule but by a two carbon chain in the procaine molecule. Hydrogen bonding occurs, therefore, in the former but not in the latter molecule. Steric interference occurs with lidocaine but not with procaine because of the presence of ortho methyl groups on the former but not on the latter molecule. Finally procaine is more ionized than lidocaine at physiological and low pHs than lidocaine because of the higher pKa of procaine (8.3 for procaine vs 7.8 for lidocaine).

2. Cardiac Glycosides

Cardiac glycosides accelerate calcium release from the SR and radically increase the death rate. Even though tachycardia and acute pulmonary oedema are present, cardiac glycosides are contraindicated, therefore, during a MH reaction.

3. Calcium Salts

Calcium salts such as calcium chloride and calcium gluconate, by raising the concentration of calcium in the extracellular fluid bathing the muscle cells, and ultimately in the myoplasm itself, aggravate MH reactions (CAMPION et al. 1971) and thereby raise mortality.

4. Sympathomimetics

Vasopressors that have a catecholamine like action must never be given during MH reactions. These drugs increase mortality to over 78%. They may exert this deleterious effect by excessively activating adenyl cyclase (BRITT et al. 1977c) and thereby indirectly increasing release of calcium from the SR. Catecholamine-stimulating drugs may also exert a similar effect by direct action on the SR (SHINEBOURNE et al. 1969).

5. Parasympatholytics

Parasympatholytic drugs such as atropine or scopolamine must be avoided as, statistically, they increase rigidity and mortality. Quinidine and its analogues have some parasympatholytic action and so are also contraindicated. Quinidine has caused fevers in some MHS patients who have received quinidine to treat arrhythmias associated with MH cardiomyopathies. The mode of action of parasympatholytic drugs on MHS muscle is uncertain but may be due to their permitting unopposed sympathetic action.

XII. Prevent Endogenous Catecholamine Release

Patients should be moved or stimulated as little as possible since any catecholamine release induced by pain or emotional tension tends to induce a recrudescence of the reaction with a return of a rising temperature and of ventricular arrhythmias. In a number of patients, for instance, ventricular fibrillation has occurred just as the patient has been transferred from the operating table to a transport trolley.

XIII. Monitoring

Monitoring during acute MH reactions should include: axillary and core temperatures; continuous electrocardiograms; heart rates; central venous pressures; urine colour, specific gravity and volume; blood urea nitrogen; blood glucose, lactate and pyruvate; serum electrolytes (sodium, potassium, chloride, calcium phosphorus and magnesium); serum enzymes (CK, HBDH, GOT, aldolase and alkaline phosphatase); serum creatinine and bilirubin; arterial and venous blood gases (oxygen tension, carbon dioxide tension, pH and base deficit); level of consciousness, pupillary size, equality and reaction, deep tendon and plantar reflexes, evidence of convulsions and skeletal muscle rigors; and skin colour, depth of colour and skin circulation.

H. Summary

Malignant hyperthermia (MH) is an autosomal dominant hereditary trait which was first described as such by Dr. Michael DENBOROUGH of Australia in 1962. It is characterized by hypercatabolic reactions induced by anaesthetic drugs or by physical or emotional stress. These reactions are characterized by:

 1. Tachycardia
 2. Arrhythmias
 3. Unstable blood pressure
 4. Skeletal muscle stiffness
 5. Hyperventilation
 6. Cyanosis
 7. Hypoxia
 8. Early elevations and late reductions in serum calcium and potassium
 9. Elevations of serum phosphorus, magnesium, blood glucose and lactate
10. Elevation after several hours, in the serum of muscle enzymes and myoglobin

Patients may die because of conversion of an ectopic ventricular arrhythmia into ventricular fibrillation, because of acute pulmonary oedema arising out of rigor of the left ventricle, because of acute disseminated intravascular coagulopathy secondary to platelet and red blood cell abnormalities, because of obstruction of the renal tubules by myoglobin or most frequently because of brain death induced by cerebral oedema.

Malignant hyperthermic reactions appear to be due to a sudden rise in the concentration of calcium in the muscle cytoplasm in the presence of triggering drugs or stresses. The source of this excess calcium is not well defined but may result from a calcium-related defect in the SR, the E-C coupling step, the transverse tubules, the sarcolemma, the adenyl cyclase part of the catecholamine receptor or even the mitochondria. The elevated myoplasmic calcium activates phosphorylase a and myosin ATPase, inhibits troponin, and uncouples oxidative phosphorylation from electron transport. There is, therefore, an acceleration of heat, water, carbon dioxide and lactic acid production and of oxygen consumption. ATP production falls while ATP hydrolysis rises. First creatine phosphate and then ATP levels in the muscle fall so that insufficient substrate remains for membrane ATPase. Potassium, magnesium and phosphorus, therefore, tend to flow out of muscle cells, while sodium and calcium, because their natural concentration gradients are in the opposite direction, leak into the muscle cells.

Prior to a reaction, a susceptible individual may exhibit a number of minor skeletal and cardiac muscle anomalies, for example excessive muscularity, joint hypermobility, skeletal muscle cramps, mitral valve prolapse, cardiomyopathy and conduction abnormalities. Platelet aggregation may be slightly impaired and red cell membranes may be slightly more vulnerable to haemolysis than normal. Diagnosis of the trait can be made by detection in isolated skeletal muscle (whole muscle fascicles, thin muscle sections, single chemically skinned fibres) of greater than normal contractures in the presence of caffeine and/or halothane, of a greater than normal depletion of muscle ATP in the presence of halothane, of less than normal uptake of radioactive calcium into SR or skeletal muscle sections, of greater than normal activation of phosphorylase a in the presence of cAMP and of abnormal skeletal muscle miroscopy.

Treatment consists of: discontinuation of triggering agents; hyperventilation with oxygen; external and if necessary, internal cooling, and administration of dantrolene sodium, and as indicated verapamil, procainamide, propanolol, sodium bicarbonate, chlorpromazine, burosemide, mannitol, insulin and/or potassium chloride.

References

Ahern CP, Somers CJ, Wilson P, McLoughlin JV (1977) The prevention of acute malignant hyperthermia in halothane sensitive Pietrain pigs by low doses of neuroleptic drugs. Proceedings of the 3rd international conference on production diseases in farm animals, Wageningen, 1976. PUDOC, Wageningen, p 169

Anderson IL, Jones EW (1976a) Porcine malignant hyperthermia: effect of dantrolene sodium on in vitro halothane-induced contraction of susceptible muscle. Anesthesiology 44:57

Anderson IL, Jones EW (1976b) Recent developments in porcine malignant hyperthermia (Abstract). Proc Int Pig Vet Soc 1976 Congress, Ames, Iowa

Anderson IL, Jones EW (1978) Dantrolene sodium in porcine MH: studies on isolated muscle strips. In: Aldrete JA, Britt BA (eds) Second international symposium on malignant hyperthermia. Grune & Stratton, New York, p 509

Anido V (1976) Malignant hyperthermia (letter to the editor). South Med J 69:1247

Auerbach VH, DiGeorge AM, Mayer BW, Hayden M, Carpenter GG, Krumperman LW, Truter TR (1973) Rhabdomyolysis and hyperpyrexia in children after administration of succinylcholine. In: Gordon RA, Britt BA, Kalow W (eds) International symposium on malignant hyperthermia. Thomas, Springfield, p 30

Bagshaw RJ, Cox R, Knight D, Detweiler DK (1978) Malignant hyperthermia in a greyhound. J Am Vet Med Assoc 172:61

Ball RA, Annis CL, Topel EG, Christian LL (1973) Clinical and laboratory diagnosis of porcine stress syndrome. Vet Med Small Anim Clin 688:1156

Barlow MB, Isaacs H (1970) Malignant hyperpyrexial deaths in a family. Reports of three cases. Br J Anaesth 42:1072

Bennett D, Cain PA, Ellis FR, Louis CF, Stanton M (1977) Calcium and magnesium contents of malignant hyperpyrexia-susceptible human muscle. Br J Anaesth 49:979

Bergera JJ, Friz RE (1971) Hyperthermic reaction during anesthesia in an infant. Case report. Plast Reconstr Surg 48:595

Berman MC, Kench JE (1973) Biochemical features of malignant hyperthermia in Landrace pigs. In: Gordon RA, Britt BA, Kalow W (eds) International symposium on malignant hyperthermia. Thomas, Springfield, p 287

Bernhardt D, Hoerder MH (1977) Anaesthesia induced myoglobinuria without hyperpyrexia – an abortive form of malignant hyperthermia? Med Klin 72:1967

Bianchi CP (1969) Pharmacology of excitation-contraction coupling in muscle – introduction: statement of the problem. Fed Proc 28:1624

Bianchi CP, Bolton TC (1967) Action of local anesthetics on coupling systems in muscle. J Pharmacol Exp Ther 157:388

Blume P, Schmidt EW, Cayuela S, Ostheimer U, Perge V, Stankovic R, Wellstein A (1978) Klinik und Laborbefunde bei maligner Hyperthermie im Kindesalter unter besonderer Berücksichtigung der Creatinkinase-Isoenzyme. Anaesthesist 27:108

Borden H, Hummer GJ, Landon CW, Paris J (1976) The use of procaine in acquired malignant hyperthermia in a patient with malignant melanoma metastatic to the parathyroid gland: a case report. Can Anaesth Soc J 23:616

Bowers E (1974) Biochemical basis of malignant hyperpyrexia. Br Med J 2:614

Bowman WC, Nott MW (1969) Actions of sympathomimetic amines and their antagonists on skeletal muscle. Pharmacol Rev 21:27

Bradley R (1976) Nutritional myodegeneration (white muscle disease) of yearling and adult cattle. Presented at the Conference on Livestock Stress and Meat Quality, September, 1976, Wageningen, Netherlands

Britt BA (1971) Malignant hyperthermia – an investigation of three patients. Ann R Coll Surg Engl 48:73

Britt BA (1973) prevention of malignant hyperthermia. In: Gordon RA, Britt BA, Kalow W (eds) International symposium on malignant hyperthermia. Thomas, Springfield, p 451

Britt BA (1976) Malignant hyperthermia: a pharmacogenetic disease of skeletal and cardiac muscle. N Engl J Med 74:1140

Britt BA (1977) Malignant hyperthermia: aetiology and pathophysiology. In: Hulsz E, Lunn JN (eds) Anaesthesiology. Proceedings of the VIth World Congress of Anaesthesiology, Mexico City, April 24–30, 1976. Excerpta Medica, Amsterdam, p 439

Britt BA (1979a) Etiology and pathophysiology of malignant hyperthermia. Fed Am Soc Exp Biol 38:44

Britt BA (1979b) Preanaesthetic diagnosis of malignant hyperthermia. Int Anesthesiol Clin 17/4:119

Britt BA (1980) Malignant hyperthermia. In: Orkin FK, Cooperman LH (eds) Complications in anaesthesiology. Lippincott, Philadelphia

Britt BA, Kalow W (1968) Hyperrigidity and hyperthermia associated with anaesthesia. Ann NY Acad Sci 151:947

Britt BA, Kalow W (1970a) Malignant hyperthermia: a statistical review. Can Anaesth Soc J 17:293

Britt BA, Kalow W (1970b) Malignant hyperthermia: aetiology unknown. Can Anaesth Soc J 17:316

Britt BA, Locher WG, Kalow W (1969) Hereditary aspects of malignant hyperthermia. Can Anaesth Soc J 16:89

Britt BA, Kalow W, Gordon A, Humphrey JG, Rewcastle NB (1973a) Malignant hyperthermia – an investigation of five patients. Can Anaesth Soc J 20:431

Britt BA, Kalow W, Endrenyi L (1973b) Malignant hyperthermia and the mitochondria in human patients. In: Gordon RA, Britt BA, Kalow W (eds) International symposium on malignant hyperthermia. Thomas, Springfield, p 387

Britt BA, Webb G, Leduc C (1974) Mild malignant hyperthermia induced by curare. Can Anaesth Soc J 21:371

Britt BA, Endrenyi L, Cadman DL, Ho MF, Fund NY-K (1975a) Porcine malignant hyperthermia – effects of halothane on mitochondrial respiration and calcium accumulation. Anesthesiology 42:292

Britt BA, Endrenyi L, Barclay RL, Cadman DL (1975b) Total calcium content of skeletal muscle isolated from humans and pigs susceptible to malignant hyperthermia. Br J Anaesth 47:647

Britt BA, Endrenyi L, Cadman DL (1975c) Calcium uptake into muscle sarcoplasmic reticulum of pigs susceptible to malignant hyperthermia: in vitro and in vivo studies with and without halothane. Br J Anaesth 47:650

Britt BA, Endrenyi L, Peters PL, Kwong FH-F, Kadijevic L (1976a) Screening of malignant hyperthermic susceptible families by CPK measurement and other clinical investigations. Can Anaesth Soc J 23:263

Britt BA, Endrenyi L, Kalow W, Peters PL (1976b) The adenosine triphosphate (ATP) depletion test: comparison with the caffeine contracture test as a method of diagnosing malignant hyperthermia susceptibility. Can Anaesth Soc J 23:624

Britt BA, Locher WG, Kalow W (1976c) Hereditary aspects of malignant hyperthermia. Can Anaesth Soc J 25:373

Britt BA, McComas AJ, Endrenyi L, Kalow W (1977a) Motor unit counting and the caffeine contracture test in malignant hyperthermia. Anesthesiology 47:490

Britt BA, Kwong FH-F, Endrenyi L (1977b) The clinical laboratory features of malignant hyperthermia management – a review. In: Henschel EO (ed) Malignant hyperthermia, current concepts. Appleton-Century-Crofts, New York, p 9

Britt BA, Kwong FH-F, Endrenyi L (1977c) Management of malignant hyperthermia susceptible patients – a review. In: Henschel EP (ed) Malignant hyperthermia, current concepts. Appleton-Century-Crofts, New York, p 63

Britt BA, Kalow W, Endrenyi L (1978a) Malignant hyperthermia – pattern of inheritance in swine. In: Aldrete JA, Britt BA (eds) Second international symposium on malignant hyperthermia. Grune & Stratton, New York, p 195

Britt BA, Shandling BR, Endrenyi L, Kent GM (1978b) Perfusion of isolated malignant hyperthermia susceptible and normal pig livers with halothane. Can Anaesth Soc J 25:373

Britt BA, Antonik A, Endrenyi L, Mickle DAG (1978c) A simplified method for measuring blood CPK in human malignant hyperthermia susceptible (MHS) patients. In: Aldrete JA, Britt BA (eds) Second international symposium on malignant hyperthermia. Grune & Stratton, New York, po 251

Britt BA, Harrison JE, McNeil KG (1979) In vivo neutron activation analysis for bone calcium (IVNAA) in malignant hyperthermia susceptible patients. Can Anaesth Soc J
26:117
Britt BA, Endrenyi L, Scott E, Frodis W (1980a) Effect of temperature, time and fascicle
size on the caffeine contracture test. Can Anaesth Soc J 27:1
Britt BA, Endrenyi L, Frodis W, Scott E, Kalow W (1980b) Comparison of effects of several
inhalation anaesthetics on caffeine-induced contractures of normal and malignant hyperthermic skeletal muscle. Can Anaesth Soc J 27:12
Bryant SH, Anderson IL (1977) Microelectrode studies of intercostal muscle fibres from ma-
lignant hyperthermia susceptible pigs. Presented at the Second International Symposium on Malignant Hyperthermia, April 1–3, 1977, Denver, Colorado
Burford GE (1940) Hyperthermia following anaesthesia. Anesthesiology 1:208
Cain PA, Ellis FR (1977) Anaesthesia for patients susceptible to malignant hyperpyrexia.
Br J Anaesth 49:941
Campion DR, Topel DG (1975) A review of the role of swine skeletal muscle in malignant
hyperthermia. J Anim Sci 41:779
Campion DR, Marsh BB, Schmidt GR, Cassens RG, Kauffman RG, Briskey EJ (1971) Use
of whole body perfusion in the study of muscle glycolysis. J Food Sci 36:545
Caropreso PR, Gittleman MA, Reilly DJ, Patterson LT (1975) Malignant hyperthermia as-
sociated with enflurane anesthesia. Arch Surg 110:1491
Casson H, Downes H (1978) Ryanodine toxicity as a model of malignant hyperthermia. In:
Aldrete JA, Britt BA (eds) Second international symposium on malignant hyperther-
mia. Grune & Stratton, New York, p 3
Cheah KS, Cheah AM (1976) The trigger for PSE condition in stress-susceptible pigs. J Sci
Food Agric 27:1137
Cheah KS, Cheah AM (1978) Calcium movements in skeletal muscle mitochondria of ma-
lignant hyperthermia pigs. FEBS Lett 95:307
Chyatte SB, Birdsong JH (1971) The use of dantrolene sodium in disorders of the central
nervous system. South med J 64:830
Chyatte SB, Birdsong JH, Roberson DL (1973) Dantrolene sodium in athetoid cerebral pal-
sy. Arch Phys Med Rehabil 54:365
Clarke IMC, Ellis FR (1975) An evaluation of procaine in the treatment of malignant hy-
perpyrexia. Br J Anaesth 47:17
Cohen PJ, Marshall BE (1968) Effect of halothane in respiratory control and oxygen consumption of rat liver mitochondria. In: Fink BR (ed) Toxicity of anesthetics. Williams
& Wilkins, Baltimore, p 24
Csongrady E (1976) Ein weiterer Fall maligner Hyperpyrexie und seine Behandlung mit Lo-
docain, Methylprednisolon und Verapamil. Anaesthesist 25:80
Cullen SC (1951) Anesthesia in general practice, 3rd edn. Year Book Publishers, Chicago,
p 88
Daniels HC, Polayes IM, Villar RV, Hehre FW (1969) Malignant hyperthermia with dis-
seminated intravascular coagulation during general anaesthesia: a case report. Current
Researchers 48:877
De Jong RH, Heavner JE, Amory DW (1974) Malignant hyperpyrexia in the cat. Anes-
thesiology 41:608
Denborough MA (1975) Serum creatine phosphokinase and malignant hyperpyrexia. Br
Med J 4:403
Denborough MA (1979) Aetiology and pathophysiology of malignant hyperthermia. Int
Anesth Clin 17/4:11
Denborough MA, Lovel RRH (1960) Letter to the Editor. Anaesthetic deaths in a family.
Lancet 1:45
Denborough MA, Forster JFA, Lovell RRH, Maplestone PA, Villiers JD (1962) Anaesthetic
deaths in a family. Br J Anaesth 34:395
Denborough MA, Forster JFA, Hudson MC, Carter NG, Zapf P (1970a) Malignant hyper-
pyrexia – a serious, preventable complication of general anaesthesia. Presented at the
Australasian Congress of Anaesthesiology, Melbourne, Australia
Denborough MH, Hudson MC, Forster JFA, Carter NG, Zapf P (1970b) Biochemical
changes in malignant hyperpyrexia. Lancet 2:1137

Denborough MA, Forster JFA, Hudson MC, Carter NG, Zapf P (1973 a) Malignant hyper-pyrexia. Br J Anaesth 45:860

Denborough MA, Hird FJR, King JO, Marginson MA, Mitchelson KR, Nayler WG, Rex, MA, Zapf P, Condron RJ (1973b) Mitochondrial and other studies in Australian Landrace pigs affected with malignant hyperthermia. In: Gordon RA, Britt BA, Kalow W (eds) International symposium on malignant hyperthermia. Thomas, Springfield, p 229

Denborough MA, Warne GL, Moulds RFW, Tse P, Martin FIR (1974) Insulin secretion in malignant hyperpyrexia. Br Med J 3:493

DePinna GA (1978) A case of osteogenesis imperfecta malignant hyperthermia susceptible anesthetic management. In: Aldrete JA, Britt BA (eds) Second international symposium on malignant hyperthermia. Grune & Stratton, New York p 409

Desmedt JE, Hainaut K (1977) Inhibition of the intracellular release of calcium by dan-trolene in barnacle giant muscle fibres. J Physiol (Lond) 265:565

Dillon JB (1968) Fulminating hyperthermia during anaesthesia. NY state J Med 68:2566

Dimarco NM, Beitz DC, Young JW, Topel DG, Christian L (1976) Gluconeogenesis from lactate in liver of stress-susceptible and stress-resistant pigs. J Nutr 106:710

Drabikowski W, Sarzala MG, Wroniszweska A, Lagwinska E, Drzewieka B (1972) Role of cholesterol in the Ca^{2+}-uptake and ATPase activity of fragmented sarcoplasmic re-ticulum. Biochim Biophys Acta 274:158

Durbin CG Jr, Rosenberg H (1979) A laboratory animal model for malignant hyperpyrexia. J Pharmacol Exp Ther 210:70

Ebashi S, Ebashi F, Kodama A (1967) Troponin as the Ca^{++} receptive protein in the con-tractile system. J Biochem (Tokyo) 62:137

Eberlein HJ (1979) Therapie der malignen Hyperthermie: vorläufige Mitteilung. Anaesthe-sist 28:247

Eighmy JJ, Williams CH, Anderson RR (1978) The fulminant hyperthermia-stress syn-drome: plasma thyroxine and triiodothyronine levels in susceptible and normal pigs. In: Aldrete JA, Britt BA (eds) Second international symposium on malignant hyperther-mia. Grune & Stratton, New York, p 161

Eikelenboom C, van Eldik P, Minkema D, Sybesma W (1976) Control of stress-susceptibil-ity and meat quality in pig breeding (Abstract). Proc Int Pig Vet Soc, 1976 Congress, Ames, Iowa

Eikelenboom G, Minkema D, van Eldick P, Sybesma W (1978) Interhitance of the malig-nant hyperthermia syndrome in Dutch Landrace swine. In: Aldrete JA, Britt BA (eds) Second international symposium on malignant hyperthermia. Grune & Stratton, New York, p 141

Elizondo G, Addis PB, Rempel WE, Madero C, Martin FB, Anderson DB, Marple DN (1976) Stress response and muscle properties in Pietrain (P), Minnesota No. 1 (M) and OxM pigs. J Anim Sci 43:1004

Ellis FR, Keaney NP, Harriman DGF, Sumner DW, Kyei-Mensah K, Tyrrell JII, Hargreaves JB, Parikh RK, Mulrooney PL (1972) Screening for malignant hyper-pyrexia. Br Med J 5:559

Ellis FR, Clarke IMC, Appleyard TN, Dinsdale RCW (1974) Malignant hyperpyrexia in-duced by nitrous oxide and treated with dexamethasone. Br med J 2:270

Ellis FR, Clarke IMC, Modgill M, Currie S, Harriman DGF (1975) Evaluation of creatine phosphokinase in screening patients for malignant hyperpyrexia. Br Med J 3:511

Ellis FR, Cain PA, Harriman DGF, Toothill C (1978a) Plasma cholinesterase and malig-nant hyperthermia. Br J Anaesth 50:1

Ellis FR, Harriman DGF, Currie S, Cain PA (1978b) Screening for malignant hyperthermia in susceptible families. In: Aldrete JA, Britt BA (eds) Second international symposium on malignant hyperthermia. Grune & Stratton, New York, p 273

Ellis KO, Bryant SH (1972) Excitation-contraction uncoupling in skeletal muscle by dan-trolene sodium. Naunyn Schmiedebergs Arch Pharmacol 274:107

Ellis KO, Carpenter JF (1972) Studies on the mechanism of action of dantrolene sodium, a skeletal muscle relaxant. Naunyn Schmiedebergs Arch Pharmacol 275:83

Ellis KO, Carpenter JF (1973) The effects of dantrolene sodium on skeletal muscle. Fed Proc 30:772

Ellis KO, Castellion AW, Honkomp LJ, Wessels FL, Carpenter JF, Halliday RP (1973) Dantrolene, a direct acting skeletal muscle relaxant. J Pharm Sci 62:948

Ellis RH, Simpson P, Tatham P, Leighton M, Williams J (1975) The cardiovascular effects of dantrolene sodium in dogs. Anaesthesia 30:318

Endo M, Blinks JR (1973) Inconsistent association of aequorin luminescence with tension during calcium release in skinned muscle fibres. Nature New Biol 246:218

Endo M, Tanaka M, Ogawa Y (1970) Calcium induced release of calcium from the sarcoplasmic reticulum of skinned skeletal muscle fibres. Nature 228:34

Faber P, Gullotta F, Koenen FW (1975) Klinische und morphologische Befunde bei maligner Hyperthermie. Dtsch Med Wochenschr 100:1

Feiglin DHI, Huckell VF, McLaughlin PR, Britt BA, Staniloff HM, Morch JE (1982) The demonstration of myocardial perfusion defects in malignant hyperthermia. In press

Feldberg W, Myers RD (1964) Effects on temperature of amines injected into the cerebral ventricles: a new concept of temperature regulation. J Physiol (Lond) 173:226

Fivehouse NR, Watson RL (1968) Hyperthermia caused by the Emerson postoperative ventilator: a solution to the problem. Anesthesiology 29:1220

Fleckenstein A (1971) Specific inhibitors and promoters of calcium action in the excitation-contraction coupling of heart muscle and their role in the prevention or production of myocardial lesions. In: Harris P, Opie L (eds) Calcium and the heart. Academic Press, London

Fleisher GA, McGonahey WM (1964) Serum creatine kinase, lactic dehydrogenase and glutamic oxalacetic transaminase in thyroid diseases and pregnancy. J Lab Clin Med 64:857

Fuchs F (1975) Thermal inactivation of the calcium regulatory mechanism of human skeletal muscle actomyosin: a possible contributing factor in the rigidity of malignant hyperthermia. Anesthesiology 42:584

Fukuchi H, Morio M, Nioh K, Ohtani M, Kawahara M, Shinozaki M (1977) Statistical review of malignant hyperthermia in Japan. Proceedings of the First Japanese Symposium on Malignant Hyperthermia. Hiroshima J Anesth 13:47

Fukuchi H, Morio M, Shinozaki M, Ishihara S (1978) Statistical considerations of malignant hyperthermia in Japan. In: Aldrete JA, Britt BA (eds) Second international symposium on malignant hyperthermia. Grune & Stratton, New York, p 483

Fukuchi H, Kuwata N, Seki Y, Morio M (1979) Preparation ad stability of parenteral solution of 0.4W/V% dantrolene sodium. Hiroshima J Anesth 15:21

Furniss P (1971) The etiology of malignant hyperpyrexia. Proc R Soc Med 64:216

Gelenberg AJ, Poskanzer DC (1973) The effect of dantrolene sodium on spasticity in multiple sclerosis. Neurology 23:1313

Gibson JA, Gardiner DM (1969) Malignant hypertonic hyperpyrexia syndrome. Can Anaesth Soc J 16:106

Greenblatt DJ, Gross PL, Harris J, Shader RI, Ciraulo DA (1978) Fatal hyperthermia following haloperidol therapy of sedative-hypnotic withdrawal. J Clin Psychiatry 39:673

Grist EM, Hall GM, Baum H (1973) The effect of procaine on calcium-induced halothane-dependent loss of respiratory control in rat liver mitochondria. Br J Anaesth 45:1234

Gronert GA (1979) Muscle contractures and ATP depletion in porcine malignant hyperthermia. Anesth Analg 58:367

Gronert GA, Heffron JJA (1979) Skeletal muscle mitochondria in porcine malignant hyperthermia: respiratory activity, calcium functions, and depression by halothane. Anesth Analg (Cleve) 58:76

Gronert GA, Theye RA (1976a) Halothane-induced porcine malignant hyperthermia: metabolic and hemodynamic changes. Anesthesiology 44:36

Gronert GA, Theye RA (1976b) Suxamethonium-induced porcine malignant hyperthermia. Br J Anaesth 48:513

Gronert GA, Milde JH, Theye RA (1976) Dantrolene in porcine malignant hyperthermia. Anesthesiology 44:488

Gronert GA, Milde JH, Theye RA (1977) Role of sympathetic activity in porcine malignant hyperthermia. Anesthesiology 47:411

Gronert GA, Mansfield E, Theye RA (1978a) Rapidly soluble dantrolene for intravenous use. In: Aldrete JA, Britt BA (eds) Second international symposium on malignant hyperthermia. Grune & Stratton, New York, p 535

Gronert GA, Theye RA, Milde JH (1978 b) Catecholamine stimulation of myocardial oxygen consumption in porcine malignant hyperthermia. Anesthesiology 49:330

Gruhl D (1971) Maligne Hyperthermie. Anaesthesist 21:229

Guedel A (1937) Postoperative hyperthermia. In: Inhalation anaesthesia. A fundamental guide. Macmillan, New York, p 133

Gulotta F, Helpap B (1975) Histologische, histochemische und elektronenmikroskopische Befunde bei maligner Hyperthermie. Virchows Arch [Pathol Anat] 367:181

Gullotta E, Wierich W, Dieckmann J (1976) Maligne Hyperthermie, chronischer Alkoholismus und tubulare Aggregate. Prakt Anaesth 11:410

Hahn MJ, Godt RE (1977) Effects of halothane on tension and calcium release in mechanically skinned porcine skeletal muscle: studies on malignant hyperthermia. Presented at the Second International Symposium on Malignant Hyperthermia, April 1–3, 1977, Denver, Colorado

Halevy S, Marx GF (1971) Hyperthermia during a second anesthesia (letter to the editor). Anesthesiology 35:44

Hall GM (1973) Calcium ion-induced loss of respiratory control in rat liver mitochondria in the presence of inhalational anaesthetic agents. Biochem Soc Trans 1:854

Hall GM (1978) Body temperature and anaesthesia. Br J Anaesth 50:39

Hall GM, Kirtland SJ, Baum H (1973) The inhibition of mitochondrial respiration by inhalational anaesthetic agents. Br J Anaesth 45:1005

Hall GM, Lucke JN, Lister D (1975) Treatment of porcine malignant hyperthermia. A review based on experimental studies. Anaesthesia 30:308

Hall GM, Bendall JR, Lucke JN, Lister D (1976 a) Porcine malignant hyperthermia. II. Heat production. Br J Anaesth 48:305

Hall GM, Masshiter K, Lucke JN, Lister D (1976 b) Hormonal changes in porcine malignant hyperthermia (letter to the editor). Br J Anaesth 48:930

Hall GM, Lucke JN, Lister D (1977) Porcine malignant hyperthermia. V. Fatal hyperthermia in the Pietrain pig, associated with the infusion of a-adrenergic agonists. Br J Anaesth 49:855

Hall GM, Lucke JN, Lovell R, Lister D (1978) Hepatic metabolism in pig malignant hyperthermia. Biochem Soc Trans 6:587

Harriman DGF (1979) Preanaesthetic investigation of malignant hyperpyrexia-microscopy. Anesth Clin 17/4:97

Harriman DGF, Ellis FR, Franks AJ, Sumner DW (1978) Malignant hyperthermia myopathy in man: an investigation of 75 families. In: Aldrete JA, Britt BA (eds) Second international symposium on malignant hyperthermia. Grune & Stratton, New York, p 67

Harris RA, Munroe J, Farmer B, Kim KC, Jenkins P (1971) Action of halothane upon mitochondrial respiration. Arch Biochem Biophys 142:435

Harrison GG (1973 a) The effect of procaine and curare on the initiation of anaesthetic-induced malignant hyperpyrexia. In: Gordon RA, Britt BA, Kalow W (eds) International symposium on malignant hyperthermia. Thomas, Springfield, p 271

Harrison GG (1973 b) Althesin and malignant hyperpyrexia. Br J Anaesth 45:109

Harrison GG (1975) Control of the malignant hyperpyrexic syndrome in MHS swine by dantrolene sodium. Br J Anaesth 47:62

Harrison GG (1977) The prophylaxis of malignant hyperthermia by oral dantrolene sodium in swine. Br J Anaesth 49:1

Harrison GG (1979) Porcine malignant hyperthermia. Int Anesth Clin 17/4:25

Harrison GG, Verburg C (1973) Erythrocyte osmotic fragility in hyperthermia-susceptible swine. Br J Anaesth 45:131

Harrison GG, Saunders SJ, Biebuyck JF, Hickman R, Dent DM, Weaver V, Terblanche J (1969) Anaesthetic induced malignant hyperpyrexia and a method for its prediction. Br J Anaesth 41:844

Hassan SZ, Meltzer HY, Cho HW, Fang VS (1978) Isoenzymes of creatine kinase in serum of families with malignant hyperpyrexia. In: Aldrete JA, Britt BA (eds) Second international symposium on malignant hyperthermia. Grune & Stratton, New York, p 233

Hausman R, Kaldi F, Burdman D (1970) Maligne (of fulminante) hyperthermie en morfologische spierveranderingen. Ned Tijdschr Geneeskd 114:1917

Heffron JJA, Isaacs H (1976) Malignant hyperthermia syndrome – evidence for denervation changes in human skeletal muscle. Klin Wochenschr 54:865

Heffron JJA, Mitchell G (1975a) Age dependent variation of serum creatine phosphokinase levels in pigs. Experientia 31:657

Heffron JJA, Mitchell G (1975b) Diagnostic value of serum creatine phosphokinase activity for the porcine malignant hyperthermia syndrome. Anesth Analg (Cleve) 54:536

Heffron JJA, Mitchell G (1976) Calcium uptake by sarcoplasmic reticulum of muscle of pigs susceptible to malignant hyperthermia (Abstract). Proc Int Pig Vet Soc, 1976 Congress, Ames, Iowa

Hess JW, MacDonald RP, Frederick RJ, Jones RN, Neely J, Gross D (1964) Serum creatine phosphokinase (CPK) activity in disorders of heart and skeletal muscle. Ann Intern Med 61:1015

Hess ML, Solaro RJ, Briggs FN (1974) Polyhydroxyl and temperature antagonism of the inhibitory effects of gram-negative endotoxin on the calcium uptake activity of cardiac sarcoplasmic reticulum. Recent Adv Stud Cardiac Struct 4:451

Hewer CL (1948) Recent advances in anaesthesia and analgesia (including oxygen therapy), 6th edn. Churchill, London

Horsey PJ (1968) Hyperpyrexia during anaesthesia. Br Med J 3:803

Howat DDC, Barker J, Vale RJ, Ellis FR (1973) Temperature regulation: a symposium on the use of induced hypothermia, the importance of normothermia in the surgical period and malignant hyperthermia. Anaesthesia 28:236

Huckell VF, Staniloff HM, Britt BA et al. (1977) A "new" cardiomyopathy associated with malignant arrhythmias and sudden death. Presented at the 26th Annual Scientific Session, American College of Cardiology, Feb. 28–March 3, 1977

Huckell VF, Staniloff HM, Britt BA, Waxman MB, Morch JE (1978a) Cardiac manifestations of malignant hyperthermia susceptibility. Circulation 58:916

Huckell VF, Staniloff HM, McLaughlin PR, Britt BA, Morch JE (1978b) Carciovascular manifestations of normothermic malignant hyperthermia. In: Aldrete JA, Britt BA (eds) Second international symposium on malignant hyperthermia. Grune & Stratton, New York, p 373

Huckell VF, Staniloff HM, Britt BA, Waxman MB, Feiglin DH, McLaughlin PR, Morch JE (1978c) Thallium-201 myocardial imaging in malignant hyperthermia: a membrane disease. Presented at the American College of Cardiology, March 6–9, 1978, Anaheim, California

Hull MJ, Webster WW, Gatz E (1971) The effects of pentobarbital on 2,4-dinitrophenol induced malignant hyperthermia during halothane general anaesthesia in dogs. J Oral Surg 29:640

Huxley HE (1965) Structural evidence concerning the mechanism of contraction in striated muscle. In: Paul WM, Daniel EE, Kay CM, Monckton G (eds) Muscle. Pergamon, Oxford, p 3

Isaacs H (1973) High serum creatine phosphokinase levels in asymptomatic members of the families of patients developing malignant hyperpyrexia – a genetic study. In: Gordon RA, Britt BA, Kalow W (eds) International symposium on malignant hyperthermia. Thomas, Springfield, p 331

Isaacs H (1981) Comments on predictive tests for malignant hyperthermia. In Press

Isaacs H, Barlow MB (1974) Central core disease associated with elevated creatine phosphokinase levels – 2 members of a family known to be susceptible to malignant hyperpyrexia. S Afr Med J 48:640

Isaacs H, Frere G, Mitchell J (1973) Histological, histochemical and ultramicroscopic findings in muscle biopsies from carriers of the trait for malignant hyperpyrexia. Br J Anaesth 45:860

Isherwood DM, Ridley J, Wilson J (1975) Creatinine phosphokinase (CPK) levels in pregnancy: a case report and a discussion of the value of CPK levels in the prediction of possible malignant hyperpyrexia. Br J Obstet Gynaecol 82:346

Itohda Y, Oda S, Nishino M et al. (1976) Anesthesia for patients with arthrogryposis multiplex congenita. Jpn J Anesth 3:697

Jaffe EC, Wedley JR (1972) Malignant hyperpyrexia, an anaesthetic hazard. Br Dent J 135:538

Jago RH, Panne MJ (1977) Malignant hyperpyrexia – the difficulty of diagnosis. Anaesthesia 32:74

James OF (1970) Hyperpyrexia and hypertonia in anaesthesia. Med J Aust 1:1154

James PO (1978) Vitamin E and malignant hyperthermia (letter to the editor). Br Med J 1:1345

Johnson PN, Inesi G (1969) The effect of methylxanthines and local anaesthetics on fragmented sarcoplasmic reticulum. J Pharmacol Exp Ther 169:308

Johnson SA, Van Horn DL, Pederson HJ (1966) The function of platelets – a review. Transfusion 6:3

Jones EW, Nelson TE, Anderson IL, Kerr DD, Burnap TK (1972) Malignant hyperthermia of swine. Anesthesiology 36:42

Kacinec J, Malatinsky J, Sadlon P, Klimasova A (1974) Syndrom malignej hypertermie. Rozhl Chir 53:734

Kalow W, Britt BA (1973) Inheritance of malignant hyperthermia. In: Gordon RA, Britt BA, Kalow W (eds) International symposium on malignant hyperthermia. Thomas, Springfield, p 67

Kalow W, Britt BA, Richter A (1977) The caffeine test of isolated human muscle in relation to malignant hyperthermia. Can Anaesth Soc J 24:678

Kalow W, Britt BA, Chan FY (1979) Epidemiology and inheritance of malignant hyperthermia. Int Anesth Clin 17/4:119

Katz D (1970) Recurrent malignant hyperpyrexia during anaesthesia. Anesth Analg (Cleve) 49:225

Kelstrup J, Hasse J, Jorni J, Reske-Nielsen R, Hanel HK (1973) Malignant hyperthermia in a family. Acta Anaesthesiol Scand 17:283

Kerr DD, Wingard DW, Gatz EE (1975) Prevention of porcine malignant hyperthermia by epidural block. Anesthesiology 42:307

Kerr DD, Wingard DW, Gatz EE (1978) Prevention of porcine malignant hyperthermia by oral dantrolene. In: Aldrete JA, Britt BA (eds) Second international symposium on malignant hyperthermia. Grune & Stratton, New York, p 83

King JO, Denborough MA (1973) Anaesthetic induced malignant hyperpyrexia in children. J Pediatr 83:37

Klein LV (1975) Case report: a hot horse. Vet Anesth 2:41

Klimanek J, Majewski W, Walencik K (1976) A case of malignant hyperthermia during epidural analgesia. Anaesthesiol Resusc 4:143

Kondo T (1971) A case of malignant hyperpyrexia. Hiroshima J Anesth 1:161

Konno J (1974) Biochemical and electromyographic study on a family of malignant hyperpyrexia. Jpn J Anesth 23:8654

Konno K (1976) Electrophysiological consideration of malignant hyperpyrexia. Anaesthesiol Resusc 12

Krebs EG, DeLange RJ, Kempf RG, Riley WDB (1966) Activation of skeletal muscle phosphorylase. Pharmacol Rev 18:163

Krzywicki K (1971) Relation of ATPase activity and calcium uptake to postmortem glycolysis. J Food Sci 36:791

Lack JA (1975) New causes of malignant hyperpyrexia. Br Med J 1:36

LaCour D, Juul-Jensen P, Reske-Nielsen E (1970) Anaestesi induceret malign hypertermi hos 4 patients efterundersogt neurofysiologisk og neuropatologisk. Nord Med 17.1636

LaCour D, Juul-Jensen P, Reske-Nielsen E (1971) Malignant hyperthermia during anaesthesia. A neurophysiological and neuropathological follow-up study of a patient and his family. Acta Anaesthesiol Scand 15:299

Larard DG, Rice CP, Robinson RW, Spencer RW, Westhead RA (1972) Malignant hyperthermia: a study of an affected family. Br J Anaesth 44:93

Lee JA (1959) A synopsis of anaesthesia, 4th edn. Wright, Bristol

Lees DE, Kim YD, Schuette W, Bull J, Whang-Peng J (1979) Causes of induced hyperthermia. Anesthesiology 50:69

Lenard HG, Kettler D (1975) Malignant hyperpyrexia and myopathy. Neuropaediatrie 6:7

Lewis E (1965) Hyperpyrexia with antidepressant drugs. Br Med J 2:1671

Lieberman P, Iaina A, David R, Agranat O, Ohry A, Ramon I, Eliahou HE (1978) Non-oliguric acute renal failure following malignant hyperthermia. Report of a case and review of the literature. In: Aldrete JA, Britt BA (eds) Second international symposium on malignant hyperthermia. Grune & Stratton, New York, p 451

Lister D (1973) Correction of adverse response to suxamethonium of susceptible pigs. Br Med J 1:208

Lister D, Hall GM, Lucke JN (1975) Malignant hyperthermia: a human and porcine stress syndrome? Lancet 1:519

Lister D, Hall GM, Lucke JN (1976) Porcine malignant hyperthermia. III. Adrenergic blockade. Br J Anaesth 48:831

Lohmann K (1934) Über die enzymatische Aufspaltung der Kreatinphosphosäure; zugleich ein Beitrag zum Chemismus der Muskelkontraktion. Biochem Z 271:264

Lucke JN (1977) Malignant hyperthermia in a parturient Poland China sow (letter to the editor). Br J Anaesth 49:1070

Lucke JN, Denny HR (1977) Anaesthetic and surgical techniques for bilateral adrenalectomy in stress sensitive pigs. Res Vet Sci 23:372

Lucke JN, Denny HR (1978) The role of the sympathetic nervous system in the pathogenesis of halothane-induced malignant hyperthermia in the Pietrain pig. Brit J Anaesth 50:75

Lucke JN, Lister D, Hall GM (1975) Malignant hyperpyrexia. Br Med J 1:454

Lucke JN, Hall GM, Lister D (1976a) Porcine malignant hyperthermia. I. Metabolic and physiological changes. Br J Anaesth 48:297

Lucke JN, Hall GM, Lister D (1976b) Body temperature and malignant hyperthermia. (letter) Lancet 2

Lucke JN, Hall GM, Lister D (1977) Anaesthesia of pigs sensitive to malignant hyperthermia. Vet Rec 100:45

Lucke JN, Denny H, Hall G, Lovell R, Lister DD (1978) Porcine malignant hyperthermia. VI. The effects of bilateral adrenalectomy and pretreatment with bretylium on the halothane-induced response. Br J Anaesth 50:241

Ludvigsen J (1953) Muscular degeneration in hogs (preliminary report). XVth Int Vet Congr Proc, 1953, p 602

Mabuchi K, Sreter FA (1977) The use of cryostat sections for measurement of Ca^{2+} uptake by sarcoplasmic reticulum. Presented at the Second International Symposium on Malignant Hyperthermia, April 1–3, 1977, Denver, Colorado

MacLennan DH (1973) Components of the calcium transport system of sarcoplasmic reticulum. In: Gordon RA, Britt BA, Kalow K (eds) International symposium on malignant hyperthermia. Thomas, Springfield, p 139

Mambo NC, Silver MD, Huckell VF, McEwan PM, Britt BA, McLaughlin PR, Morch JE (1981) Malignant hyperthermia susceptibility: a light and electron microscopic study of endomyocardial biopsies from nine patients. Hum Pathol 11:381

Marx GF (1969) Malignant hyperthermia. Anesthesiology 31:585

Masoro EJ (1976) Effects of cold on cellular metabolism: enzymes and other cellular changes. Prog Biometeorol [D] 1:19

Mayer BW, Auerbach VH, Arby JB, Mestre GM (1978) Malignant hyperthermia complicated by Sanarelli-Shwartzman phenomenon. In: Aldrete JA, Britt BA (eds) Second international symposium on malignant hyperthermia. Grune & Stratton, New York, p 427

McCrimmon A, Lewin E (1967) Serum creatine phosphokinase: a useful tool in muscle disease. Am J Med Technol 33:269

McIntosch D, Berman MC (1974) Neutral lipid and phospholipid composition of normal and myopathic skeletal muscle of pigs. S Afr Med J 48:1221

Meltzer H (1969) Muscle enzyme release in the acute psychoses. Arch Gen Psychiatry 21:102

Milton AS, Wendlandt S (1971) The effect of different environmental temperatures on the hyperpyrexia produced by the intraventricular injection of pyrogen, 5-hydroxytryptamine and prostaglandin E_1 in the conscious cat. J Physiol (Paris) 63:340

Mitchelson KR, Hird FJR (1973) Effect of pH and halothane on muscle and liver mitochondria. Am J Physiol 225:1393

Modell JH (1966) Septicemia as a cause of immediate postoperative hyperthermia. Anesthesiology 27:329

Moulds RFW (1977) A comparison of the effects of sodium thiocyanate and dantrolene sodium on an isolated mammalian skeletal muscle. Br J Pharmacol 59:129

Moulds RFW (1978) The site of the abnormality in MH muscle: a comparison of MH muscle and denervated muscle. In: Aldrete JA, Britt BA (eds) Second international symposium on malignant hyperthermia. Grune & Stratton, New York, p 49

Moulds RFW, Denborough MA (1974a) Biochemical basis of malignant hyperpyrexia. Br Med J 2:241

Moulds RFW, Denborough MA (1974b) Identification of susceptibility to malignant hyperpyrexia. Br Med J 2:245

Moulds RFW, Denborough MA, Anderson RM, Dennett X (1974) Studies on muscle in malignant hyperpyrexia. Aust NZ J Med 4:106

Mount LE (1976) Effects of heat and cold on energy metabolism of the pig. Prog Biometeorol [D] 1:227

Murray BRP, Wiliams PAD (1969) Malignant hyperpyrexia during anaesthesia for colectomy. Br Med J 1:488

Nakajima H, Hoshiyama M, Yamashita A, Kiyomoto A (1976) Electrical and mechanical response to diltiazem in potassium depolarized myocardium of the guinea pig. Jpn J Pharmacol 26:571

Nakamura Y, Schwartz A (1972) The influence of hydrogen ion concentration on calcium binding and release by skeletal muscle sarcoplasmic reticulum. J Gen Physiol 59:22

Nayler WG, Szeto J (1972) Effect of verapamil on contractility, oxygen utilization, and calcium exchangeability in mammalian heart muscle. Cardiovasc Res 6:120

Nelson TE (1973) Porcine stress syndrome. In: Gordon RA, Britt BA, Kalow W (eds) International symposium on malignant hyperthermia. Thomas, Springfield, p 191

Nelson TE (1976) Animal model: porcine malignant hyperthermia. Am J Pathol 84:199

Nelson TE (1978) Excitation-contraction coupling: a common etiologic pathway for malignant hyperthermia susceptible muscle. In: Aldrete JA, Britt BA (eds) Second international symposium on malignant hyperthermia. Grune & Stratton, New York, p 23

Nelson TE, Flewellen EH (1979) Rationale for dantrolene vs. procainamide for treatment of malignant hyperthermia. Anesthesiology 50:118

Nelson TE, Jones EW, Venable JH, Kerr DD (1972) Malignant hyperthermia of Poland China swine. Studies of a myogenic etiology. Anesthesiology 36:52

Nelson TE, Jones EW, Bedell DM (1973) Porcine malignant hyperthermia: a study of the triggering effects of succinylcholine. Anesth Analg (Cleve) 52:908

Nelson TE, Jones EW, Henrickson RL, Falk SN, Kerr DD (1974) Porcine malignant hyperthermia: observations on the occurrence of pale, soft, exudative musculature among susceptible pigs. Am J Vet Res 35:347

Nelson TE, Bedell DM, Jones EW (1975) Porcine malignant hyperthermia: effects of temperature and extracellular calcium concentration on halothane-induced contracture of susceptible skeletal muscle. Anesthesiology 42:301

Nicholson MJ (1969) Hyperthermia during anesthesia. Anesth Analg (Cleve) 48:792

Nicholson MJ (1971) Malignant hyperthermia with subsequent uneventful general anesthesia. Anesth Analg 50:1104

Nygren A (1965) Muscular involvement in acutely intoxicated alcoholics revealed by elevated serum CPK activity. Opusc Med 10:329

Oda S, Itohda Y, Nishino M et al. (1977) Ten cases of malignant hyperthermia in Nagasaki. Hiroshima J Anesth 13:11

Ojima T, Takamatsu O, Henmi M, Honda M (1971) A case of abnormal hyperpyrexia developing during anesthesia. Hiroshima J Anesth 7:67

Okumura F, Kuro M (1975) The etiology of malignant hyperthermia. Jpn J Anesth 24:525

Opie JH (1978) Myocardial metabolism and heart disease. Jpn Cir J 42:1223

Perry SV (1965) Muscle proteins in contractions. In: Paul WM (ed) Muscle. Pergamon, Oxford, p 29

Pinsky L, Levy EP (1973) Malignant hyperpyrexia or the XX-XY Turner phenotype? (letter to the editor). J Pediatr 83:896

Pollock RA, Turner JS (1974) Malignant hyperthermia in the otolaryngologic patient. Laryngoscope 84:2113

Pollock RA, Standefer JC, Hildebrand PK, Goodwin B, Li TK (1973) Malignant hyperthermia in the American Landrace pig. In: Gordon RA, Britt BA, Kalow W (eds) International symposium on malignant hyperthermia. Thomas, Springfield, p 224

Popinigis J (1973) Physiological control of energy-producing processes in mitochondria and the possibility of its disturbances in malignant hyperthermia syndrome caused by anaesthetics. Anaesthesiol Resusc 1:63

Purkis IE, Horrelt O, DeYoung G, Fleming RAP, Langley GR (1967) Hyperpyrexia following anaesthesia in a second member of a family, with associated coagulation defect. Can Anaesth Soc J 14:183

Puschel K, Schubert-Thile I, Hirth L, Benkmann H, Brinkmann B (1978) Maligne Hyperthermie in der 13. Vollnarkose. Anaesthesist 27:488

Rabinowitz M, Desalles L, Meisler J, Lorand L (1965) Distribution of adenyl cyclase activity in rabbit skeletal muscle fractions. Biochim Biophys Acta 97:29

Raitt DG, Merrifield AJ (1974) Dexamethasone in malignant hyperpyrexia. Br Med J 4:656

Reske-Nielsen E (1973) Ultrastructure of human muscle in malignant hyperthermia. Acta Pathol Microbiol Scand [A] 81:585

Reske-Nielsen E (1978) Malignant hyperthermia in Denmark – survey of a family study and investigations into muscular morphology in ten additional cases. In: Aldrete JA, Britt BA (eds) Second international symposium in malignant hyperthermia. Grune & Stratton, New York, p 287

Reske-Nielsen E, Haase J, Kelstrup J (1975) Malignant hyperthermia in a family. The ultrastructure of muscle biopsies of healthy members. Acta Pathol Microbiol Scand [A] 83:651

Roberts JT, Ali HH, Ryan JF (to be published) A tourniquet test for malignant hyperthermia. Anesth Analg (Cleve)

Rosenberg H (1978) Sites of action of halothane on skeletal muscle. In: Aldrete JA, Britt BA (eds) Second international symposium on malignant hyperthermia. Grune & Stratton, New York, p 11

Ryan JF (1977) Abnormalities of myofibrillar ATPase function and sarcoplasmic calcium uptake: 14 patients. Presented at the Second International Symposium on Malignant Hyperthermia, April 1–3, 1977, Denver, Colorado

Ryan JF (1979) Treatment of Acute Hyperthermia Crises. Int Anesth Clin 17/4:153

Ryan JF, Papper EM (1970) Malignant fever during and following anaesthesia. Anesthesiology 32:196

Sage RE, Hall RJ (1972) Severe fibrinolysis in fatal malignant hyperpyrexia. Med J Aust 1:755

Saikawa T, Nagamoto Y, Arita M (1977) Electrophysiologic effects of diltiazem, a new slow channel inhibitor, on canine cardiac fibers. Jpn Heart J 18:235

Sandow A (1970) Skeletal muscle. Annu Rev Physiol 32:1040

Satnick JH (1969) Hyperthermia under anaesthesia with regional muscle flaccidity. Anesthesiology 30:472

Schanus EG, Addis PB, Rempel WE, McGrath C, Lovrien RE (1981) (to be published) A molecular basis for malignant hyperthermia

Schmitt J, Schmidt K, Ritter H (1974) Hereditary malignant hyperpyrexia associated with muscle adenylate kinase deficiency. Humangenetik 24:253

Schweizer O, Howland WS, Ryan GM, Goldiner PL (1971) Hyperpyrexia in the operative and immediate postoperative period. Anesth Analg (Cleve) 50:906

Shibata M, Sakai Y, Tanaka I, Shida C (1971) A case considered to be malignant hyperpyrexia. Hiroshima J Anesth 7:129

Shinebourne EA, Hess ML, White RJ, Hamer J (1969) The effect of noradrenaline on the calcium uptake of the sarcoplasmic reticulum. Cardiovasc Res 3:113

Short CE (1978) The significance of MH in animal anesthesia. In: Aldrete JA, Britt BA (eds) Second international symposium on malignant hyperthermia. Grune & Stratton, New York, p 175

Short CE, Paddleford RR, McGrath CJ (1976) Preanaesthetic evaluation and management of MH in pig experimental model. Anesth Analg (Cleve) 55:653

Smith JB, Willis AL (1971) Aspirin selectively inhibits prostaglandin production in human platelets. Nature New Biol 231:235

Snow JC (1970a) Malignant hyperthermia during anesthesia and surgery. Arch Opthalmol 84:407

Snow JC (1970b) Malignant hyperpyrexia. ENT Monthly 49:427

Snow JC, Healy GB, Vaughan CW, Kripke BJ (1972) Malignant hyperthermia during anesthesia for adenoidectomy. Arch Otolaryngol 95:442

Solomons CC, Myers DN (1973) Hyperthermia of osteogenesis imperfecta and its relationship to malignant hyperthermia. In: Gordon RA, Britt BA, Kalow W (eds) International symposium on malignant hyperthermia. Thomas, Springfield, p 319

Solomons CC, Tan S, Aldrete JA (1978) Platelet metabolism in MH. In: Aldrete JA, Britt BA (eds) Second international symposium on malignant hyperthermia. Grune & Stratton, New York, p 221

Stanec A, Spiro AJ, Lent RW (1978) Malignant hyperthermia associated with hypocalcaemia. In: Aldrete JA, Britt BA (eds) Second international symposium on malignant hyperthermia. Grune & Stratton, New York, p 437

Stanley B, Pal NR (1964) Fatal hyperpyrexia with phenelzine and imipramine. Br Med J 4:1011

Stephen CR (1967) Fulminant hyperthermia during anaesthesia and surgery. JAMA 202:106

Steward DJ (1979) Malignant hyperpyrexia: the acute crisis. Int Anesth Clin 17/4:1

Steward DJ, Thomas TA (1973) Intracellular calcium metabolism and malignant hyperpyrexia. In: Gordon RA, Britt BA, Kalow W (eds) International symposium on malignant hyperthermia. Thomas, Springfield, p 409

Stovner J (1968) Muskelrigiditet, hyperpyrexia of metabolsk acidose utlost av succinylkolin. Tidsskr Nor Laegeforen 1:646

Sutherland EW, Rall RW (1960) The relation of adenosine-3′,5′-phosphate and phosphorylase to the actions of catecholamines and other hormones. Pharmacol Rev 12:265

Sutherland EW, Rall RW, Menon T (1962) Adenyl cyclase. I. Distribution, preparation and properties. J Biol Chem 237:1220

Takagi A (1977) Increased release of calcium from sarcoplasmic reticulum (SR) by halothane in malignant hyperthermia (MH). Hiroshima J Anesth 13:155

Tan S, Aldrete JA, Solomons CC (1978) Correlation of serum creatine phosphokinase and pyrophosphate during surgery in patients with malignant hyperthermia susceptibility. In: Aldrete JA, Britt BA (eds) Second international symposium on malignant hyperthermia. Grune & Stratton, New York, p 389

Tanabe R, Nishino K, Yoshioka H, Hanaki C, Morio M (1971) Studies on hyperthermia during anesthesia. I. Hyperthermia produced by warming. Hiroshima J Anesth 7:147

Theilade D, Rosendal T (1978) Malignant hyperpyrexia. Anaesthesia 33:606

Thomford NR, Hamelberg WE, Wiederholt WC (1969) Sudden hyperpyrexia during general anaesthesia. Surgery 66:850

Thompson DEA, Tallack JA (1973) Coexistent muscle disease and malignant hyperpyrexia. In: Gordon RA, Britt BA, Kalow W (eds) International symposium on malignant hyperthermia. Thomas, Springfield, p 309

Thorens S, Endo M (1975) Calcium-induced calcium release and "depolarization"-induced calcium release: their physiological significance. Proc Jpn Acad 51:473

Thorpe W, Seeman P (1973) Drug-induced contracture of muscle. In: Gordon RA, Britt BA, Kalow W (eds) International symposium on malignant hyperthermia. Thomas, Springfield, p 152

Tobias MA, Miller CG (1970) Malignant hypertonic hyperpyrexia. Anaesthesia 25:253

Tonogai R, Kokubo S, Yamada Y, Kohyama A, Inagaki M, Saito T (1978) A case of malignant hyperthermia during anaesthesia. Hiroshima J Anesth 14:163

Tuttle JP (1900) Heat-stroke as a post-operative complication. JAMA 35:1685

Uchida Y (1976) Effect of diltiazem, a new anti-Ca^{++} agent, on left ventricular function in patients with and without angina pectoris: a study using ultrasonic analogue conversion system: Jpn Heart J 17:599

Van Wormer DE, Armstrong MS, Solomons C (1975) Laboratory screening test for malignant hyperpyrexia. Am J Clin Pathol 63:593

Wade JG (1973) The late treatment of malignant hyperthermia. In: Gordon RA, Britt BA, Kalow W (eds) International symposium on malignant hyperthermia. Thomas, Springfield, p 441

Wakabayashi T, Ebashi S (1968) Reversible change in physical state of troponin induced by calcium ion. J Biochem (Tokyo) 64:731)

Waltemath CL (1973) The pathological physiology of hyperthermia. In: Gordon RA, Britt BA, Kalow W (eds) International symposium on malignant hyperthermia. Thomas, Springfield, p 16

Williams CH (1976) Some observations on the etiology of the fulminant hyperthermia-stress syndrome. Perspect Biol Med 20:120

Williams CH, Galvez TL, Brucker RF (1971) Malignant hyperthermia in swine. Fed Proc 30:1208

Williams CH, Houchins C, Shanklin MD (1975) Pigs susceptible to energy metabolism in the fulminant hyperthermia stress syndrome. Br Med J 3:411

Williams CH, Shanklin MD, Hedrick HB et al. (1978) The fulminant hyperthermia-stress syndrome: genetic aspects, hemodynamic and metabolic measurements in susceptible and normal pigs. In: Aldrete JA, Britt BA (eds) Second international symposium on malignant hyperthermia. Grune & Stratton, New York, p 113

Williams ER, Bruford A (1967) Creatine phosphokinase in motor neurone disease. Clin Chim Acta 69:53

Willner JH, Cerri CJ, Wood DS (1979) Malignant hyperthermia: abnormal cyclic AMP metabolism in skeletal muscle. Neurology 29:557

Willner JH, Wood DS, Cerri C, Britt BA (1980) Increased Myophosphorylase A in Malignant Hyperthermia. N Engl J Med 303:138

Wilson JW (1978) Malignant hyperthermia. South Med J 71:1454

Wilson RD, Nichols RJ, Dent TE, Allen CR (1966) Disturbances of the oxidative-phosphorylation mechanisms as a possible etiological factor in sudden unexplained hyperthermia. Anesthesiology 26:232

Wilson RD, Dent TE, Traber DL, McCoy NR, Allen CR (1967) Malignant hyperpyrexia with anaesthesia. JAMA 202:183

Winckler C, Greco J, Bazin G, Echinard K (1971) A propos d'un cas d'hyperthermie maligne sous anesthesie generale. Anesth Analg (Paris) 28:37

Wingard DW (1977) Malignant hyperthermia – acute stress syndrome of man? In: Henschel EO (ed) Malignant hyperthermia, current concepts. Appleton-Century-Crofts, New York, p 79

Wingard DW (1978) Some observations on stress-susceptible patients. In: Aldrete JA, Britt BA (eds) Second international symposium on malignant hyperthermia. Grune & Stratton, New York, p 363

Wolfe BM, Gaston LW, Keltner RM (1973) Malignant hyperthermia of anaesthesia. Am J Surg 126:717

Wood DS (1978) Sarcoplasmic reticulum function and caffeine sensitivity in human malignant hyperthermia. Presented at the IVth International Congress on Neuromuscular Diseases, 1978, Montreal, Quebec

Woolf N, Hall L, Thorne C, Down M (1970) Serum creatine phosphokinase levels in pigs reacting abnormally to halogenated anaesthetics. Br Med J 3:386

Yamazaki Y, Nakazaki K, Sekomoto T, Sugawara S, Tanaka H (1971) Malignant hyperpyrexia during anaesthesia – a case report. Hiroshima J Anesth 7:103

Yana J, Kitamura E, Sha N, Nagata N, Tatekawa S, Nishimura K, Fujimori M (1977) Myoglobinuria associated with anesthesia. Hiroshima J Anesth 13:35

Yoh K, Suzuki A, Matsuura S, Ishihara T, Tsuchioka H (1974) A case of malignant hyperpyrexia and the review of aetiology. Hiroshima J Anesth 10:47

Zsigmond EK (1975) Vererbung der malignen Hyperthermie und Veränderungen der Krea-tin-Phospokinase. In: Bergmann H, Blauhut B (eds) Maligne Hyperthermie, Akupunk-tur, biomedizinische Technik, abdominelle Intensivtherapie. Springer, Berlin Heidel-berg New York, p 42

Zsigmond EK, Starkweather WH, Duboff GS, Flynn KA (1972a) Abnormal creatine-phos-phokinase isoenzyme pattern in families with malignant hyperpyrexia. Anesth Analg (Cleve) 51:827

Zsigmond EK, Starkweather WH, Duboff GS, Flynn K (1972b) CPK and malignant hyper-thermia. Anesth Analg 51:220

Zsigmond EK, Kothary SP, Penner J, Duboff GS (1978) Normal erythrocyte fragility and abnormal platelet aggregation in MH families. In: Aldrete JA, Britt BA (eds) Second international symposium on malignant hyperthermia. Grune & Stratton, New York, p 213

CHAPTER 18

Febrile Convulsions

J. B. P. STEPHENSON and C. OUNSTED

A. Introduction

In this chapter we take a fresh look at childhood febrile convulsions, hoping to provoke new paths of exploration in an exciting territory which is still surprisingly unknown. We will present new material in preference to reiterating the older evidence.

The most recent comprehensive review which is recommended reading is that by LENNOX-BUCHTHAL (1973); other monographs with a major emphasis on febrile convulsions include McGREAL (1957), OUNSTED et al. (1966), MILLICHAP (1968) and BRAZIER and COCEANI (1976).

B. Definitions: Tautology and Bogus Dichotomy

There is a deceptive simplicity about the term "febrile convulsion". However one constructs one's definition, it can be agreed that seizures with fever are common in young children. Beyond that, one runs immediately into difficulties. Because so often a seizure or convulsion (we will discuss the meaning of these terms later) follows upon a fever without any other obvious explanation, it is easy to embrace the concept of a "true" febrile convulsion. Then follow various exclusive definitions, and their respective self-fulfilling prophecies. For example, one may exclude children with "acute neurologic illness" (NELSON and ELLENBERG 1976) "such as meningitis, lead encephalopathy, marked systemic dehydration and seizures after immunization procedures". From this definition it follows that meningitis cannot be a cause of febrile convulsions, and therefore a lumbar puncture is never necessary – a disastrous fallacy! Excluding seizures after dehydration and immunization procedures assumes an underlying encephalopathy in each case, whereas in the one the convulsions may be metabolic (STEPHENSON 1971) and in the other syncopal (STEPHENSON 1979a).

The concept of benign or "simple" febrile convulsions was strongly championed by LIVINGSTONE (1954); in its extreme tautological form this definition includes "no sequelae" (McGREAL 1957) – all simple febrile convulsions are then harmless.

"Febrile convulsions apply to convulsions occurring solely with fever" was LENOX-BUCHTHAL's definition (1973), logically excluding the possibility of epilepsy as a sequela. Later (LENNOX-BUCHTHAL 1976) she admitted that her first definition was "blatantly false", and thereby gave a clue to the diverse nature of febrile convulsions which will be elaborated below. Nevertheless, like most authors, she will exclude children whose first seizure is without fever. She will also assume a genetic trait and not willingly attach the febrile convulsions label to a child with preceding brain damage or malformation: such an approach will magnify the importance of neurological sequelae.

Finally, barring McGreal (1956, 1957), Gastaut and Gastaut (1957, 1958), and the authors of earlier eras (see Temkin 1971), it has been assumed by all that febrile convulsions are *epileptic* seizures, that is, involve hypersynchronous massive discharges of populations of cerebral neurones (sudden excessive excitation of cortical grey matter). Gastaut (1974) has pointed out that seizures may be epileptic, anoxic, toxic, metabolic, or psychic. This is no mere semantic quibble. If a febrile seizure is epileptic, then a series of later afebrile seizures would suggest epilepsy. In contrast, if the febrile convulsions were anoxic or syncopal (Stephenson 1978 d), then one might expect convulsive syncope – fainting fits – as a sequela. Aside from the differing prognostic implications, the mechanisms and the pharmacology must clearly be quite distinct in these two seizure types: only the epileptic mechanism has so far received the pharmacologists' attention.

C. Difficulties in Definition

Fever or pyrexia is the easiest part of any definition of febrile convulsions. But inevitably the level of elevated temperature chosen and where this is measured are arbitrary. Also, it is unusual to know the degree of fever until after the convulsion has occurred, sometimes not for several hours or even days in some countries. The term convulsion is commonly applied to any febrile seizure (that is, loss of consciousness with fever) whether convulsive (stiff, jerking) or not. Non-convulsive seizures (atonic, absence) occur with loss of consciousness but without obvious motor accompaniments. Episodes of jerking or trembling during fever, with preservation of consciousness are not generally regarded as febrile convulsions. Hence a working definition of a "febrile convulsion" is loss of consciousness (usually but not necessarily with motor phenomena) and a temperature of say 38 °C recorded within say six hours. Even with this apparently all-embracing definition, it should be recognized that some infants with fever-associated convulsions will escape recognition, and other will be falsely diagnosed (see Meldrum, 1978, discussing fever *induced* by experimental epileptic status). A good example is the convulsions which often followed acute infantile hypernatraemia (Stephenson 1971). Such infants frequently have fever secondary to water loss, but their biochemical imbalance inhibits seizures until body fluids are diluted by rehydration several hours later.

D. Cerebral Pathology

I. Acute

The most important acute illness which affects the brain and may be associated with fever and convulsions is bacterial meningitis. Seizures are much more common in young children with this disease, and their occurrence adversely affects the prognosis (Ounsted 1951). The seizures are presumed to be epileptic in type, with no genetic component (OUNSTED 1976). Penicillin given in the treatment of bacterial meningitis may itself appear to cause epileptic convulsions, not merely through absolute overdose but speculatively because of breakdown of the blood–cerebrospinal fluid/brain barrier (MARKS and HIRSHFELD, 1968). It has always been surprising that this penicillin-induced epileptic status, if such it were, never caused brain damage in febrile children. The explanation seems to be that the asymmetrical stimulus-sensitive multifocal myoclonus induced by penicillin is not epileptic status at all, but a convincing mimic of it. Evidence from its occurrence in a brain-dead adult is convincing that the muscle twitching results from neuronal discharges no higher than the caudal brain-stem and possibly in the spinal cord itself (SACK-ELLARES and SMITH 1979).

II. Chronic

Malformation of the brain, or damage to it before, during, or after birth may be followed by presumably epileptic seizures during childhood febrile illnesses. If the cerebral pathology is sufficiently gross, it will be apparent on prospective neuro-developmental examination before the first febrile convulsion (NELSON and ELLEN-BERG 1976, 1978) or inferred from the medical history and examination findings after the convulsion. Lesser degrees of chronic cerebral pathology may be undetectable by these means. Although it is impossible to exclude pre-existing small cerebral lesions, it is reasonable to use data from children with definite or probable cerebral pathology as internal controls to compare and contrast with those whose febrile convulsions appear to require a specific genetic predisposition without obvious structural defect. We will do this in a later section.

Mention should be made of the small cell collections (variously called alien tissue, hamartia, or hamartomata) which have been found in temporal lobectomy specimens. In the biographies of these patients with temporal lobe epilepsy, some, with hamartia or hamartomata only, have no history of earlier febrile convulsions. This prenatal cerebral pathology does not of itself imply that an individual will experience seizures during the inevitable febrile illness of childhood. However, in a small proportion of those with mesial temporal sclerosis found on temporal lobectomy, hamartia, or hamartomata are present *in addition* (OUNSTED unpublished).

While it is known that prolonged febrile convulsions may do the damage which the pathologist later calls mesial temporal sclerosis, it is not known how often such febrile convulsions owe their existence and localization to a preceding malformation such as we have described.

E. Mechanisms of Febrile Convulsions

From their description, febrile seizures could be anoxic (syncopal), epileptic, or a combination of the two (STEPHENSON 1978 d). At the time of writing, the onset of spontaneous natural febrile convulsions has not been recorded polygraphically, so conclusions about their nature must be inferential. Best known is the epileptic mechanism, which will be discussed first.

I. Epileptic Seizure Mechanism

Epileptic seizures commonly result from hypersynchronous discharges of populations of cerebral neurones (GASTAUT and BROUGHTON 1972). In clonic or tonic–clonic convulsive seizures there is no bradycardia or asystole, but rather tachycardia at the onset (GASTAUT and BROUGHTON 1972). Recently a different polygraphic appearance has been described in certain tonic seizures. In these so-called "generalized cortical electrodecremental events" there is a suppression and desynchronization of the electroencephalogram (EEG) coupled with bradycardia or even asystole (FARIELLO et al. 1979).

Rarely, epileptic febrile seizures have been induced in children experimentally and recorded polygraphically. In one such example the injection of sulphur oil into a genetically susceptible 7-year-old led to fever and an atonic seizure at 39.2 °C with generalized spike and wave, and tachycardia without asystole (GASTAUT and TASSINARI 1966, p. 92–94). It is presumed that the febrile convulsions in children with acute or chronic cerebral pathology, are intrinsically cerebral and therefore epileptic in type (STEPHENSON 1978 d, 1979 a). The same applies to hemiclonic seizures, although in such children no evidence of gross underlying pathology may be detected on computerized X-ray tomography (CT scan) of the brain (GASTAUT and GASTAUT 1977).

Indirect evidence comes from studies of the factors which predict later epilepsy. A suspect neurodevelopmental examination, implying an abnormal brain, is the most powerful predictor (NELSON and ELLENBERG 1976; ANNEGERS et al. 1979). Of the features of the febrile seizure itself, lateralization (hemiconvulsion) is the most important (NELSON and ELLENBERG 1976). When a convulsion continues sufficiently long to persist after arrival in hospital – febrile status epilepticus – the epileptic component of the seizure can be established with certainty (AICARDI and CHEVRIE 1970), although the mode of onset can only be guessed at.

We shall present evidence to show that, although EEG spikes (brief high-voltage discharges) do not predict later epilepsy (LENNOX-BUCHTHAL 1973), they may reflect, at least in part, an epileptic mechanism for the febrile convulsions in such children. Such EEG spikes appear during development, and are much more frequently detected after the age of three years than before (LENNOX-BUCHTHAL 1973; TSUBOI and ENDO 1977; TSUBOI 1978; this chapter Sect. F.II, F.IV).

II. Anoxic Seizure Mechanism

Although it is perhaps naive to assume anoxia to be responsible, it has been known for many years that sudden reduction in cerebral circulation would cause convulsive seizures or syncope (COOPER 1836; KUSSMAUL and TENNER 1959; LASLETT 1909). "Anoxic" seizures have since been extensively studied, whether caused by breath-holding (BRIDGE et al. 1943; GAUK et al. 1963; LIVINGSTON 1970; RENDLE-SHORT 1972), reflex asystole (ACKER et al. 1973; FADEN et al. 1977; GAUSTAUT and GAUSTAUT 1957, 1958; GASTAUT 1968, 1974; GASTAUT and FISCHER-WILLIAMS 1957; GASTAUT et al. 1961; KELLAWAY and DRUCKMAN, cited in MEYER and WALTZ 1961; LAXDAL et al. 1969; LOMBROSO and LERMAN 1967; MAULSBY and KELLAWAY 1964; RASMUSSEN et al. 1978; SCHLESINGER 1973; SCHLESINGER et al. 1977; STEPHEN-

SON 1978 a, b, c, 1979 b) or vena caval obstruction (PAMPIGLIONE and WATERSTON 1961).

In the EEG department, "anoxic" seizures due to cardiac asystole can be reproduced by ocular compression which activates the vagal-mediated oculocardiac reflex (LOMBROSO and LERMAN 1967; STEPHENSON 1978 a, b). In such anoxic seizures there may be gross slowing of the EEG, or flattening if the child is young or the cardiac asystole long. The observer may note a constellation of seizure phenomena (STEPHENSON 1980 b). First there is flexion of the upper limbs with upward eye deviation and then a series of downward eye jerks. One or two extension jerks may follow, with snorting, sometimes tongue biting, and large pupils. Urinary incontinence, if it occurs, is during or at the conclusion of the EEG flattening. Then a further burst of downward eye jerks is followed by awakening, sometimes with disorientation or agitation for several seconds. No colour change is necessarily observed, but pallor, or flushing followed by pallor, or a tinge of cyanosis followed by pallor, are common.

In these anoxic seizures of vagocardiac origin, the manifestations at any age are related to duration of asystole but the relationship is not exact and we do not know if electromechanical dissociation can occur as is reported after acute myocardial infarction (MARSHALL 1978) – if that were the case electrocardiographic (ECG) complexes would be seen on the tracing but propulsive ventricular contraction would be weak or absent. It is our experience (STEPHENSON 1980 b) that crying or hyperventilation before ocular compression makes it unlikely that cardiac asystole may be induced, while rebreathing to bring the partial pressure of carbon dioxide (pCO_2) back to normal will restore vagal sensitivity. This is in line with other evidence on the modification of bradycardia by respiration (GANDEVIA et al. 1978 a, b; ANONYMOUS 1978; DALY and ANGELL-JAMES 1979) and the long-known point that acidaemia blocks the inhibitory action of vagal acetycholine on the heart (GESSEL et al. 1944).

Although it is self-evident that the anoxic seizures induced by ocular compression under polygraphic control are due simply to cardiac arrest, it is more difficult to establish the nature of naturally occurring reflex anoxic seizures such as follow surprising pain. Five related pieces of evidence support the assertion that they also result from vagal-mediated cardiac standstill (STEPHENSON 1978 a).

1) The natural attacks closely resemble the experimental seizures induced when ocular compression leads to cardiac asystole either sitting (GASTAUT and GASTAUT 1958; GASTAUT et al. 1961; GASTAUT 1974) or supine (LOMBROSO and LERMAN 1967; STEPHENSON 1978 a).

2) If ocular compression induces an anoxic seizure in a particular child, the parent witnessing it recognizes it to be identical to the child's regular attacks (GASTAUT and GASTAUT 1958; LOMBROSO and LERMAN 1967; STEPHENSON 1978 a).

3) Even if an anoxic seizure is not induced by ocular compression, asystole of four seconds or more is likely (LOMBROSO and LERMAN 1967; STEPHENSON 1978 a).

4) When naturally occurring reflex anoxic seizures have been witnessed or recorded, extreme bradycardia or asystole hase been observed at the onset (BRIDGE et al. 1943; MAULSBY and KELLAWAY 1964; LOMBROSO and LERMAN 1967 – Fig. 10).

5) Atropine prevents both the naturally occuring seizures and the abnormal oculocardiac response (MAULSBY and KELLAWAY 1964; LOMBROSO and LERMAN

1967). This applies both to atropine sulphate 0.01 mg kg^{-1} day^{-1} and to atropine methonitrate 0.3–0.6 mg kg^{-1} day^{-1} (Stephenson 1979 b).

It is worth commenting that vagal-mediated cardiac asystole, blocked by atropine, has been implicated in both primary cerebral and cardiac dysfunction. Accompanying the seizures of cerebral origin induced by electroconvulsive therapy (ECT), atropine-sensitive bradyarrhythmias have long been recognised (Bankhead and Towens 1950; Richardson et al. 1957). A similar atropine-reversible asystole has also been described in both acute and chronic "sick sinus syndrome" (Shaw 1979) but one suspects that in some of the chronic cases (Mendel et al. 1972; Scarpa 1976) the diagnosis of structural disease of the heart was tenuous and that pharmacological studies would have suggested alternative machanisms (Dighton 1974).

Although reflex vagal-mediated cardiac asystole is generally regarded as benign and reversible (Lombroso and Lerman 1967; Stephenson 1978 a), one fatal case of what is almost certainly the same condition has been reported (Paulson 1963) and an animal model with catastrophic potential has been described (Branch et al. 1977). In the fatal case, the child vomited, was given mouth-to-mouth respiration, and taken erect to hospital in a car. The resulting irreversible cortical destruction was attributed, speculatively, to a combination of pulmonary aspiration and cerebral hypoperfusion exacerbated by gravity.

A recent example of near fatal reflex anoxic seizures and their prevention by a atropine methonitrate will be of interest to pharmacologists (Stephenson 1979 b).

Case Report. A girl aged 2 years 7 months, weight 12 kg, had a history of holding her breath without crying immediately after every painful stimulus since infancy. Her father had been similarly affected. After a bath she bumped, took a breath, went limp and glazed and white, with eyes rolling and large pupils. She then went stiff straight out in her mother's arms and jerked and frothed. After this, and just as her eyes were beginning to follow, she vomited, then stopped breathing and became limp and motionless. Her mother, a trained nurse, put her onto the floor on her side, sucked and then breathed into her mouth. She thought the child was already dead. When the ambulance arrived, an airway was put in, and both, mother and child were whisked off to the intensive care unit. Then the child cried and spoke to her mother.

Two days later ocular compression supine induced 9.8 s asystole, general gross slowing of the EEG, and an anoxic seizure with upper limb flexion and dazed appearance. After waking, she was pale and slept for four hours. Her heart rate had been approximately 126/min before the ocular compression. Her mother insisted that she be atropinized and that ocular compression studies be used to confirm protection against future attacks.

She was treated with atropine methonitrate drops 0.8 mg five times daily (4 mg/day, 0.33 mg kg^{-1} day^{-1}. The next day she had fever, which then disappeared spontaneously. Three days later, ocular compression induced asystole of 2.3 s with no after-pallor or sleepiness: heart rate was 102–140/min beforehand. No atropine side effects were evident. Twenty-four hours later, on 1.6 mg atropine methonitrate five times daily (8 mg/day; 0.66 mg kg^{-1} day^{-1}), and 3¾ h after the last dose, ocular compression still only induced 2.3 s asystole, with no respiratory arrest or pallor. The heart rate beforehand had been 102–136/min, and dryness of the mouth was evident. The child went home on this dose, with her mother.

The following day the child fell off a table; she held her breath but had no other vagal signs. Five days later the mother's confidence was much improved, but the child was awakening at night because of dryness of the nostrils and her lips were cracking; pupils were normal, heart rate 132–140/min. The dose of atropine methonitrate was then tailed down to 4 mg/day in four doses, and side effects disappeared with clinical control remaining.

That *febrile* convulsions could be anoxic or ischaemic seizures is not a new idea. More recently than Hippocrates (quoted in TEMKIN 1971) an anoxic mechanism was proposed by KUSSMAUL and TENNER (1859) and again by McGREAL (1956, 1957), and GASTAUT and GASTAUT (1957, 1958). Twenty years later, a review of the history of children with vagocardiac reflex anoxic seizures (STEPHENSON 1978a) disclosed that, in addition to pain and other well-known precipitations, fever appeared to have been responsible for identical seizures in 14% – this incidence was much greater ($P < 0.002$) than the 3.4% expected (NELSON and ELLENBERG 1976). A prospective study of 100 children with febrile convulsions supported the concept of an anoxic mechanism (STEPHENSON 1978d) and this is further strengthened by new data presented in a later series.

III. Combined Anoxic and Epileptic Mechanism

While an anoxic mechanism may of itself account for a brief tonic febrile seizure with immediate recovery it cannot be the whole story in a fevered child who stiffens and then has 30 min of clonic jerking. We have seen an epileptic seizure precipitated by an anoxic seizure which was itself induced by ocular compression (STEPHENSON, personal observation, in a girl with septo-optic dysplasia). That such a combined mechanism may be operating in certain febrile convulsions will be elaborated below. It has been suggested independently that the febrile seizures in cerebral malaria are anoxic in origin, even though their continuation may be clearly due to an epileptic mechanism (BRUETON 1978). BRUETON found that the critical determinant was the level of haemoglobin ($P < 0.001$). He also observed that the group of children with falciparum parasitaemia, anaemia, and convulsions had features in common with genetic febrile convulsions: age was between six months and four years, male: female ratio was high, and there was an increased past and family history of febrile convulsions.

One may speculate that so-called stress convulsions (FRIIS and LUND 1974), when they are not simply convulsive syncope, involve a combination of the anoxic and epileptic mechanisms. In this way they may resemble febrile convulsions to which they are genetically closely linked.

A note of caution is worthwhile in regard to the analysis of anoxic and epileptic mechanisms. A recent paper (ZIEGLER and LIN 1978) suggested that the convulsive syncope which may abruptly follow blood donation in the supine position must be of primarily cerebral origin and not caused by cardiac asystole, because the research nurse never detected an absent pulse. Since cardiac contractions normally resume at the onset of anoxic seizures, only prospective monitoring will detect the cardiac component.

F. Ocular Compression Study of Febrile Convulsion Phenotypes and Genotypes

In this section we present original data from four related studies of the oculocardiac response in febrile convulsions and related paroxysmal disorders. These studies were generated after analysis of 118 children who had ocular compression, 58

Table 1. Syncope (105 children over the age of eight years): relation to previous febrile convulsions

	Previous history of febrile convulsions	No febrile convulsions	Total (% FC)
Type of syncope			
Simple syncope	3	69	72 (4%)
Convulsive syncope	8	25	33 (24%)
Oculocardiac reflex			
Asystole under 2 s on OC	0	47	47 (0%)
2 s or more asystole on OC	11	47	58 (19%)

$P = 0.006$ (between simple and convulsive syncope)
$P = 0.005$ (between asystole under 2 s and 2 s or more asystole on OC)

OC = Ocular compression; FC = Febrile convulsions

of them after reflex anoxic seizures (Stephenson 1978 a). Since then approximately 3,000 ocular compressions have been undertaken using the same technique (Stephenson, personal observations).

I. Syncope: Relation to Previous Febrile Convulsions

This first study is a retrospective analysis of older children with syncope. All children over eight years of age at the time of test, who had had ocular compression (OC) under EEG and ECG control, and who had clear diagnoses of syncope or convulsive syncope (fainting with stiffness, and perhaps jerking, i.e. a motor anoxic seizure), were coded for type of syncope, duration of asystole on OC and previous history of febrile convulsions. None had EEG spikes (this was a finding, not a criterion).

Table 1 displays the results. It is evident that in simple syncope, presumed to be of vasovagal mechanism without cardiac asystole, the incidence of previous febrile convulsions does not differ from that in the general population (Nelson and Ellenberg 1976). By contrast, a quarter of those with convulsive syncope had a history of earlier febrile convulsions ($P = 0.006$). Such a finding is consistent with the hypothesis that both the convulsive syncope of the older child and the febrile convulsion have an "anoxic" mechanism in the form of vagal-mediated cardiac asystole. In accord with this, it was found that all children with previous febrile convulsions and syncope, convulsive or otherwise, had asystole on OC of 2 s or over ($P = 0.005$).

II. Febrile Convulsion Trial

The criteria for entry to this trial were any seizure or seizures with fever, no exclusions, all under eight years of age when tested.

A total of 630 children were admitted to the trial (indicated by the symbol FC 630 in the tables). All children had documented fever of 38 °C or over within

6 h of the febrile seizures; none were excluded except on grounds of age (over eight years). All had ocular compression, with EEG and ECG running. On each occasion, before OC, clinical diagnosis was made as follows:

Classification was made into three groups on basis of description of febrile convulsion and physical examination of the child, without reference to the EEG:

I. "Anoxic" (syncopal).
II. "Encephalopathic" (acute or chronic cerebral pathology or hemiconvulsions).
III. Unclassified ("others" including anoxic–epileptic combinations, and seizures not convincingly I or II).

I. The "anoxic" type of febrile convulsion was defined as: the seizures with fever conform to one or more of these descriptions:
   1. Tonic only.
   2. Tonic with one or two jerks.
   3. Indistinguishable by history from ordinary reflex anoxic seizures.
   4. Resemble the reflex anoxic seizures induced by other stimuli in the same child.

   The seizure descriptions suggested anoxic seizures in 111 cases in all.

II. The second category of febrile convulsions, "encephalopathic", was employed in two situations:
   1. Cerebral pathology (with or without hemiconvulsions)
      a) Acute (bacterial meningitis, viral encephalitis, e.g. herpes, etc.)
      b) Chronic (cerebral palsies, evidence of cerebral malformations, mental handicap with dysmorphic features but excluding unaccompanied developmental delay).
   2. Hemiconvulsions (hemiclonic or lateralized convulsive seizures, suggesting focal epileptic origin, but without other evidence of focal pathology, and excluding generalised non-focal seizures followed by hemisyndrome, e.g. Todd's paralysis or hemiplegia).

   The seizures in such children are presumed to be epileptic, irrespective of the EEG appearances. Of the total, 30 had evidence of acute or chronic cerebral pathology as detailed in Table 2; the remaining 72 had lateralized convulsions or hemiconvulsions.

III. The remaining 417 children, the "others", could not be classified as "anoxic" or "encephalopathic" by the clinical method used. Such seizures might have an "anoxic" onset, but many clonic jerks thereafter.

   Included were:
   1. Generalized (bilateral) clonic seizures followed by Todd's hemiparesis, or permanent hemiplegia.
   2. Minor deviations such as left- or right-handedness in the first year of life.
   3. Any febrile seizure with inadequate description for classification purposes.

The composition of the series is displayed in Table 3. Of note is the male predominance except in hemiconvulsions, EEG spikes in all types but most in the encephalopathic group, and the clustering of prolonged asystole and first degree family history of febrile convulsions into the "anoxic" group and less so into the "others".

Table 4 shows that the median asystole on OC was significantly long in the "anoxic" group: this table will be discussed further in Sect. III (Pertussis immunisa-

Table 2. Details of cerebral pathology in 30 consecutive children with febrile seizures (FC 630)

Intractable multifocal epilepsy, MH-presumed prenatal malformation
First seizure with meningococcal meningitis at six months
Congenital right hemiplegia
Sotos syndrome (cerebral gigantism)
Severe birth asphyxia, microcephaly, tetraplegia
Spastic diparesis
Fractured skull and right subdural, craniotomy (battered baby)
Neonatal DIC + hypoglycaemia; dysequilibrium–disparesis; hydrocephalus
Congenital right hemiparesis
Trigonocephaly, hypotonia, severe MH
Neonatal *E. Coli* meningitis–left hemiparesis
Asymmetrical tetraplegia ? malformation
Dysmorphic MH–prenatal malformation
Neonatal asphyxia and status epilepticus
Meningomyelocele: shunted hydrocephalus
Post-neonatal listeria monocytogenes meningitis
Acute herpes simplex encephalitis
Acute herpes simplex encephalitis
"Arrested hydrocephalus"
Birth asphyxia–cerebral palsy
Congenital right hemiparesis
Haemophilus influenzae meningitis recently
Neonatal status epilepticus
Neonatal right hemiconvulsions and right hemisyndrome
Meningomyelocele: hydrocephalus
? Cerebral venous thrombosis post-neonatal: left hemiparesis
Clinical meningoencephalitis (acute)
Prenatal cerebral malformation presumed–MH
Hydrocephalus + meningocele
Global delay; left hemisyndrome; Sotos syndrome

MH = Mental handicap; DIC = Disseminated intravascular coagulation

Table 3. Composition of febrile convulsion trial (FC 630)

	Anoxic	Encephalopathic		Unclassified (others)	Total
		Hemi-	Cerebral pathology		
Number of children	111	72	30	417	630
Males	70	33	17	258	378
Females	41	39	13	159	252
Male: female ratio	1.71	0.85	1.31	1.62	1.50
EEG spikes	5 (4.5%)	8 (11.1%)	4 (13%)	21 (5.0%)	38 (5.9%)
7 s asystole on OC[a]	25 (22.5%)	1 (1.4%)	1 (3%)	22 (5.3%)	49 (7.8%)
lst degree relative with FC	21 (18.9%)	4 (5.6%)	0 (0%)	50 (12.0%)	75 (11.9%)

[a] 7 s asystole on OC is chosen as abnormally long because 70% with asystole of 7 s or more had anoxic seizures induced, while none was induced after less than 7 s asystole

Table 4. Febrile convulsion groups (FC 630) compared with pertussis immunization convulsions (12)

Type of FC	Number of children	Median asystole on OC (s)	Median age at test (months)	Number with FC in 1st degree relative	Number with Todd's paralysis or hemiplegia after FC
Anoxic	111	3.6	35	21 (18.9%)	0 (0%)
Encephalopathic	102	1.2	24	4 (3.9%)	16 (15.7%)
Unclassified (others)	417	1.6	30	50 (12.0%)	6 (1.4%)
Total	630	1.7	30	75 (11.9%)	22 (3.5%)
PIC	12	3.7	$25\frac{1}{2}$	2 (17%)	0 (0%)

PIC = Pertussis immunization convulsions

Table 5. Median asystole on OC in febrile convulsions subgroups (FC 630)

	Number	Duration(s)
Hemiconvulsions	72	1.2
Cerebral pathology	30	1.0
Unclassified–1st-degree relative with FC	50	3.5
No 1st-degree relative with FC	367	1.4
Total–1st-degree relative with FC	75	3.4
–Parent[a] with FC	34	3.4
–Sibling[a] with FC	47	3.8

[a] Six with both parent and sibling affected

Table 6. Prolonged asystole on ocular compression related to first degree family history of febrile convulsions (FC 630)

	Asystole on OC 7 s or over	
FH of FC	16 (21.3%)	75
FH negative	33 (5.9%)	555
	49 (7.8%)	630

First-degree $\chi^2 = 19.7$; $P < 0.0001$
OC = Ocular compression; FH = Family history

tion convulsions). In Table 5, further subdivision of the material reveals that a prolonged median asystole on OC is a feature of children who have a first-degree relative, i.e. parent or sibling, affected by febrile convulsions. Taking 7 s as representing a very long asystole on OC (because 70% of children having 7 s or more asystole on OC had anoxic seizures thereby induced, but *no* anoxic seizures resulted

Table 7. Todd's paresis or hemiplegia after febrile convulsions (FC 630)

Sex	Side of post-ictal weakness		
	Right	Left	
Male	6	3	9
Female	1	12	13
	7	15	22

$P = 0.01$ (Fisher's exact test)

Table 8. Todd's paresis or hemiplegia related to type of febrile convulsion (FC 630)

Anoxic		0/111	(0%)
Encephalopathic	Cerebral pathology	4/30	(13.3%)
	Hemiconvulsions	12/72	(16.7%)
Unclassified	lst-degree relative with FC	0/50	(0%)
(Others)	No FC in lst-degree relative	6/367	(1.6%)[a]

[a] Abnormal handedness in three; 7 s or more asystole on OC in two

Table 9. Spikes in EEG more common after the age of three years in febrile seizures except "cerebral pathology" (FC 630)

FC group	Under three years		Three years or over		Total children
	Spikes	No. of children	Spikes	No. of children	
Unclassified	8 (3.2%)	252	13 (7.9%)	165	417
Anoxic	0 (0%)	57	5 (9.3%)	54	111
Hemi-	2 (4.3%)	46	6 (23.1%)	26	72
Cerebral pathology	3 (17.6%)	17	1 (7.7%)	13	30
	13 (3.5%)	372	25 (9.7%)	258	630

Less than three years vs three years or over–$\chi^2 = 9.25$, $P < 0.005$
Omitting cerebral pathology–$\chi^2 = 11.9$, $P < 0.001$

from asystole of less than 7 s, Table 6 confirms that having an affected first-degree relative increases the likelihood of an excessive oculocardiac reflex very highly significantly ($P < 0.0001$).

Of the 630 children, 22 had Todd's paresis (temporary hemiparesis) or permanent hemiplegia. This was left-sided, implying right cerebral hemisphere pathology, in 12 of 13 girls, and right-sided in 6 of 9 boys (Table 7). This confirms the results of studies previously reported (Taylor 1969; Taylor and Ounsted 1971; Ounsted 1976).

Table 8 further analyses these children with transient or permanent weakness. Most hemipareses followed hemiconvulsions with or without obvious pre-existing cerebral pathology. The few who had generalized bilateral clonic febrile seizures and post-ictal unilateral weakness are insufficient for statistical analysis, but they did have histories of preceeding minor abnormalities of handedness (e.g. being left-handed aged eight months) and a tendency to prolonged asystole on OC quite different from that recorded in the "encephalopathic" group.

It may be speculated that in these six children a combination of fever-induced anoxic seizure, a subclinical pre-existing cerebral lesion, and a long secondary epileptic seizure interacted to the injury of the vulnerable segment of brain.

Finally, Table 9 confirms previous findings (LENNOX-BUCHTHAL 1973; TSUBOI and ENDO 1977, TSUBOI 1978) that in children with febrile convulsions EEG spikes are much more common over the age of three years. However, in the small number in the subgroup with cerebral pathology, we found no increased incidence of spikes with age.

III. Pertussis Immunization Convulsions

Pertussis vaccine is highly reactogenic (BARKIN and PICHICHERO 1979) and innoculations which contain the pertussis vaccine, are more likely to be followed by convulsions (usually febrile) than are diphtheria and tetanus vaccines (EHERENGUT 1974). Despite convincing evidence of its protective value (CHURCH 1979), acceptance in a number of countries has declined with the growth of the belief in the pertussis vaccine as a direct cause of death or of a damaging irreversible encephalopathy (KUHLENKAMPFF et al. 1974; STEWART 1977). This belief is not supported by any recent study (WILLIAMS 1976; MELCHIOR 1977, FUKUYAMA et al. 1977; Tsucbiya et al. 1978; GRIFFITH 1978; BELLMAN et al. 1979).

However, the mechanism of the vaccine-associated convulsions is important. If they can be damaging, pharmacological prophylaxis deserves investigation. If not, then this should be made clear for public reassurance.

Over 2 years, 12 consecutive children with a history of at least one seizure within 48 h of pertussis-containing immunization were investigated by OC (STEPHENSON 1979a).

In each case the child satisfied the definition of febrile convulsions given in Sect. II (Febrile Convulsion Trial). The individual asystole readings on OC in order of magnitude were: 0.6, 2.4, 2.4, 2.8, 3.4, 3.6, 3.8, 4.5, 6.5, 12.6, 13.4, and 19.6 s. Three children with febrile convulsions after whooping cough who were examined concurrently had asystole readings of 0.4, 0.5, and 1.3 s, significantly lower values ($P = 0.02$, two-tailed Wilcoxon or Mann–Whitney U test). A summary of the findings in pertussis immunization convulsions is given in Table 4 and Fig. 1. The apparent similarity between the results and those in "anoxic" febrile convulsions is confirmed by multiple linear regression analysis which also strengthens the significance of the difference between the pertussis immunization convulsions and "encephalopathic" febrile convulsions ($P = 0.01$).

On this evidence it is suggested that convulsions after pertussis immunization have a vagal-mediated "anoxic" mechanism, while convulsions after the disease pertussis may be truly encephalopathic.

IV. Genetic Analysis: Febrile Convulsions and/or Reflex Anoxic Seizures

In this section we try to disentangle the mechanism and genetics of febrile convulsions further, by looking at a large number of children identified by an excessive

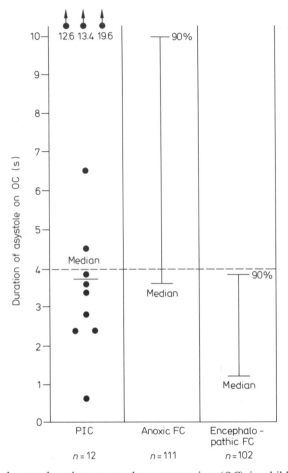

Fig. 1. Individual asystole values on ocular compression (*OC*) in children with pertussis immunization convulsions (*PIC*) compared with median and 90th percentile for two types of febrile convulsions (*FC*)

Table 10. Ocular compression induced 7 s asystole or more and an anoxic seizure in these children with a history of febrile convulsions, reflex anoxic seizures, or a combination of both

Age at test (years)	History			Number of children (families)
	Febrile convulsions	Febrile convulsions and reflex anoxic seizures or syncope	Reflex anoxic seizures	
≥ 3	24 (23)	21 (20)[a]	36 (35)[a]	81 (78)[a]
< 3	20	7	35 (34)[a]	62 (61)[a]
	44 (43)	28 (27)[a]	71[b] (69)[a]	143 (139)[a]

[a] in parentheses ( ): number of families–where two siblings both tested
[b] Includes five children from three sets of identical twins with reflex anoxic seizures

Table 11. Ocular compression induced 7 s or more asystole but no anoxic seizure in these children with a history of febrile convulsions, reflex anoxic seizures, or a combination of both

| Age at test (years) | History | | | Number of children/ families [a] |
	Febrile convulsions	Febrile convulsions and reflex anoxic seizures or syncope	Reflex anoxic seizures	
≥ 3	14	8	4	26
< 3	14	4	5	23
	28	12	9	49

[a] No sibling pairs were tested, so number of children = number of families

Table 12. Sex ratios in febrile convulsions and reflex anoxic seizures contrasted (OC 7+)

| | Type of seizure, by history | | | |
	Male	Female	Total	M:F ratio
Febrile convulsions [a]	41	31	72	1.32
Both febrile convulsions and reflex anoxic seizures or syncope	20	20	40	1.00
Reflex anoxic seizures [a]	28	52	80	0.54
Total	89	103	192 [b]	

[a] $\chi^2 = 6,5$; $P = 0,01$
[b] From 188 families

oculocardiac reflex. These children had a history of either febrile convulsions, or reflex anoxic seizures or both. The majority (139 children from 143 families) had anoxic seizures induced by ocular compression (Table 10). The remainder (49 children from 49 families) had prolonged asystole without any apparent seizure occurring (Table 11). The first genetic point is that there were three pairs of identical twins concordant for reflex anoxic seizures (Table 10); five of these children are in this series, the sixth had an asystole between 6 and 7 s and is therefore excluded (i.e. she had a history of reflex anoxic seizure but one was not provoked by ocular compression).

The sex ratio shows distinct differences ($P = 0.01$) between male-dominated febrile convulsions and the strong female preponderance in "pure" reflex anoxic seizures (Table 12). The group with both febrile seizures and afebrile anoxic seizures or syncope are intermediate, with no sex difference.

Spikes on EEG were seen in 10% of the series. As in the febrile convulsion trial described in the previous section, spikes were not common till the age of three years or over (Table 13). Two children with cerebral pathology and spikes were excluded from this analysis since we found previously that their spikes were not related to age. We then looked at the children in this series who had febrile convulsions (whether or not they *also* had reflex anoxic seizures or syncope) and were of the

Table 13. EEG spikes more common after the age of three years in children with febrile convulsions and abnormal oculocardiac reflex (OC 7+)

Age at test (years)	Spikes	No spikes	Total with 7 s asystole on OC
≥ 3	10 (14.9%)	56	66
< 3	1 (2.3%)	43	44
	11 (10.0%)	99	110[a]

$P = 0.02$ (Fisher's exact test)
[a] Two children with cerebral pathology excluded

Table 14. EEG spikes relate to clonic (unclassified and hemiclonic) rather than pure "anoxic" febrile convulsions in children age three years or over with excessive oculocardiac reflex (OC 7+)

Type of febrile convulsion	Spikes	No spikes	Total
Anoxic	2 (5.6%)	34	36
Remainder excluding cerebral pathology[a] (Unclassified and hemiclonic)	8 (26.7%)	22	30
	10 (15.2%)	56	66

$P = 0.017$ (Fisher's exact test)
[a] Two children

Table 15. First-degree relative with seizure or syncope is equally likely whether or not an anoxic seizure is induced, in series of children with 7 s or more asystole on OC, and history of febrile convulsions and or reflex anoxic seizures

	First-degree relative affected	Number of families
Anoxic seizure induced by OC	36 (25.9%)	139
No anoxic seizures on OC	13 (26.5%)	49
Total	49 (26.0%)	188

OC = ocular compression

age three years or over, to see whether the appearance of spikes in the EEG was related to the type of febrile convulsion. It was (Table 14). Spikes were seen in only about 5% of those with febrile convulsions which by history sounded to be "anoxic" but in more than a quarter of those with clonic (generalized or hemi-) febrile convulsions.

Lastly we made some preliminary observations on the genetics. In 49 of the 188 families, a first-degree relative of the proband had a history of seizures or syncope (Table 15). The incidence of affected first-degree relatives was the same in those in

Table 16. No effect of age at test on likelihood of first-degree relative with seizure or syncope, in series of children with 7 s or more asystole on OC, and history of febrile convulsions and/ or reflex anoxic seizures

Age at test (years)	First degree relative affected	Number of families
≥ 3	28 (26.9%)	103
< 3	21 (24.7%)	85
Total	49 (26.1%)	188

Table 17. First-degree family history of seizures or syncope is related to type of seizure disorder (children with 7 s or more asystole on OC)

Seizure disorder	First-degree relative affected	Number of families
Reflex anoxic seizures (RAS)	10 (12.8%)	78
Febrile convulsions (FC)	19 (26.8%)	71
Both febrile convulsions and reflex anoxic seizures or syncope in the same child (FCRASS)	20 (51.3%)	39
Total	49 (26.1%)	188

RAS vs FC–$\chi^2 = 3.71$, $P \simeq 0.05$
FC vs FCRASS–$\chi^2 = 5.57$, $P < 0.02$
RAS vs FCRASS–$\chi^2 = 18.5$, $P < 0.0001$

whom an anoxic seizure was actually induced as in the remainder with asystole on OC of 7 c or over (Table 15). Therefore, all were included in further analyses.

It was guessed that probands under three years of age might have less affected first-degree relatives than the older children, but again, as shown in Table 16, there was no difference, so all ages are included in the final analyses.

Table 17 displays the striking increase in the proportion of children with a first-degree relative affected by any type of seizure or syncope as one proceeds from pure reflex anoxic seizures, through pure febrile convulsions, to febrile convulsions and reflex anoxic seizures or syncope in the same child. The percentage doubles at each step. Examining the history of seizure or syncope in the first-degreee relative more closely it is evident that there is strong concordance between the type of seizure in the proband and in the first-degree relative (Table 18). Febrile convulsions are recorded in first-degree relatives of a fifth of the probands with febrile convulsions, but in none of the relatives of those with pure reflex anoxic seizures (Table 19). Most interesting is the group of children with a history of a combination of febrile convulsions and afebrile reflex anoxic seizures or syncope. Their affected relatives segregate into febrile convulsions alone, febrile convulsions with reflex anoxic seizures and/or syncope, and syncope (convulsive or otherwiese).

Table 18. Type of seizure or syncopal disorder in affected first-degree relatives of children with febrile convulsions, reflex anoxic seizures, or a combination in the same child (OC 7+)

One or more 1st-degree relatives affected by:	Diagnosis in proband by history			Total number of families
	Febrile convulsions	Combination of febrile convulsions and reflex anoxic seizures or syncope	Reflex anoxic seizures	
Febrile convulsions	14	8		22
Combination of febrile convulsions and reflex anoxic seizures or syncope		6		6
Reflex anoxic seizures			7	7
Syncope or convulsive syncope	1	4	2	7
Convulsive breath-holding	1			1
Stress convulsions	1			1
Childhood fits	1			1
Convulsions		1		1
?Temporal lobe epilepsy		1		1
Epilepsy			1	1
Febrile convulsions in one parent syncope in the other	1			1
Total number of families	19	20	10	49

Table 19. First-degree family history of febrile convulsions is common when proband has febrile convulsions but not seen in cases of pure afebrile reflex anoxic seizures (OC 7+)

Diagnosis in proband by history	Febrile convulsions in 1st-degree relative	Total number of families
Febrile convulsions only	15 (21.1%)	71
Afebrile reflex anoxic seizures only	0 (0%)	78

$\chi^2 = 15.7$, $P < 0.0001$

V. Clinical Example: Genetic Anoxic Seizures, Syncope, and Febrile Convulsions

As an illustration of the type of history obtained in a child with "combined febrile convulsions and reflex anoxic seizures or syncope" we include a brief case report. Although it will be seen that this child had an anoxic seizure in the EEG laboratory, she did not have 7 s asystole on ocular compression and so was not included in the series analysed above.

Case report (The phraseology of the parents is indicated by quotation marks). A girl was born in September 1965. At the age of three, she split her chin and when the stitches came out she "had a faint" and was incontinent ("wet"). At three and a half she was unwell with a fever and was feeling sick and "walked through" and fell down and became "awful stiff". She had a total of three such episodes with fever before the age of five and also two similar episodes when her mother was brushing her hair. They were all about the same. When she went to school at five the school doctor asked questions and she went to hospital, had an EEG and started phenobarbitone. Since then she has had occasional "turns", about once in nine months. Most have been precipitated by emotional situations such as going to a doctor or a dentist, but one was in the night on the stairs when the mother found a pool of water on the carpet and a bruise on her face, and once the child said "I think I'm going to faint" for no apparent reason. The general sequence of events was that the child would feel sweaty and her head "going funny and dizzy and feeling sleepy" and she would "go out" with eyes rolling and rigidity and incontinence of urine and then afterwards grab her mother and want to sleep, being a "terrible colour", grey, and staying grey for about half an hour afterwards. In September 1976, she "took a turn" in the doctor's consulting room and also in the EEG department, where there was tonic rigidity and apparent cardiac arrest from an EEG point of view for about 30 s (the EEG was flat for more than 25 s). Later that month she felt unwell in the hospital waiting room and was taken outside, sat on a wall and then "went out" with rigidity, foaming, eyes rolling, incontinence, and "twitching in the middle", i.e. a "definite convulsion". Her pulse was said to be "very low" afterwards, by the consultant. She went home in an ambulance. In December 1976, when standing at a bus stop she said "Mum, I'm not feeling well", then "went right down" twitching, incontinent, "stiff just like a convulsion." She has had no episodes since but was still on phenobarbitone, down from 30 mg three times daily to 30 mg twice daily, and was not allowed to go to the swimming baths because "she is on tablets for epilepsy."

Father came into the EEG room and at the sight of the EEG paper went white and sat down and sweated and then said "I have been fighting this all my life, it is awfully embarrassing." He said that if over-excited or if he went to doctors or hospitals he used to faint but can now "get it" when standing and may "get dizzy" when getting up from sitting. The fainting was much more prominent when he was a young child.

The EEG was reported thus. She was awake and cooperative. There was moderately responsive but well organized alpha rhythm of 8–9 c/s with a normal amount of random slower activity and prominent frontal fast activity. Hyperventilation caused her considerable distress because she expected to be able to induce an attack but no abnormality occurred. Stroboscopic activation was not carried out.

Ocular compression was done under EEG and ECG control. The resting ECG showed a marginally long P–R interval of just over 0.2 s. Ocular compression on one occasion induced asystole of no more than 1.2 s followed by facial pallor, tachycardia, and sweating slow artifact on the EEG which developed within 20–30 s. The EEG itself was not slowed. A second ocular compression induced an asystole of about 2.3 s with complete atrioventricular block. She then vomited.

Cardiac investigation later was totally negative. Anti-epileptic medication was stopped, and improvement was such that antisyncopal drugs were not required.

VI. Summary of Results from Ocular Compression Studies

From the initial study of reflex anoxic seizures it was shown that febrile convulsions of similar character were present in 14%.

The syncope study revealed that there was a similar association between convulsive syncope, or syncope with excessive asystole on OC, with febrile convulsions.

The febrile convulsion trial confirmed certain previous work: the male preponderance except in hemiconvulsions, the sex difference in determining which cerebral hemisphere was affected, and the appearance of EEG spikes after the age of three years (except in cerebral pathology cases).

New findings were: confirmation of preliminary work showing that prolonged asystole on OC is a feature of febrile convulsions which appear to be "anoxic", a high proportion of children with "anoxic" febrile convulsions with affected first-degree relatives, evidence that in the large bulk of febrile convulsions prolonged asystole on OC is associated with a first-degree family history. Limited data suggested that an "anoxic" mechanism and minor preceding cerebral abnormality might interact to induce unilateral cerebral damage or dysfunction after a generalized febrile convulsion.

The study of pertussis immunization convulsions suggested that these had an "anoxic" mechanism, with a tendency to prolonged asystole on ocular compression, whereas pertussis convulsions could be encephalopathic, as previously thought.

The analysis of children with prolonged asystole on OC and a history of febrile convulsions, reflex anoxic seizures, or a combination of the two (febrile convulsions and reflex anoxic seizures or syncope in the same child) illuminated the genetics further, but also raised further questions. The male predominance in pure febrile convulsions was as expected, but the female preponderance in ordinary reflex anoxic seizures is unexplained (possibly excessive pain sensitivity from diminished endorphins). The sex ratio is unity in children with both types of seizure.

Spikes on EEG were only common at the age of three years or over, and when they appeared they were unevenly distributed within those who had febrile convulsions. Spikes were rare in "anoxic" febrile convulsions, but common in clonic febrile convulsions.

The genetic contribution, as judged by the percentage of affected first-degree relatives, increased exponentially from the pure reflex anoxic seizure group, through pure febrile convulsions, to the group with both febrile convulsions and reflex anoxic seizures or syncope. In the first two groups the majority of families showed concordance in the type of seizure between proband and first-degree relative, but in the combined group there was segregation. Interestingly, no child with febrile convulsions (pure or combined) had a first-degree relative with pure reflex anoxic seizures and no child with *pure* reflex anoxic seizures had a first-degree relative with febrile convulsions.

G. Genetics

Genetic studies of seizure disorders universally assume them to be epileptic, and experimentally employ animal epilepsies (e.g. NAQUET 1975). New studies will be needed to explore the genetic basis of the separate anoxic and epileptic mechanisms and their interactions. Meanwhile it is satisfying that previous work (TAYLOR 1969; TAYLOR and OUNSTED 1971; OUNSTED 1976) ties in well with the results of the ocular compression studies discussed earlier.

Genetic testing is difficult with the available methods. We have tested one father of a child with febrile convulsions and prolonged asystole on OC. The father suffered from "stress convulsions" (FRIIS and LUND 1974), and OC induced an anoxic seizure in him.

Of the genetic hypotheses, autosomal dominance with incomplete penetrance (LENNOX-BUCHTHAL 1973) is most popular. Polygenic inheritance is another alternative championed by TSUBOI (1977), TAY (1979) and FUKUYAMA et al. (1979). The heterogeneity of febrile convulsions makes it unlikely that the final genetic solution will be simple.

One piece of information has not so far been integrated into any genetic analysis. This is the finding of CALLAWAY (1978) that in three generations of a family with D/G translocation Down's syndrome, all 7/7 carriers of the translocation had severe febrile convulsions, while none of those without this chromosome translocation had febrile convulsions. A similar family has recently been found in Oxford, with presumed mesial temporal sclerosis resulting in temporal lobe epilepsy in the child, with a history of very long febrile convulsions and 14/21 translocation karyotype.

It is of considerable interest that the prognosis for remission in temporal lobe epilepsy (TLE) preceded by febrile convulsions in childhood is strongly related to the family history (LINDSAY et al. 1980). A first-degree relative with febrile convulsions negates the adverse prognostic factors previously delineated for non-genetic TLE (LINDSAY et al. 1979) and instead allows 50% remission and a high chance of a drug-free, independent adult life. On the basis of this work (which was of course started before febrile convulsions were classified as "anoxic" or "encephalopathic"), it has been proposed that a common gene is involved in both ordinary genetic febrile convulsions and TLE. One hypothesis for the action of this gene would be a propensity to inhibit epileptic seizures (LINDSAY et al. 1980). Another hypothesis would propose some kind of biochemical maturation, with a damping of cholinergic activity both in the amygdala and in the heart, with the passage of time.

H. Brain Damage from Febrile Convulsions

There is much evidence that prolonged and particularly long unilateral febrile convulsions (febrile status) may lead to permanent brain damage, with temporal lobe epilepsy, hemiparesis, and learning disorder (AICARDI 1977; AICARDI and BARATON 1971; AICARDI and CHEVRIE 1976; CHEVRIE and AICARDI 1975, 1978; LINDSAY et al. 1979; OUNSTED et al. 1966; WALLACE and CULL 1979). The fact that febrile status is much less damaging in the long run when a first-degree relative is affected (LINDSAY et al. 1979, 1980) suggests that predominantly non-genetic mechanisms ("encephalopathy"?) may be operating in the damaged children. Experimentally, young rats with heat-induced *epileptic* seizures performed less well later in life (NEALIS et al. 1978) but the experimental effect of anoxic seizures from brief asystole is not known.

The results of experimental seizures in adolescent baboons have been summarised in MELDRUM (1978), but important though these studies are the seizures were all *epileptic*. Brain swelling has been shown on CT scan shortly after febrile status (GASTAUT and GASTAUT 1977) – the best pharmacological approach to this cerebral oedema (if it is that) is not yet clear, but some solutions have been suggested in a general review (MILLER 1979).

The large prospective study with 7-year follow-up of over 50000 pregnancies did not suggest that long febrile convulsions were damaging, at least not to children who were neurodevelopmentally normal before the first seizure (ELLENBERG and NELSON 1978; NELSON and ELLENBERG 1978). Unfortunately, although huge, this study would need to have been ten times larger to clarify the factors operating in children whose long febrile seizures seemed to damage their brains.

J. Prophylactic Drug Therapy of Febrile Convulsions

Because febrile convulsions might sometimes be dangerous and could come without warning, drug prophylaxis was introduced. FAERØ et al. (1972) published the first trial suggesting that phenobarbitone with adequate plasma concentration prevented *recurrence* of febrile convulsions. *First* febrile convulsions cannot be prevented (OUNSTED 1978), except in meningitis (OUNSTED 1951). HECKMATT et al. (1976) showed that high levels of phenobarbitone were *not* preventative of recurrences. However, several trials have agreed that daily phenobarbitone *reduces* recurrences of febrile convulsions whether "simple" (resembling our anoxic seizures) or "complex" (encephalopathic) (THORN 1975; WALLACE 1975; WOLF 1977a, b; WOLF et al. 1977). These trials were criticized on the grounds that no placebo was used and intermittent therapy by intelligent parents was dismissed (CAMFIELD and CAMFIELD 1978). Later CAMFIELD et al. (1980) remedied the first defect by showing that phenobarbitone was superior to placebo at the $P = 0.03$ level. CAMFIELD mixed a riboflavin tracer with both drug and placebo to give urine fluorescence in this double-blind trial. Phenobarbitone given acutely was found to be effective by PEARCE et al. (1977). It might be that phenobarbitone had won the day here, a thought echoed by FREEMAN (1978) in "Febrile seizures: an end to confusion". FISHMAN (1979) summarized the published trials of phenobarbitone and added them together to give a reduction of recurrences from 30%–10% ($P < 0.0001$). He concluded by recommending phenobarbitone therapy to all those whose febrile convulsions began before the age of 18 months [i.e. 50% of the seizure population – LENNOX-BUCHTHAL (1973)] together with any who had unusual seizures, development, or family history. If his recommendations were carried out, getting on for 2% of the child population would be having repeated measurements of the plasma phenobarbitone for 2½ years. A paediatrician caring for the children within a population of 200000 would need to take at least 15 specimens from young children every week. 10% of the children would have recurrences of febrile convulsions anyway, (FISHMAN 1979) and 20% of the remainder would not tolerate the drug (HECKMATT et al. 1976; WOLF and FORSYTHE 1978; FISHMAN 1979).

One might add that some of the parents, and perhaps the doctors, would be concerned by the reports of impaired brain growth and development in rat pups given phenobarbitone without "toxic" serum levels (DIAZ et al. 1977; DIAZ and SCHAIN 1978).

Some success has been reported with higher dose phenobarbitone administration at the time of fevers (PEARCE et al. 1977). Going further, KNUDSEN and VES-

TERMARK (1978) found no difference between the prophylactic effect of continuous phenobarbitone and intermittent rectal diazepam – previously shown to be absorbed very rapidly (AGURELL et al. 1975). Concluding this brief survey of the use of phenobarbitone, it must be emphasized that even the strongest protagonists of this drug admit that there is no evidence that it influences the long-term prognosis (WOLF 1979).

Of other antiepileptic drugs, only sodium valproate (dipropylacetate) has been used in controlled trials. Although it may reduce recurrences (CAVAZZUTI 1975; WALLACE and SMITH 1980; NGWANE and BOWER 1980), the escalating list of side effects of this drug (BATALDEN et al. 1979; GERBER et al. 1979; COULTER and ALLEN 1980; JACOBI et al. 1980) is likely to make doctors wary of prescribing it (STEPHENSON 1980a).

A recent suggestion (KEINANEN-KIUKAANNIEMIS et al. 1979) has been the use of rectally administered diazepam combined with the prostaglandin-synthetase-inhibiting antipyretic acetominophen (paracetamol, 4-acetamidophenol). A trial of this combination during childhood fevers is no doubt already under way.

K. Special Cases: Familial Dysautonomia and Down's Syndrome

Two conditions deserve special mention because of the light they may throw on the general question of febrile convulsions. In familial dysautonomia (Riley–Day syndrome) febrile convulsions and anoxic seizures are exceedingly common (AXELROD et al. 1974), whereas in mongolism (Down's syndrome) febrile seizures are said to be rare (KIRMAN 1951). In both syndromes there are unusual pharmacological responses, in the one to cholinergics, in the other to cholinergic blockade by atropine.

Familial dysautonomia (AXELROD et al. 1974) is a rare autosomal recessive disorder confined to Ashkenazi Jews. Afflicted childred have frequent fevers and inappropriate temperature control, so that, for instance, fever may be higher after immunization than after serious infections such as pneumonia. Remarkably, about 40% of these children have seizures (shaking or stiffening associated with loss of consciousness) (AXELROD et al. 1974). Of these, 60% have seizures with high fever (febrile convulsions), 20% with severe "breath-holding", and 20% with hypoxia as from pneumonia or mucus plugs in bronchi. The description of the "breath-holding" attacks resembles that of the reflex anoxic seizures from cardiac asystole described elsewhere in this chapter, but their mechanism has not been established with certainty. The combination of febrile convulsions and reflex anoxic seizures, which both remit at the age of five years suggests a common mechanism. There is no increase in incidence of these convulsive disorders in the siblings of patients with familial dysautonomia, so we are apparently dealing with a genocopoy which may nevertheless allow insights into common genetic febrile convulsions and reflex anoxic seizures. Among other defects, patients with familial dysautonomia appear to have (at least at certain locations) a deficiency of the enzyme choline acetyltransferase (MITTAG et al. 1974) and presumably defective cholinergic transmission. A cholinergic denervation effect is suggested by the exaggerated response to methacholine and bethanechol (AXELROD et al. 1972, 1974). Although vagovagal reactions may be massive and sometimes fatal in the condition (AXELROD, 1979, personal communication), there is no cardiac slowing on carotid massage (Axel-rod 1979, personal communication), or on ocular compression (Stephenson, un-published observation). Since there is also extensive sympathetic denervation, an-other theoretical mechanism for cerebral hypoxia could be a defect in pulmonary vasomotor control and so lack of autoregulation in response to alveolar hypo-ventilation. Other aspects of abnormal respiratory and circulatory responses to hypoxia in this condition are to be found in the literature (Filler et al. 1965; Edel-man et al. 1967).

In Down's syndrome (mongolism) due to an excess of genetic material carried on chromosome 21, febrile convulsions are reported to be rare or non-existent (Gibbs et al. 1964; Veall 1974).

Other non-febrile seizures or convulsions are also rare under the age of four years (Veall 1974). Such epileptic seizures as do occur in the young mongol are infantile spasms which are distinctive in being sometimes pyridoxine-responsive (Wolcott and Chun 1973). Such seizures may be precipitated by the administra-tion of 5-hydroxytryptophan (Coleman 1971). As the mongol approaches old age the situation changes and epileptic seizures become extremely commong (Veall 1974; Tangye 1979), possibly because of the premature development of Alzhei-mer's disease and its structural and neurochemical basis. It is pertinent to the thesis developed in this chapter that in Down's syndrome there is a remarkable sensitivity to atropine, which may easily cause death. The excessive reaction of the pupils of the mongol's eye was demonstrated by the group led by Kirman (Berg et al. 1959). Later it was shown that, although the vagomimetic effect of small doses of atropine was normal in Down's syndrome (adult white males were tested), the cardio-accel-erator effect of larger doses was more than doubled (Harris and Goodman 1968). That this latter effect could be prevented by treatment with the β-adrenoreceptor blocking drug propranolol suggests that excessive sympathetic drive is operating. There is no evidence on the oculo-cardiac reflex in Down's syndrome, but the re-sponse to ocular surgery for strabismus should allow this deficiency to be cor-rected. It should be mentioned in passing that in dogs (Gandevia et al. 1978 b) and presumably in humans (Stephenson 1979b) atropinization does not totally block the oculocardiac reflex, which involves sympathetic inhibition as well as vagal ac-tivation.

It is of considerable interest that in a single family briefly reported from Aus-tralia (Calloway 1978) all seven carriers of D/G translocation (involving mis-placement of genetic material from chromosome 21), in three generations had se-vere febrile convulsions. If these carriers were unbalanced, with a genetic deficiency on chromosome 21, this would hint at the locus of at least one of the genes involved in febrile convulsions and would go some way to explaning the protective effect of the extra chromosome 21 genetic material in Down's syndrome itself. A similar family, with 14/21 translocation and febrile convulsions, is under investigation in Oxford.

Thus we have two genetic conditins with distinctive but different autonomic control and contrasting incidence of those early childhood convulsions which we postulate to have a "reflex anoxic" basis. Further study of these models of nature may elucidate the mechanisms and even the genetic loci of the more common gen-eral febrile convulsions and reflex anoxic seizures.

Since this section was written, it has been determined that in Down's syndrome there is a 3% incidence of febrile convulsions (evidently non-genetic), and 2% of reflex anoxic seizures (STEPHENSON, unpublished observations).

L. New Pharmacological Aspects of Febrile Convulsions

In this section we mention some aspects of pharmacology which might be developed with profit to affected children. Some of the threads may in due course tie together, but are at present disconnected.

First there is a point regarding input and output to and from the brain. SIEMES et al. (1978) presented evidence of a reduction of blood–cerebrospinal fluid barrier after febrile convulsions. TRIMBLE (1978) demonstrated increased serum prolactin in epilepsy, but had not yet tested children with febrile convulsions. In any future studies, differentiation of "anoxic" from encephalopathic/epileptic seizures would add meaning to the results.

Next there is a paradox in the action of carbamazepine, the solution of which might help in the management of "anoxic" febrile convulsions should these be shown to result from cardiac asystole. BEERMAN and EDHAG (1978) found carbamezepine to depress idioventricular and therefore escape cardiac rhythms. Theoretically, the drug might prevent early restoration in reflex asystole. However, JACOBSON and RUSSELL (1979) used carbamezepine to treat glossopharyngeal neuralgia with syncope from asystole. More work is needed to clarify these observations.

Finally, there is the large question of acetylcholine in brain and heart, and its relation to febrile convulsions and their prevention. This question looms larger with the suggestion that a vagal-mediated atropine-sensitive cholinergic mechanism might be involved in certain febrile seizures. The central cerebral cholinergic mechanisms of pyrexia have been discussed in some detail by TANGRI et al. (1976). Outside the field of pyrexia, it is known that focal neostigmine may activate spike discharges in the amygdala (GIRGIS 1978), an effect partly reversed by atropine or scopolamine (hyoscine). Choline administration modifies the central action of atropine (WECKER et al. 1978). Experimentally, atropine prevents febrile convulsions in the rat (MILLICHAP et al. 1960; MILLICHAP 1968, pp. 155–156), and inhibits the convulsions expected after withdrawal from forced sodium barbital drinking (WAHLSTROM 1978). In humans, although the tonic epileptic seizures with EEG flattening and bradycardia known as "generalized cortical electrodecremental events" may respond to methylphenydate (FARIELLO et al. 1979), identical episodes – described as apnoeic spells – have been successfully treated with atropine (HOOSHMAND 1972).

Cholinesterase is located in the sinus node and atrioventricular node of the heart (JAMES and SPENCE 1966) as well as in the brain. Vagocardiac cholinergic activity can be investigated using prostigmine and atropine (DIGHTON 1974), and we know from clinical experiments that atropine sulphate or atropine methonitrate can prevent spontaneous and ocular compression-induced reflex anoxic seizures (STEPHENSON 1979 b). We know nothing of the location of the cholinergic mechanisms of febrile convulsions (if they exist) nor do we know how to block them safely. But if we consider these questions at all, we may have advanced.

The fact that atropine sulphate and scopolamine (hyoscine) enter the brain while atropine methonitrate does not should help to test hypotheses on the mechanism of febrile convulsions and refine preventative methods. If convulsions involve excessive acetylcholine mechanism at muscarinic receptors in brain and heart, then atropine sulphate should be more effective than atropine methonitrate. By contrast, if convulsions are mediated purely through vagocardiac ischaemic anoxia, then atropine mehtonitrate will be as effective as atropine sulphate.

In relation to therapy, while atropine sulphate may reverse the muscarinic component of the central cholinergic mechanisms of temperature reduction, atropine methonitrate – not getting to brain – will not influence this. Atropine methonitrate will of course, like the sulphate, inhibit sweating by its direct peripheral action, but will not slow heat loss if the ambient temperature is kept low. Therefore, atropine methonitrate deserves a trial in the prevention of febrile convulsions where a vagal "anoxic" mechanism is proposed, as in pertussis immunization convulsions (Stephenson 1979 a, b) where it could be given at the time of the immunization dose.

Lastly, if cholinergic mechanisms are involved in the genetic temporal lobe epilepsy linked to febrile convulsions, then scopolamine (hyoscine) which enters the brain strongly is worthy of investigation. The primate model of Girgis (1978) is an intriguing one for all who wish to discern and to modify for the better the neurochemical links between brain and behaviour and paroxysmal events.

M. Hypotheses

1) The "anoxic" convulsive threshold is low in early childhood.
2) In genetic febrile convulsions, fever triggers such "anoxic" seizures.
3) The sensitivity of the vagocardiac mechanism is a measure of the gene dose.
4) A further genetic mechanism is responsible for EEG spike generation in the absence of cerebral pathology.
5) Interaction occurs between these "anoxic" and "epileptic" mechanism.
6) Further interactions may occur when underlying cerebral pathology is also present, antedating the first febrile convulsion.

References

Acker D, Boehm FH, Askew DE, Rothman H (1973) Electrocardiogram changes with intrauterine contraceptive device insertion. Am J Obstet Gynecol 115:458–461
Agurell S, Berlin A, Ferngren H, Hellstrom B (1975) Plasma levels of diazepam after parentral and rectal administration in children. Epilepsia 16:277–283
Aicardi J (1977) Post-natal seizures: clinical effects. In: Berenberg SR (ed) Brain, fetal and infant. Nijhoff, The Hague, pp 295–301
Aicardi J, Baraton J (1971) A pneumoencephalographic demonstration of brain atrophy following status epilepticus. Dev Med Child Neurol 13:660–667
Aicardi J, Chevrie JJ (1970) Convulsive status epilepticus in infants and children. A study of 239 cases. Epilepsia 11:187–197
Aicardi J, Chevrie JJ (1976) Febrile convulsions: neurological sequelae and mental retardation. In: Brazier MA, Coceani F (eds) Brain dysfunction in infantile febrile convulsions. Raven, New York, pp 247–257
Annegers JF, Hauser WA, Elveback LR, Kurland LP (1979) The risk of epilepsy following febrile convulsions. Neurology (NY) 29:297–303

Anonymous (1978) Breathing and control of heart rate. Br Med J 2:1663–1664

Axelrod FB, Branon N, Mecker M, Nachtigal R, Dancis J (1972) Treatment of familial dysautonomia with bethanecol (Urecholine). J Pediatr 81:573–578

Axelrod FB, Nachtigal R, Dancis J (1974) Familial dysautonomia: diagnosis pathogenesis and management. Adv Pediatr 21:75–96

Bankhead AJ, Towens JK (1950) The anticipation and prevention of cardiac complications in electroconvulsive therapy. Am J Psychiatry 106:911–917

Barkin RM, Pichichero ME (1979) Diphtheria-pertussis-tetanus vaccine: reactogenicity of commercial products. Pediatrics 63:256–260

Batalden PB, Vandyne BJ, Cloyd JA (1979) Pancreatitis associated with valproic acid therapy. Pediatrics 64:520–522

Beerman B, Edhag O (1978) Depressive effect of carbamazepine on idioventricular rhythm in man. Br Med J 2:171–172

Bellman MH, Miller DL, Poore PD, Ross EM (1979) National childhood encephalopathy study – a preliminary report. Arch Dis Childh 54:970

Berg JM, Brandon MW, Kirman BH (1959) Atropine in mongolism, Lancet 2:441–442

Branch CE, Robertson BT, Beckett SD, Walds AL, James TN (1977) An animal model of spontaneous syncope and sudden death. J Lab Clin Med 90:592–603

Brazier MAB, Coceani F (eds) (1976) Brain dysfunction in infantile febrile convulsions. Raven, New York

Bridge EM, Livingston S, Tietze C (1943) Breath-holding spells. J Pediatr 23:539–561

Brueton MJ (1978) The neurological complications of plasmodium faciparum malaria in childhood. MD Thesis, University of London

Callaway BG (1978) Febrile convulsions and DG translocation. Med J Aust 2:115

Camfield P, Camfield C (1978) Phenobarbital and febrile seizures. Pediatrics 61:940

Camfield PR, Camfield CS, Shapiro SH, Cummings C (1980) The first febrile seizure – antipyretic instruction plus either phenobarbitone or placebo to prevent recurrence. J Pediatrics 97:16–21

Cavazzuti G (1975) Prevention of febrile convulsions with dipropylacetate (Depakine). Epilepsia 16:647–648

Chevrie JJ, Aicardi J (1975) Duration and lateralisation of febrile convulsions. Etiological factors. Epilepsia 16:781–789

Chevrie JJ, Aicardi J (1978) Convulsive disorders in the first year of life: neurological and mental outcome and mortality. Epilepsia 19:67–74

Church MA (1979) Evidence of whooping-cough – vaccine efficacy from the 1978 whooping-cough epidemic in Hertfordshire. Lancet 2:188–190

Coleman M (1971) Infantile spasms associated with 5-hydroxytryptophan administration in patients with Down's Syndrome. Neurology (NY) 21:911–919

Cooper Sir Astley (1836) Some experiments and observations on tying the carotid and vertebral arteries, and the pneumogastric, phrenic and sympathetic nerves. Guys Hosp Rep 1:457–475

Coulter DL, Allen RJ (1980) Pancreatitis associated with valproic acid therapy for epilepsy. Ann Neurol 7:92

Daly MdeB, Angell-James JE (1979) Role of carotid-body chemoreceptors and their reflex interactions in bradycardia and cardiac arrest. Lancet 1:764–767

Diaz J, Schain RJ (1978) Phenobarbital: effects of long-term administration on behaviour and brain of artificially reared rats. Science 199:90–91

Diaz J, Schain RJ, Baily BG (1977) Phenobarbital – induced brain growth retardation in artificially reared rat pups. Biol Neonate 32:77–82

Dighton DH (1974) Sinus bradycardia: autonomic influences and clinical assessment. Br Heart J 36:791–797

Edelman NH, Richards EC, Fishman AP (1967) Abnormal ventilatory and circulatory responses to hypoxia in familial dysautonomia. J Clin Invest 46:1051

Eherengut W (1974) Über konvulsive Reaktionen nach Pertussis-Schutzimpfung. Dtsch Med Wochenschr 99, 273–2279

Ellenberg JH, Nelson KB (1978) Febrile seizures and later intellectual performance. Arch Neurol 35:17–21

Faden A, Spire JP, Faden R (1977) Fits, faints and the I.U.D. Ann Neurol 1:305–306
Faerø Kastrup KW, Nielsen EL, Melchior JC, Thorn I (1972) Successful prophylaxis of febrile convulsions with phenobarbital. Epilepsia 13:279–285
Fariello RG, Doro JM, Forster FM (1979) Generalised cortical electrodicremental event. Clinical and neurophysiological observations in patients with dystonic seizures. Arch Neurol 36:285–291
Filler J, Smith AA, Stone S, Dancis J (1965) Respiratory control in familial dysautonomia. J Pediatr 66:509–516
Fishman MA (1979) Febrile seizures: the treatment controversy. J Pediatr 94:177–184
Freeman JM (1978) Febrile seizures: an end to confusion. Pediatrics 61:806–808
Friis ML, Lund M (1974) Stress convulsions. Arch Neurol 31:155–159
Fukuyama Y, Tomori N, Sugitate M (1977) Critical evaluation of the role of immunisation as an etiological factor of infantile spasms. Neuropädiatrie 8:224–237
Fukuyama Y, Kagawa K, Tanaka K (1979) A genetic study of febrile convulsions. Eur Neurol 18:166–182
Gandevia SC, McCloskey DI, Potter EK (1978 a) Inhibition of baroreceptor and chemoreceptor reflexes on heart rate by afferents from the lungs. J Physiol (Lond) 276:369–381
Gandevia SC, McCloskey DI, Potter EK (1978 b) Reflex bradycardia occurring in response to diving, nasopharyngeal stimulation and ocular pressure, and its modification by respiration and swallowing. J Physiol (Lond) 276:383–394
Gastaut H (1968) A physiopathogenic study of reflex anoxic cerebral seizures in children (syncopes, sobbing spasms and breath-holding spells). In: Kellaway P, Petersen I (eds) Clinical electroencephalography of children. Grune & Stratton, New York, pp 257–274
Gastaut H (1974) Syncopes: generalised anoxic cerebral seizures. In: Vinken PJ, Gruyn GW (eds) Handbook of clinical neurology, vol 15. North-Holland, Amsterdam, 815–835
Gastaut H, Broughton R (1972) Epileptic seizures. Thomas, Springfield
Gastaut H, Fischer-Williams M (1957) Electroencephalographic study of syncope. Lancet 2:1018–1025
Gastaut H, Gastaut J-L (1977) Computerized axial tomography in epilepsy. In: Penry JK (ed) Epilepsy, the eighth international symposium. Raven, New York, pp 5–15
Gastaut H, Gastaut Y (1957) Syncopes et convulsions. A propos de la nature syncopale de certains spasms du sanglot et de certaines convulsions essentielles hyperthermiques ou à froid. Rev Neurol (Paris) 96:158–163
Gastaut HH, Gastaut Y (1958) Electroencephalographic and clinical study of anoxic convulsions in children. Electroencephhalogr Clin Neurophysiol 10:607–620
Gastaut H, Tassinari CA (1966) Triggering mechanisms in epilepsy: the electro-clinical point of view. Epilepsia 7:85–138
Gastaut H, Fischer-Williams M, Gibson W, El Ouahchi S (1961) Clinicoelectroencephalographic study of reflex vaso-vagal syncope provoked by ocular compression. In: Gastaut H, Mayer JS (eds) Cerebral anoxia and the electroencephalogram. Thomas, Springfield, pp 535–553
Gauk EW, Kidd L, Pichard JS (1963) Mechanism of seizures associated with breath-holding spells. N Engl J Med 268:1436–1441
Gerber N, Dickinson RG Harland RC, Lynn RK, Houghton D, Antonias JI, Schimschock JC (1979) Reye-like syndrome associated with valproic acid therapy. J Pediatr 95:142–144
Girgis M (1978) Neostigmine activated epileptiform discharges in the amygdala: electrographic – behavioural correlations. Epilepsia 19:521–530
Griffith AH (1978) Reactions after pertussis vaccine: a manufacturer's experiences and difficulties since 1964. Br Med J 1:809–814
Harris WS, Goodman RM (1968) Hyper-reactivity to atropine in Down's syndrome. Engl J Med 279:407–410
Heckmatt JZ, Houston AB, Clow DJ, Stephenson JBP, Dodd KL, Lealman GT, Logan RW (1976) Failure of phenobarbitone to prevent febrile convulsions. Br Med J 1:559–561
Hooshmand H (1972) Apneic spells treated with atropine. Neurology (NY) 22:1217–1221
Jacobi G, Thorbeck R, Ritz A, Janssen W, Schmidts H-L (1980) Fatal hepatotoxicity in child on phenobarbitone and sodium valproate. Lancet 1:712–713

Jacobson RR, Russell R (1979) Glossopharyngeal neuralgia with cardiac arrhythmia: a rare but treatable cause of syncope. Br Med J 1:379–380

James TN, Spence CA (1966) Distribution of cholinesterase within the sinus node and A-V node of the human heart. Anat Rec 155:151–161

Keinanen-Kiukaanniemis S, Luoma P, Kangas L, Saukkonen A-L (1979) Antipyretic effect and plasma concentrations of rectal acetaminophen and diazepam in children. Epilepsia 20:607–612

Kellaway P, Druckman R (1961) The anoxic basis of certain seizures in young children. Presented at the American Electroencephalographic Society, June 13, 1959, Hotel Claridge, Atlantic City, NJ Quoted on p 315 in Meyer JS, Waltz AG: Relationship of cerebral anoxia to functional and electroencephalographic abnormality. In: Gastaut H, Meyer JS (eds) Cerebral anoxia and the electrocephalogram. Thomas, Springfield, pp 307–328

Kirman BH (1951) Epilepsy in mongolism. Arch Dis Child 26:501–503

Knudsen FU, Vestermark S (1978) Prophylactic diazepam or phenobarbitone in febrile convulsions: a prospective controlled study. Arch Dis Child 53:660–663

Kuhlenkampff M, Schwartzman JS, Wilson J (1974) Neurological complications of pertussis innoculation. Arch Dis Child 49:46–49

Kussmaul A, Tenner A (1859) On the nature and origin of epileptiform convulsions caused by profuse bleeding, and also those of true epilepsy (translated by Bronner E). Selected monographs. The New Sydenham Society, London

Laslett EE (1909) Syncopal attacks, associated with prolonged arrest of the whole heart. QJ Med 2:347–355

Laxdal T, Gomez MR, Reitset J (1969) Cyanotic and pallid syncopal attacks in children (breath-holding spells). Dev Med Child Neurol 755–763

Lennox-Buchthal MA (1973) Febrile convulsions: a reappraisal. Elsevier, Amsterdam

Lennox-Buchthal MA (1976) A summing up: clinical session. In: Brazier MAB, Coceano F (eds) Brain dysfunction in infantile febrile convulsions. Raven, New York, pp 327–351

Lindsay J, Ounsted C, Richards P (1979) Long-term outcome in children with temporal lobe seizures. I. Social outcome and childhood factors. Dev Med Child Neurol 21:285–298

Lindsay J, Ounsted C, Richards P (1980) Long-term outcome in children with temporal lobe seizures. IV. Genetic factors, febrile convulsions and the remission of seizures. Dev Med Child Neurol 22:429–439

Livingston S (1954) The diagnosis and treatment of convulsive disorders in children. Thomas, Springfield, pp 79–80

Livingston S (1970) Breath-holding spells in children: differentiation from epileptic attacks. JAMA 212:2231–2239

Lombroso CT, Lerman P (1967) Breath-holding spells (cyanotic and pallid infantile syncope) Pediatrics 39:563–581

Marshall AJ (1978) Repetitive cardiac arrest from electromechanical dissociation. Br Med J 2:97–98

Marks MI, Hirshfeld S (1968) Neurotoxicity of penicillin. N Engl J Med 279:1002–1003

Maulsby R, Kellaway PO (1964) Transient hypoxic crises in children. In: Kellaway P, Petersen I (eds) Neurological and electroencephalographic correlative studies in infancy. Grune & Stratton, New York, pp 349–360

Melchior JC (1977) Infantile spasms and early immunisation against whooping cough. Arch Dis Child 52:134–137

Meldrum B (1978) Physiological changes during prolonged seizures and epileptic brain damage. Neuropädiatrie 9:203–212

Mendel WJ, Hayakawatt AHN, Danzig R, Kermaier AL (1972) Assessment of sinus node function in patients with the sick sinus syndrome. Circulation 46:761–769

Meyer JS, Waltz AG (1961) Relationship of cerebral anoxia to functional and electroencephalographic abnormality. In: Gastaut H, Meyer JS (eds) Cerebral anoxia and the electroencephalogram. Thomas, Springfield, pp 307–328

Miller JD (1979) The management of cerebral oedema. Br J Hosp Med 21:152–164

Millichap JG (1968) Febrile convulsions. Macmillan, New York London

Millichap JG, Hernandez P, Zales MR, Halpern LA, Kramer BI (1960) Studies in febrile seizures. IV. Evaluation of drug effects and development of potential new therapy (Pyrietal). Neurology (NY) 10:578–583

Mittag TW, Mindel JS, Green JP (1974) Choline acetyltransferase in familial dysautonomia. Ann NY Acad Sci 228:301–306

McGreal DA (1956) Observations on febrile convulsions. Am J Dis Child 92:504–505

McGreal DA (1957) Convulsions in childhood. A clinical and electroencephalographic study of 500 cases in children under the age of seven. MD thesis, University of St. Andrews

Naquet R (1975) Genetic study of epilepsy: contributions of different models, especially the photosensitive Papio papio. In: Brazier MAB (ed) Growth and development of the brain. Raven, New York, pp 219–230

Nealis JGT, Rosman NP, De Piero TJ, Ouellelte EM (1978) Neurological sequelae of experimental febrile convulsions. Neurology (NY) 28:246–250

Nelson KB, Ellenberg JH (1976) Predictors of epilepsy in children who have experienced febrile seizures. N Engl J Med 295:1029–1033

Nelson KB, Ellenberg JH (1978) Prognosis in children with febrile seizures. Pediatrics 61:720–727

Ngwane E, Bower BA (1980) Continous sodium valproate or phenobarbitone in the prevention of "simple" febrile convulsions. Arch Dis Child 55:171–174

Ounsted C (1951) Significance of convulsions in children with purulent meningitis. Lancet 1:1245–1248

Ounsted C (1976) Genetic messages and convulsive behaviour in pyrexia. In: Brazier MAB, Coceani F (eds) brain dysfunction in infantile febrile convulsions. Raven, New York, pp 279–290

Ounsted C (1978) Preventing febrile convulsions. Dev Med Child Neurol 20:799–805

Ounsted C, Lindsay J, Norman R (1966) Biological factors in temporal lobe epilepsy. Heinemann, London

Pampiglione G, Waterston DJ (1961) EEG observations during changes in venous and arterial pressure. In: Gastaut H, Meyer JS (eds) Cerebral anoxia and the electroencephalogram. Thomas, Springfield, pp 250–255

Paulson G (1963) Breath-holding spells: a fatal case. Dev Med Child Neurol 5:246–251

Pearce JL, Sharman JR, Foster RM (1977) Phenobarbital in acute management of febrile convulsions. Pediatrics 60:569–572

Rasmussen V, Hauns S, Skagen K (1978) Cerebral attacks due to excessive vagal tone in heavily trained persons. Acta Med Scand 204:401–405

Rendle-Short J (1972) The physiopathology of breath-holding attacks: a hypothesis. Aust Paediatr J 8:92–94

Richardson DJ, Lewis WH, Gahagan LH, Sheehan D (1957) Etiology and treatment of cardiac arrhythmias under anaesthesia for electroconvulsive therapy. NY State J Med 57:881–886

Sackellares JC, Smith DS (1979) Myoclonus with electrocerebral silence in a patient receiving penicillin. Arch Neurol 36:851–858

Scarpa WJ (1976) The sick sinus syndrome. Am Heart J 92:648–660

Schlesinger Z (1973) Life-threatening "vagal reactions" to physical fitness test. JAMA 226:1119

Schlesinger Z, Bazilay J, Stryjer D, Almog CH (1977) Life-threatening "vagal reaction" to emotional stimuli. Isr J Med Sci 13:59–61

Shaw DB (1979) Bradycardias. Medicine 19:959–966

Siemes H, Siegert M, Hanefield F (1978) Febrile convulsions and bloodcerebrospinal fluid barrier. Epilepsia 19:57–66

Stephenson JBP (1971) Uraemia as a determinant of convulsions in acute infantile hypernatraemia. Arch Dis Child 46:676–679

Stephenson JBP (1978 a) Reflex anoxic seizures ("white breath-holding"): non-epiletpic vagal attacks. Arch Dis Child 53:193–200

Stephenson JBP (1978 b) Ocular compression in reflex anoxic seizures. Arch Dis Child 53:693

Stephenson JBP (1978c) Non-epileptic television syncope. Br Med J 1:1622

Stephenson JBP (1978d) Two types of febrile seizure: anoxic (syncopal) and epileptic mechanisms differentiated by oculocardiac reflex. Br Med J 2:726–728

Stephenson JBP (1979a) Pertussis immunisation convulsions are not evidence of encephalopathy. Lancet 2:416–417

Stephenson JBP (1979b) Atropine methonitrate in management of near-fatal reflex anoxic seizures. Lancet 2:955

Stephenson JBP (1980a) Prophylaxis against febrile convulsions. Br Med J 1:642–643

Stephenson JBP (1980b) Reflex anoxic seizures and ocular compression. Dev Med Child Neurol 22:380–386

Stewart GT (1977) Vaccination against whooping-cough. Efficiency versus risks. Lancet 1:234–237

Tangri KK, Misra N, Bhargara KP (1976) Central cholinergic mechanisms of pyrexia. In: Brazier MAB, Coceani F (eds) Brain dysfunction in infantile febrile convulsions. Raven, New York, pp 89–106

Tangye SR (1979) The EEG and incidence of epilepsy in Down's syndrome. J Ment Defic Res 23:17–24

Tay JS (1979) Dermatoglyphics in children with febrile convulsions. Br Med J 1:660

Taylor DC (1969) Differential rates of cerebral maturation between sexes and between hemispheres. Lancet 2:140–142

Taylor DC, Ounsted C (1971) Biological mechanisms influencing the outcome of seizures in response to fever. Epilepsia 12:33–45

Temkin I (1971) The falling sickness, 2nd edn. John Hopkins Press, Baltimore, pp 53, 280, 284, 316

Thorn I (1975) A controlled study of prophylactic long-term treatment of febrile convulsions. Acta Neurol [Suppl] 60:67–73

Trimble MR (1978) Serum prolactin in epilepsy and hysteria. Br Med J 2:1682

Tsuboi T (1977) Genetic aspects of febrile convulsions. Hum Genet 38:169–173

Tsuboi T (1978) Correlation between EEG abnormality and age in childhood. Neuropädiatrie 9:229–238

Tsuboi T, Endo SL (1977) Febrile convulsions followed by non-febrile convulsions. A clinical, electroencephalographic and follow-up study. Neuropädiatrie 8:209–223

Tsucbiya S, Kagawa K, Fukuyama Y (1978) Critical evaluation of the role of immunisation as an etiological factor in infantile spasms (second report). Brain Dev (Tokyo) 3:171

Veall RM (1974) The prevalence of epilepsy among mongols related to age. J Ment Defic Res 18:99–106

Wahlstrom G (1978) The effects of atropine on the tolerance and the convulsions seen after withdrawal from forced barbital drinking in the rat. Psychopharmacology (Berlin) 59:123–128

Wallace SJ (1975) Continuous prophylactic anticonvulsants in selected children with febrile convulsions. Acta Neurol Scand [Suppl] 60:62–65

Wallace SJ, Cull AM (1979) Long-term psychological outlook for children whose first fit occurs with fever. Dev Med Child Neurol 21:28–40

Wallace SJ, Smith JA (1980) Successful prophylaxis against febrile convulsions with valproic acid or phenobarbitone. Br Med J 1:353–354

Wecker L, Deltbarn W-D, Schmidt DE (1978) Choline administration: modification of the central actions of atropine. Science 199:86–87

Williams AL (1976) Sudden death in infancy syndrome. Med J Aust 2:188

Wolcott GJ, Chun RMW (1973) Myoclonic seizures in Down's Syndrome. Dev Med Child Neurol 15:805–808

Wolf SM (1977a) The effectiveness of phenobarbital in the prevention of recurrent febrile convulsions in children with and without a history of pre-, peri- and postnatal abnormalities. Acta Paediatr Scand 66:585–587

Wolf SM (1977b) Effectiveness of daily phenobarbital in the prevention of febrile seizure recurrence in "simple" febrile convulsions and "epilepsy triggered by fever". Epilepsia 18:95–99

Wolf SM (1979) Controversies in the treatment of febrile convulsions. Neurology (NY) 29:287–290

Wolf SM, Forsythe A (1978) Behaviour disturbance, phenobarbital and febrile seizures. Pediatrics 61:728–731

Wolf SM, Carr A, Davis DC et al. (1977) The value of phenobarbital in the child who has had a single febrile seizure: a controlled prospective study. Pediatrics 59:378–385

Ziegler DK, Lin J (1978) Convulsive syncope: relationship to cerebral ischaemia. Ann Neurol 4:173–174

CHAPTER 19

The Pyrogenic Responses
of Non-mammalian Vertebrates

W. W. REYNOLDS and M. E. CASTERLIN

A. Thermoregulation in Non-mammalian Vertebrates

Vertebrate animals can be classified on the basis of their thermoregulatory mechanisms into endotherms and ectotherms. Endotherms produce a significant quantity of internal heat through relatively high and controllable rates of aerobic metabolism, while at the same time having a relatively low but variable thermal conductance, so that their major source of body heat is internal (REYNOLDS 1979). The only non-mammalian vertebrate class which is primarily endothermic is the class Aves, the birds. Some fishes (tunas and lamnid sharks), and some large varanid lizards and brooding pythons among the reptiles also show a limited degree of endothermy; but by and large, lower vertebrates (Reptilia, Amphibia, Osteichthyes, Chondrichthyes, Agnatha) are ectothermic (REYNOLDS 1979). Ectotherms have relatively low rates of metabolic heat production and relatively high thermal conductance (i.e. poor thermal insulation), so that most metabolic heat is rapidly lost to the environment. The major source of body heat is external; i.e. the body temperature differs little from the temperature of the environment.

In ectotherms as well as in endotherms, blood flow and breathing (ventilation of gas exchange structures, either gills or lungs) affect rates of heat exchange between the body core and the environment (REYNOLDS 1977a; REYNOLDS and CASTERLIN 1978a). Vasomotor phenomena constitute a major thermoregulatory mechanism in birds and mammals, but do not significantly affect body core temperatures of ectotherms under steady-state conditions (REYNOLDS et al. 1976b). Endotherms can alter rates of heat production and heat exchange to a much greater extent than can ectotherms, but in evolving such mechanisms, the endotherms capitalized on features already present at a rudimentary level in many ectotherms.

One form of thermoregulation which exists in both ectotherms and endotherms, and probably in most or all motile animals, is behavioural thermoregulation (REYNOLDS and CASTERLIN 1979). This form of thermoregulation evolved very long ago in very primitive animals (NAKAOKA and OOSAWA 1977) and still persists in the endothermic birds and mammals (ADAIR 1974; CRAWSHAW and STITT 1975). In fact, behavioural thermoregulatory responses apparently develop earlier in ontogeny in mammals (SATINOFF et al. 1976) and in birds (MYHRE 1978) than do physiological mechanisms. Thus, physiological mechanisms complement, rather than replace behavioural thermoregulatory mechanisms in the higher vertebrates. In fact, other things being equal, behavioural means are usually employed to avoid the necessity of utilizing the more vigorous physiological thermoregulatory mechanisms of sweating or shivering. When possible, a mammal will tend to remain within its thermoneutral zone where neither sweating nor shivering are required. An ectotherm will attempt to remain at its preferred temperature (PT) or *thermal preferendum* (Reynolds and Casterlin 1979), which is species specific.

Behavioural thermoregulation can take a number of forms, depending on the nature of the thermal environment. For terrestrial animals (i.e. those dwelling in air), radiation and evaporation are effective means of heat exchange. Accordingly, postural orientations to the sun and wind are important. The thermal environment in air is complex, and air temperature is only part of it: sun and shade, wind speed and direction, and relative humidity are also important factors which offer numerous possibilities for behavioural as well as physiological exploitation for regulating body temperatures. Many terrestrial ectotherms, such as lizards, are often referred to as "heliotherms" because they make extensive use of solar radiation to regulate their body temperatures with a high degree of precision during daylight hours, particularly in arid environments with little cloud cover. (For extensive reviews of thermoregulation in reptiles and amphibians, see Huey and Stevenson 1979; Smith 1979; Brattstrom 1979.)

In water, evaporation and radiation are not effective means of heat exchange; heat is transferred by conduction and convection. Thus, the thermal environment of an aquatic ectotherm is fully characterized by water temperature alone (Reynolds and Casterlin 1979). Possibilities for behavioural thermoregulation are limited to preference and avoidance responses (Reynolds 1977b) along thermal gradients, i.e. selecting favourable water temperatures (subject to constraints of availability in time and space) and avoiding unfavourable or lethal water temperatures. Postural orientations are generally ineffective and evaporative heat loss is impossible while the animal is fully immersed in water. Most aquatic ectotherms breathe by means of gills, and owing to the high thermal conductance and specific heat of water surrounding the animal and passing over its gills, the body core temperature generally does not differ greatly from the ambient water temperature (Reynolds et al. 1976b) unless ambient temperatures are changing very rapidly (Reynolds 1977a). Ectotherms exhibit neither shivering nor non-shivering thermogenesis, and if an aquatic ectotherm increases aerobic heat production by increasing activity, it also increases the rate of heat loss to the water through the gills and body surface, so that the slight "excess" core temperature may actually decrease (Stevens and Fry 1970, 1974; Dean 1976; Mueller 1976; Reynolds and Casterlin 1980). A few species of tuna fishes have evolved counter-current *retia mirabilia* for thermal isolation of active red swimming muscles (Dizon and Brill 1979), giving a considerable degree of regional endothermy to these specialized fast-swimming fishes, but these are the exception among aquatic gill-breathers. Most fishes must simply choose the best available water temperature in order to control their body temperatures. By this means, however, many fishes are able to control their body temperatures with a surprising degree of precision under favourable circumstances (Reynolds and Casterlin 1976, 1977, 1978b, 1979), as can fish-like amphibian tadpole larvae (Casterlin and Reynolds 1977a, 1978a), sharks (Reynolds and Casterlin 1978c; Casterlin and Reynolds 1979), and lampreys (McCauley et al. 1977; Reynolds and Casterlin 1978d).

Some evidence suggests that all vertebrates possess a common and homologous central nervous system (CNS) thermoregulatory control centre in the preoptic/anterior hypothalamic (PO/AH) region of the brain, sometimes referred to as the rostral brain-stem (CRAWSHAW and HAMMEL 1973, 1974). For example, placement of thermodes in the PO/AH, and use of these to heat or cool the region, similarly affect thermoregulatory responses of sharks (CRAWSHAW and HAMMEL 1973), bony fishes (HAMMEL et al. 1969; CRAWSHAW and HAMMEL 1974), reptiles (HAMMEL et al. 1967) and mammals (HAMMEL et al. 1973). The input (sensory) and integrative (CNS) portions of the thermoregulatory control circuit appear to be basically similar among the vertebrates, the major difference arising in the effector side of the circuit where endotherms have added on physiological refinements (KLUGER 1978, 1979).

A thermoregulatory phenomenon which all vertebrates seem to share is the febrile response to pyrogens, which will be the subject of the remainder of this chapter. In terms of control theory (HAMMEL 1968; KLUGER 1978, 1979), a fever is a rise in body temperature resulting from an increase in the thermoregulatory "set-point" above the normothermic level. This is distinct from hyperthermia, in which the set-point is not raised, and the effector mechanisms attempt to return the temperature to normothermia. In fever, the temperature is regulated about the increased set-point by the effector mechanisms. Pyrogens are agents which raise the set-point. Antipyretics are agents which do not usually alter the set-point by themselves, but rather prevent pyrogens from raising the set-point by interfering with the neuropharmacological mechanisms mediating the febrile response.

B. Febrile Responses of Birds

Birds (class Aves) are, like mammals, homeoendotherms or heteroendotherms, although they evolved to endothermy independently from a different group of reptiles than the mammals arose from. Do birds become febrile? Studies on fever in birds have been limited.

VAN MIERT and FRENS (1968) induced fever in chickens (*Gallus domesticus*) by intravenous (i.v.) injection of *Escherichia coli* endotoxin. PITTMAN et al. (1976) induced fever in chickens by injection of *Salmonella abortus-equi* endotoxin into the anterior hypothalamus, and also by injection of prostaglandin E_1 (PGE_1) into the anterior hypothalamus. NISTICO and ROTIROTI (1978) induced fever in chickens by infusion of PGE_1, PGE_2, or O-antigen into the third cerebral ventricle. Fevers induced by O-antigen were abolished or reduced by intravenous (i.v.), intramuscular (i.m.) or intracerebroventricular (i.c.v.) injection of the antipyretics indomethacin, aspirin, or ibuprofen, but PGE fever was unaffected by the antipyretics..

D'ALECY and KLUGER (1975) injected pigeons (*Columba livia*) with the Gram-negative bacterium *Pasteurella multocida*, the agent of fowl cholera, and found a complex dose-dependent febrile response which was attenuated by sodium salicylate. Salicylate alone lowered body temperatures by 0.32 °C. Intraperitoneal (i.p.) injections of live *P. multocida* resulted in terminal hyperpyrexia and death, while i.p. injections of 5×10^7–5×10^{10} killed *P. multocida* cells caused fevers ranging from 0.09° to 1.06 °C without mortality.

C. Febrile Responses of Reptiles

Fever was first demonstrated in the lizard *Dipsosaurus dorsalis* by VAUGHN et al. (1974), induced by intracardiac injection of killed Gram-negative bacteria, *Aeromonas hydrophila*. Fever has also been induced in *D. dorsalis* by intracardiac injection of *Pasteurella haemolytica* and *Citrobacter diversus* (KLUGER 1978, 1979). KLUGER (1978, 1979) also reported induction of fever in *Iguana iguana* by intracardiac injection of *A. hydrophila*. BERNHEIM and KLUGER (1977) induced fever in *D. dorsalis* by intracardiac injection of lizard or rabbit-derived endogenous or leucocytic pyrogen (LP).

KLUGER et al. (1975) showed that fever enhances survival of *D. dorsalis* infected with live *A. hydrophila*, which causes haemorrhagic septicaemia. BERNHEIM and KLUGER (1976a) showed that the antipyretic salicylate blocks the febrile response of *D. dorsalis*, and (1976b) that this antipyretic action reduces survival by preventing fever in the infected animals.

Lizards are generally heliothermic, thermoregulating by shuttling between sun and shade during the day; at night their body temperatures fall to ambient burrow temperatures. They can develop fever only during the day, by spending more time in the sun (or near a radiant heat source in the laboratory). MALVIN and KLUGER (1979) showed that the green iguana (*I. iguana*) does not increase its metabolic heat production or oxygen consumption when injected with bacteria and prevented from thermoregulating behaviourally. However, despite the fact that fever in heliothermic lizards is necessarily a strictly diurnal phenomenon, survival from infections is enhanced (KLUGER et al. 1975; KLUGER 1978). BERNHEIM et al. (1978) have suggested that febrile enhancement of survival of infected lizards is attributable in part to more rapid movement of macrophages to the site of infection due to increased blood flow, while KLUGER and ROTHENBURG (1979) have demonstrated a reduction in bacterial growth resulting from an interaction of fever and reduced iron availability.

D. Febrile Responses of Amphibians

CASTERLIN and REYNOLDS (1977a), and REYNOLDS and COVERT (1977) reported the discovery of febrile responses to intraperitoneal (i.p.) injection of killed *A. hydrophila* in two species of anuran amphibian tadpole larvae, *Rana catesbeiana* and *R. pipiens*. These aquatic larvae thermoregulate in water behaviourally as do fishes; when febrile, they select a higher than normal water temperature, thereby raising their body temperatures. KLUGER (1977) induced fever in the adult tree frog *Hyla cinerea* with *A. hydrophila*. MYHRE et al. (1977) reported febrile responses in adult *R. esculenta* to several pyrogens, including *Mycobacterium xenopi*, *M. ranae*, and *M. aquae II*, prostaglandin E_1, and endogenous pyrogen (LP). Thus, either aquatic tadpoles or terrestrial adults of four different anuran amphibian species develop fever in response to various pyrogens.

E. Febrile Responses of Fishes

Behavioural fever was first demonstrated in bony fishes (class Osteichthyes) by REYNOLDS et al. (1976a), who found that i.p. injection of 4×10^9 killed *A. hydro-*

phila cells induced a 1°–3 °C increase in preferred temperature of bluegill sunfish (*Lepomis macrochirus*) and largemouth bass (*Micropoterus salmoides*). Fever was later found in goldfish, *Carassius auratus* (REYNOLDS and COVERT 1977; COVERT and REYNOLDS 1977; REYNOLDS et al. 1978c). Tests have not yet been conducted to determine whether sharks and lampreys also exhibit fever.

The antipyretic acetaminophen (paracetamol) prevents fever in bluegills (REYNOLDS 1977c). Fever can be induced in bluegills or goldfish not only by killed or live *A. hydrophila* (REYNOLDS et al. 1976a; REYNOLDS and COVERT 1977; COVERT and REYNOLDS 1977) – the pyrogenic agent presumably being the lipopolysaccharide endotoxin from the Gram-negative bacterial cell wall – but also by lyophilized *E. coli* endotoxin (Difco Labs strain 055:B5; REYNOLDS et al. 1978c) and by killed Gram-positive *Staphylococcus aureus*, which lacks endotoxin (REYNOLDS et al. 1978a). The magnitude of the fever depends on the pyrogen and administered dosage, and also apparently on the "febrile scope" between the normothermic thermal preferendum of the species and its ultimate upper incipient lethal temperature, which is greater for goldfish than for the other two species tested (REYNOLDS and CASTERLIN 1980).

The goldfish and the bass, but not the bluegill, exhibit diel thermoregulatory rhythms (REYNOLDS and CASTERLIN 1976, 1978e; REYNOLDS et al. 1978b). The rhythm is maintained during fever, cycling about a higher febrile set-point (COVERT and REYNOLDS 1977). Because of the rhythm of preferred temperature, 24-h mean temperatures before and after administration of pyrogens are compared to determine whether a febrile response has occurred (REYNOLDS et al. 1976a) to avoid difficulties of interpretation caused by the rhythm.

A fish placed in a homogeneous thermal environment (a tank of water at a single temperature) cannot thermoregulate and cannot develop fever. When injected with pyrogens, a fish shows no significant increase in core body temperature or in oxygen consumption as compared with control fish injected only with sterile pyrogen-free saline (handling and injection procedures do induce greater locomotor activity compared with undisturbed fish) (REYNOLDS and CASTERLIN 1980; REYNOLDS et al. 1980). Increased movement, blood flow and gill ventilation rates actually serve to decrease the body core "excess" (above ambient water) temperature, since heat losses exceed any augmentation in heat production by the skeletal muscles. Thus a fish cannot develop fever by other than behavioural means, as is true of most ectotherms and even neonatal rabbits (SATINOFF et al. 1976). NAGAI and IRIKI (1978) have reported an autonomic response of fish to bacterial pyrogen, but this is of doubtful thermoregulatory significance (it may, however, presage the later evolution of physiological thermoregulatory mechanisms in endotherms; REYNOLDS 1977a; REYNOLDS and CASTERLIN 1978a).

F. Pyretic and Antipyretic Agents

CLARK and LIPTON (1974) observed that "agents which alter the set-point for physiological thermoregulatory activity produce a complementary shift in the behavioural set-point as well." POLK and LIPTON (1975) further observed that "to characterize drug actions on thermoregulatory processes it is necessary to know whether compounds which alter body temperature also cause changes in thermoregulatory motivation." CLARK and LIPTON (1974) found, for example, that tetrodotoxin (produced by pufferfishes, family Tetraodontidae) and saxitoxin lowered the set-point(s) for behavioural and physiological thermoregulation in the cat.

It is our purpose here to review the literature regarding effects of various substances on thermoregulation in non-mammalian vertebrates. While not all of these substances may strictly fit the definition of pyretics or antipyretics, it is useful to catalogue those substances which have been found not to be pyretics or antipyretics as well as those which are, so that future investigations need not duplicate existing knowledge. Some relevant information has been published, for example, in the fisheries literature rather than in biomedical journals, and may be missed in literature searches limited in scope. We will include data on substances which have been shown to affect body temperature in either an upward or a downward direction in various species, although the emphasis will be on pyretics and antipyretics. In many cases, the neuropharmacological mode of action of the substances is not known or not given in the literature; in other cases, the mode of action is speculative.

I. Bacterial Pyrogens

Various kinds of bacteria, both Gram-negative and Gram-positive, have been found to induce fever in non-mammalian vertebrates, just as they do in mammals. Gram-negative *A. hydrophila*, either live or killed, induces fever when injected by various routes into fishes (REYNOLDS et al. 1976a, 1978a, c, 1979, 1980; REYNOLDS 1977c; REYNOLDS and Covert 1977), amphibians (CASTERLIN and REYNOLDS 1977a; REYNOLDS and COVERT 1977; KLUGER 1977), and reptiles (VAUGHN et al. 1974; KLUGER et al. 1975; BERNHEIM and KLUGER 1976a, b, 1977; KLUGER 1978, 1979; MALVIN and KLUGER 1979). Presumably, it is the lipolysaccharide (LPS) endotoxin in the cell wall of Gram-negative bacteria which is the major pyrogen, since *E. coli* endotoxin induces fever in fish (REYNOLDS et al. 1978c) and in birds (VAN MIERT and FRENS 1968). However, endotoxin is not the only bacterial pyrogen, for Gram-positive bacteria which lack endotoxin, such as *Staphylococcus aureus*, also induce fever (REYNOLDS et al. 1978a). Other bacteria or bacterial products which induce fever in non-mammalian vertebrates include *Pasteurella multocida* (birds; D'ALECY and KLUGER 1975) and *P. haemolytica* (lizards; KLUGER 1978, 1979), *Citrobacter diversus* (lizards; KLUGER 1979), *Mycobacterium* spp. (frogs; MYHRE et al. 1977), and *Salmonella abortus-equi* endotoxin (birds; PITTMAN et al. 1976).

II. Endogenous Leucocytic Pyrogen

Bacterial and other exogenous pyrogens are thought to induce fever by stimulating leucocytes of the host organism to produce endogenous leucocytic pyrogen (LP), which differs from endotoxin in being proteinaceous and thus thermolabile. BERNHEIM and KLUGER (1977) have identified an endogenous pyrogen-like substance in the lizard *Dipsosaurus dorsalis* which behaves similarly to mammalian LP: it is thermolabile, and induces a monophasic fever of short latency.

MYHRE et al. (1977) presented evidence for the existence of an endogenous pyrogen in the frog *Rana esculenta*. It has not yet been determined whether fishes produce a similar substance, but it seems not unlikely that they do.

III. Prostaglandins

It has been hypothesized that a further stage in the mediation of fever involves the production of prostaglandins, particularly those of the E series (MILTON and WENDLANDT 1970, 1971; VANE 1971; BLIGH and MILTON 1972; COCEANI 1974; CRAWSHAW and STITT 1975; ZIEL and KRUPP 1976; VEALE et al. 1977; ELATTAR 1978), although this has been disputed (CRANSTON et al. 1976). PGE_1 induces fever in mammals (CRAWSHAW and STITT 1975), frogs (MYHRE et al. 1978), and even arthropods (CASTERLIN and REYNOLDS 1978 b; CASTERLIN et al. 1978; REYNOLDS et al. 1979; Chap. 20, this volume). The PGE fever is of relatively short latency and duration. PGE is rapidly inactivated in vivo by enzymes (COCEANI 1974, 1976; BISHAI and COCEANI 1976), and so must be injected directly into the brain in order to induce fever in vertebrates. Intraperitoneal injection of PGE_1 does not induce fever in fish, probably because it does not reach the brain before being inactivated (REYNOLDS and CASTERLIN, unpublished data). In arthropods, however, PGE_1 can be injected directly into the haemocoel of the open circulatory system (see Chap. 20, this volume).

NISTICO and ROTIROTI (1978) induced fever in the chicken *Gallus domesticus* by infusing PGE_1 or PGE_2 into the third cerebral ventricle. The fever so induced was not blocked by antipyretics. PITTMAN et al. (1976) also induced fever in the chicken by injecting PGE_1 into the anterior hypothalamus.

IV. Antipyretics

Antipyretics are thought to prevent fever by interfering with PG synthesis (VANE 1971; ZIEL and KRUPP 1976; VEALE et al. 1977). Salicylate has been found to be antipyretic in lizards (BERNHEIM and KLUGER 1976a, b), and acetaminophen is antipyretic in fish (REYNOLDS 1977c). Both substances are antipyretic in mammals as well. NISTICO and ROTIROTI (1978) found that aspirin (salicylate), indomethacin and ibuprofen prevent induction of fever in birds by O-antigen, but do not affect PGE fever.

Antipyretics supposedly do not alter body temperature by themselves, but rather interfere with the effects of pyrogens. SATINOFF (1972) disputed this, presenting evidence that salicylate can lower the body temperature of rats. However, acetaminophen alone did not significantly affect the PT of fish (REYNOLDS 1977c) or of crayfish (see Chap. 20, this volume).

GREEN and LOMAX (1976, 1977) reported that the histamine antagonist pyrilamine blocked the induction of fever by histamine in the damselfish *Chromis chromis* but had no effect by itself.

V. Parietalectomy

Parietalectomy increases the preferred temperatures of lizards (ENGBRETSON and HUTCHISON 1976; ROTH and RALPH 1977; RALPH et al. 1979), as compared with normal or with sham-operated animals. The effect of the pineal–parietal complex may be mediated through neural mechanisms or via control of brain electrolytes (RALPH et al. 1979), or by means of the hormone melatonin, which is secreted by the pineal complex (HUTCHISON, personal communication).

VI. Hormones

LOUW et al. (1976) injected monitor lizards (*Varanus albigularis*) with daily subcutaneous doses of L-thyroxine Na (200 µg/100 g body weight/day) for seven days, and found that this induced a 27% increase in resting metabolic rate and a 63% increase in the thermal gradient between core and ambient temperature, at the normothermic preferred temperature of 35 °C. Since the body temperature was held constant at 38 °C during these tests in a temperature-controlled chamber, the increased core–peripheral thermal gradient implies that the ambient temperature was lower to compensate for the increased metabolic rate of the thyroxine-treated animals. The authors noted also that, by six weeks after treatment and metabolic rate measurements, the PT of the lizards was re-measured in a photothermal gradient and proved to be lower by 1.3 °C (33.6 °C) compared with similar tests before thyroxine treatment (34.9 °C). REYNOLDS, CASTERLIN and SPIELER (1982) found a similar decrease in PT of bluegill sunfish and goldfish following addition of thyroxine to the water, but did not measure metabolic rates. Possibly the lowered PT offset the increased metabolic heat production in *Varanus*, but LOUW et al. (1976) provided no data on the PT immediately following the seven-day thyroxine treatment, when the metabolic rates were measured. It is worthy of note that the monitor lizard family Varanidae approaches endothermy more closely than any other reptile group (BARTHOLOMEW and TUCKER 1964), in terms of "tachymetabolic" response to thyroxine (reaching about a third of the metabolic rate of an equivalent sized mammal). *V. albigularis* did not display any metabolic response to noradrenaline (although heart rate decreased), however, indicating the absence of non-shivering thermogenesis (LOUW et al. 1976). BLIGH et al. (1976) reported no effect of i.c.v. injections of noradrenaline on the panting response of *Varanus* to high temperature.

TONQUE (1977) investigated the effects of thyrotropin releasing hormone (TRH) and other hormones on behavioural thermoregulation in neonatal chickens (*Gallus domesticus*). Many neonatal birds, like some neonatal mammals (SATINOFF et al. 1976), are largely ectothermic and thermoregulate primarily by behavioural means (MYHRE 1978). TRH, as well as thyroid stimulating hormone (TSH), are secreted more actively in response to a cold stimulus in mammals, and TRH is known to have effects on the CNS distinct from its TSH-releasing function (TONQUE 1977). Intraventricular injection of TRH blocked thermoregulatory behaviour (heat-seeking) of chicks, although similar injections of LHRH, constituent amino acids of TRH, or i.p. injections of TSH or thyroxine did not affect the chick's thermoregulatory behaviour. i.p. injection of TRH was ineffective unless preceded by i.p. thyroxine pre-treatment; i.p. injection of somatostatin blocked the thermoregulatory behaviour unless preceded by thyroxine pre-treatment. The minimum dose of intraventricular TRH which blocked thermoregulatory behaviour was 0.5 µg. TONQUE (1977) inferred from these results that TRH plays some central

(CNS) role in mediating behavioural thermoregulation in chicks, noting also that thyroxine influences the CNS distribution of TRH.

There are interesting interactions of hormones and other substances involved in the acclimatization responses of ectothermic vertebrates to changes in temperature (acclimatization being an alternative and complementary strategy to thermoregulation in ectotherms; REYNOLDS 1979). The thyroid apparently participates in the mediation of compensatory changes in oxidative metabolism during temperature acclimatization (LAGERSPETZ et al. 1974), and LAGERSPETZ et al. (1974) suggest that control of the thyroid in the acclimatization process may occur either directly by catecholamines, or by TSH, the release of which may be affected by the neurochemical changes found during temperature acclimatization. HARRI (1974) concluded that thyroid hormones may be important in regulating the responsiveness to catecholamines in amphibians, affecting sensitivity to adrenaline. HULBERT (1978) suggested that the mode of action of thyroid hormones in thermal acclimatization involved alteration of the level of unsaturation of membrane fatty acids, affecting membrane fluidity and function. WODTKE (1978) reported changes in lipid composition of liver mitochondrial membranes in carp during thermal acclimatization. YAKOVLEVA and KOMACHKOVA (1978) reported that the response of sturgeon (*Acipenser guldenstadti*) to a decrease in water temperatures follows the pattern of stress reaction, and noted changes in number, growth and differentiation of neurosecretory cells in the dorsal part of the preoptic nucleus of the fish. BROWN et al. (1978) noted that stress due to physical injury elevated plasma thyroxine in rainbow trout (*Salmo gairdneri*). PETER and McKEOWN (1975) report that thyroxine has a negative feedback effect on both the pituitary and the hypothalamus in goldfish (*Carassius auratus*).

Diel fluctuations of serum levels of triiodothyronine and thyroxine are complementary to diel rhythms of prolactin and preferred temperature in goldfish (REYNOLDS 1977 d; SPIELER et al. 1977; REYNOLDS et al. 1978 b; SPIELER and NOESKE 1979). WIGHAM et al. (1977) noted that in the tilapia *Sarotherodon mossambicus*, TRH inhibited prolactin release but not synthesis. PETER and McKEOWN (1975) state that there are afferent pathways to the hypothalamus from the preoptic-thalamic region that tend to stimulate prolactin secretion, "presumably by inhibiting hypothalamic PIF [prolactin release-inhibiting factor] activity." MEIER (1970) found that thyroxine phases the circadian fattening response to prolactin. TAKAHARA et al. (1977) found that PGE_1 stimulates the release of prolactin from the pituitary, while HORSEMAN and MEIER (1978) hypothesize that some of prolactin's osmoregulatory effects in fishes are mediated by stimulation of prostaglandin synthesis, based on their finding that indomethacin or aspirin, which inhibit prostaglandin synthesis (VANE 1971), prevent elevation of plasma chloride following prolactin injection into the teleost fish *Fundulus grandis*. PGE_1 induced increases in plasma chloride concentrations in fish treated with indomethacin or aspirin. TAKAHARA et al. (1977) deduced that indomethacin might block the release of prolactin and other pituitary hormones. LAGERSPETZ et al. (1974) reported that daily injections of adrenaline stimulated thyroid activity in frogs (*Rana temporaria*), but injections of 5-hydroxytryptamine (5-HT) did not affect the thyroid.

Prolactin levels in the serum of goldfish rise and fall (McKEOWN and PETER 1976) in a daily rhythm which roughly parallels the diel thermoregulatory rhythm

(REYNOLDS 1977 d), with the peak of both rhythms occurring during the latter part of scotophase (pre-dawn). The rhythmic conjunction of behaviourally mediated thermocycle and exogenously controlled photoperiod was found to maximize growth and reproductive potential of the goldfish (SPIELER et al. 1977, REYNOLDS et al. 1978 b; REYNOLDS 1977 d). However, the causal relationships among these factors remain as yet unclear, for neither hypophysectomy nor injection of pro-lactin (REYNOLDS and CASTERLIN, unpublished data) affect the preferred tempera-ture of goldfish. It is perhaps worthy of note, however, that prolactin is known to have osmoregulatory effects in fishes, and that salinity of the ambient water effects the PT of some fishes (GARSIDE and MORRISON 1977, GARSIDE et al. 1977). Ratios of Ca^{2+} and Na^+ ions in the brain are reported to affect thermoregulation (MEYERS et al. 1976; MYERS 1977; SAXENA 1976), suggesting a possible connection.

From all of the above, it is apparent that thyroxine, prolactin and other hor-mones have some relation to thermal acclimatization and thermoregulation, but the web of causes and effects is intricately woven and requires further study.

VII. Pesticides

1. Organochlorines

Organochlorine pesticides affect axonal transmission in the central and peripheral nervous systems (DOMANIK and ZAR 1978). DDT and related compounds (DDD, DDE, and methoxychlor) increase the PT of Atlantic salmon (*Salmo salar*) by 4°–5 °C when present in the ambient water at concentrations of 0.03–0.05 ppm (*pp'*DDT), 0.16–0.30 ppm (*op'*DDT), 0.04–0.10 ppm (*pp'*DDD), 0.50–2.00 ppm (*pp'*DDE), and 0.04–0.05 ppm (methoxychlor), according to PETERSON (1976). OGILVIE and ANDERSON (1965) reported that higher doses of DDT raised the PT of *S. salar* by 6°–10 °C, while lower doses (down to 5 ppb) decreased PT by 2 °C. JAVAID (1972) reported that DDT raised the PT by as much as 10 °C, or lowered it by as much as 8 °C, depending on dosage, in various salmonid fishes. GARDNER (1973) reported similar findings for the brook trout *Salvelinus fontinalis*, over a concentration range of 20–50 ppb. A five-fold decrease in the concentration of DDT necessary to induce a 4°–5 °C increase in the PT of *S. salar* (PETERSON 1973 a, 1976) induces a decrease in PT (ANDERSON 1971).

Aroclor (a polychlorinated biphenyl, or PCB) caused no change in PT of two salmonid species (PETERSON 1973 a, b, 1976; MILLER and OGILVIE 1975). Sodium pentachlorophenate (NaPCP) induced a 5 °C decrease in PT of *S. salar* at a con-centration of 1 ppm (PETERSON 1976). Lindane produced a 1 °C increase at 0.01–0.03 ppm, but the change was not statistically significant (PETERSON 1976). Aldrin at 0.05–0.15 ppm lowered PT of *S. salar* by 3 °C; concentrations of 0.01–0.025 ppm of dieldrin, or 5–25 ppb of heptachlor produced insignificant decreases of about 1 °C (PETERSON 1976). Thus organochlorines can either raise or lower the PT of fishes, depending on the compound and the dosage.

2. Organophosphates

Organophosphate pesticides are acetylcholinesterase inhibitors (DOMANIK and ZAR 1978). Concentrations of 0.05–1.0 ppb in the ambient water induced dose- and age-dependent decreases of 1.9–4.3 °C in PT of adult shiners (*Notropis cornutus*) with lesser effects in younger individuals (DOMANIK and ZAR 1978). Concentrations of 25–50 ppb induced a 2 °C decrease in PT of *S. salar* (PETERSON 1976). Fenitrothion induced a similar decrease at 0.4–1.0 ppm, but this was reportedly not statistically significant (PETERSON 1976). Azinphosphorethyl (Guthion) at 2–3 ppb lowered PT of *S. salar* by 4 °C (PETERSON 1976), as did 100–250 ppb of chlorpyrifos (Dursban) and 150–300 ppb of naled (Dibrom). It therefore appears that this class of compounds, unlike organochlorines, tends to lower but not raise the PT of fishes.

3. Other Pesticides

Carbaryl (Sevin), a carbamate pesticide, was found by PETERSON (1976) to have no effect on PT of *S. salar* at concentrations of 0.25–1.00 ppm. ANDERSON (1971) reported that potassium cyanide (KCN) at 20–40 ppb lowered the PT of *S. salar* by 5 °C. MILLER and OGILVIE (1975) reported that 10 ppm of phenol lowered the PT of *Salvelinus fontinalis* by 3 °C.

VIII. Heavy Metals and Their Salts

OPUSZYNSKI (1971) reported that copper sulphate ($CuSO_4$) lowered the preferred temperature of fathead minnows (*Pimephales promelas*) previously exposed to 0.20–0.25 ppm by 5 °C, while PETERSON (1976) found that 15–30 ppb lowered the PT of *S. salar* by 2 °C. Cadmium sulphate ($CdSO_4$) at 2 ppb produced an insignificant 1 °C decrease in PT of *S. salar*, while zinc sulphate ($ZnSO_4$) at 0.4 ppm produced no change (PETERSON 1976). The apparent tendency for heavy metals is to produce a decrease in PT, so they are not pyrogenic.

IX. Inorganic Ions (Salinity)

Concentrations of ions in the brain have been hypothesized to play a role in mammalian thermoregulation (see, for example, MYERS 1977). If this is true for other vertebrates, it may offer an explanation for the effects of ambient water salinity on PT of several fish species (GARSIDE and MORRISON 1977; GARSIDE et al. 1977). Three-spined sticklebacks (*Gasterosteus aculeatus*) collected from seawater exhibited final preferenda of 18 °C in seawater, and 16 °C in freshwater; preferenda were higher in brackish water (10.5 ‰ salinity) than in seawater or freshwater (GARSIDE et al. 1977). The marine mummichog (*Fundulus heteroclitus*) preferred 3°–6 °C higher temperatures in seawater than in freshwater, while the freshwater killifish *F. diaphanus* preferred 5°–8 °C higher temperatures in freshwater than in seawater (GARSIDE and MORRISON 1977). GARSIDE et al. (1977) interpreted these results in terms of osmoregulatory load. Changes in cerebrospinal fluid (CSF) or hypothalamic $Ca^{2+}:Na^+$ ion ratio could also mediate such an effect (MYERS et al. 1976). Sodium and calcium ions have also been found to affect the temperature setpoint of the pigeon (SAXENA 1976).

X. Nutritive Substances

Nutritional status has been found to affect the body temperatures of endotherms and the preferred temperatures of ectotherms (REGAL 1966, 1967; JAVAID and ANDERSON 1967; BUSTARD 1967; LILLYWHITE et al. 1973; GATTEN 1974; STUNTZ and MAGNUSON 1976; REYNOLDS and CASTERLIN 1979). Reptiles reportedly exhibit a thermophilic response after feeding which is supposed to facilitate the rate of digestion (REGAL 1966, 1967; BUSTARD 1967; GATTEN 1974), and starvation is reported to lower the preferred temperatures of fishes (JAVAID and ANDERSON 1967; STUNTZ and MAGNUSON 1976; REYNOLDS and CASTERLIN 1979). The mechanisms mediating these thermoregulatory effects of nutritional status are not yet known.

XI. Other Substances Affecting Thermoregulation

OGILVIE and FRYER (1971) found that exposing guppies (*Poecilia reticulata*) to a subanaesthetic dose of 300 ppb of sodium pentobarbitol (nembutal) lowered their PT by 6 °C. Later, FRYER and OGILVIE (1974) reported that exposing *S. gairdneri* (rainbow trout) to 480 ppb significantly raised the PT, whereas 300 ppb significantly lowered the PT of *S. salar*. Thus it is apparent that this substance raises or lowers the PT of fishes according to dosage and species, but it is difficult to separate the dosage effects from species effects. Pentobarbitol affects thermoregulation in mammals by acting on the hypothalamus (WEISS and LATIES 1963; FELDBERG 1970).

    GREEN and LOMAX (1976, 1977) exposed damselfish (*Chromis chromis*) to various pharmacological agents that modify cholinergic or histaminergic activity in the brain. Cholinergic stimulation, both muscarinic and nicotinic, lowered the thermoregulatory (upper avoidance temperature) set-point. Oxotremorine significantly lowered the set-point (4 °C) when injected intracerebrally (0.1–1.0 µg) or when added to the ambient water (systemic exposure by the "contamination technique") at 1 ppm (1 mg/l), (GREEN and LOMAX 1976); 1 ppm of atropine blocked this effect, but hyoscine was ineffective. Nicotine at 0.1 ppm significantly lowered the set-point by 3.3 °C, but a greater concentration of 1 ppm was ineffective. The cholinesterase inhibitors neostigmine (1 ppm) and physostigmine (0.1–1.0 ppm) had no effect at the concentrations tested. Histamine (0.01–0.1 ppm) raised the set-point significantly by 1.8°–2.4 °C. The histamine antagonist pyrilamine (1.0 ppm) blocked this pyrogenic effect of histamine, but had no effect by itself (thus acting as an antipyretic) as has already been noted. The histamine metabolite imidazole acetic acid had no effect on the set-point. The route of administration indicates that there is little blood–brain barrier in fish to histamine passage. The effect of histamine was interpreted by GREEN and LOMAX (1976) as an action of the H_1 receptors. L-Dopa significantly raised the set-point by 3.4 °C at 10 ppm concentration, but was ineffective at 30, 1.0, or 0.1 ppm; GREEN and LOMAX (1976) suggested that this might be explained by a changing balance between antagonistic dopaminergic and noradrenergic effects of L-dopa. In general, GREEN and LOMAX (1976) concluded, "biogenic amine activity in the fish appears to modulate the thermostats in the central nervous system in a manner similar to that found in endotherms when due allowance is made for species differences."

FRYER and OGILVIE (1978) exposed guppies to 20–120 ppm concentrations of 5-HT, a putative neurotransmitter in the CNS thermoregulatory centre, and found that lower doses decreased, and higher doses significantly increased, the PT. Injections of 5-HT (2 µg/g, ip) induced first a decrease of 4 °C, and then a subsequent increase of 1.5 °C compared with the normothermic temperature in Atlantic salmon (FRYER and OGILVIE 1978). This work also indicated that the blood–brain barrier of fish does not prevent entry of 5-HT into the brain. The pattern of temperature change observed in salmon is similar to that resulting from systemic or central injection of 5-HT in rabbits (JACOB et al. 1972). Both 5-HT and catecholamines have been found in the brains of fishes (VON EULER 1961; WELSH 1968).

BLIGH et al. (1976) injected noradrenaline (a putative neurotransmitter as well as a hormone) and carbachol (a cholinometic substance) into the cerebral ventricles of the monitor lizard *Varanus albigularis*, and found that noradrenaline or physiological saline injections i.c.v. had no effect on panting thresholds, but that carbachol inhibited panting and disrupted thermoregulatory behaviour. The inhibitory effect of carbachol on panting in this lizard parallels similar results for sheep, goats, and rabbits (BLIGH et al. 1971), but the lack of effect of noradrenaline contrasts with the effect on these mammals; however, effects of these substances vary even among mammalian species (BLIGH 1973), and BLIGH et al. (1976) postulate that the species differences may be due to transmitters acting at more than one synaptic point in the neuronal network controlling thermoregulation.

Morphine induces hypothermia in doves (ZIEHUISEN 1895), as well as in mammals, probably through some central action involving neurotransmitters (LOTTI 1973).

G. Survival Value of Fever in Non-mammalian Vertebrates

Fever has been found to enhance survival in lizards (KLUGER et al. 1975) and fishes (COVERT and REYNOLDS 1977) infected with live *A. hydrophila*. Preventing fever by eliminating opportunities to thermoregulate behaviourally, or by administration of antipyretics (BERNHEIM and KLUGER 1976b), reduces survival. The enhanced survival cannot be explained by differences in agglutinating antibody titres (COVERT and REYNOLDS 1977) nor by the effects of temperature alone on bacterial growth as measured in vitro (KLUGER et al. 1975; COVERT and REYNOLDS 1977). However, serum levels of reduced iron also fall during fever, and a combination of reduced iron availability and increased temperature significantly reduces bacterial growth (KLUGER and ROTHENBURG 1979). Serum levels of other metals change also: zinc decreases, and copper increases in availability (KLUGER, personal communication). These may also affect bacterial growth; $CuSO_4$ is widely used as an algicide to limit growth of blue-green algae (Cyanobacteria), and to combat parasitic diseases of fishes as well.

Another mechanism by which fever may help an organism to fight infection is by enhancing blood flow and thereby speeding the movements of blood leucocytes to the site of infection. REYNOLDS (1977a) and REYNOLDS and CASTERLIN (1978a) showed that blood flow in fishes is increased by a rise in temperature, and BERNHEIM et al. (1978) showed that such enhanced blood flow does in fact speed the movement of leucocytes to the site of infection in lizards. Thus a febrile rise in temperature, whether produced by behavioural or by physiological means, works in conjunction with other host defense (immune) reactions to help combat infections in at least two different ways.

The fact that the febrile response can be traced far back into evolutionary time (or alternatively, that it might have arisen independently many times in diverse groups of animals, including invertebrates) suggests that fever does serve a very important adaptive function in helping to combat infection (STERN 1977).

H. Summary of Agents Found to Induce Fever in Non-mammalian Vertebrates

In addition to such influences as feeding, parietalectomy, and salinity variations, the following agents have been found to induce fever (an increase in preferred or body temperatures) at some dosages in some species of non-mammalian vertebrates, and therefore are at least sometimes pyretic in a broadly defined sense:

Bacteria (live, killed, Gram-negative, or Gram-positive)
Endotoxin from Gram-negative bacteria (LPS)
Endogenous leucocytic pyrogen (LP)
O-antigen
Prostaglandins (E_1, E_2)
Histamine
Sodium pentobarbital
DDT and related organochlorines (DDD, DDE, methoxychlor)
L-dopa
5-HT (serotonin).

J. Summary of Antipyretics Found to Block Fever in Non-mammalian Vertebrates

These substances have been reported to prevent the induction of fever by pyretic agents in some species of non-mammalian vertebrates, while generally producing no effect on thermoregulation by themselves:

Salicylate (aspirin)
Acetaminophen (paracetamol)
Indomethacin
Ibuprofen
Pyrilamine (histamine antagonist; blocks histamine-induced fever).

References

Anderson JM (1971) Assessment of the effects of pollutants on physiology and behavior. II. Sublethal effects and changes in ecosystems. Proc R Soc Lond [Biol] 77:307–320

Adair ER (1974) Hypothalamic control of thermoregulatory behavior. In: Lederis K, Cooper KE (eds) Recent studies of hypothalamic function. Karger, Basel pp 341–358

Bartholomew GA, Tucker VA (1964) Size, body temperature, thermal conductance, oxygen consumption and heart rate in Australian varanid lizards. Physiol Zool 37:341–354

Bernheim HA, Kluger MJ (1976a) Fever and antipyresis in the lizard *Dipsosaurus dorsalis*. Am J Physiol 231:198–203

Bernheim HA, Kluger MJ (1976b) Fever: effect of drug-induced antipyresis on survival. Science 193:237–239

Bernheim HA, Kluger MJ (1977) Endogenous pyrogen-like substance produced by reptiles. J Physiol (Lond) 267:659–666

Bernheim HA, Bodel PT, Askenase PW, Atkins E (1978) Effects of fever on host defense mechanisms after infection in the lizard *Dipsosaurus dorsalis*. Br J Exp Pathol 59:76–84

Bishai I, Coceani F (1976) Presence of 15-hydroxy prostaglandin dehydrogenase, prostaglandin-Δ^{13}-reductase and prostaglandin E-9-keto(α)-reductase in the frog spinal cord. J. Neurochem 26:1167–1174

Bligh J (1973) Temperature regulation in mammals and other vertebrates. North-Holland, Amsterdam

Bligh J, Milton AS (1972) The thermoregulatory effects of prostaglandin E_1 when infused into a lateral cerebral ventricle of the Welsh mountain sheep at different ambient temperatures. J Physiol (Lond) 229:30–31P

Bligh J, Cottle WH, Maskrey M (1971) Influence of ambient temperature on the thermoregulatory responses to 5-hydroxytryptamine, noradrenaline and acetylcholine injected into the lateral cerebral ventricles of sheep, goats and rabbits. J Physiol (Lond) 212:377–392

Bligh J, Louw G, Young BA (1976) Effect of cerebroventricular administration of noradrenaline and carbachol on behavioural and autonomic thermoregulation in the monitor lizard *Varanus albigularis albigularis*. J Therm Biol 1:241–243

Brattstrom BH (1979) Amphibian temperature regulation studies in the field and laboratory. Am Zool 19:345–356

Brown S, Fedoruk K, Eales JG (1978) Physical injury due to injection or blood removal causes transitory elevations of plasma thyroxine in rainbow trout, *Salmo gairdneri*. Can J Zool 56:1998–2003

Bustard HR (1967) Activity cycle and thermoregulation in the Australian gecko *Gehyra variegata*. Copeia 1967:753–758

Casterlin ME, Reynolds WW (1977a) Behavioral fever in anuran amphibian larvae. Life Sci 20:593–596

Casterlin ME, Reynolds WW (1978a) Behavioral thermoregulation in *Rana pipiens* tadpoles. J Therm Biol 3:143–145

Casterlin ME, Reynolds WW (1978b) Prostaglandin E_1 fever in the crayfish *Cambarus bartoni*. Pharmacol Biochem Behav 9:593–595

Casterlin ME, Reynolds WW (1979) Shark thermoregulation. Comp Biochem Physiol [A] 64:451–453

Casterlin ME, Reynolds WW, Covert JB (1978) Prostaglandin E_1- and bacterial pyrogen-induced fever in aquatic ectotherms. Fed Proc 37:427

Clark WG, Lipton JM (1974) Complementary lowering of the behavioural and physiological thermoregulatory set-points by tetrodotoxin and saxitoxin in the cat. J Physiol (Lond) 238:181–191

Coceani F (1974) Prostaglandins and the central nervous system. Arch Intern Med 133:119–129

Coceani F (1976) Prostaglandin system in developing and mature central nervous tissue. In: Brazier MAB, Coceani E (eds) Brain dysfunction in infantile febrile convulsion. Raven, New York, pp 55–67

Covert JB, Reynolds WW (1977) Survival value of fever in fish. Nature 267:43–45

Cranston WI, Duff GW, Hellon RF, Mitchell D, Townsend Y (1976) Evidence that brain prostaglandin synthesis is not essential in fever. J Physiol (Lond) 259:239–249

Crawshaw LI, Hammel HT (1973) Behavioral temperature regulation in the California horn shark, *Heterodontus francisci*. Brain Behav Evol 7:447–452

Crawshaw LI, Hammel HT (1974) Behavioral regulation of internal temperature in the brown bullhead, *Ictalurus nebulosus*. Comp Biochem Physiol [A] 47:51–60

Crawshaw LI, Stitt JT (1975) Behavioural and autonomic induction of prostaglandin E_1 fever in squirrel monkeys. J Physiol (Lond) 244:197–206

D'Alecy LG, Kluger MJ (1975) Avian febrile response. J Physiol (Lond) 253:223–232

Dean JM (1976) Temperatures of tissues in freshwater fishes. Trans Am Fish Soc 105:709–711

Dizon AE, Brill RW (1979) Thermoregulation in tunas. Am Zool 19:249–265

Domanik AM, Zar HJ (1978) The effect of malathion on the temperature selection response of the common shiner, *Notropis cornutus*. Bull Environ Contam Toxicol 7:193–206

Elattar TMA (1978) Prostaglandins: physiology, biochemistry, pharmacology and clinical applications. J Oral Pathol 7:239–282

Engbretson GA, Hutchison VH (1976) Parietalectomy and thermal selection in the lizard *Sceloporus magister*. J Exp Zool 198:29–38

Feldberg W (1970) Monoamines of the hypothalamus as mediators of temperature regulation. In: The hypothalamus. Academic Press, New York

Fryer JN, Ogilvie DM (1974) Temperature selection response of Atlantic salmon, *Salmo salar*, and rainbow trout, *Salmo gairdneri*, after exposure to pentobarbitol. Comp Gen Pharmacol 5:111–116

Fryer JN, Ogilvie DM (1978) Alteration of thermoregulatory behavior in fish by 5-hydroxytryptamine. Pharmacol Biochem Behav 8:129–132

Gardner DR (1973) The effect of some DDT and methoxychlor analogs on temperature selection and lethality in brook trout fingerlings. Pestic Biochem Physiol 2:437–440

Garside ET, Morrison GC (1977) Thermal preferences of mummichog, *Fundulus heteroclitus* L., and banded killifish, *F. diaphanus* (LeSueur), (Cyprinodontidae) in relation to thermal acclimation and salinity. Can J Zool 55:1190–1194

Gatten RE Jr (1974) Effect of nutritional status on the preferred body temperature of the turtles *Pseudemys scripta* and *Terrapene ornata*. Copeia 1974:912–917

Green MD, Lomax P (1976) Behavioural thermoregulation and neuroamines in fish (*Chromis chromis*). J Therm Biol 1:237–240

Green MD, Lomax P (1977) Fish (*Chromis chromis*) as a model for the study of thermoregulatory behavior. In: Cooper KE, Lomax P, Schönbaum E (eds) Drugs, biogenic amines and body temperature. Karger, Basel, pp 74–76

Hammel HT (1968) Regulation of internal body temperature. Ann. Rev Physiol 30:641–710

Hammel HT, Caldwell FT Jr, Abrams RM (1967) Regulation of body temperature in the blue-tongued lizard. Science 156:1260–1262

Hammel HT, Strømme SB, Myhre K (1969) Forebrain temperature activates behavioral thermoregulatory response in arctic sculpins. Science 165:83–85

Hammel HT, Crawshaw LI, Cabanac HP (1973) The activation of behavioral responses in the regulation of body temperature in vertebrates. In: Schönbaum E, Lomax P (eds) The pharmacology of thermoregulation. Karger, Basel, pp 124–141

Harri MNE (1974) The relation between thyroid activity and responsiveness to adrenaline during cold acclimation in the frog, *Rana temporaria*. Comp Gen Pharmacol 5:305–309

Horseman ND, Meier AH (1978) Prostaglandin and the osmoregulatory role of prolactin in a teleost. Life Sci 22:1485–1490

Huey RB, Stevenson RD (1979) Integrating thermal physiology and ecology of ectotherms: a discussion of approaches. Am Zool 19:357–366

Hulbert AJ (1978) The thyroid hormones: a thesis concerning their action. J Theor Biol 73:81–100

Jacob J, Girault JM, Peindaries R (1972) Actions of 5-hydroxytryptamine and 5-hydroxytryptophan injected by various routes on the rectal temperature of the rabbit. Neuropharmacology 11:1–16

Javaid MY (1972) Effect of DDT on temperature selection of some salmonids. Pak J Sci Ind Res 15:171–172

Javaid MY, Anderson JM (1967) Influence of starvation on selected temperatures of some salmonids. J Fish Res Board Can 24:1515–1519

Kluger MJ (1977) Fever in the frog *Hyla cinerea*. J Therm Biol 2:79–81

Kluger MJ (1978) The evolution and adaptive value of fever. Am Sci 66:38–43

Kluger MJ (1979) Fever in ectotherms: evolutionary implications. Am Zool 19:295–304

Kluger MJ, Rothenburg BA (1979) Fever and reduced iron: their interaction as a host defense response to bacterial infection. Science 203:374–376

Kluger MJ, Ringler DH, Anver MR (1975) Fever and survival. Science 188:166–168

Lagerspetz KYH, Harri MNE, Okslahti R (1974) The role of the thyroid in the temperature acclimation of the oxidative metabolism in the frog *Rana temporia*. Gen Comp Endocrinol 22:169–176

Lillywhite HB, Licht P, Chelgren P (1973) The role of behavioral thermoregulation in the growth energetics of the toad, *Bufo boreas*. Ecology 54:375–383

Lotti VJ (1973) Body temperature responses to morphine. In: Schönbaum E, Lomax P (eds) The pharmacology of thermoregulation. Karger, Basel, pp 236–244

Louw G, Young BA, Bligh J (1976) Effect of thyroxine and noradrenaline on thermoregulation, cardiac rate and oxygen consumption in the monitor lizard *Varanus albigularis albigularis*. J Therm Biol 1:189–193

Malvin MD, Kluger MJ (1979) Oxygen uptake in green iguana (*Iguana iguana*) injected with bacteria. J Therm Biol 4:147–148

McCauley RW, Reynolds WW, Huggins NH (1977) Photokinesis and behavioral thermoregulation in adult sea lampreys (*Petromyzon marinus*). J Exp Zool 202:431–437

McKeown BA, Peter RE (1976) The effects of photoperiod and temperature on the release of prolactin from the pituitary gland of the goldfish. Can J Zool 54:1960–1969

Meier AH (1970) Thyroxin phases the circadian fattening response of goldfish to prolactin. Proc Soc Exp Biol Med 133:1113–1116

Miller DL, Ogilvie DM (1975) Temperature selecton in the brook trout (*Salvelinus fontinalis*) following exposure to DDT, PCB and phenol. Bull Environ Contam Toxicol 14:545–551

Milton AS, Wendlandt S (1970) A possible role of prostaglandin E_1 as a modulator for temperature regulation in the central nervous system of the cat. J Physiol (Lond) 207:76–77P

Milton AS, Wendlandt S (1971) Effects on body temperature of prostaglandins of the A, E, and F series on injection into the third ventricle of unanaesthetized cats and rabbits. J Physiol (Lond) 218:325–336

Mueller R (1976) Investigations on the body temperature of freshwater fishes. Arch Fischereiwiss 27:1–28

Myers RD (1977) New aspects of the role of hypothalamic calcium ions, 5-HT and PGE during normal thermoregulation and pyrogen fever. In: Cooper KW, Lomax P, Schönbaum E (eds) Drugs, biogenic amines and body temperature. Karger, Basel, pp 374–386

Myers RD, Simpson CW, Higgins D, Natterman RA, Rice JC, Redgrave P, Metcalf G (1976) Hypothalamic Na^+ and Ca^{++} ions and temperature set-point: new mechanisms of action of a central of peripheral thermal challenge and intrahypothalamic 5-HT, NE, PGE_1 and pyrogen. Brain Res Bull 1:301–327

Myhre K (1978) Behavioral temperature regulation in neonate chick of bantam hen (*Gallus domesticus*). Poultry Sci 57:1369–1375

Myhre K, Cabanac M, Myhre G (1977) Fever and behavioural temperature regulation in the frog *Rana esculenta*. Acta Physiol Scand 101:219–229

Nagai M, Iriki M (1978) Autonomic response of the fish to pyrogen. Experientia 34:1177–1178

Nakaoka Y, Oosawa F (1977) Temperature-sensitive behavior of *Paramecium caudatum*. J Protozool 24:575–580

Nistico G, Rotiroti D (1978) Antipyretics and fever induced in adult fowls by prostaglandins E_1, E_2 and O somatic antigen. Neuropharmacology 17:197–204

Ogilvie DM, Anderson JM (1965) Effect of DDT on temperature selection by young Atlantic salmon, *Salmo salar*. J Fish Res Board Can 22:503–512

Ogilvie DM, Fryer JN (1971) Effect of sodium pentobarbitol on the temperature selection response of guppies (*Poecilia reticulata*). Can J Zool 49:949–951

Opuszynski K (1971) Temperature preference of fathead minnow (*Pimephales promelas* Raf.) and its changes induced by copper salt $CuSO_4$. Pol Arch Hydrobiol 18:401–408

Peter RE McKeown BA (1975) Hypothalamic control of prolactin and thyrotropin secretion in teleosts, with special reference to recent studies on the goldfish. Gen Comp Endocrinol 25:153–165

Peterson RH (1973 a) Temperature selection of juvenile Atlantic salmon (*Salmo salar*) and
    brook trout (*Salvelinus fontinalis*) as influenced by various chlorinated hydrocarbons.
    J Fish Res Board Can 30:1091–1097
Peterson RH (1973 b) Temperature selection of juvenile Atlantic salmon (*Salmo salar* L.)
    exposed to some pesticides. Fish Res Board Can MS Rep Ser 1251:1–9
Peterson RH (1976) Temperature selection of juvenile Atlantic salmon (*Salmo salar*) as in-
    fluenced by various toxic substances. J Fish Res Board Can 33:1722–1730
Pittman OJ, Veale WL, Cockeram AW, Cooper KE (1976) Changes in body temperature
    produced by prostaglandins and pyrogens in the chicken. Am J Physiol 230:1284–1287
Polk DK, Lipton JM (1975) Effects of sodium salicylate, aminopyrine and chlorpromazine
    on behavioral temperature regulation. Pharmacol Biochem Behav 3:167–172
Ralph CL, Firth BT, Turner JS (1979) The role of the pineal body in ectotherm thermoregu-
    lation. Am Zool 19:273–293
Regal PJ (1966) Thermophilic response following feeding in certain reptiles. Copeia
    1966:588–590
Regal PJ (1967) Voluntary hypothermia in reptiles. Science 155:1551–1553
Reynolds WW (1977 a) Thermal equilibration rates in relation to heartbeat and ventilatory
    frequencies in largemouth blackbass, *Micropterus salmoides*. Comp Biochem Physiol
    [A] 56:195–201
Reynolds WW (1977 b) Temperature as a proximate factor in orientation behaviour. J Fish
    Res Board Can 34:734–739
Reynolds WW (1977 c) Fever and antipyresis in the bluegill sunfish, *Lepomis macrochirus*.
    Comp Biochem Physiol [C] 57:165–167
Reynolds WW (1977 d) Circadian rhythms in the goldfish *Carassius auratus* L.: preliminary
    observations and possible implications. Rev Can Biol 36:355–356
Reynolds WW (1979) Perspective and introduction to the symposium: thermoregulation in
    ectotherms. Am Zool 19:193–194
Reynolds WW, Casterlin ME (1976) Thermal preferenda and behavioral thermoregulation
    in three centrarchid fishes. In: Esch GW, McFarlane RW (eds) Thermal ecology II. US
    National Technical Information Service, Springfield, Va, pp 185–190
Reynolds WW, Casterlin ME (1977) Temperature preferences of four fish species in an elec-
    tronic thermoregulatory shuttlebox. Prog Fish-Cult 39:123–125
Reynolds WW, Casterlin ME (1978 a) Estimation of cardiac output and stroke volume from
    thermal equilibration and heartbeat rates in fish. Hydrobiologia 57:49–52
Reynolds WW, Casterlin ME (1978 b) Behavioral thermoregulation and diel activity in
    white sucker (*Catostomus commersoni*). Comp Biochem Physiol [A] 59:261–262
Reynolds WW, Casterlin ME (1978 c) Thermoregulatory behavior in the smooth dogfish
    shark, *Mustelus canis*. Fed Proc 37:427
Reynolds WW, Casterlin ME (1978 d) Behavioral thermoregulation by ammocoete larvae
    of the sea lamprey (*Petromyzon marinus*) in an electronic shuttlebox. Hydrobiologia
    61:145–147
Reynolds WW, Casterlin ME (1978 e) Complementarity of thermoregulatory rhythms in
    Micropterus salmoides and *M. dolomieui*. Hydrobiologia 60:89–91
Reynolds WW, Casterlin ME (1979) Behavioral thermoregulation and the "final prefer-
    endum" paradigm. Am Zool 19:211–224
Reynolds WW, Casterlin ME (1980) The role of fever in aquatic vertebrates. In: Cox B,
    Lomax P, Milton AS, Schönbaum E (eds) Thermoregulatory mechanisms and their
    therapeutic implications. Karger, Basel, pp 148–151
Reynolds WW, Covert JB (1977) Behavioral fever in aquatic ectothermic vertebrates. In:
    Cooper KE, Lomax P, Schönbaum E (eds) Drugs, biogenic amines and body temper-
    ature. Karger, Basel, pp 108–110
Reynolds WW, Casterlin ME, Covert JB (1976 a) Behavioural fever in teleost fishes. Nature
    259:41–42
Reynolds WW, McCauley RW, Casterlin ME, Crawshaw LI (1976 b) Body temperatures
    of behaviorally thermoregulating largemouth blackbass (*Micropterus salmoides*). Comp
    Biochem Physiol [A] 54:461–463
Reynolds WW, Casterlin ME, Covert JB (1978 a) Febrile responses of bluegill (*Lepomis ma-
    crochirus*) to bacterial pyrogens. J Therm Biol 3:129–130

Reynolds WW, Casterlin ME, Matthey JK Millington ST, Ostrowski AC (1978 b) Diel patterns of preferred temperature and locomotor activity in the goldfish *Carassius auratus*. Comp Biochem Physiol [A] 59:225–227

Reynolds WW, Covert JB, Casterlin ME (1978 c) Febrile responses of goldfish *Carassius auratus* to *Aeromonas hydrophila* and to *Escherichia coli* endotoxin. J Fish Dis 1:271–273

Reynolds WW, Casterlin ME, Covert JB (1979) Comparative thermoregulatory and febrile behavior of aquatic ectothermic vertebrates and arthropods. Fed Proc 38:1053

Reynolds WW, Casterlin ME, Covert JB (1980)Behaviorally mediated fever in aquatic ectotherms. In: Lipton JM (ed) Fever. Raven, New York, pp 207–212

Reynolds WW, Casterlin ME, Spieler RE (1982) Thyroxine: effect on behavioral thermoregulation in fishes. Can J Zool 60:926–928

Roth JJ, Ralph CL (1977) Thermal and photic preferences in intact and parietalectomized *Anolis carolinensis*. Behav Biol 19:341–348

Satinoff E (1972) Salicylate: action on normal body temperature in rats. Science 176:532–533

Satinoff E, McEwen GN Jr, Williams BA (1976) Behavioral fever in newborn rabbits. Science 193:1139–1140

Saxena PN (1976) Sodium and calcium ions in the control of temperature set-point in the pigeon. Br J Pharmacol 56:187–192

Smith EN (1979) Behavioral and physiological thermoregulation of crocodilians. Am Zool 19:239–247

Spieler RE, Noeske TA (1979) Diel variations in circulating levels of triiodothyronine and thyroxine in goldfish. Can J Zool 57:665–669

Spieler RE, Noeske TA, deVlaming VL, Meier AH (1977) Effects of thermocycles on body weight gain and gonadal growth in the goldfish, *Carassius auratus*. Trans Am Fish Soc 106:440–444

Stern RC (1977) Pathophysiologic basis for sympatric treatment of fever. Pediatrics 59:92–98

Stevens ED, Fry FEJ (1970) The rate of thermal exchange in a teleost, *Tilapia mossambica*. Can J Zool 48:221–226

Stevens ED, Fry FEJ (1974) Heat transfer and body temperatures in non-thermoregulatory teleosts. Can J Zool 52:1137–1145

Stuntz WE, Magnuson JJ (1976) Daily ration, temperature selection and activity of bluegill. In: Esch GW, McFarlane RW (eds) Thermal ecology II. US National Technical Information Service, Springfield, VA, pp 180–184

Takahara J, Mori M, Ofuji N et al. (1977) Effects of prostaglandin E$_1$ and indomethacin on ACTH, prolactin, GH and LH from the rat pituitary in vitro. Endocrinol Jpn 24:97–103

Tonque T (1977) TRH: a possible mediator of behavioral thermoregulation in neonatal chicken. Proc Int Union Physiol Sci 13:757

Vane JR (1971) Inhibition of prostaglandin synthesis as a mechanism of action for aspirin-like drugs. Nature 231:232–235

Van Miert ASJPAM, Frens J (1968) The reaction of different animal species to bacterial pyrogens. Zentral Veterinaer med 15:532–543

Vaughn LK, Bernheim HA, Kluger MJ (1974) Fever in the lizard *Dipsosaurus dorsalis*. Nature 252:473–474

Veale WL, Cooper KE Pittman QJ (1977) Role of prostaglandins in fever and temperature regulation. In: Ramwell PW (ed) The prostaglandins, vol 3. Plenum, New York, pp 145–167

Von Euler US (1961) Occurrence and distribution of catecholamines in the fish brain. Acta Physiol Scand 52:62–64

Weiss B, Laties VG (1963) Effects of amphetamines, chlorpromazine and pentobarbitol on behavioral thermoregulation. J Pharmacol Exp Ther 140:1–7

Welsh JH (1968) Distribution of serotonin in the nervous system of various animal species. Adv Pharmacol 6:71–88

Wigham T, Nishioka RS, Bern HA (1977) Factors affecting in vitro activity of prolactin cells in the euryhaline teleost *Sarotherodon mossambicus (Tilapia mossambica)*. Gen Comp Endocrinol 32:120–131

Wodtke E (1978) Lipid adaptation in liver mitochondrial membranes of carp acclimated to different environmental temperatures: pholospholipid composition, fatty acid pattern, and cholesterol content. Biochim Biophys Acta 529:280–291

Yakovleva IV, Komachkova ZK (1978) Hypothalamo-hypophyseal neurosecretory system and the thyroid in the parr of the sturgeon *Acipenser guldenstadti* during variation in environmental temperature. Zh Evol Biokhim Fiziol 14:175–179

Ziel R, Krupp P (1976) Mechanisms of action of antipyretic drugs. In: Brazier MAB, Coceani F (eds) Brain dysfunction in infantile febrile convulsions. Raven, New York, pp 153–160

Zeihuisen H (1895) Beiträge zur Lehre der Immunität und Idiosynkrasie. I. Über den Einfluß der Körpertemperatur auf die Wirkung einiger Gifte an Tauben. Arch Exp Pathol Pharmakol 35:181–212

CHAPTER 20

The Pyrogenic Responses of Invertebrates

M. E. CASTERLIN and W. W. REYNOLDS

A. Thermoregulatory Responses of Invertebrates

Thermoregulatory responses of invertebrates have been much less thoroughly studied than have those of the vertebrates. It is our purpose here briefly to review background information on thermoregulatory responses of normothermic invertebrates, before discussing febrile responses to pyrogenic agents.

With the exception of some facultatively endothermic insects (HEINRICH 1973; MAY 1979) most invertebrates are ectotherms (REYNOLDS 1979). As such, they thermoregulate primarily by behavioural means. In terrestrial ectotherms, behavioural thermoregulation can take the form of postural orientations to the sun (heliothermy), substratum (thigmothermy), or wind (evaporative cooling). Radiation and evaporation, as well as conduction and convection, are important means of heat exchange in air, allowing complex possibilities for thermoregulatory strategies. For aquatic ectotherms, which remain immersed in water, routes of thermal exchange are much more limited. Radiation and evaporation are not viable means of thermal exchange in water, so heat exchange is limited to conduction and convection. Behavioural thermoregulatory strategies cannot make effective use of postural orientations in water, so ectotherms are limited to seeking out appropriate water temperatures by responding to thermal gradients (REYNOLDS 1977a; REYNOLDS and CASTERLIN 1979a). Behavioural thermoregulatory responses of aquatic ectotherms, including motile aquatic and marine invertebrates, are characterized by preference (seeking out a suitable or "optimal" water temperature for a particular physiological function or state) and/or avoidance (moving away from lethal or suboptimal temperatures) responses along thermal gradients. Ability to thermoregulate behaviourally in water is, of course, limited by the availability of suitable choices of water temperatures. The body core temperatures of small ectotherms (less than 1 kg) differ little from ambient water temperatures under steady-state conditions (REYNOLDS et al. 1976b), although physiological functions such as changes in blood flow or gill ventilation rate can alter rates of heat exchange under changing ambient conditions (SPAARGAREN 1976; REYNOLDS 1977b; REYNOLDS and CASTERLIN 1978).

Little information is available on thermoregulatory responses of invertebrates other than arthropods. Some work has been published on temperatures preferred and avoided by the starfish (Echinodermata) *Asterias forbesii* (CASTERLIN and REYNOLDS, 1980d), by the whelk (Mollusca) *Nassarius trivittatus* (CASTERLIN and REYNOLDS 1980a), by the archiannellid (Annelida) *Protodrilus symbioticus* (GRAY 1965), and by the protozoan *Paramecium caudatum* (NAKAOKA and OOSAWA 1977).

However, most published data on invertebrate thermoregulation have dealt with the great Phylum Arthropoda, a vast and diverse assemblage of highly evolved groups including the primitive chelicerates such as scorpions and the horseshoe "crab" *Limulus polyphemus*, and the mandibulate classes Insecta (some of which are facultative endotherms) and Crustacea. Insect thermoregulation has recently been reviewed by several authors including HEINRICH (1973) and MAY (1979). We will review here primarily what is known of thermoregulatory behaviour of aquatic and marine crustaceans, and of primitive chelicerates exemplified by *Limulus*, for it is in these groups that the phenomenon of behavioural fever has been found to occur among the invertebrates. Other groups remain to be tested for pyrogenic responses.

The horseshoe "crab" *Limulus polyphemus* is a primitive marine chelicerate arthropod, more closely allied with the scorpions and spiders, and with the extinct ancient eurypterids and trilobites, than with the true crabs. Tested in an Ichthyotron electronic shuttlebox (REYNOLDS 1977c), which permits an animal to control water and body temperatures by means of normal unconditioned locomotor movements, *Limulus* is an imprecise thermoregulator compared with other animals similarly tested (REYNOLDS et al. 1979; CASTERLIN and REYNOLDS 1980b), voluntarily occupying a 25 °C span of temperatures (out of a potential 50 °C range) but avoiding temperatures below 15 °C or above 40 °C (REYNOLDS and CASTERLIN 1979b,c), and prefering temperatures between 25° and 30 °C under normothermic conditions. *Limulus* has proved to be a very useful animal biomedically, as its blood amoebocytes contain a substance which coagulates upon contact with bacterial endotoxin, giving rise to the widely used *Limulus* amoebocyte lysate (LAL) laboratory test for the presence of endotoxin.

Among the mandibulate arthropods, the insects (HEINRICH 1973; MAY 1979) and the curstaceans have been most thoroughly studied with respect to thermoregulation. Some work has been done on planktonic microcrustaceans (ACKEFORS and ROSEN 1970), but the decapod macrocrustaceans have received the most attention. In the following discussion we will focus attention on the Decapoda and on *Limulus*, in which febrile responses have been found. Febrile responses have not yet been reported among the insects.

Thermoregulatory behaviour has been studied in several freshwater crayfish species, including *Orconectes immunis* (CRAWSHAW 1974), *O. causeyi* (LORING and HILL 1976), *O. obscurus* (HALL et al. 1978), and *Cambarus bartoni* (CASTERLIN and REYNOLDS 1977, 1978, 1980c; REYNOLDS et al. 1979). Marine Decapoda whose thermoregulatory behaviours have been characterized include the spiny lobster *Panulirus argus* (REYNOLDS and CASTERLIN 1979f; CASTERLIN and REYNOLDS 1979b, 1980b), the American lobster *Homarus americanus* (REYNOLDS and CASTERLIN 1979d), the pink shrimp *Penaeus duorarum* (REYNOLDS and CASTERLIN 1979c), and the grass shrimp *Palaemonetes vulgaris* (CASTERLIN and REYNOLDS 1979). *Homarus*, *Palaemonetes*, and *Cambarus* are the more precise thermoregulators, followed by the less precise *Panulirus*, *Penaeus*, and *Limulus* (REYNOLDS et al. 1979; CASTERLIN and REYNOLDS 1979b, 1980b). The first three species thermoregulate with a degree of precision similar to that exhibited by similarly tested bony fishes and other aquatic lower vertebrates (REYNOLDS et al. 1979), generally voluntarily occupying a 10°–11 °C range of temperature or less when permitted to control water temperatures in an electronic shuttlebox, or allowed to choose temperatures in a linear gradient (CASTERLIN and REYNOLDS 1979). Most species select a sharply defined, species-specific modal thermal preferendum (REYNOLDS 1977 a; REYNOLDS and CASTERLIN 1979 a). That is to say, when normothermic (afebrile and not in cold torpor), each species selects a particular environmental temperature (final thermal preferendum) which is characteristic of that species and which is unaffected by the previous thermal exposure of that individual (whereas acute or short-term thermal preferenda, as measured within less than two hours in a gradient or shuttlebox, are dependent largely upon previous thermal acclimation; REYNOLDS and CASTERLIN 1979 a). Febrile responses to pyrogens are measured against that normothermic species-specific final preferendum.

B. Febrile Responses of Invertebrates

Because thermoregulation is mediated entirely by behaviour in aquatic arthropods, the same is true of febrile responses. A fever is generated entirely by behavioural means in these animals; thus the term "behavioural fever" (REYNOLDS et al. 1976 a). A behavioural fever is defined as a statistically significant increase in preferred temperature above the normothermic species-specific final preferendum (REYNOLDS et al. 1976 a). Operationally, following initial acclimatization to the final preferendum (REYNOLDS and CASTERLIN 1979 a), the mean preferred temperature is compared statistically for 24 h before and after administration of a pyrogen, and any significant increase is evidence of a behavioural fever. Periods of 24 h are used before and after treatment because some species exhibit circadian rhythms of preferred temperature (REYNOLDS et al. 1978 a; COVERT and REYNOLDS 1977); the 24-h mean would be unaffected by such thermoregulatory rhythms, and reflect only the effect of the administered pyrogen. We have standardized our procedures accordingly, even though not all species exhibit thermoregulatory rhythms (REYNOLDS and CASTERLIN 1979 b).

Most of the experimental work to date on behavioural fever in arthropods has been conducted in our laboratory. However, recently CABANAC (personal communication) discovered a febrile response in several species of scorpions (chelicerate arthropods related to *Limulus*), and UNESTAM (personal communication) has observed infected crayfish to crawl out onto the stream bank to sun themselves (a heliothermic febrile response, apparently).

Behavioural fever in invertebrate animals was first reported by CASTERLIN and REYNOLDS (1977), who discovered that injection of killed *Aeromonas hydrophila* (a Gram-negative bacterium ubiquitous in freshwater environments) induced a febrile response (increase of 1.8 °C above the normothermic 22.1 °C final thermal preferendum) in the crayfish *Cambarus bartoni*. It was subsequently found (CASTERLIN and REYNOLDS 1978, 1980 c) that *C. bartoni* also exhibited a febrile response when injected with prostaglandin E_1, which is known to induce fever in mammalian vertebrates (CRAWSHAW and STITT 1975). PGE_1 was also found to induce fever in the marine decapods *Penaeus duorarum* and *Homarus americanus*, and also in *Limulus* (CASTERLIN and REYNOLDS 1979 b, 1980 b, c). CABANAC (personal communication) reports that PGE_1 is also pyrogenic in scorpions.

A number of antipyretics are thought to counteract the fever-inducing action of various pyrogens by interfering with prostaglandin synthesis (Vane 1971; Ziel and Krupp 1976). The fact that PGE_1 induces fever in various arthropods suggests that prostaglandins may also play a role in mediating febrile reactions of these invertebrates. If so, we would expect that antipyretics would prevent fever in arthropods as they do in the vertebrates (Ziel and Krupp 1976; Bernheim and Kluger 1976; Reynolds 1977 d). Indeed, Casterlin and Reynolds (1980 c) recently discovered that the antipyretic acetaminophen (paracetamol) does in fact prevent the febrile response of C. bartoni to bacterial pyrogens, while not affecting normothermic thermoregulation. The discoveries that prostaglandins as well as bacterial endotoxins induce fever in arthropods, and that antipyretics such as acetaminophen prevent the induction of fever but do not affect normal thermoregulation in afebrile animals, suggests the possibility that common neuropharmacological mechanisms may be operating in both arthropod and vertebrate febrile mechanisms. Because these phylogenetic lineages (protostome and deuterostome, respectively) diverged from one another more than 600 million years ago, it is reasonable to infer that, to the extent that these mechanisms do prove to be similar, they either evolved independently in two separate evolutionary lines, or the basic febrile mechanisms must have evolved very long ago indeed, in very primitive metazoan animals (or possibly even in the Protozoa?). Until the emergence of the homeoendothermic higher vertebrates (birds and mammals), fever (and thermoregulation generally) had to by mediated by means of behavioural effector mechanisms. However, the sensory and integrative mechanisms controlling these behavioural responses may have evolved long ago, since all motile animals that have been studied apparently respond behaviourally (thermoregulate) to temperature. That the phenomenon of fever is found so widespread phylogenetically, in groups as otherwise divergent as arthropods and vertebrates, suggests that fever must have some general adaptive function which presumably helps the organism to combat infectious pathogens. The mechanisms by which fever enhances survival are not yet fully known, but preliminary results with ectothermic lower vertebrates suggest how this might occur. Kluger and Rothenburg (1979) found that bacterial growth is retarded when temperatures are elevated and trace metals such as iron are simultaneously reduced; zinc levels in the blood of febrile animals are also lowered, while copper is elevated (Kluger, personal communication). Bernheim et al. (1978) also found that blood flow is enhanced in lizards during fever, speeding the movement of leucocytes to the site of infection. Covert and Reynolds (1977) found that febrile goldfish (Carassius auratus) survive infection better than afebrile goldfish, presumably by similar mechanisms. While comparable experiments have not yet been performed with any invertebrates, the fact that arthropods exhibit fever is in itself an indication that the response is in some way beneficial to the animals. It seems likely that the survival value of fever in invertebrates arises through mechanisms similar to those operating in the vertebrates, although the beneficial effects of fever have not yet been fully uncovered even in mammals (Kluger and Rothenburg 1979), so much experimental work with both vertebrates and invertebrates remains to be performed.

C. Doses and Routes of Administration

A principal pyrogenic component of Gram-negative bacteria (such as *A. hydrophila*) which is known to induce fever in vertebrates (REYNOLDS et al. 1978 b), is bacterial endotoxin, a lipopolysaccharide component of the cell wall. This endotoxin also initiates clotting of the blood of *Limulus* and other arthropods, which is the basis of the LAL test for endotoxin. Because endotoxin induces rapid clotting of the blood, followed by death of the animal, bacteria cannot be injected directly into the haemocoel (these animals have an open circulatory system, in which the haemocoel is a large blood sinus filling the body cavity). Rather, fever is induced by injecting bacteria either into the gill chamber or into the abdomen, which is filled with muscles. A dose of the order of 10^9 killed *A. hydrophila* cells administered by this route induces fever in *C. bartoni*, with no other discernible effects on the animal. Sterile, pyrogen-free saline administered in this way does not alter thermoregulation.

Prostaglandin (PGE_1) can be injected directly into the haemocoel without inducing mortality (except at very high dosages). PGE_1 is likely rapidly inactivated in vivo, so relatively large doses (of the order of 0.1 mg, plus or minus an order of magnitude) are injected into the haemocoel to induce fever. In vertebrates, PGE_1 is injected directly into the brain near the thermoregulatory centre in the preoptic/anterior hypothalamic (PO/AH) region (CRAWSHAW and STITT 1975). However, the precise location of the thermoregulatory centre in arthropods is as yet unknown, but because of the open circulatory system, injecting large doses of PGE_1 into the haemocoel permits sufficient PGE_1 to reach the thermoregulatory centre and induce fever before being catabolized by enzymes. The febrile response is dose dependent at least over a dosage range of 0.05–0.5 mg in *C. bartoni*, inducing fevers ranging in magnitude from 1.0°–3.4 °C (CASTERLIN and REYNOLDS 1978), compared with 1.8 °C in response to a dose of 10^9 killed *A. hydrophila* injected into the gill chambers (CASTERLIN and REYNOLDS 1977, 1980c). The febrile response tends to peak at about 6 (4–8) h after PGE_1 injection in various arthropods (*Cambarus*, *Penaeus*, *Homarus*, *Limulus*), at peak amplitudes of nearly +15 °C at higher doses in *Limulus* and *Homarus* (which have the largest scope for fever between the normal final thermal preferendum and the ultimate upper incipient lethal temperature; CASTERLIN and REYNOLDS 1979 b, 1980c). Part of the latency is due to thermal lag in the Ichthyotron shuttlebox, so the response is a bit slower and of longer duration than is typical of mammals. The magnitude of the febrile response to PGE_1 begins to decline after 4–8 h, but the response is sufficiently great that there is a significant increase in the 24-hour mean temperature compared with the 24 h prior to PGE_1 injection. At larger dosages, some animals appear immobilized for varying periods following injection with PGE_1. Also, some animals expired within several days after the testing period was concluded, but the cause of such delayed mortality is unknown. We are uncertain how much PGE_1 actually reached the thermoregulatory centres of the injected arthropods; furthermore, the precise location of the thermoregulatory centre, and normal physiological PGE_1 concentrations in the thermoregulatory centre, are as yet unknown. It is known, however, that prostaglandins are synthesized and accumulated in the tissues of various invertebrates (Bito 1972; Morse et al. 1978; Ogata et al. 1978).

The antipyretic acetaminophen was administered not by injection, but rather via the "contamination route" (Green and Lomax 1977), which consists of dissolving the substance in the ambient water, from whence it is presumably taken up through the gills of the animal (Casterlin and Reynolds 1980c). A 325 mg acetaminophen (paracetamol) tablet was placed in the water in each of the two chambers of the shuttlebox (each containing 50 l water). This dosage and route of administration effectively prevented induction of fever by *A. hydrophila* injection, but did not interfere with normothermic thermoregulation in *C. bartoni* (Casterlin and Reynolds 1980c). It is not unlikely that this antipyretic effect was mediated by interference with PGE_1 biosynthesis, as is thought to occur in vertebrate antipyresis (Vane 1971; Ziel and Krupp 1976; Veale et al. 1977).

D. Similarities of Febrile Responses of Vertebrates and Invertebrates

Invertebrates, exemplified by arthropods, generate a fever behaviourally in response to pyrogens, as do the lower ectothermic vertebrates and even some neonatal mammals (Satinoff et al. 1976). Substances which induce fever in mammals, bacterial endotoxin and prostaglandin, are also pyrogenic in arthropods. Substances which are antipyretic in mammals, interfering with the pyretic action of pyrogens (e.g. acetaminophen), also prevent fever in arthropods. No obvious differences have emerged from experimental data available to date, although a great deal of further work is needed to elucidate fully the nature of neuropharmacological mechanisms mediating fever in arthropods and other animals.

References

Ackefors H, Rosen C-G (1970) Temperature preference experiments with *Podon polyphemoides* Leuckart in a new type of alternative chamber. J Exp Mar Biol Ecol 4:221–228

Bernheim HA, Kluger MJ (1976) Fever and antipyresis in the lizard *Dipsosaurus dorsalis*. J Physiol (Lond) 231:198–203

Bernheim HA, Bodel PT, Askenase PW, Atkins E (1978) Effects of fever on host defense mechanisms after infection in the lizard *Dipsosaurus dorsalis*. Br J Exp Pathol 59:76–84

Bito LZ (1972) Comparative study of concentrative prostaglandin accumulation by various tissues of mammals and marine vertebrates and invertebrates. Comp Biochem Physiol [A] 43:65–82

Casterlin ME, Reynolds WW (1977) Behavioral fever in crayfish. Hydrobiologia 56:99–101

Casterlin ME, Reynolds WW (1978) Prostaglandin E_1 fever in the crayfish *Cambarus bartoni*. Pharmacol Biochem Behav 9:593–595

Casterlin ME, Reynolds WW (1979a) Behavioral thermoregulation in the grass shrimp, *Palaemonetes vulgaris* (Say). Rev Can Biol 38:45–46

Casterlin ME, Reynolds WW (1979b) Fever induced in marine arthropods by prostaglandin E_1. Life Sci 25:1601–1604

Casterlin ME, Reynolds WW (1980a) Behavioral response of the New England dog whelk, *Nassarius trivittatus*, to a temperature gradient. Hydrobiologia 69:79–81

Casterlin ME, Reynolds WW (1980b) Behavioral thermoregulation and febrile responses of aquatic arthropods. In: Thermoregulatory mechanisms and their therapeutic implications. Karger, Basel

Casterlin ME, Reynolds WW (1980c) Fever and antipyresis in the crayfish *Cambarus bartoni*. J Physiol (Lond) 303:417–421

Casterlin ME, Reynolds WW (1980 d) Behavioral response of the starfish *Asterias forbesii* to a thermal gradient. Hydrobiologica 71:265–266

Covert JB, Reynolds WW (1977) Survival value of fever in fish. Nature 267:43–45

Crawshaw LI (1974) Temperature selection and activity in the crayfish, *Orconectes immunis*. J Comp Physiol 95:315–322

Crawshaw LI, Stitt JT (1975) Behavioral and autonomic induction of prostaglandin E_1 fever in squirrel monkeys. J Physiol (Lond) 244:197–206

Gray JS (1965) The behavior of *Protodrilus symbioticus* (Giard) in temperature gradients. J Anim Ecol 34:455–461

Green MD, Lomax P (1977) Behavioural thermoregulation and neuroamines in fish (*Chromus chromus*). J Therm Biol 1:237–240

Hall LW Jr, Cincotta DA, Stauffer JR Jr, Hocutt CH (1978) Temperature preference of the crayfish *Orconectes obscurus*. Arch Environ Contam Toxicol 7:379–383

Heinrich B (1973) Mechanisms of insect thermoregulation. In: Wieser W (ed) Effects of temperature on ectothermic organisms: ecological implications and mechanisms of compensation. Springer, Berlin Heidelberg New York, pp 139–150

Kluger MJ, Rothenburg BA (1979) Fever and reduced iron: their interaction as a host defense response to bacterial infection. Science 203:374–376

Loring MW, Hill LG (1976) Temperature selection and shelter utilization of the crayfish, *Orconectes causeyi*. Southwest Nat 21:219–226

May ML (1979) Insect thermoregulation. Annu Rev Entomol 24:313–349

Morse DE, Kayne M, Tidyman M, Anderson S (1978) Capacity for biosynthesis of prostaglandin-related compounds: distribution and properties of the rate-limiting enzyme in hydrocorals, gorgonians, and other coelenterates of the Caribbean and Pacific. Biol Bull 154:440–452

Nakaoka Y, Oosawa F (1977) Temperature-sensitive behavior of *Paramecium caudatum*. J Protozool 24:575–580

Ogata H, Nomura T, Hata M (1978) Prostaglandin biosynthesis in the tissue homogenates of marine animals. Bull Jpn Soc Sci Fish 44:1367–1370

Reynolds WW (1977a) Temperature as a proximate factor in orientation behavior. J Fish Res Board Can 34:734–739

Reynolds WW (1977b) Thermal equilibration rates in relation to heartbeat and ventilatory frequencies in largemouth blackbass, *Micropterus salmoides*. Comp Biochem Physiol [A] 56:195–201

Reynolds WW (1977c) Fish orientation behavior: an electronic device for studying simultaneous responses to two variables. J Fish Res Board Can 34:300–304

Reynolds WW (1977d) Fever and antipyresis in the bluegill sunfish, *Lepomis macrochirus*. Comp Biochem Physiol [C] 57:165–167

Reynolds WW (1979) Perspective and introduction to the symposium: thermoregulation in ectotherms. Am Zool 19:193–194

Reynolds WW, Casterlin ME (1978) Estimation of cardiac output and stroke volume from thermal equilibration and heartbeat rates in fish. Hydrobiologia 57:49–52

Reynolds WW, Casterlin ME (1979a) Behavioral thermoregulation and the "final preferendum" paradigm. Am Zool 19:211–224

Reynolds WW, Casterlin ME (1979b) Thermoregulatory behavior of the primitive arthropod *Limulus polyphemus* in an electronic shuttlebox. J Therm Biol 4:165–166

Reynolds WW, Casterlin ME (1979c) Thermoregulatory behavior and diel activity of *Limulus polyphemus*. In: Cohen E (ed) Biomedical applications of the horseshoe crab (Limulidae). Liss, New York, pp 47–59

Reynolds WW, Casterlin ME (1979d) Behavioral thermoregulation and locomotor activity in the lobster *Homarus americanus*. Comp Biochem Physiol [A] 64:25–28

Reynolds WW, Casterlin ME (1979e) Thermoregulatory behavior of the pink shrimp *Penaeus duorarum* Burkenroad. Hydrobiologia 67:141–143

Reynolds WW, Casterlin ME (1979f) Behavioral thermoregulation in the spiny lobster *Panulirus argus* (Latreille). Hydrobiologia 66:141–143

Reynolds WW, Casterlin ME, Covert JB (1976a) Behavioural fever in teleost fishes. Nature 259:41–42

Reynolds WW, McCauley RW, Casterlin ME, Crawshaw LI (1976b) Body temperatures of behaviorally thermoregulating largemouth blackbass (*Micropterus salmoides*). Comp Biochem Physiol [A] 54:461–463

Reynolds WW, Casterlin ME, Matthey JK, Millington ST, Ostrowski AC (1978a) Diel patterns of preferred temperature and locomotor activity in the goldfish *Carassius auratus*. Comp Biochem Physiol [A] 59:225–227

Reynolds WW, Covert JB Casterlin ME (1978b) Febrile responses of goldfish (*Carassius auratus*) to *Aeromonas hydrophila* and to *Escherichia coli* endotoxin. J Fish Dis 1:271–273

Reynolds WW, Casterlin ME, Covert JB (1979) Comparative thermoregulatory and febrile behavior of aquatic ectothermic vertebrates and arthropods. Fed Proc 38:1053

Satinoff E, McEwen GN Jr, Williams BA (1976) Behavioral fever in newborn rabbits. Science 193:1139–1140

Spaargaren DH (1976) On stroke volume of the heart and cardiac output in aquatic animals. Neth J Sea Res 10:1–43

Vane JR (1971) Inhibition of prostaglandin synthesis as a mechanism of action for aspirin-like drugs. Nature 231:232–235

Veale WK, Cooper KE, Pittman QJ (1977) Role of prostaglandins in fever and temperature regulation. In: Ramwell PW (ed) The prostaglandins, vol 3. Plenum, New York, pp 145–167

Ziel R, Krupp P (1976) Mechanisms of action of antipyretic drugs. In: Brazier MAB, Coceani F (eds) Brain dysfunction in infantile febrile convulsions. Raven, New York, pp 153–160

Subject Index

Handbook of Experimental Pharmacology

Continuation of "Handbuch der experimentellen Pharmakologie"

Editorial Board
G.V.R.Born, A.Farah,
H.Herken, A.D.Welch

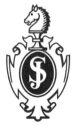

Springer-Verlag
Berlin
Heidelberg
New York

Handbook of Experimental Pharmacology

Continuation of "Handbuch der experimentellen Pharmakologie"

Editorial Board
G.V.R.Born, A.Farah, H.Herken, A.D.Welch

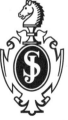

Springer-Verlag
Berlin
Heidelberg
New York